Inflammatory Disorders
of the Nervous System

CURRENT CLINICAL NEUROLOGY

Daniel Tarsy, MD, SERIES EDITORS

Inflammatory Disorders of the Nervous System

Pathogenesis, Immunology, and Clinical Management

Edited by

Alireza Minagar, MD
J. Steven Alexander, PhD

Louisiana State University Health Science Center
Shreveport, LA

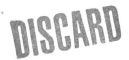

HUMANA PRESS ✴ TOTOWA, NEW JERSEY

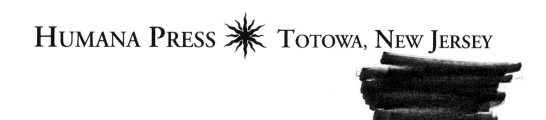

© 2005 Humana Press Inc.
999 Riverview Drive, Suite 208
Totowa, New Jersey 07512

humanapress.com

Due diligence has been taken by the publishers, editors, and authors of this book to assure the accuracy of the information published and to describe generally accepted practices. The contributors herein have carefully checked to ensure that the drug selections and dosages set forth in this text are accurate and in accord with the standards accepted at the time of publication. Notwithstanding, as new research, changes in government regulations, and knowledge from clinical experience relating to drug therapy and drug reactions constantly occurs, the reader is advised to check the product information provided by the manufacturer of each drug for any change in dosages or for additional warnings and contraindications. This is of utmost importance when the recommended drug herein is a new or infrequently used drug. It is the responsibility of the treating physician to determine dosages and treatment strategies for individual patients. Further it is the responsibility of the health care provider to ascertain the Food and Drug Administration status of each drug or device used in their clinical practice. The publisher, editors, and authors are not responsible for errors or omissions or for any consequences from the application of the information presented in this book and make no warranty, express or implied, with respect to the contents in this publication.

This publication is printed on acid-free paper. ∞
ANSI Z39.48-1984 (American Standards Institute) Permanence of Paper for Printed Library Materials.

Production Editor: Robin B. Weisberg
Cover design by Patricia F. Cleary

Cover illustration: Cerebral endothelial cells. Photograph by Dr. J. Steven Alexander.

For additional copies, pricing for bulk purchases, and/or information about other Humana titles, contact Humana at the above address or at any of the following numbers: Tel.: 973-256-1699; Fax: 973-256-8341; E-mail: orders@humanapr.com; or visit our Website: www.humanapress.com

Printed in the United States of America. 10 9 8 7 6 5 4 3 2 1

eISBN: 1-59259-905-2

Library of Congress Cataloging-in-Publication Data

Inflammatory disorders of the nervous system : pathogenesis, immunology, and clinical management / edited by Alireza Minagar, J. Steven Alexander.
    p. ; cm. -- (Current clinical neurology)
Includes bibliographical references and index.
ISBN 1-58829-424-2 (alk. paper)
1. Neuritis. 2. Nervous system--Pathophysiology. 3. Inflammation.
[DNLM: 1. Inflammation. 2. Nervous System Diseases. WL 140 I43 2005]
I. Minagar, Alireza. II. Alexander, J. Steven. III. Series.
RC416.I546 2005
616.8'56--dc22

2004020033

Series Editor's Introduction

The critical role of the inflammatory response in the pathophysiology of certain nervous system disorders has been appreciated for quite some time. Currently, rapidly accelerating knowledge of new molecular mechanisms known to be involved in systemic inflammatory disorders has extended to the investigation of a number of peripheral and central neurological disorders. Many of those discussed in this volume have been the usual suspects for immune-mediated, inflammatory neurological disorders such as, for example, multiple sclerosis, acute disseminated encephalomyelitis, optic neuritis, transverse myelitis, central nervous system (CNS) vasculitis, and neuropsychiatric systemic lupus erythematosis. Importantly, possible inflammatory mechanisms are now also undergoing scrutiny in chronic neurological diseases traditionally classified as neurodegenerative disorders, such as Alzheimer's and Parkinson's diseases.

In *Inflammatory Disorders of the Nervous System,* Drs. Minagar and Alexander have gathered an impressive group of investigators who review the basic principles of neuroinflammation and their emerging role in the more common inflammatory disorders of the nervous system. The first group of chapters review new and emerging research in neuroinflammation, while the rest explore the diseases cited above as well as other disorders where the role of the immune system and inflammation is currently less well understood, such as neurosarcoidois, HIV-associated dementia, and HTLV-associated neurological disorders. As the authors of these chapters point out, the central nervous and immune systems have a known special relationship, disturbances in which may account for some aspects of neuroinflammation. The role of microglia in inflammatory CNS disease has never been fully understood and now comes under scrutiny as possibly mediating maladaptive inflammatory responses. On the other hand, a balance appears to exist between the useful and protective vs possibly damaging effects of various neuroinflammatory mechanisms. The extent to which neuroinflammation is either a primary, etiological cause or a more passive, associated bystander in the pathophysiology of neurological disorders probably varies considerably among various conditions. Sorting all of this out remains for future research that should be ably assisted by this outstanding overview of the current state of knowledge in this area.

Daniel Tarsy, MD
Department of Neurology
Beth Israel Deaconess Medical Center
Harvard Medical School
Boston, MA

Preface

The last decade witnessed vast scientific advances in our understanding of molecular mechanisms of the inflammatory cascade involved in pathogenesis of diverse neurological disorders. Endothelial cells, activated leukocytes, resident immune cells within the central nervous system (CNS), and many classes of inflammatory mediators, especially chemokines and cytokines, are the major components of this complex and largely unsolved pathological puzzle. Through innumerable experiments, we have learned more about the role of each one of these players in the course of the inflammatory response, and have become able to apply some of our knowledge toward the development of more effective treatments with fewer adverse effects.

The objective of *Inflammatory Disorders of the Nervous System: Pathogenesis, Immunology, and Clinical Management* is to provide readers with a highly detailed review of the basic principles of neuroinflammation and extensive updates on the latest findings on common neuroinflammatory disorders. Emerging concepts in the field of inflammation such as "endothelial and leukocyte microparticles" and "gene microarray technology" are introduced and provide important links between CNS and general inflammation processes. Our book should be of interest to a broad range of both basic research and clinical scientists with a core interest in neuroinflammation. It is our impression that neuroinflammation is among the most rapidly growing fields in inflammation research, and our knowledge of new developments in this field will enable scientists and clinicians around the globe to better diagnose and treat some of these untreatable and exigent neurological conditions.

We are greatly indebted to the contributors, who made *Inflammatory Disorders of the Nervous System: Pathogenesis, Immunology, and Clinical Management* a reality by providing their superior knowledge and expertise in this rapidly developing field. We are also grateful to Richard Lansing, Robin Weisberg, and Damien DeFrances of Humana Press who provided their invaluable editorial expertise and technical advice for the publication of this book. We hope that our scientist colleagues find this book a useful resource in their unrelenting research into the mechanisms of inflammation.

Alireza Minagar
J. Steven Alexander

Contents

Contributors

YEON S. AHN, MD • Wallace H. Coulter Platelet Laboratory, Department of Medicine, University of Miami School of Medicine, Miami, FL

DEBORAH ALEMAN-HOEY, MD • Division of Neurology, Department of Medicine, University of Texas Health Science Center at San Antonio, San Antonio, TX

J. STEVEN ALEXANDER, PhD • Department of Cellular and Molecular Physiology, Louisiana State University Health Sciences Center, Shreveport, LA

CRYSTAL S. ANGLEN, PhD • Department of Cellular and Molecular Physiology, The Scripps Research Institute, La Jolla, CA

ROHIT BAKSHI, MD • Center for Neurological Imaging, Brigham & Women's Hospital, Harvard Medical School, Boston, MA

ROBIN L. BREY, MD • Division of Neurology, Department of Medicine, University of Texas Health Science Center at San Antonio, San Antonio, TX

STALEY A. BROD, MD • Department of Neurology, University of Texas Health Science Center at Houston, Houston, TX

MONICA J. CARSON, PhD • Division of Biomedical Sciences, University of California, Riverside, CA

WADE DAVIS, PhD • Department of Statistics, Baylor University, Waco, TX

DEEPA M. DESHPANDE • Transverse Myelitis Center, Department of Neurology, Johns Hopkins University School of Medicine, Baltimore, MD

PAUL D. DREW, PhD • Department of Neurobiology and Developmental Sciences, University of Arkansas for Medical Sciences, Little Rock, AR

ELDA M. DURAN, MS •Departments of Psychiatry and Behavioral Sciences, University of Miami School of Medicine, Miami, FL

MARJORIE R. FOWLER, MD • Department of Pathology, Louisiana State University Health Sciences Center, Shreveport, LA

FABRIZIO GIULIANI, MD • Department of Clinical Neurosciences, University of Calgary, Calgary, Alberta, Canada

EDUARDO GONZALES-TOLEDO, MD, PhD • Department of Radiology, Louisiana State University Health Sciences Center, Shreveport, LA

DAKSHINAMURTY GULLAPALLI, MD • Veterans Administrations Hospital, Salem, VA

LAWRENCE L. HORSTMAN, BS • Wallace H. Coulter Platelet Laboratory, Department of Medicine, University of Miami School of Medicine, Miami, FL

JOAQUIN J. JIMENEZ, MD • Wallace H. Coulter Platelet Laboratory, Department of Medicine, University of Miami School of Medicine, Miami, FL

WENCHE JY, PhD • Wallace H. Coulter Platelet Laboratory, Department of Medicine, University of Miami School of Medicine, Miami, FL

ADAM I. KAPLIN, MD, PhD • Department of Psychiatry and Behavioral Sciences, Johns Hopkins University School of Medicine, Baltimore, MD

WILLIAM J. KARPUS, PhD • Department of Pathology, Feinberg School of Medicine, Northwestern University, Chicago, IL

TONI KAZIC, PhD • Departments of Computer Science and Health Management Informatics, University of Missouri, Columbia, MO

ROGER E. KELLEY, MD • Department of Neurology, Louisiana State University Health Sciences Center, Shreveport, LA

DOUGLAS A. KERR, MD, PhD • Transverse Myelitis Center, Department of Neurology, Johns Hopkins University School of Medicine, Baltimore, MD

TAMMY KIELIAN, PhD • Department of Neurobiology and Developmental Sciences, University of Arkansas for Medical Sciences, Little Rock, AR

CHITRA KRISHNAN, MHS • Transverse Myelitis Center, Department of Neurology, Johns Hopkins University School of Medicine, Baltimore, MD

MICHAEL D. LAIRMORE, DVM, PhD • Center for Retrovirus Research and Department of Veterinary Biosciences; Department of Molecular Virology, Immunology, and Medical Genetics, Comprehensive Cancer Center, The Arthur G. James Cancer Hospital and Solove Research Institute, Ohio State University, Columbus, OH

DOUGLAS J. LANSKA, MD • Veterans Affairs Medical Center, Tomah, WI and Department of Neurology, University of Wisconsin, Madison, WI

BINDHU MICHAEL, BVSc & AH, MSc, MS, PhD • Center for Retrovirus Research and Department of Veterinary Biosciences, Ohio State University, Columbus OH

ALIREZA MINAGAR, MD • Department of Neurology, Louisiana State University Health Sciences Center, Shreveport, LA

SHARIQ MUMTAZ, MD • Department of Neurology, Memorial University New Foundland, NL, Canada

AMRITHRAJ NAIR, BVSc & AH • Center for Retrovirus Research and Department of Veterinary Biosciences, Ohio State University, Columbus OH

CARLOS A. PARDO, MD • Transverse Myelitis Center, Department of Neurology, Johns Hopkins University School of Medicine, Baltimore, MD

LAWRENCE H. PHILLIPS, II, MD • Department of Neurology, University of Virginia Health Sciences Center, Charlottesville, VA

SEAN J. PITTOCK, MD • Department of Neurology, Mayo Clinic College of Medicine, Rochester, MN

CORINNE PLOIX, PharmD, PhD • Department of Molecular Biology, The Scripps Research Institute, La Jolla, CA

RAMAN SETH, MBBS, MS • Departments of Computer Science and Health Management Informatics, University of Missouri, Columbia, MO

PAUL SHAPSHAK, PhD • Departments of Psychiatry and Behavioral Sciences, Neurology, Pathology, Comprehensive Drug Research Center, and Pediatrics McDonald Foundation Gene Team, University of Miami School of Medicine, Miami, FL

WILLIAM A. SHEREMATA, MD • Multiple Sclerosis Center, University of Miami School of Medicine, Miami, FL

LEE SILVERMAN, DVM • Center for Retrovirus Research and Department of Veterinary Biosciences, Ohio State University, Columbus OH

DEAN M. WINGERCHUK, MD • Department of Neurology, Mayo Clinic College of Medicine, Scottsdale, AZ

V. WEE YONG, PhD • University of Calgary, Departments of Clinical Neurosciences and Oncology, Calgary, Alberta, Canada

RANA ZABAD, MD • Department of Clinical Neurosciences, University of Calgary, Calgary, Alberta, Canada

FABIANA ZIEGLER, MD • Departments of Psychiatry and Behavioral Sciences, University of Miami School of Medicine, Miami, FL

ROBERT ZIVADINOV, MD, PhD • Department of Neurology, State University of New York at Buffalo School of Medicine and Biomedical Sciences; Buffalo Neuroimaging Analysis Center, The Jacobs Neurological Institute, Buffalo, NY

Continuing Medical Education

RELEASE DATE
May 1, 2005

EXPIRATION DATE
May 1, 2007

ESTIMATED TIME TO COMPLETE
5 hours

ACCREDITATION
This activity has been planned and implemented in accordance with the essential areas and policies of the Accreditation Council for Continuing Medical Education (ACCME) through the joint sponsorship of The American Society of Contemporary Medicine and Surgery and Humana Press/eXtensia. The American Society of Contemporary Medicine and Surgery is accredited by the Accreditation Council for Continuing Medical Education to provide continuing medical education for physicians.

CREDIT DESIGNATION
The American Society of Contemporary Medicine and Surgery designates this educational activity for a maximum of five category 1 credits toward the AMA Physician's Recognition Award. Each physician should claim only those credits that he/she actually spent in the activity.

METHOD OF PARTICIPATION AND FEE
The American Society of Contemporary Medicine and Surgery is pleased to award category 1 credit(s) toward the AMA Physician's Recognition Award for this activity. By reading the chapters and completing the CME questions, you are eligible for up to five category 1 credits toward the AMA/PRA. Following that, please complete the Answer Sheet and claim the credits. A minimum of 75% correct must be obtained for credit to be awarded. Finally, please complete the Activity Evaluation on the other side of the Answer Sheet. Please submit the Answer Sheet/Activity Evaluation according to the information printed on the top of that page. Your test will be scored within 4 weeks. You will then be notified of your score with a certificate of credit, or you will receive an additional chance to pass the posttest. Credit for the activity is available until May 1, 2007. There is no fee for this activity.

FACULTY AND DISCLOSURE
Faculty for CME activities are expected to disclose to the activity audience any real or apparent conflict(s) of interest related to the content of the material they present. The faculty for this activity report no conflicts of interests or relationships to disclose.

PROVIDER DISCLOSURE
The American Society of Contemporary Medicine and Surgery is an independent organization that does not endorse specific products of any pharmaceutical concern and therefore has nothing to disclose. Humana Press/ eXtensia are independent organizations that do not endorse specific products of any pharmaceutical concern and therefore have nothing to disclose.

INTENDED AUDIENCE

This activity is intended for neurologists and other physicians who treat inflammatory disorders of the nervous system.

OVERALL GOAL

The overall goal of this activity is to update the knowledge of clinicians on strategies and techniques needed to comprehensively manage patients with inflammatory disorders of the nervous system.

LEARNING OBJECTIVES

After completing this CME activity, participants should have improved their overall knowledge and attitudes in regard to inflammatory disorders of the nervous system. Specifically, participants should be able to:

- Distinguish the pathogenesis of inflammation
- Discuss the details of interactions among activated leukocytes, endothelial cells, and inflammatory mediators (i.e., cytokines, chemokines, adhesion molecules, etc.) in the context of inflammatory disorders of the central nervous system
- Describe how the central nervous system and immune system communicate and interact during inflammation of the nervous system
- Assess the modern concepts behind the phenomenon of inflammation, such as endothelial microparticles, gene microarray expression, and failure of endothelial barrier function
- Understand the pathogenesis and clinical manifestations, as well as management, of some of the most common and least understood inflammatory disorders of the central nervous system, such as multiple sclerosis, neuro-sarcoidosis, HIV-associated-dementia, Devic's disease, and West Nile virus encephalitis
- Demonstrate assessment strategies for patients with a variety of inflammatory disorders of the central nervous system

UNLABELED/ UNAPPROVED USE DISCLOSURE

In accordance with ACCME standards for Commercial Support, the audience is advised that this CME activity may contain references to unlabeled or unapproved uses of drugs or devices.

Endothelial Cell–Leukocyte Interactions During CNS Inflammation

J. Steven Alexander and Alireza Minagar

1. INTRODUCTION

Inflammation is a reactive response to infection or injury that involves many complex interactions between formed blood elements, vascular and tissue cells, which is controlled by the release and synthesis of several classes of soluble mediators in response to tissue injury, bacterial, or viral products. Some mediators are stored within several cell types (e.g., histamine, 5-hydroxytryptamine, proteases, and cationic proteins), whereas others are synthesized or induced cell-derived factors (e.g., prostanoids, leukotrienes, platelet-activating factor, and cytokine/chemokines), as well as products of proteolytic cascades in plasma (complement products, blood-coagulation cascade products, kinins). The extent, timing, and specificity of this response is related to the lability, metabolism, and scavenging/inactivation of these mediators. The recruitment of leukocytes to the sites of injury or infection is a central event in the inflammatory response, and often results in "bystander" tissue dysfunction and damage from leukocyte oxidants, proteases, and other mediators in several disease states.

The steps in leukocyte recruitment include capture and rolling of activated leukocyte by the endothelium, leukocyte adhesion to the endothelial lining of the vessel wall, transendothelial migration of activated leukocytes to the inflammatory focus, and passage through the extracellular matrix. Endothelial cells are critical regulators and participants in this process and interact with leukocytes, particularly following exposure to inflammatory mediators. This chapter highlights recent advances in our understanding of the mechanisms of leukocyte–endothelial adhesive interactions at the level of cell-surface protein–protein binding events and in intracellular signal transduction pathways that regulate leukocyte egress out of the vascular space and into epithelial-lined tissues and their relevance to inflammation of the central nervous system (CNS).

2. VASCULAR LEAKAGE

One of the earliest inflammatory responses to the release of several acutely acting mediators (e.g., histamine, kinins, prostanoids, etc.) is an acutely increased microvascular (usually postcapillary venular) permeability to water and plasma proteins. This leak is thought to reflect reorganization and/or contraction of endothelial adherens and *tight* junctions *(1)*. Vascular endothelial (VE) cadherin (VE-cadherin) or *cadherin-5* has been shown to be a major component of the endothelial adherens junction *(2,3)* with N- and P-cadherins *(4,5)*, which maintain and regulate

From: *Current Clinical Neurology: Inflammatory Disorders of the Nervous System:
Pathogenesis, Immunology, and Clinical Management*
Edited by: A. Minagar and J. S. Alexander © Humana Press Inc., Totowa, NJ

vascular permeability along with several components of tight junctions, which include junctional adhesion molecules (JAMs) *(6)*, occludin *(7)*, and members of the *claudin* family of proteins *(8)*.

It is still unclear how these proteins reorganize when the barrier is altered; however, endocytosis *(9)*, or a similar form of cadherin internalization, has been demonstrated in endothelial cells exposed to several vasoactive mediators *(10)*. Redistribution or contraction of junctional proteins *(11)* might also increase endothelial solute permeability by disintegrating the seal created by these proteins, or by changing the amount of proteins in cells or their expression at the cell surface. Additionally, active junction remodeling may play an important role in controlling how leukocytes pass across the endothelium into tissues during inflammation. Although leukocyte recruitment during inflammation is often associated with increased solute leakage, this probably reflects both the number of leukocytes recruited and migrated, and the extent of their activation, because leukocytes can often migrate across the endothelium without significant perturbation of this solute barrier *(12)*. In the CNS, this increased endothelial solute leakage delivers plasma-borne inflammatory mediators to the CNS and presents a more serious problem. The interruption of the blood–brain barrier (BBB) even transiently can lead to extensive nervous system disturbances, including altered nerve conduction, irreversible damage to neurons, loss of myelin sheath, and loss of other CNS-resident cells. This increased vascular permeability in the BBB is now recognized as an underlying mechanism in many CNS disease processes.

Mechanistically the increased solute leakage serves at least two purposes: first, to deliver opsonizing antibodies to sites of inflammation and second, the solute leakage from vessels may hemoconcentrate plasma to slow blood flow below the critical velocity, favoring a close approach of leukocytes to the underlying endothelium, an initial step in leukocyte recruitment. The actual tethering or capture events between leukocytes and activated endothelium are mediated by the selectin family of adhesion molecules and their sulfated, sialylated, and fucosylated, glycoprotein ligands *(13,14)*.

2.1. Selectins

Selectins are a group of calcium-dependent, type-I transmembrane glycoproteins that bind to sialylated carbohydrate moieties on target proteins. The selectin family consists of three structurally related molecules: L-selectin, E-selectin, and P-selectin *(15–17)*. Genes encoding selectin adhesion molecules are located on chromosome 1. Each selectin molecule contains an amino-terminus C-type lectin domain, which plays a central role in adhesion of selectin to its ligand. C-type lectin domains recognize carbohydrate structures in a Ca^{2+}-dependent manner. This region is followed by an epidermal growth factor (EGF)-like motif, which modulates selectin binding to its ligands by maintaining the lectin domain in a proper orientation for ligand binding *(18,19)*. The EGF-like domain is followed by various numbers of consensus repeat (CR) domains. The selectin molecule is anchored in the membrane by a single transmembrane domain and contains a short cytoplasmic tail. The number of CR domains is the major structural difference between selectin molecules.

2.2.1. L-Selectin

L-selectin (CD62L), which initially was identified as a lymphocyte homing receptor, is exclusively expressed by leukocytes (neutrophils, monocytes, some subgroups of natural killer[NK] cells, and naïve T and B lymphocytes). L-selectin supports rolling in vivo and in vitro *(20)* and is expressed at the tips of leukocyte microvilli, which mediate early capture of leukocytes. L-selectin mediates lymphocyte recruitment and attachment to the high endothelial venules of the lymphatic tissue. Additionally, L-selectin plays a major role in recruitment of leukocytes into the inflammatory foci *(21)*. Upon activation of the leukocytes by fMet-Leu-Phe (fMLP) or interleukin (IL)-8, L-selectin is shed from leukocytes in what appears to be a metalloproteinase-dependent cleavage.

2.2.2. P-Selectin

P-selectin (CD62P), which is synthesized and stored in endothelial Weibel-Palade and platelet α-granules, can be rapidly (<1 min) mobilized to the cell surface to support endothelial/platelet adhesion.

This surface expression can be triggered by diverse mediators, including histamine, tumor necrosis factor (TNF)-α, thrombin, and lipopolysaccharide (LPS). P-selectin synthesis can also be increased by endothelial exposure to IL-4 and IL-13 *(22)*. P-selectin mediates leukocyte rolling and has a major role in their recruitment to the inflammatory foci. Once P-selectin is expressed on the endothelial surface, it can be rapidly re-internalized by endocytosis. Capture and rolling of leukocytes are reversible and transient events. To stop rolling and arrest a leukocyte, the low-affinity transient interactions of rolling must be substituted by high-affinity adhesion reactions between the leukocyte and the underlying endothelium.

2.2.3. E-Selectin

E-selectin (CD62E) is not constitutively expressed by resting endothelial cells. However, stimulation of endothelial cells by TNF-α, IL-1, bacterial LPS, or other inflammatory chemoattractants, endothelial expression of E-selectin molecules is elevated at the transcriptional and translational levels. E-selectin functions as a rolling adhesion receptor. Upregulation of E-selectin expression by endothelial cells on stimulation with stimuli, e.g., TNF-α is mediated by activation of the transcription factor nuclear factor-κB (NF-κB), which is dissociated from its inhibitor I-κ-B. Expressed E-selectin molecules on the endothelial surface support leukocyte rolling. Interestingly, in models of cerebral inflammation, such as experimental autoimmune encephalomyelitis (EAE), E- and P-selectins may not play dominant roles *(23)*.

2.2.4. Selectin Ligands

Some of the important ligands for selectins include P-selectin glycoprotein ligand-1 (PSGL-1), heparin derivatives, CD34, CD24, and mucosal addressin cell adhesion molecule-1 (MAdCAM-1). Selectins bind carbohydrate residues on sialylCD15, sialyl-Lewis X, and serine/threonine-rich mucins, e.g., PSGL-1, GlyCAM-1, and CD34 *(24)*.

2.3. Rolling Mechanics

Leukocytes roll along the endothelium when selectin-type molecular bonds are formed before the initially formed bonds are broken. Rolling will cease if cells do not encounter further endothelial ligands to support rolling. Rolling does not use metabolic activity and can continue in the presence of metabolic inhibitors. Rolling also encourages leukocyte encounters with endothelial integrin ligands, platelet-aggregating factor (PAF), and chemokines that lead to slower rolling and eventual cell arrest.

2.4. PAF/Chemokines/Cytokines

PAF can be rapidly formed by activated endothelial cells and is mobilized to the endothelial cell surface, where neutrophils brought into close approach with the endothelium increase their level of activation (priming). Leukocyte cytosolic Ca^{2+} is also increased, via inside out signaling β2-integrins, which make them more prone to degranulation and reorganization of PSGL-1 at the cell surface *(25)*. Besides PAF, endothelial cells synthesize many other signal molecules during inflammation e.g., IL-8 (a CXC chemokine). IL-8 is formed by active endothelial cells and released at the cell surface, where it interacts with matrix molecules. IL-8 activates β2-integrins and promotes polymorphonuclear leukocyte (PMN) adhesion to the endothelium. Another endothelial CX3C cytokine, termed *fractalkine*, can also bind to, and activate monocytes at the endothelial surface. Platelets may participate in leukocyte adhesion, both by binding to expressed PSGL-1, which may lead to more adhesive cell aggregates, and by releasing chemokines that bind to CXCR2 receptors on PMNs *(25)*. Together, cytokines and chemokines, along with several other mediators. including prostanoids, PAF, complement, growth factors, and nitric oxide (NO), regulate many leukocyte- and endothelial-dependent adhesive events in inflammation.

3. LEUKOCYTE ARREST

3.1. Integrins

Integrins are a large group of cell-surface heterodimer glycoproteins, which adhere cells to proteins in the extracellular matrix or to ligands on other cells. Integrins are composed of noncovalently linked dimers of α- and β-subunits, where the NH2-terminus globular heads of the β-subunits participate in interchain linking and ligand binding.

3.1.1. Leukocyte Integrins

Several leukocyte integrins have important roles in inflammation. Integrins consist of homodimers of α- and β-subunits of which more than 25 have been described; however, only a few are found in leukocytes. Some $\beta 2$-containing integrins include $\alpha L\beta 2$ (lymphocyte function-associated antigen-1 [LFA-1]), $\alpha M\beta 2$ [Mac-1], $\alpha x\beta 2$ [150/95]) and $\alpha d\beta 2$.

3.1.2. β_2-Integrins

β_2-integrins are exclusively expressed on leukocytes and, upon activation, undergo a conformational change involving the phosphorylation of the β-subunit. β_2-integrins participate in four important heterodimers: CD11a/CD18 LFA-1/$\alpha_L\beta_2$, CD11b/CD18 (Mac-1), exclusive to granulocytes and monocytes, CD11c/CD18, and CD11d/CD18. LFA-1/$\alpha_L\beta_2$ is expressed by mature leukocytes and binds to surface ligands, especially *intercellular adhesion molecule* (ICAM). LFA-1 participates in leukocyte adhesion, activation, and transendothelial migration and also serves as a costimulatory molecule in T-cell activation.

3.1.3. β_1-Integrins

The most significant member of the β_1-integrin subfamily is $\alpha_4\beta_1$ (VLA-4), expressed on lymphocytes, hematopoietic stem cells, eosinophils, neutrophils, and NK cells and binds to vascular cell adhesion molecule (VCAM-1). In addition to its ability to mediate firm leukocyte adhesion to the endothelium, $\alpha_4\beta_1$ also binds fibronectin and osteopontin, and may influence leukocyte homing and rolling. Another important leukocyte integrin, $\alpha_4\beta_7$ (lymphocyte Peyer's patch adhesion molecule [LPAM-1]) is a ligand for MAdCAM-1, and mediates leukocyte homing to the gut and, apparently, the inflamed cerebrum in models of multiple sclerosis (MS) *(23,26,28)*. In patients with MS, a monoclonal antibody against $\alpha 4$-integrin, "Antegren" (which blocks VLA-4/VCAM-1 and a4b7integrin/MAdCAM-1 binding) has been used as a novel therapy *(27,29)*.

3.2. Immunoglobulin Superfamily Ig-CAMs

Several immunoglobulin cell adhesion molecules (Ig-CAMs) are expressed on leukocytes and endothelial and epithelial cells and mediate important binding interactions in inflammation and host defense *(30)*. Members of the Ig-CAMs superfamily exhibit Ig-like structures and include ICAM-1, ICAM-2, VCAM-1, and platelet-endothelial cell adhesion molecule-1 (PECAM-1), as well as neural cell adhesion molecule (N-CAM). These molecules function not only as adhesion molecules, but also act as part of a transmembrane-signaling system which helps control leukocyte diapedesis and other inflammatory responses *(31)*.

3.2.1. ICAM-1 and ICAM-2

ICAM-1 is constitutively expressed by endothelial cells and its expression can be further increased by cytokine exposure. ICAM-1 is also expressed on several other cell types, including epithelia. ICAM-2 is a truncated form of ICAM-1 that does not appear to be induced by inflammatory stimuli *(32)* but is expressed at higher basal levels than ICAM-1. ICAM-1 serves as a ligand for Mac-1 and LFA-1 and can also be shed from the endothelial surface as soluble ICAM-1 (sICAM-1). Although sICAM-1 has been used as an index of inflammation, it is not clear if it blocks ICAM-1/$\beta 2$-integrin binding. Additionally, ICAM-2-gene-deficient mice show a less severe inflammatory phenotype than ICAM-1-knockout mice despite the fact that it's not a "regulated" type of Ig-CAM.

3.2.2. VCAM-1

VCAM-1 and its ligand $\alpha_4\beta_1$ (VLA-4) form another important adhesion system in inflammation that has been associated with several forms of chronic inflammation (e.g., arthritis, dermatitis, and neuritis). VCAM-1 expression by endothelial cells is induced by cytokine stimulation, and its expression by resting endothelium is minimal. Upregulation of VCAM-1 expression by endothelial cells also requires post-transcriptional events involving the NF-κB-transcription system. Other cells also expressing VCAM-1 include epithelial cells, Kupffer cells, and dendritic cells.

3.2.3. MAdCAM-1

MAdCAM-1 and its ligands $\alpha_4\beta_7$ and L-selectin form a significant adhesion system associated with induction of intestinal inflammation. MAdCAM-1-dependent leukocyte adhesion has also been demonstrated in brain inflammation (e.g., EAE and possibly MS). MAdCAM-1 is expressed at the surface of high endothelial venules in gut, Peyer's patches, mesenteric lymph nodes, the lamina propria of both the small and large intestine, and mammary gland. In addition to its role in lymphocyte trafficking to mucosal lymphoid tissue, MAdCAM-1 is dramatically increased in IBD *(33)* and EAE *(27,34)*.

3.2.4. JAMs

Junctional adhesion molecules-(JAM) 1–3 are recent additions to the Ig superfamily and are tight junctional components that help regulate leukocyte emigration. Since JAMs appear to be downregulated by inflammatory cytokines, the loss of junctional integrity produced by cytokines may reflect, in part, disintegration of the restrictive barrier to leukocyte exchange partially formed by JAMs. It is interesting to note that JAM-1 has been shown to be a ligand for the β2 integrin LFA-1, which functions in leukocyte migration *(35)*. JAM-2 is restricted to high endothelial venules and lymph nodes and is important in the recruitment of NK, dendritic, and T-cells to these locations through binding of JAM-2 to JAM-3 expressed on these cells *(36)*.

3.3. Vascular Adhesion Protein-1 (VAP-1)

VAP-1 *(37)* is an additional selectin-independent adhesion element that supports binding of lymphocytes to endothelial cells at lymph nodes and inflammation sites *(38)*. VAP-1 mediates the specific binding of CD8$^+$ T cells and NK cells to high endothelial venules independent of L-selectin, PSGL-1, and α4 integrins. Although VAP-1 is not an autonomous lymphocyte adhesive determinant, it cooperates with LFA-1, Mac-1, and L-selectin ligands to confer specific binding of CD8$^+$ lymphocytes to lymph nodes and inflamed endothelia. Together with peripheral node addressins, VAP-1 seems to be a major determinant of the flux of lymphocytes that occurs in some of the healthy vascular beds (e.g., lymphoid tissue) and inflamed tissue. It is possible that VAP-1 (in conjunction with ICAM-1), mediates the adhesion of tumor-infiltrating lymphocytes into carcinomas; thus, VAP-1 may participate in normal antitumor defenses *(39)*.

4. TRANSENDOTHELIAL MIGRATION

The process of transendothelial migration of leukocytes (known as *diapedesis*) is a highly complex and regulated process, i.e., inflammation. In the inflamed BBB, increased lymphocyte traffic is a central and early event in several inflammatory and immune-mediated CNS diseases. Migration likely involves multiple levels of endothelial-leukocyte communication and remodeling of adhesion molecules, cytoskeletal features, and cell-cell junctions (e.g., LFA-1, PECAM-1) *(40)*.

4.1. PECAM-1

PECAM-1 is a highly *N*-glycosylated membrane protein constitutively expressed by nearly all endothelial cells, which regulates leukocyte movement out of blood vessels (extravasation). The extracellular region of PECAM-1, composed of six C-2-type domains, is heavily *N*-glycosylated, with carbohydrate residues accounting for 40% of its apparent molecular weight (130 kDa). PECAM-1 is also expressed by platelets, monocytes, neutrophils, NK cells and T-lymphocyte subsets *(41)*. The interendothelial junction is one of the major sites of PECAM-1 expression, where PECAM-1 supports cell-cell adhesion in a homophilic, Ca^{2+}-dependent manner. Mamdouh et al *(42)* have described membrane cycling of PECAM-1 as a mechanism for leukocyte-transendothelial migration. PECAM-1 may also mediate the movement of leukocytes through tissues in a heterophilic manner *(43)*. Ligation of leukocyte PECAM results in an upregulation of leukocyte-integrin function and which may modify the transendothelial migration of activated leukocytes *(40)*. Elevated plasma levels of insoluble PECAM-1 are shed into the circulation as a membrane-bound form of these adhesion molecules, known as *endothelial microparticles*, and have been reported in MS and several other pathological conditions *(44)*. This particle shedding, remodeling of junctions, and the underlying matrix may also occur with contributions from several proteases (e.g., elastase *[45,46]*, metalloproteinases [MMPs] *[47]*).

Transendothelial migration of activated leukocytes during inflammatory responses occurs mostly at small-diameter postcapillary venules, where the endothelium expresses high levels of adhesion molecules during inflammation. At least two forms of leukocyte migration have been characterized: PECAM-independent (type I) and PECAM-independent (type II). PECAM-1 is involved in some, but not all forms of leukocyte migration, possibly in cell traction *(48)*.

It has been reported that leukocyte penetration of the BBB is mediated by cytokine-induced ECAM expression (type II migration) *(49)*, particularly via VCAM-1-mediated endothelial adhesion, and perhaps to a lesser extent, adhesion mediated by ICAM-1, PECAM-1, and E-selectin; VCAM-1 apparently has less of a direct role in lymphocyte extravasation. E-selectin expression in response to cytokines appears to be lower in brain microvessels than in peripheral, extra-CNS vascular tissues *(50)*. In the brain, PECAM-1 appears to have an essential function in chronic cerebral inflammation, and blocking PECAM-1 prevents antigen-specific T-cell homing to the CNS *(51)*. Both PECAM-1 and VE-cadherin may be regulated by mitogen-activated protein kinase (MAPK) activity, with both molecules concomitantly downregulated following persistent MAP kinase kinase (MEK)-1 activation e.g., in inflammation *(52)*.

The described rolling, arrest, and migration of leukocytes are controlled by several classes of mediators, which control the presentation, expression, and activation of adhesive determinants in each of these steps. The mediators controlling these processes are far too numerous to describe in great detail, but with respect to CNS pathology, we will consider the roles of several cytokines and chemokines.

4.2. Cytokines

Cytokines are regulatory proteins released between cells, which are powerful modifiers of cell activity, particularly in immune and inflammatory responses. Cytokines are not pre-formed zymogens but are rapidly synthesized and secreted. Cells often secrete multiple cytokines in a network fashion to enhance, limit, or modify cellular responses, frequently through activation of transcription. Cytokines exhibit a variety of biological activities and have roles in the immune response, hematopoiesis, neurogenesis, embryogenesis, and oncogenesis. In inflammation, cytokines regulate the activity of phagocytes and other immune system and vascular cells. Cytokines control expression of adhesion molecules, the inducible nitric oxide synthase (iNOS), and several other mediators of inflammation and, hence, leukocyte emigration into tissues.

In cerebral inflammation, there is abundant evidence that leukocyte infiltration, BBB loss, and tissue injury are directly associated with cytokine action, particularly via overexpression of cytokines. For example, the cytokine "storm" seen in MS is an important example of a cytokine-mediated inflammatory response in the CNS. Additionally, cytokines like TNF-α, IL-1β and IFN-γ are also implicated in Alzheimer's disease (AD) and AIDS-related CNS pathology. Cytokines are classified as proinflammatory (Th1) or antiinflammatory (regulatory, Th2). These molecules mediate their effects through binding to receptors on target cells. In inflammation, some of the most injurious cytokines are the Th1 cytokines, as well as several growth factors. Pro-inflammatory cytokines include IL-1, IL-6, IFN-γ TNF-α. Some important Th-2 cytokines would include IL-4, 5, 10, and 14, which promote antibody responses and can modify or limit responses to inflammatory cytokines.

IL-1 and its close relative IL-18 are proinflammatory cytokines that support many events in the inflammatory cascade. IL-1 also activates antigen-presenting cells (APC) and CD4$^+$ lymphocytes. Some of the important genes activated by IL-1α and IL-1β include cyclooxygenase-2 (COX-2), phospholipase A$_2$, and iNOS *(53)*. The activity of these genes yields several inflammatory products, including PGE$_2$, PAF, and high levels of NO/NO$_x$ species. IL-18 also reinforces effects of IL-12 and IL-15, especially in driving the production of IFN-γ and inhibiting angiogenesis. IL-2 stimulates proliferation and activation of B cells and T cells. IL-15, like IL-2, increases lymphocyte (especially NK-cell) activity and stimulates cytokine production by CD4$^+$ cells. IL-21 also supports lymphocyte proliferation, NK- and B-cell maturation. IL-6 produces many similar effects as IL-2 and is produced by T cells, macrophages, and monocytes.

IL-10, one of the most important Th2 cytokines, produced by T and B cells and represses secretion of proinflammatory cytokines, and as well, modulates responses by TB, and NK cells; monocytes; and neutrophils. IL-22 is produced by activated T cells during acute inflammation. IL-22 is similar to IL-10, but IL-22 does not block monocyte-derived inflammatory cytokine production as IL-10 does. IL-19 exhibits many of the properties associated with IL-10.

Another Th2 cytokine, IL-5 stimulates B-cell differentiation and thus antibody production, as well as alterations in Ig-class expression. IL-4 plays an important role in the growth and differentiation of Th2 cells, IgE induction (in allergic responses), and in the switching of antibody isotypes. IL-4 also enhances antigen processing and presentation. IL-5 stimulates the production and maturation of eosinophils during inflammation.

IL-12 provides a critical link between innate immunity and adaptive immunity, activates Th1 induction and leukocyte maturation, and enhances the cytolytic activity of NK cells and macrophages. IL-12 also increases the release of IFN-γ by T cells and NK cells.

4.3. Interferons

Interferons modulate many events in the immune system and during inflammation. There are more than 20 type I IFNs, including IFN-α, IFN-β, IFN-o and IFN-τ; IFN-γ is a type II interferon. IFN-α, IFN-β, and IFN-γ are released early on in the inflammatory response. IFN-α and IFN-β promote NK-cell proliferation, stimulate innate and adaptive immune responses specific to viral infections, and also exert some antiparasitic activity. Activated NK cells release IFN-γ, which induces macrophage secretion of cytokines, activating T-cell responses.

TNF-α and TNF-β activate macrophages and inhibit apoptosis of neutrophils and eosinophils. Most importantly, TNF-α promotes vascular endothelial expression of several adhesion molecules that bind leukocytes and other formed blood elements. One difference between TNF-α and IL-1 is that TNF-receptor signaling may promote apoptosis, whereas IL-1β does not, and actually is a hematopoietic factor, as well as an EGF *(54)*, through its induction of COX-2 *(55)*. As already described IL-1, IL-18, and TNF-α can, however, induce the expression of endothelial cell-adhesion molecules *(53)* to promote leukocyte adhesion.

4.4. Growth Factors

It is now well recognized that microvascular proliferation and remodeling is a central phenomenon in the inflammatory process. Several VEGFs can be classified within the cytokine family and have been shown to be significantly increased during inflammation, where they increase solute permeability and promote new vessel formation *(56)*. Some also behave like some Th1 cytokines in that they can increase the expression of some adhesion molecules (e.g., ICAM-1 but perhaps not other ECAMs) *(57)*.

Although largely regarded as only inflammatory molecules, cytokines have now been recognized as important signaling molecules in the CNS outside of disease process and appear to participate in the onset of sleep, diurnal rhythm, and nerve conduction *(58)*. Additionally, antiinflammatory cytokine (IL-10, TGF-β1) expression also reportedly regulates neuronal and glial function in the CNS outside of episodes of inflammation *(58)*; therefore, what is regarded as CNS inflammation may be the result of an excessive or inappropriate level of signaling that is neuroregulatory at normal levels.

4.5. Chemokines

As previously described, chemokines are small chemotactic polypeptides formed by activated macrophages, microglia, astrocytes, and inflammatory cells, often in response to cytokine exposure, which modulate leukocyte adhesion and migration. Some examples of chemokines are IL-8, MIP-1α, MIP-1β, MCP-1, MCP-2, MCP-3, Gro-A, GRO-b, RANTES, and exotaxin. Chemokines and their receptors represent important adhesion/signaling systems that control leukocyte motility and activation in inflammation *(59)*. Chemokines (or chemoattractant cytokines) are the major *in situ* regulators of integrin activity on endothelium-recruited leukocytes. Chemokines are generally displayed at endothelial sites of leukocyte migration *(60)*, where they signal through transmembrane receptors linked to the α subunit of heterodimeric Gi-proteins on the endothelium-binding leukocyte *(61)*. Chemokine receptors are also altered during immune activation with naïve T-cells expressing CXCR4 and CXCR7 and activated T cells expressing CXCR3, CCR5, and CXCR3 *(62)*. Rolling of activated leukocytes on the endothelium, is influenced by chemokines and assists them in tethering to the underlying endothelium where they come into close proximity with selectin ligands and potential ligands for costimulatory receptors.

4.5.1. IL-8

IL-8, a CXC chemokine, is synthesized by monocytes, macrophages, and endothelial cells during inflammation. IL-8 is a potent chemotactic factor that attracts and activates neutrophils, basophils, and T cells and increases their adhesion at sites of inflammation. IL-8 is formed by actived endothelial cells and released at the cell surface and interacts with components of the matrix. Cerebrospinal fluid (CSF)-chemokine and leukocyte-chemokine-receptor expression patterns appear to be closely correlated with disease activity and staging in MS *(63)*. IL-8 activates $β_2$ integrins and promotes neutrophil adhesion to the endothelium. Another endothelial CX3C cytokine, termed *fractalkine* (FKN, CX3CL1; see 4.5.3.) can also bind and activate monocytes at the endothelial surface (*see* below).

4.5.2. CXCL10/CXCR3

During EAE, lymphocyte migration into the inflamed cerebrum appears to be mediated by CXCL10 binding to CXCR3 expressed on CNS-homing lymphocytes, but it is not completely clear whether this drives CNS inflammation, since blocking CXCL10 also appears to worsen this disease *(64)*. The chemokine receptors CCR3 and CXCR4 are expressed by activated cerebral endothelial cells and may be important as (1) HIV-1 coreceptors, (2) in endothelial chemotaxis during angiogenesis, and (3) in promoting leukocyte penetration of the brain *(65)*. Biernacki et al *(66)* have demonstrated that in a model of MS, allogeneic or myelin basic protein reactive T-cell supernatants stimulate brain endothelium to secrete the chemokines CXCL10/IP-10, CCL2/MCP-1, CXCL8/IL-8 and also increase endothelial expression of ICAM-1. IFN-γ was necessary but insufficient to reproduce these effects and Th2 supernatants did not block this effect. Although junctional integrity and permeability were not Th1/Th2 cytokine-dependent, ZO-1 and ZO-2 expression were modified under these conditions. Most important, prior migration of either cell type (Th1 or Th2) encouraged increased extravasation and vascular leakage. This suggests that in the brain, lymphocyte entry into the tissue may lead to a persistent activation of some immune responses regardless of the type of polarization.

4.5.3. Fractalkine

Fractalkine (FKN) is a novel chemokine that exists in two forms: secreted and membrane-anchored. FKN promotes adhesion, chemotaxis, and activation of leukocytes (e.g., macrophages, microglia) *(67)*. FKN is normally produced by neurons, particularly during cell stress, and is associated with HIV-associated dementias (HAD). Fractalkine signaling triggers the formation of several neurologically active factors through binding to the CX3CR1 receptor. Activation of CX3CR1 activates the transcription factors Elk-1, TCF, SRF, c-Jun, and ATF-2 in macrophages and microglia that make MIP-1b and IL-8. Additionally, another important role of FKN in HAD and other forms of neuroinflammation may be that it acts as a prosurvival (antiapoptotic) factor for activated microglia, protecting them against Fas-mediated apoptosis *(68)*.

4.6. Prostanoids

Prostanoids are thought to have important functions in the development of Alzheimer's disease (AD), based on several studies that show benefit from chronic use of nonsteroidal anti-inflammatory drugs (NSAIDs). However, other studies using selective COX-2 inhibitors have not universally reproduced these findings. It is anticipated that CNS-specific COX-1 inhibitors may therefore be the most beneficial NSAIDs for future AD therapy.

4.7. Other Chemoattractants

Activation of the classic or alternate complement pathways also can remodel endothelial junctions, form leukocyte chemoattractants, and contribute to tissue injury during inflammation. C3a and C5a are both vasodilators, and contribute to mast-cell activation. C5a is particularly important as a chemoattractant for leukocytes and also increases the activation of integrins to promote leukocyte motility. C3b and C3bi are also potent stimuli for leukocyte phagocytosis *(69)*. Interestingly, a new model by Heit et al. *(70)* suggests that at least neutrophils exhibit a hierarchical prioritization to different chemotactic stimuli, with bacterial and complement (fMLP, C5a) dominating over tissue derived mediators (LTB$_4$, IL-8) and using Mac-1 versus LFA-1 respectively.

4.8. Nitric Oxide

NO has extraordinarly complex and varied roles in leukocyte-dependent injury and migration that depends on the its level of NO flux, its source, and the biochemical environment under which it is formed. For example, the relatively low NO fluxes generated by endothelial NOS are thought to block leukocyte platelet adhesion to the endothelium and their accompanying injury *(71)*, whereas the higher levels of NO formed by iNOS are often associated with an enhancement of tissue injury *(72)*.

5. LEUKOCYTE MIGRATION AND MATRIX REMODELING

Leukocyte migration through basal lamina and extracellular matrix toward sites of inflammation may be related to the elevation in proteases, e.g., matrix metalloproteases (MMPs). During exacerbations of MS, elevated levels of MMP-9 and other MMPs have been reported in the CSF (MMP-9) and in MS plaques, respectively *(63)*. Similarly, it is has been shown that one of the therapeutic mechanisms of IFN-β in MS consists of lowering the MMP-9/tissue inhibitor of MMP-1 (TIMP-1) ratio, which in turn may limit leukocyte migration *(73)*. Neutrophil elastase degrades junctional cadherins *(74)*, and elastase may have a similar role in neutrophil migration *(45)*.

As mentioned previously, Biernacki et al. *(66)* found that lymphocyte penetration of the brain microvasculature, irrespective of Th1/Th2 polarity, caused a subsequent increase in solute leakage and cell trafficking. Sallusto et al. *(62)* showed that T-cell receptor stimulation of either Th1 or Th2 cells produced equivalent expression of chemokines (e.g., RANTES, MIP-1b, I-309, IL-8), which may support lymphocyte migration into the CNS. Recently, Wolf et al. *(75)* examined T-cell motility

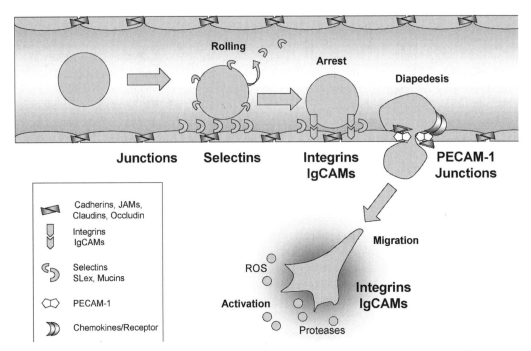

Fig. 1. A model for the interaction between activated leukocytes and the inflamed endothelium. This interaction includes the release of acute and chronic activators of leukocyte rolling, adhesion and emigration. Acutely, the mobilization of P-selectin and PAF as well as complement and chemoattractants (fMLP, LTB4) drive leukocyte infiltration of tissues. The adhesion and migration of leukocytes across and through tissues involves various adhesion molecules (selectins, integrins, and PECAM-1). Chronic inflammation is associated with upregulation of cytokines and chemokines and the synthesis and expression of additional adhesion molecules by endothelial cells in response to these mediators which support leukocyte homing, adhesion and emigration.

through fibrillar collagen and found that despite production of MMP-9, MT1-MMP, MT4-MMP, cathepsin, uPA, ADAM-9,10,11,15 and 17 by these cells, there was no dependence of guidance or motility on these enzymes *(75)*.

5.1. Ischemic Stress and Neuroinflammation

The interruption of blood flow also triggers an inflammatory response in the postischemic cerebrum and is characterized by extensive leukocyte (especially granulocyte, monocyte) adhesion *(76)*, infiltration, formation of cytokines and chemokines, and a form of progressive tissue injury that is leukocyte dependent. Additionally, this injury is also associated with the release of prostanoids and PAF, the induction of endothelial adhesion molecules *(77)* and MMPs *(78)*, and the promotion of an exogenous (leukocyte dependent) and endogenous (endothelial, glial) *(79)* tissue injury and loss of blood brain barrier.

5.2. Alzheimer's Disease (AD)

AD, the most common form of dementia, affects 1% of individuals ages 65 and older. Several markers in AD are related to inflammation (e.g., apolipoprotein E, the formation of proinflammatory cytokines) *(80)*. The brain is extensively infiltrated by leukocytes in many forms of inflammation, but in AD, neuroinflammation appears to involve activation of microglia (derived from monocytes), with leukocyte infiltration occurring only after microglial activation. The presence of active microglia within degenerating plaques is one of the hallmark neuropathological features of AD. The activation of these cells is induced by IFN-γ and other inflammatory cytokines *(81)*. These cells express MHC-class II molecules (HLA-DR), β-2 integrins (CD11b), leukocyte-common antigen, and the Ig receptor Fc-γ RI, consistent with activation of cells in the monocyte lineage.

Highly active microglia are phagocytic and may actively remove β-amyloid, which is beneficial *(82)*; however, active glia also release several products that may trigger inflammation, particularly reactive oxygen metabolites and NO-derived products, which account for the high degree of oxidant-stress markers in the AD plaque. McGeer et al. *(80)* state that complement, acute phase proteins, cytokines, chemokines, prostanoids, and proteases are all important mediators released near or by active microglia in AD. The cytokines associated with AD initiation include IL-1α, IL-1β, IL-6, TGF-β and TNF-α. In AD, some of the chemokines detected include IL-8, MCP-1, MIP-1α, MIP-1β, CXC-R2, CC-R3 and CC-R5; however, in AD, the CXCR3 receptor and its ligand fractalkine may have a dominant function in disease development. Fractalkine is produced by neurons undergoing stress, and antibody blockade of fractalkine is protective against LPS-induced stress. Hypertrophic and GFAP-expressing astrocytes are also present in the AD plaque and may help segregate the plaque from normal tissue. These activated astrocytes also express ICAM-1, making them adhesive for leukocytes. *(83)* T cells also appear to contribute to the inflammation seen near AD plaques. T cells have been observed in these plaques, which are CD45+ and express LFA-1, but their absolute magnitude is not very high in AD plaques.

5.3. HIV-Associated Dementia

HAD is characterized by neuroinflammation, particularly activation of macrophages and monocytes, astrogliosis, and neuronal cell injury, which produces the typical loss in cognitive impairment and delirium that are seen in in the condition. Some of the viral products secreted by HIV-infected cells, (e.g., Tat-1) seem ideally designed as inflammatory mediators. For example, we have reported that Tat-1 diminish the endothelial barrier by downregulating intercellular junctions *(84)*, as well as upregulating E-selectin *(85,86)* to increase leukocyte integration within tissues, binding to tissues, and penetration of tissue barriers (e.g., the BBB). Tat-1 is now also recognized as a ligand for the Flk-1/KDR-VEGF receptor *(87)*, which may provoke endothelial activation and proliferation-dependent CNS changes. Many other nonendothelial cells also express VEFG-R2 and respond to VEGF, including dendritic cells and monocytes/macrophages, and might be functionally altered in HIV-associated inflammation.

5.4. MS

The pathogenesis of MS represents an ongoing neuroinflammatory response that may arise from an immune-mediated response to components in the myelin sheath and leads to leukocyte-dependent injury and loss of BBB. The "storm" of cytokines associated with exacerbations of MS creates several forms of vascular injury, including disruption of BBB (seen as gadolinium-enhancing lesions), which contribute to the development of neurological deficits by impairing normal impulse conduction. The cytokines associated with MS include a parallel upregulation of proinflammatory (IFN-γ, TNF-α, TNF-β, and IL-12) and antiinflammatory cytokines (TGF-β and IL-10), as well as mobilization of IL-6 and perforin. MMPs clearly have a role in pathogenesis of MS through multiple mechanisms, including destruction of the extracellular matrix, proteolysis of endothelial junctional elements, and proteolysis of IFN-β (which is used for MS treatment). It is highly likely that the abundant Th1 cytokines in MS support the production of MMPs, particularly MMP-9, which targets the proteins described above.

6. SUMMARY

Inflammation, both within and outside of the CNS, encompasses a similar set of mediators, cells, mechanisms, and relationships, but the controlled access of the CNS compartments to the immune and circulatory system components and their interactions with CNS immune components (astrocytes, microglia) creates a unique set of inflammatory events in several neurological diseases. The balance between proinflammatory and antiinflammatory cytokines clearly has an essential function in normal CNS physiology *(58)*. Given the described roles of cytokines in inflammation, their imbalance in CNS pathology exhibits many features associated with inflammatory events elsewhere in the body and will likely provide the basis for many future therapies. The following chapters of this volume expand on specific inflammatory components in CNS disease and how these components are used both prognostically and therapeutically.

REFERENCES

1. Rabiet MJ, Plantier JL, Rival Y, Genoux Y, Lampugnani MG, Dejana E. Thrombin-induced increase in endothelial permeability is associated with changes in cell-to-cell junction organization. Arterioscler Thromb Vasc Biol 1996;16:488–496.
2. Dejana E. Endothelial adherens junctions: implications in the control of vascular permeability and angiogenesis. J Clin Invest 1996;98:1949–1953.
3. Lampugnani MG, Resnati M, Raiteri M, et al. A novel endothelial specific membrane protein is a marker of cell-cell contacts. J Cell Biol 1992;118:1511–1522.
4. Liaw CW, Cannon C, Power MD, Kiboneka PK, Rubin LL. Identification and cloning of two species of cadherins in bovine endothelial cells. EMBO J 1990;9:2701–2708.
5. Alexander JS, Blaschuk OW, Haselton FR. An N-cadherin-like protein contributes to solute barrier maintenance in cultured endothelium. J Cell Physiol 1993;156:610–618.
6. Bazzoni G. The JAM family of junctional adhesion molecules. Curr Opin Cell Biol 2003;15:525–530.
7. Furuse M, Hirase T, Itoh M, Nagafuchi A, Yonemura S, Tsukita S, Tsukita S. Occludin: a novel integral membrane protein localizing at tight junctions. J Cell Biol 1993;123:1777–1788.
8. Furuse M, Fujita K, Hiiragi T, Fujimoto K, Tsukita S. Claudin-1 and -2: novel integral membrane proteins localizing at tight junctions with no sequence similarity to occludin. J Cell Biol 1998;141:1539–1550.
9. Kevil CG, Ohno N, Gute D, et al. Hydrogen peroxide induces cadherin endocytosis in vitro: role in barrier regulation. Free Radic Biol Med 1998;24:1015–1022.
10. Alexander JS, Alexander BC, Eppihimer LA, et al. Inflammatory mediators induce sequestration of VE-cadherin in cultured human endothelial cells. Inflammation 2000;24:99–113.
11. Dudek SM, Garcia JG. Cytoskeletal regulation of pulmonary vascular permeability. J Appl Physiol 2001;91:1487–1500.
12. Huang AJ, Furie MB, Nicholson SC, Fischbarg J, Liebovitch LS, Silverstein SC. Effects of human neutrophil chemotaxis across human endothelial cell monolayers on the permeability of these monolayers to ions and macromolecules. J Cell Physiol 1988;135:355–366.
13. Etzioni A, Doerschuk CM, Harlan JM. Of man and mouse: leukocyte and endothelial adhesion molecule deficiencies. Blood 1999;94:3281–3288.
14. Vestweber D, Blanks JE. Mechanisms that regulate the function of selectins and their ligands. Physiol Rev 1999;79:181–213.
15. Bevilacqua MP, Nelson RM, Mannori G, Cecconi O. Endothelial-leukocyte adhesion molecules in human disease. Annu Rev Med 1994;45:361–378.
16. Kahn J, Ingraham RH, Shirley F, Migaki GI, Kishimoto TK. Membrane proximal cleavage of L-selectin: identification of the cleavage site and a 6-kD transmembrane peptide fragment of L-selectin. J Cell Biol. 1994 Apr;125(2):461–470.
17. Patel KD, Cuvelier SL, Wiehler Shahina. Selectins: critical mediators of leukocyte recruitment. Semin Immunol 2002;14:73–81.
18. Ley K. The role of selectins in inflammation and disease. Trends Mol Med 2003;9:263–268.
19. Hodivala-Dilke KM, McHugh KP, Tsakiris DA, et al. Beta$_3$-integrin-deficient mice are a model for Glanzmann thrombasthenia showing placental defects and reduced survival. J Clin Invest 1999;103:229–238.
20. Jones DH, Schmalstieg FC, Dempsey K, Krater SS, Nannen DD, Smith CW, Anderson DC. Subcellular distribution and mobilization of MAC-1 (CD11b/CD18) in neonatal neutrophils. Blood 1990;75:488–498.
21. Zakrzewicz A, Grafe M, Terbeek D, et al. L-selectin-dependent leukocyte adhesion to microvascular but not to macrovascular endothelial cells of the human coronary system. Blood 1997;89:3228–3235.
22. Woltmann G, McNulty CA, Dewson G, Symon FA, Wardlaw AJ. Interleukin-13 induces PSGL-1/P-selectin-dependent adhesion of eosinophils, but not neutrophils, to human umbilical vein endothelial cells under flow. Blood 2000;95:3146–3152.
23. Engelhardt B, Vestweber D, Hallmann R, Schulz M. E- and P-selectin are not involved in the recruitment of inflammatory cells across the blood-brain barrier in experimental autoimmune encephalomyelitis. Blood 1997;90:4459–72.
24. Rosen SD. Ligands for L-selectin: homing, inflammation, and beyond. Annu Rev Immunol 2004;22:129–156.
25. Zimmerman GA, Dixon DA, McIntyre TM, Prescott SM, Weyrich AS. Endothelial cell interactions with polymorphonuclear leukocytes (PMNs): a paradigm for juxtacrine signaling. In: Molecular Basis for Microcirculatory Disorders. Schmid-Schonbein GS, Granger DN (eds.), Springer-Verlag, New York, 2003.

26. Engelhardt B, Conley FK, Kilshaw PJ, Butcher EC. Lymphocytes infiltrating the CNS during inflammation display a distinctive phenotype and bind to VCAM-1 but not to MAdCAM-1. Int Immunol 1995;7:481–491.

27. Kanwar JR, Kanwar RK, Wang D, Krissansen GW. Prevention of a chronic progressive form of experimental autoimmune encephalomyelitis by an antibody against mucosal addressin cell adhesion molecule-1, given early in the course of disease progression. Immunol Cell Biol 2000;78:641–645.

28. Kanwar JR, Kanwar RK, Krissansen GW. Simultaneous neuroprotection and blockade of inflammation reverses autoimmune encephalomyelitis. Brain 2004;127(Pt 6):1313–1331.

29. Miller DH, Khan OA, Sheremata WA, et al. International Natalizumab Multiple Sclerosis Trial Group. A controlled trial of natalizumab for relapsing multiple sclerosis. N Engl J Med 2003;348:15–23.

30. Hopkins AM, Baird AW, Nusrat A. ICAM-1: targeted docking for exogenous as well as endogenous ligands. Adv Drug Deliv Rev 2004;56:763–778.

31. Cook-Mills JM. VCAM-1 signals during lymphocyte migration: role of reactive oxygen species. Mol Immunol 2002;39:499–508.

32. Vallien G, Langley R, Jennings S, Specian R, Granger DN. Expression of endothelial cell adhesion molecules in neovascularized tissue. Microcirculation 2000;7:249–258.

33. Sasaki M, Elrod JW, Jordan P, Itoh M, Joh T, Minagar A, Alexander JS. CYP450 dietary inhibitors attenuate TNF-alpha-stimulated endothelial molecule expression and leukocyte adhesion. Am J Physiol Cell Physiol 2004;286:C931–939.

34. Kanwar JR, Harrison JE, Wang D, Leung E, Mueller W, Wagner N, Krissansen GW. Beta7 integrins contribute to demyelinating disease of the central nervous system. J Neuroimmunol 2000;103:146–152.

35. Ostermann G, Weber KS, Zernecke A, Schroder A, Weber C. JAM-1 is a ligand of the beta(2) integrin LFA-1 involved in transendothelial migration of leukocytes. Nat Immunol 2002;3:151–158.

36. Liang TW, Chiu HH, Gurney A, et al. Vascular endothelial-junctional adhesion molecule (VE-JAM)/JAM 2 interacts with T, NK, and dendritic cells through JAM 3. J Immunol 2002;168:1618–1626.

37. Salmi M, Jalkanen S. A 90-kilodalton endothelial cell molecule mediating lymphocyte binding in humans. Science 1992;257:1407–1409.

38. Salmi M, Kalimo K, Jalkanen S. Induction and function of vascular adhesion protein-1 at sites of inflammation. J Exp Med. 1993;178:2255–2260.

39. Yoong, KF, McNab G, Hubscher SG, Adams DH. Vascular adhesion protein-1 and ICAM-1 support the adhesion of tumor-infiltrating lymphocytes to tumor endothelium in human hepatocellular carcinoma. J Immunol 1998; 160:3978–3988.

40. Sandig M, Korvemaker ML, Ionescu CV, Negrou E, Rogers KA. Transendothelial migration of monocytes in rat aorta: distribution of F-actin, alpha-catnin, LFA-1, and PECAM-1. Biotech Histochem 1999;74:276–293.

41. Moore KL, Stults NL, Diaz S, Smith DF, Cummings RD, Varki A, McEver RP. Identification of a specific glycoprotein ligand for P-selectin (CD62) on myeloid cells. J Cell Biol 1992;118:445–456.

42. Mamdouh Z, Chen X, Pierini LM, Maxfield FR, Muller WA. Targeted recycling of PECAM from endothelial surface-connected compartments during diapedesis. Nature 2003;421:748–753.

43. Muller WA, Randolph GJ. Migration of leukocytes across endothelium and beyond: molecules involved in the trans-migration and fate of monocytes. J Leukoc Biol 1999;66:698–704.

44. Minagar A, Jy W, Jimenez JJ, et al. Elevated plasma endothelial microparticles in multiple sclerosis. Neurology 2001;56:1319–1324.

45. Ionescu CV, Cepinskas G, Savickiene J, Sandig M, Kvietys PR. Neutrophils induce sequential focal changes in endothelial adherens junction components: role of elastase. Microcirculation 2003;10:205–220.

46. Cepinskas G, Noseworthy R, Kvietys PR. Transendothelial neutrophil migration. Role of neutrophil-derived proteases and relationship to transendothelial protein movement. Circ Res 1997;81:618–626.

47. Faveeuw C, Preece G, Ager A. Transendothelial migration of lymphocytes across high endothelial venules into lymph nodes is affected by metalloproteinases. Blood 2001;98:688–695.

48. Radi ZA, Kehrli ME Jr, Ackermann MR. Cell adhesion molecules, leukocyte trafficking, and strategies to reduce leukocyte infiltration. J Vet Intern Med 2001;15:516–529.

49. Wong D, Prameya R, Dorovini-Zis K. In vitro adhesion and migration of T lymphocytes across monolayers of human brain microvessel endothelial cells: regulation by ICAM-1, VCAM-1, E-selectin and PECAM-1. J Neuropathol Exp Neurol 1999;58:138–152.

50. Stins MF, Gilles F, Kim KS. Selective expression of adhesion molecules on human brain microvascular endothelial cells. J Neuroimmunol 1997;76:81–90.

51. Qing Z, Sandor M, Radvany Z, et al. Inhibition of antigen-specific T cell trafficking into the central nervous system via blocking PECAM1/CD31 molecule. J Neuropathol Exp Neurol 2001;60:798–807.

52. Wu J, Sheibani N. Modulation of VE-cadherin and PECAM-1 mediated cell-cell adhesions by mitogen-activated protein kinases. J Cell Biochem 2003;90:121–137.

53. Dinarello CA. The IL-1 family and inflammatory diseases. Clin Exp Rheumatol 2002;20(5 Suppl 27):S1–13.

54. Amano K, Okigaki M, Adachi Y, et al. Mechanism for IL-1 beta-mediated neovascularization unmasked by IL-1 beta knock-out mice. J Mol Cell Cardiol 2004;36:469–480.

55. Kuwano T, Nakao S, Yamamoto H, Tsuneyoshi M, Yamamoto T, Kuwano M, Ono M. Cyclooxygenase-2 is a key enzyme for inflammatory cytokine-induced angiogenesis. FASEB J 2004;18:300–310.

56. Carmeliet P. Manipulating angiogenesis in medicine. J Intern Med 2004. ;255:538–561.

57. Lu M, Perez VL, Ma N, Miyamoto K, Peng HB, Liao JK, Adamis AP. VEGF increases retinal vascular ICAM-1 expression in vivo. Invest Ophthalmol Vis Sci 1999;40:1808–1812.

58. Vitkovic L, Bockaert J, Jacque C. "Inflammatory" cytokines: neuromodulators in normal brain? J Neurochem 2000; 74:457–471.

59. Olson TS, Ley K. Chemokines and chemokine receptors in leukocyte trafficking. Am J Physiol Regul Integr Comp Physiol 2002;283:R7–28.

60. Stein JV, Rot A, Luo Y, et al. The CC chemokine thymus-derived chemotactic agent 4 (TCA-4, secondary lymphoid tissue chemokine, 6Ckine, exodus-2) triggers lymphocyte function-associated antigen 1-mediated arrest of rolling T lymphocytes in peripheral lymph node high endothelial venules. J Exp Med 2000;191:61–76.

61. Thelen M. Dancing to the tune of chemokines. Nat Immunol 2001;2:129–134.

62. Sallusto F, Kremmer E, Palermo B, et al. Switch in chemokine receptor expression upon TCR stimulation reveals novel homing potential for recently activated T cells. Eur J Immunol 1999;29:2037–2045.

63. Sellebjerg F, Sorensen TL. Chemokines and matrix metalloproteinase-9 in leukocyte recruitment to the central nervous system. Brain Res Bull 2003;61:347–355.

64. Klein RS. Regulation of neuroinflammation: the role of CXCL10 in lymphocyte infiltration during autoimmune encephalomyelitis. J Cell Biochem 2004;92:213–222.

65. Berger O, Gan X, Gujuluva C, et al. CXC and CC chemokine receptors on coronary and brain endothelia. Mol Med 1999;5:795–805.

66. Biernacki K, Prat A, Blain M, Antel JP. Regulation of cellular and molecular trafficking across human brain endothelial cells by Th1- and Th2-polarized lymphocytes. J Neuropathol Exp Neurol 2004;63:223–232.

67. Cotter R, Williams C, Ryan L, Erichsen D, Lopez A, Peng H, Zheng J. Fractalkine (CX3CL1) and brain inflammation: implications for HIV-1-associated dementia. J Neurovirol 2002;8:585–598.

68. Boehme SA, Lio FM, Maciejewski-Lenoir D, Bacon KB, Conlon PJ. The chemokine fractalkine inhibits Fas-mediated cell death of brain microglia. J Immunol 2000;165:397–403.

69. Wright SD, Silverstein SC. Receptors for C3b and C3bi promote phagocytosis but not the release of toxic oxygen from human phagocytes. J Exp Med 1983;158:2016–2023.

70. Heit B, Tavener S, Raharjo E, Kubes P. An intracellular signaling hierarchy determines direction of migration in opposing chemotactic gradients.J Cell Biol 2002;159:91–102.

71. Li H, Forstermann U. Nitric oxide in the pathogenesis of vascular disease. J Pathol 2000;190:244–254.

72. Laroux FS, Pavlick KP, Hines IN, et al. Role of nitric oxide in inflammation. Acta Physiol Scand 2001;173:113–118.

73. Waubant E, Goodkin D, Bostrom A, Bacchetti P, Hietpas J, Lindberg R, Leppert D. IFNbeta lowers MMP-9/TIMP-1 ratio, which predicts new enhancing lesions in patients with SPMS. Neurolog. 2003;60:52–57.

74. Carden D, Xiao F, Moak C, Willis BH, Robinson-Jackson S, Alexander S. Neutrophil elastase promotes lung microvascular injury and proteolysis of endothelial cadherins. Am J Physiol 1998;275(2 Pt 2):H385–392.

75. Wolf K, Muller R, Borgmann S, Brocker EB, Friedl P. Amoeboid shape change and contact guidance: T-lymphocyte crawling through fibrillar collagen is independent of matrix remodeling by MMPs and other proteases. Blood 2003;102:3262–3269.

76. Campanella M, Sciorati C, Tarozzo G, Beltramo M. Flow cytometric analysis of inflammatory cells in ischemic rat brain. Stroke 2002;33:586–592.

77. Stanimirovic D, Satoh K. Inflammatory mediators of cerebral endothelium: a role in ischemic brain inflammation. Brain Pathol 2000;10:113–126.

78. Lo EH, Wang X, Cuzner ML. Extracellular proteolysis in brain injury and inflammation: role for plasminogen activators and matrix metalloproteinases. J Neurosci Res 2002;69:1–9.

79. Fukuda S, Fini CA, Mabuchi T, Koziol JA, Eggleston LL Jr, del Zoppo GJ. Focal cerebral ischemia induces active proteases that degrade microvascular matrix. Stroke 2004;35:998–1004.

80. McGeer EG, McGeer PL. Inflammatory processes in Alzheimer's disease. Prog Neuropsychopharmacol Biol Psychiatry 2003;27:741–749.

81. Gasic-Milenkovic J, Dukic-Stefanovic S, Deuther-Conrad W, Gartner U, Munch G. Beta-amyloid peptide potentiates inflammatory responses induced by lipopolysaccharide, interferon-gamma and 'advanced glycation endproducts' in a murine microglia cell line. Eur J Neurosci 2003;17:813-821.

82. Frackowiak J, Wisniewski HM, Wegiel J, Merz GS, Iqbal K, Wang KC. Ultrastructure of the microglia that phagocytose amyloid and the microglia that produce beta-amyloid fibrils. Acta Neuropathol (Berl) 1992;84:225–233.

83. Akiyama H, Kawamata T, Yamada T, Tooyama I, Ishii T, McGeer PL. Expression of intercellular adhesion molecule (ICAM)-1 by a subset of astrocytes in Alzheimer disease and some other degenerative neurological disorders. Acta Neuropathol (Berl) 1993;85:628–634.

84. Oshima T, Laroux FS, Coe LL, et al. Interferon-gamma and interleukin-10 reciprocally regulate endothelial junction integrity and barrier function. Microvasc Res 2001;61:130–143.

85. Cota-Gomez A, Flores NC, Cruz C, et al. The human immunodeficiency virus-1 Tat protein activates human umbilical vein endothelial cell E-selectin expression via an NF-kappa B-dependent mechanism. J Biol Chem 2002;277:14390–14399.
86. Ichikawa H, Wolf RE, Au TY, et al. Exogenous xanthine promotes neutrophil adherence to cultured endothelial cells. Am J Physiol 1997;273:G342–G347.
87. Rusnati M, Urbinati C, Musulin B, et al. Activation of endothelial cell mitogen activated protein kinase ERK(1/2) by extracellular HIV-1 Tat protein. Endothelium 2001;8:65–74.

CME QUESTIONS

1. Which statement about leukocyte–endothelium interaction is correct?
   A. This interaction in the context of inflammation involves upregulation of expression of adhesion molecules.
   B. Complement and cytokines play a role in this interaction.
   C. During inflammatory cascade, chemokines guide the activated leukocytes toward sites of inflamed endothelium.
   D. All of the above are correct.

2. Which statement about transendothelial migration of leukocytes is correct?
   A. Transendothelial migration of activated leukocytes during inflammatory response occurs mostly at small-diameter postcapillary venules, where the endothelium expresses high levels of adhesion molecules during inflammation.
   B. Transendothelial migration of leukocytes occurs mostly at the arteriolar level.
   C. Transendothelial migration of leukocytes occurs only at lymphatic vessels.
   D. Transendothelial migration of leukocytes takes place only at large veins.

3. Which of the following statements about chemokines is correct?
   A. Chemokines (or chemoattractant cytokines) are the major *in situ* regulators of integrin activity on endothelium-recruited leukocytes.
   B. Chemokines are generally displayed on endothelial sites of leukocyte migration, where they can signal through transmembrane receptors linked to the α subunit of heterodimeric Gi proteins on the endothelium-adherent leukocyte.
   C. Chemokines and chemokine receptors play a significant role in pathogenesisof inflammatory disorders, such as multiple sclerosis.
   D. All of the above are correct.

4. Which statement about VCAM-1 is incorrect?
   A. VCAM-1 and its ligand $\alpha_4\beta_1$ (VLA-4) are another important adhesion system in inflammation that has been associated with several forms of chronic inflammation (e.g., arthritis, dermatitis, neuritis).
   B. VCAM-1 expression by endothelial cells is induced by cytokine stimulation, while its expression by resting endothelium is minimal.
   C. Upregulation of expression of VCAM-1 by endothelial cells requires posttranscriptional events involving the NF-κB-signaling system.
   D. A monoclonal antibody (natalizumab) binds $\alpha_4$integrin on the surface of activated lymphocytes and monocytes effectively, blocks their adhesion to VCAM-1 and MAdCAM-1 on activated endothelium, and has been used successfully in treatment of systemic lupus erythematosus.

2

Multiple Sclerosis

A Disease of Miscommunication Between the Immune and Central Nervous Systems?

Monica J. Carson, Crystal S. Anglen, and Corinne Ploix

1. IMMUNE PRIVILEGE

1.1. The Problem

A functional central nervous system (CNS) is essential for mammalian survival; therefore, the CNS must be defended from insults and other pathogens. The molecules (e.g., free radicals, cytokines, proteases) produced in vast quantities by the activated immune system to combat pathogens have the demonstrated potential to disrupt CNS function *(1–3)*. To balance these opposing needs, (sufficient defense of the CNS without loss of CNS function), the CNS and immune system have developed a unique relationship referred to as immune privilege. Disruptions in this unique relationship leading to disregulated CNS inflammation are now thought to contribute to the onset and progression of many diverse types of CNS pathology, including CNS autoimmune diseases such as multiple sclerosis (MS), Rasmussen's encephalitis, and narcolepsy; neurodegenerative diseases such as Alzheimer's disease, Parkinson's disease, and stroke; and the secondary neurodegeneration associated with spinal cord injury *(3–10)*.

Currently, the following three issues concerning the pathogenesis of CNS autoimmune and neurodegenerative diseases are under substantial debate:

1. Is the CNS really an immune-privileged site? Specifically, to what extent is the CNS passive in its interactions with the immune system, and to what extent is the CNS an active regulator of inflammatory responses?
2. Is all inflammation within the CNS maladaptive, or can CNS inflammation be beneficial for CNS function?
3. Do microglia, the resident macrophages of the brain, perform different functions from macrophages that acutely infiltrate the CNS in response to pathogenic signals?

In this chapter, we explore these three broad issues by focusing on the pathogenesis of a chronic demyelinating CNS inflammatory disease: MS. MS most frequently presents as a relapsing–remitting pathology, suggesting that its pathology may result from offsetting detrimental and protective/regenerative interactions between the CNS and immune systems *(11,12)*. Further, we examine the CNS mechanisms that contribute to maintaining immune privilege and promoting successful resolution of acute inflammatory responses. We specifically examine the potential for microglia to play key functions in MS pathogenesis because of their ability to regulate and be regulated by both the CNS and immune systems and to develop both neuroprotective and neurotoxic effector functions *(13)*.

From: *Current Clinical Neurology: Inflammatory Disorders of the Nervous System: Pathogenesis, Immunology, and Clinical Management*
Edited by: A. Minagar and J. S. Alexander © Humana Press Inc., Totowa, NJ

1.2. Immune Privilege Defined

More than 60 yr ago, Medawar illustrated in an elegant series of experiments that showed that the CNS was immunologically distinct from other peripheral tissues *(14)*. When Medawar placed allografts (tissue grafts from the same species but expressing a different major histo-compatibility complex [MHC] haplotype) into peripheral tissue sites, the allografts were rapidly destroyed by the immune system. By contrast, allografts placed within the CNS were not immediately rejected and survived for substantially longer periods. Subsequent experiments from numerous groups confirmed the following two key tenets that define the current concept of CNS immune privilege:

1. The threshold for initiating T-cell responses against antigens found primarily within the CNS is much higher than for antigens found primarily outside the CNS *(9,15)*.
2. The types of immune cells recruited to a tissue by inflammatory insults (e.g., lipopolysaccharide, viral infection, mechanical damage to stroma) and the kinetics of recruitment differ when the insult occurs in the CNS as opposed to other peripheral tissue sites. Within the CNS, the kinetics of inflammation are delayed, and there is a tendency for fewer granulocytes to be recruited than outside the CNS *(9,16)*.

1.3. How Are Immune Responses Initiated in Nonimmune-Privileged Sites?

Before we can explore how immune privilege is maintained in the healthy CNS and overcome in MS, we need to define how T-cell responses are initiated outside of the CNS. In nonimmune-privileged sites, T-cell responses to pathology are shaped by the profile and progression of the innate immune response (e.g., macrophages, granulocytes, fibroblasts, stromal cells) *(17,18)*. In brief, tissue macrophages/immature dendritic cells become activated by any of several non-specific danger signals (e.g., tumor necrosis factor [TNF]-α, cell debris) produced by damaged and distressed tissue cells and pathogen-associated molecular patterns (PAMPs) (e.g., endotoxin, peptidoglycans, guanine and cytosine-rich oliognucleotides/CpGs) recognized by pattern-recognition receptors *(17,18)*. On activation, tissue macrophages/immature dendritic cells are stimulated to produce cytokines, chemokines, and free radicals, and to capture anti-gen from pathogens and cellular debris. Because T cells do not recognize whole proteins, macrophages/immature dendritic cells must proteolytically process the captured antigen by reducing the protein into antigenic peptides.

After antigen capture, tissue macrophages/tissue dendritic cells migrate to the draining lymph nodes, where they present antigen to T cells and initiate primary induction of T-cell-effector function *(17,18)*. Acting as antigen-presenting cells (APCs), macrophages/dendritic cells activate CD4+ T cells by presenting antigen in the binding cleft of MHC class II and CD8+ T cells by presenting antigen within the cleft of MHC class I. Once activated by antigen presentation, T cells leave the lymph nodes and circulate throughout the body in search of their target antigen. After entering the target tissue, the target antigen must be re-presented to the infiltrating T cell by resident and infiltrat-ing macrophages/dendritic cells. In the absence of APCs, the T cell is blind to the presence of its target antigen, even when it is immersed in its target antigen. Without local antigen presentation, the T cell will leave the tissue to continue searching for its target.

1.4. Is Immune Privilege Equivalent to Immune Isolation?

In the decades immediately following Medawar's seminal experiments, the immune privilege of the CNS was assumed to be caused by the immune system's inability to detect antigens within the CNS *(19)*. The presence of the blood–brain barrier (BBB) and the absence of a lymphatic sys-tem that can passively drain CNS antigens into lymph nodes coupled with the absence of a resi-dent population of APCs capable of presenting antigen or migrating to the lymph nodes were together presumed to sequester the CNS from the immune system. If the immune system became aware of CNS antigens by a rupture in the BBB, the subsequent drainage of CNS antigens into the cervical lymph nodes, and/or the intrusion of APCs into the CNS, the immediate result was presumed to be the initiation of destructive CNS autoimmune inflammation. Conversely, anti-CNS immune responses could be initiated outside the CNS by viruses or other pathogens expressing an antigen target similar in molecular structure to an endogenous CNS antigen (a molecular mimic) *(20,21)*. If a sufficiently strong anti-CNS immune response was initiated outside the CNS, the activated immune cells were presumed to breach the BBB, encounter their CNS antigen targets, and launch destructive CNS autoimmunity. In this paradigm, the CNS is a passive victim of the immune system; thus, the damage to CNS myelin and neurons observed in the histopathology of MS was previously viewed as the inevitable and sequential result of failing to prevent macrophages and T cells from infiltrating the CNS and becoming aware of CNS antigens.

Currently, a very different view of CNS–immune system interactions has begun to evolve that alters our view of the pathogenesis of CNS inflammatory diseases *(3,22–24)*. First, immunocompetent T cells, macrophages and dendritic cells do readily cross the BBB and transverse the healthy CNS in the absence of neuropathology and clinical symptoms *(5)*. Second, several classes of viral infection can be cleared from the CNS by an acute self-resolving CNS inflammation without evidence of any long-lasting bystander effects and without induction of chronic CNS autoimmunity *(25)*. Third, brain injuries (e.g., stroke, blunt injury, axotomies) do not initiate destructive CNS autoimmunity *(3,22–24)*. Yet, these forms of injury do cause the release of CNS antigens into circulation and are associated with infiltration of CNS auto-reactive T cells and MHC-expressing APCs into the sites of CNS injury. Fourth, microglia have demonstrated potential to act as a resident CNS-specific type of APC that serves to limit, redirect, and even terminate proinflammatory T-cell responses *(26,27)*. Finally, new data indicate that in some situations, CNS-autoimmunity may serve to limit neurodegeneration and perhaps promote neuroprotection. In this paradigm, MS histopathology is likely a consequence not only of an inappropriately activated peripheral immune system but also of failures in the active immunosuppressive and neuroprotective mechanisms operating within the CNS.

2. MULTIPLE SCLEROSIS: THE STEREOTYPIC DISEASE OF CNS INFLAMMATION

2.1. What is Multiple Sclerosis?

MS has been actively studied for more than a century, but much about MS, including its cause, remains a mystery. What is known? MS is one of the first chronic CNS neurodegenerative diseases recognized to have an inflammatory component driving pathogenesis and clinical disability *(11,12)*. Although MS-initiating agents/events remain a subject of speculation, pedigree and epidemiological studies indicate that MS susceptibility has both environmental and genetic components. On the genetic level, the MHC class II locus has been most consistently correlated with MS susceptibility, although many loci appear to have roles in modulating MS risk and pathogenesis. From these observations, inappropriate activation of myelin-specific CD4[+] T cells are suspected to have causative roles in MS pathogenesis. Interestingly, epidemiology studies also suggest that encounters with unknown environmental factors around puberty prime individuals to develop MS 10 to 20 yr later. Furthermore, researchers have speculated that MS susceptibility may result from early encounters with viruses or bacteria that prime the immune system to generate destructive antimyelin-T-cell responses at later ages in response to reactivating signals (e.g., pathogens, bacteria, viruses) *(11,12,20)*.

Clinically, onset of MS symptoms most often occurs between 20 and 40 yr of age *(11,28)*. About 85% of persons experience a relapsing–remitting form of MS in which periods of full or partial symptom remission follow clinical episodes of disability. The frequency, severity, and types of clinical episodes vary widely between individuals. Initial symptoms can include transient bouts of extreme fatigue, vertigo, optic neuritis, weakness, and/or numbness in the extremities. With time, symptoms become much more severe and debilitating and can include ataxia, paraparesis, painful limb spasms, and cognitive impairment. After several years, the disease progression tends to convert from an episodic to a progressive neurological deterioration. Approximately 15% of persons experience a progressive deterioration from the initial onset of symptoms.

Because none of these symptoms are unique to MS, the diagnosis of MS is based on the occurrence of two or more episodes of clinical disability coupled with finding two or more lesions within CNS-white-matter tracts disseminated in time and location *(11,28)*. Furthermore, because a definitive laboratory test for MS does not exist, the diagnosis of MS can be made only if all other potential causes of these clinical signs have been excluded. For example, diseases with viral, bacterial, or even parasitic causes (e.g., acute disseminated encephalomyelitis, sarcoidosis, disseminated Lyme disease), can all initially present with symptoms similar to MS.

2.2. Does Multiple Sclerosis Have Variable Pathogenesis or a Collection of Related Syndromes?

The extreme heterogeneity of disease onset, progression, clinical symptoms, and histopathology has also raised the possibility that MS in not a single disease with a single cause but a collection of symptomatically related syndromes that may have multiple causes. For example, tropic spastic paraparesis (TSP) (also known as human T-cell lymphoma/leukemia virus [HTLV]-associated myelopathy) was originally defined as a form of MS *(29)*; however, once TSP was identified as one of the many clinical consequences of HTLV-1 infection, its unique histopathology was distinguished from other forms of MS *(29,30)*. With continued epidemiology and research, some current subtypes of MS may eventually be recognized as distinct diseases with causes and pathologies that differ from those of MS.

Likewise, it should be cautioned that the heterogeneous nature of MS in itself is not a conclusive indication that MS is more than one disease. For example, immunization of susceptible rodent strains with myelin antigens in the presence of strong adjuvants triggers a T-cell-dependent demyelinating disease called *experimentally induced autoimmune encephalomyelitis* (EAE) *(31)*; however, the clinical symptoms, kinetics, severity, and histopathology of EAE are highly dependent on the type of adjuvant and the genetic background of the treated animal *(32)*. For example, the same antigenic peptide from the myelin oligodendrocyte glycoprotein (MOG) *(92–106)* has been used to immunize SJL/J and A.SW mice, two different mouse strains expressing the same MHC class II haplotype (H-2^s) but with different propensities for generating CD4$^+$ T-cell phenotypes *(33)*. SJL/J mice lack natural killer (NK)1.1 T cells and are more prone to generate T-helper type 1 (Th1)-CD4$^+$ T-cell responses (interleukin [IL]-2 and interferon [IFN; producing T cells]), whereas A.SW mice have a normal complement of NK1.1 T cells and are more prone to generate Th2 CD4$^+$ T-cell responses (IL-4, IL-10 [producing T cells]). Immunizing SJL/J mice with MOG in the presence of complete Freud's adjuvant (CFA; the oil and water immersion of killed mycobacterium tuberculosis) leads to a relapsing–remitting form of EAE. By contrast, immunizing A.SW mice with the same protocol leads to a primary progressive model of EAE. Addition of pertussis toxin (PT) treatment to the immunization protocol failed to alter the long-term disease progression observed in the SJL/J mice but did convert clinical disease from a primary progressive to a secondary progressive form in A.SW mice.

Histologically, the pathology induced by the identical causative agents also differed in the two mouse strains *(33)*. In SJL/J mice, only mild demyelination occurred and was accompanied by T-cell infiltration. In the A.SW mice, large areas of demyelination developed accompanied by neutrophil infiltration and minimal T-cell infiltration. In immunized A.SW mice without PT treatment, immunoglobin (Ig) deposition was detected in the CNS and high titers of MOG antibodies were detected in the serum. These results raise the question of which mouse model is the correct model of MS but also highlight that the apparent heterogeneity of MS could also be largely a function of the polymorphic immunological genotypes of those persons with this disease.

2.3. Multiple Sclerosis Pathogenesis

Early in the study of MS, the pathogenomonic feature of the disease was the appearance within the CNS of demyelinated lesions often infiltrated with lymphocytes and activated macrophages *(11,28)*. Although numerous studies have documented the extreme heterogeneity of lesion types, it remains unclear to what extent lesion heterogeneity is caused by the evolution of lesions with disease progression or whether it reflects distinct pathogenic processes.

2.3.1. Classification of Multiple Sclerosis Lesions

Recently, Lucchinetti et al. performed a large-scale analysis of MS lesions from biopsy and autopsy material *(34)*. Although many of their observations confirmed those of previous investigators, they made a notable addition. All of the analyzed lesions could be grouped into four distinct patterns, and all lesions from a single individual belonged to only one pattern. Owing to the small amount of tissue taken for biopsy analysis, there has been some discussion of whether the authors would have been able to detect lesion heterogeneity within a single individual. Despite this caveat, the primary implication from their study is that symptomatic MS results from at least four distinct types of pathogenic mechanisms.

Interestingly, the authors note that both type I and II MS lesions shared features with those detected in EAE. In both type I and II MS lesions, myelin loss was predominantly seen in perivenous locations and the edges of the lesions were sharply demarcated. Areas of active demyelination were associated with lymphocytic and myeloid inflammation. As noted by previous investigators, remyelination and preservation of oligodendrocytes were also readily apparent in these areas of active destruction. The primary difference between patterns I and II was the deposition of Ig G and activated complement in pattern II lesions and the absence of such deposition in pattern I lesions. Of the four described lesion types, type I was the most frequent and was most associated with the relapsing–remitting form of MS.

By contrast, the pathologies of pattern III and IV lesions were noted to be reminiscent of viral- or toxin-induced models of oligodendroctye dystrophy. Most notably, type III lesions, unlike type I and II lesions, were not centered around veins and lesion borders were diffuse and irregular. In addition, oligodendrocyte death was quite prominent in both type III and IV lesions. The apparent method of death differed between the two lesions. In type III lesions, oligodendrocytes displayed nuclear condensation and fragmentation characteristic of apoptotic death, while those in type IV lesions displayed features suggesting necrotic death. Deposition of IgG and activated complement were not detected in either type III or IV lesions, although both lesion types contained lymphocytes and activated myeloid cells.

2.3.2. Axonal Damage Underlies Progressive and Permanent Multiple Sclerosis-Associated Disability

Although generally described as a disease of demyelination, MS is also a disease of axonal damage and neuronal dysfunction *(35–39)*. Indeed, magnetic resonance imaging, magnetic resonance spectroscopy, and positron emission tomography examinations of MS patients during disease progression indicate that accumulating permanent clinical dysfunction correlates more closely with axonal damage than with infiltration of activated immune cells. Histological analysis has confirmed that neurons are damaged during the earliest stages of MS. Axonal damage and transection have even been detected in neurons with apparently intact healthy myelin sheaths and in brain regions without overt inflammation.

Within lesions, progressive irreversible axonal damage is likely the consequence of sustained demyelination and exposure to neurotoxic products produced during the inflammatory process. The cause of neuronal damage in apparently healthy brain regions distant from inflammation is less clear *(40)*. It is likely that this latter form of neuronal damage is owing in part to Wallerian degeneration of neurons damaged within inflamed lesions. Of unknown significance is the microglia clustering and global expression of microglial-activation markers in cells with an unactivated ramified morphology observed coincident with neuronal damage in otherwise normal-appearing brain regions *(40–42)*. Are these merely microglial responses to neuronal pathology with little consequence for the progression of disease, or do these microglial responses prime these healthy brain regions for autoimmune attack? Alternatively, as some have suggested, are these activated microglia initially attempting to save stressed neurons, perhaps by the production of growth factors *(43,44)*?

Ultimately, attempting to interrupt MS pathogenesis requires identifying sites of intervention prior to the accumulation of substantial irreversible axonal damage. Thus, the key question is: which comes first? Does dysfunction of microglia and/or astrocytes inappropriately recruit lymphocytes, macrophages and dendritic cells across the BBB? Does microglial activation increase the ability of microglia to present antigen to T cells and promote detrimental T-cell responses? Do CNS-infiltrating T cells and macrophages directly and indirectly activate microglia and astrocytes? Conversely, does neuronal pathology and/or oligodendrocyte dysfunction lead to inappropriate activation of microglia and astrocytes?

3. AUTOIMMUNITY

3.1. How Is Autoimmunity Initiated?

Before we can address how the immune-privileged status of the CNS is breached in MS, we need to understand how autoimmunity is initiated against nonimmune-privileged targets.

3.1.1. How Is Autoimmunity Initiated Against Nonimmune-Privileged Organs?

Peripheral organs are largely protected from autoimmune attack because T cells with high affinity for antigens expressed by peripheral organs (e.g., pancreas, liver, kidney) are deleted from the T-cell population during development *(18,45,46)*. Despite the removal of these self-reactive T cells, T cells autoreactive for peripheral organ antigens (and CNS antigens) are readily detected in all adult mammalian species. Furthermore, simply transferring high-affinity autoreactive T cells specific for peripheral organ antigens is by itself insufficient to trigger autoimmunity. For example, transfer of T cells specific for the influenza hemagglutinin (HA) into mice expressing the HA antigen in their pancreatic islets (Ins-HA mice) is insufficient to cause pancreatic autoimmune diabetes *(45,46)*. This is not because the HA-T cells fail to detect and respond to their target antigen. After transfer into Ins-HA mice, the transferred T cells proliferate and a few T cells even accumulate around the islets. These results indicate that induction of destructive proinflammatory T-cell-effector function requires more than just antigen presentation. For instance, to induce autoimmune diabetes in Ins-HA mice, HA-specific T cells must be primed by homeostatic or adjuvant signals in addition to antigenic signals *(47)*.

3.1.2. What Are Homeostatic and Adjuvant Signals, and Why Do They Promote Autoimmunity?

The numbers of T cells in circulation are maintained at a species-specific and strain-specific homeostatic set point. T cells sense the total numbers of T cells in circulation by competing for survival factors (CCL21 for CD4[+] T cells and IL-15 for CD8[+] T cells) *(47,48)*. When T cell numbers are low (because of partial depletion of T cells by genetic or environmental factors), high concentrations of these survival factors become available, and T cells begin to proliferate and acquire a semiactivated phenotype (capable of crossing the BBB) in the absence of antigen presentation *(47)*. Homeostatic proliferation/activation by itself is insufficient to drive the differentiation of T-cell-effector function *(47,48)*. However, when homeostatic proliferation is coupled with antigen presentation, all aspects of T-cell activation are dramatically accelerated and augmented *(47)*. Similarly, strong adjuvants such as CFA, the oil–water immersion homogenate of killed mycobacterium tuberculosis, or PT have many effects on T cells, APCs, and stromal cells *(17)*. The net result of these adjuvants is to bypass and/or amplify the receptor pathways triggered by these homeostatic survival factors, leading to accelerated and augmented T-cell responses to antigenic signals.

3.1.3. Do Homeostatic and Adjuvant Signals Have a Role in Spontaneous Autoimmunity?

During development, the number of T cells maintained in circulation is primarily determined by thymic production of T cells. With increasing age, thymic output declines, and homeostatic mechanisms begin to significantly contribute to the number of T cells maintained in circulation *(49,50)*. Strikingly, two separate studies have suggested that thymic output of T cells is dramatically decreased in patients with either MS or autoimmune rheumatoid arthritis (RA) *(49,50)*. In both studies, the thymic T-cell output of rheumatoid arthritis and MS patients was reduced to that observed in healthy individuals who were 30 yr older. Thus, it is likely that in these MS patients, circulating T cells were subject to strong homeostatic (autoimmune-priming) signals.

Increased homeostatic proliferation is not only a risk factor for lymphopenic (T-cell deficient) individuals but also may be a risk factor in those with normal levels of T cells. Abnormal increases in the production of survival factors would also inappropriately induce homeostatic T-cell proliferation. For example, transgenic overexpression of CCL21 outside the CNS induced homeostatic $CD4^+$ T-cell proliferation in non-lymphopenic mice *(47)*. Without other amplifying factors, CCL21 overexpression was sufficient to prime autoreactive T cells to inititiate destructive autoimmunity against peripheral organs. Suggestively, CCL21 expression is induced in the CNS and pancreas during the preclinical stages of rodent EAE and autoimmune diabetes, respectively *(51,52)*. Taken together, these data strongly imply that homeostatic signals can have a role in priming the immune system for destructive autoimmune responses.

Although MS patients are quite unlikely to have been subjected to CFA or PT treatments prior to the onset or relapse of symptoms, several groups have correlated the impact of systemic infections with the onset and progression of MS. Although this remains an area of substantial debate, one epidemiological study found that the risk of MS relapse was nearly threefold higher following systemic infections, typically upper respiratory tract infections *(53)*. Data derived from transgenic mouse models provide some support for systemic infections acting as nonspecific adjuvants able promote CNS inflammation. For example, mice in which nearly the entire circulating T-cell population has been transgenically engineered to be specific for myelin basic protein (MBP) do not develop CNS autoimmunity if maintained in a clean, specific pathogen-free animal colony *(54)*; however, when these transgenic mice were maintained in a dirty colony and presumably became infected with common murine pathogens, the mice developed EAE symptoms and pathology.

3.2. Are Homeostatic and Adjuvant Signals Sufficient to Enable Destructive CNS Autoimmunity?

Our discussion of homeostatic and adjuvant signals has focused primarily on the priming of the immune system—and not the CNS—in autoimmunity. Because homeostatic signals do not alter the CNS, it is unlikely that homeostatic signals by themselves are sufficient to induce CNS autoimmunity. It is highly likely that the effectiveness of adjuvants at promoting CNS autoimmunity is dependent on their ability to regulate both the CNS and immune system. At least four types of observations support this conclusion. First, autoreactive T cells are readily detected in the bloodstream of healthy people and rodents *(55,56)*. Yet, systemic infection does not automatically result in CNS autoimmune destruction. Second, treating mice with CFA alone and not with immunizing antigen leads to a rapid and robust accumulation of T cells within the CNS *(57–59)*. Yet, these cells are not retained within the CNS, nor do clinical and/or histopathological signs develop. Third, even when CCL21 and other strong T-cell chemoattractants are transgenically overexpressed within the murine CNS, T cells fail to accumulate within the CNS, and CNS autoimmune destruction does not occur *(60)* (Ploix and Carson, unpublished results). Finally, humans with autoimmune diabetes develop robust proinflammatory T-cell responses against a variety of antigens expressed in both the pancreas and the CNS (such as glutamic acid decarboxylase [GAD65], glial fibrillary acidic protein, IA-2 antigen) *(61–64)*. Despite the presence of activated T cells autoreactive for CNS antigens, diabetic individuals do not have a higher incidence of encephalitis than the population at large.

The existence of a much higher threshold for initiating autoreactive immune responses against the CNS (as compared to other tissues) is reaffirmed by a close comparison of just the immune responses to GAD65 between individuals with autoimmune diabetes and stiff-man's syndrome, a form of CNS autoimmune-induced ataxia *(63)*. GAD is the biosynthesizing enzyme of the inhibitory neurotransmitter γ-aminobutyric acid and is highly expressed in pancreatic islet cells and a subpopulation of CNS neurons. Analysis of first-degree "at-risk" relatives of patients with autoimmune diabetes reveals that antibody and T-cell responses against GAD65 not only are strong predictors of incipient autoimmune diabetes but also that these responses can be detected years before the onset of clinical autoimmune diabetes. Although 60 to 80% of persons with autoimmune diabetes have strong detectable GAD65 responses, the risk of their developing stiff-man's syndrome is rare *(62)*. Stiff man's syndrome's incidence in persons with autoimmune diabetes is less than 0.001%. Surprisingly, the reverse is not true. Approximately 30% of individuals with stiff-man's syndrome develop a mild form of diabetes in adulthood. Individuals with stiff man's syndrome also have anti-GAD antibodies with a higher titer and increased epitope recognition as compared with those detected in individuals with autoimmune diabetes *(62)*. These data imply that the initiation of CNS autoimmune disease requires a stronger immune response than that required to initiate autoimmune destruction.

4. CAN THE HEALTHY CNS SUPPORT ANTIGEN-SPECIFIC T-CELL RESPONSES?

The previous discussion demonstrates that chemokine induction, homeostatic signals, and/or peripheral immune responses are sufficient to initiate destructive autoimmunity against peripheral tissues; however, these same signals are by themselves insufficient to initiate CNS autoimmunity. Consequently, it has been proposed that the CNS lacks an effective resident APC population capable of effectively recruiting, retaining, or activating T-cell responses. From this viewpoint, initiation of CNS autoimmunity (and MS) would be dependent on one of two events: the infiltration of sufficient numbers of peripheral APCs (macrophages and dendritic cells) into the CNS or the induction of inappropriate APC function by CNS cells.

4.1. Microglia Are the Resident Tissue Macrophages of the CNS

Of all the cells in the CNS, only microglia are hemopoetically derived and readily able to express sufficient levels of MHC class I, MHC class II, and the costimulatory molecules required to fully activate both CD4+ and CD8+ T cells *(13,16,26,65,66)*. Microglia comprise between 5 and 15% of the cells in the CNS. Found in all regions of the CNS, microglia are strategically situated to control the onset and progression of autoreactive T-cell responses; however, under nonpathological conditions, microglia in the CNS of healthy rodents and humans are largely MHC class I- and II-negative. In their inactivated state, microglial expression of costimulatory molecules B7.2 and CD40 is low to negligible. Therefore, in the absence of other signals, microglia are incapable of acting as APCs and thus of retaining or locally activating T cells within the CNS.

Microglia do appear poised to transform rapidly into APCs *(13,16,26,65,66)*. In response to a wide array of signals (e.g., age, mechanical injury, bacterial or viral exposure), microglia rapidly express MHC. Exposure to proinflammatory cytokines produced by activated T cells and/or damaged cells, such as interferon (IFN)-γ and TNF-α, dramatically increases microglial expression of intercellular adhesion molecule (ICAM)-1, CD40, B7.2, and B7.1. Direct interactions between microglia and T cells can also amplify the ability of microglia to become APCs. The outcome of these interactions is in part dependent on T-cell activation state.

Activated T cells express CD154, the ligand for CD40, a receptor expressed on activated microglia and other potential APCs. Recently, several studies have demonstrated that CD40-triggered microglia express higher levels of MHC class II, CD40, B7.2, and B7.1 and begin to produce IL-12 and IL-23 *(67–69)*. The production of IL-12 and IL-23 in turn increases T-cell production of IFN-γ. CD40-triggered microglia are also primed to respond more robustly to other environmental cues. For example, CD40 ligation dramatically increases the β-amyloid and IFN-γ-induced production of TNF-α by microglia *(67–69)*. T cells can even selectively cross-regulate microglial expression of costimulatory molecules. For example, in organotypic cultures, Th1 (IFN-γ-, TNF-α producing) T cells were able to selectively increase microglial expression of B7.1, while selectively decreasing expression of B7.2. Th2 (IL-10-, IL-4-producing) cells could only decrease B7.2 without increasing B7.1 expression *(70)*. By contrast, Th2 cells, but not Th1 cells, decreased microglial expression of ICAM-1 and thus decreased the efficiency of antigen-presentation by microglia. In summary, as one of their most universal responses to pathology in general and to exposure of activated cytokine-producing T cells in particular, microglia acquire the potential to interact with T cells in an antigen-specific manner. Microglial ability to function as an APC is in turn modified by antigen-activated T cells.

CNS astrocytes have also occasionally been postulated to have a role in antigen-presentation to CD4[+] T cells. Although astrocytes can be induced to express MHC class II in vitro, several studies have failed to detect astrocytic expression of MHC class II in either rodent models of demyelination or in biopsy/autopsy CNS tissue from patients with MS *(71,72)*. Taken together, these data suggest that the potential for astrocytes to act as APCs to CD4[+] T cells does exist; however, in all pathologies currently characterized, microglia are likely to be the only CNS resident cell able to act as a potent APC to CD4[+] T cells in vivo. By contrast, nearly all cells in the CNS have been detected to express MHC class I in at least some forms of CNS pathology *(71,72)*. Thus, all cells in the CNS have the potential to present antigen to CD8[+] T cells and, in turn, to be harmed by the induced cytotoxic functions of activated CD8[+] T cells. For the remainder of this chapter, we focus primarily on antigen-presentation to CD4[+] T cells because linkage studies have consistently implicated an MHC class II locus as a MS susceptibility factor, CD4[+] T-cell responses are required for antibody mediated responses, and CD4[+] T cells have pivotal roles in CD8[+] T-cell-induced demyelination.

4.2. Are Microglia or Infiltrating Immune Cells Acting as Antigen-Presenting Cells in Multiple Sclerosis Lesions?

The identities of the myeloid cells within MS lesions are uncertain. Frequently, the characterization of lesion-associated myeloid cells as either activated microglia or CNS-infiltrating macrophages has been based primarily on their morphology. Cells with ramified morphologies have generally been labeled as microglia, and those with amoeboid morphologies are labeled macrophages. The imprecision of morphologically based criteria to determine cell type has been experimentally demonstrated. When fluorescently labeled rodent microglia were placed on cultured rodent brain slices, they developed both ramified and amoeboid morphologies that appeared dependent on brain region and type of tissue damage *(73)*. Conversely, ramified morphologies do not necessarily represent microglia. When fluorescently labeled myeloid dendritic cells are injected into the CNS parenchyma, they retain a ramified morphology even after migration into the CNS *(74)*. Similarly, in autoimmune responses outside of the CNS, both macrophages and dendritic cells can display ramified rather than amoeboid morphologies *(47)*.

4.3. Is It Relevant to Distinguish Microglia From Central Nervous System-Infiltrating Macrophages?

At present, there are no definitive markers that distinguish activated microglia from macrophages in histological sections. Activated microglia express all of the common macrophage markers, including Fc receptor, CD11b, F4/80, CD14, and CD45 *(8,26,75,76)*. Therefore, from histological sections alone, neither the identity of the myeloid cells in the MS lesions nor their relative functions can be determined. However, this overlap in markers and morphology does not necessarily indicate that microglia and macrophages have identical functions.

For example, several studies have indicated that microglia initially seed the CNS at least as early as embryonic day 15 in rodents. Under most conditions, the parenchymal microglial population is self-renewing, receiving little contribution from the bone marrow *(77–79)*. This is in contrast to what occurs in all other tissues. In nonimmune-privileged tissues, tissue macrophage populations are continually replaced by bone marrow stem cells throughout the life of the individual. The rate and extent that the bone marrow replaces tissue macrophage populations has been determined using irradiation bone marrow chimeric rodents. In these animals, the bone marrow of a recipient animal is killed by lethal irradiation and replaced by donor bone marrow expressing markers such as green fluorescent protein. In peripheral tissues, the replacement half-life ranges from days (liver) to months (skin, heart), varying in a tissue-specific manner. Irradiation bone marrow chimeric mice have also revealed that parenchymal microglia are phenotypically distinct from the macrophage populations located in nonparenchymal CNS sites *(77–79)*. Although often referred to as microglia, macrophages located in the meninges, subarachnoid spaces, choroids plexus, and perivascular regions are replaced within weeks by donor bone marrow and are thus phenotypically distinct from parenchymal microglia.

These phenotypic differences between parenchymal microglia and nonparenchymal macrophages have largely been confirmed in humans, most notably, in bone marrow transplant studies *(1,80)*. On occasion, bone marrow donor cells that are well matched for histocompatibility antigens are mismatched by gender. For instance, when male donor cells are transplanted into female recipients, donor cells can be identified by *in situ* hybridization analysis using Y-chromosome-specific probes. When cerebral spinal fluid (CSF) and brain tissue were examined by these methods after donor-cell reconstitution of the peripheral immune system, parenchymal microglia were found to be of the recipient genotype, whereas cells in nonparencyhmal sites and in the CSF were found to be of the donor genotype.

Flow cytometric analysis and quantitative real-time polymerase chain reaction analysis of rodent material have further revealed that parenchymal microglia differ by their relative expression of CD45 from other tissue macrophages or macrophages that acutely infiltrate the CNS in response to pathogenic signals *(65,76,81)*. In comparison to the other macrophage populations, parenchymal microglia express very low levels of CD45 (also called *leukocyte common antigen*), a protein tyrosine phosphatase expressed by all nucleated cells of hemopoetic lineage. All other differentiated hemopoetically derived cells in the mature adult animal (lymphocytes, macrophages, granulocytes) express high levels of CD45. In response to chronic pathology or robust in vivo inflammatory signals, the CD45 levels on both microglia and other macrophages increase; however, even after activation, microglial levels of CD45 tend to remain at an intermediate level between that of unactivated microglia and mature macrophages *(65,76,81)*. Although these fine gradations in expression can be measured in flow cytometric analysis of cell suspensions, differentiation of activated microglia and macrophages by differential expression of CD45 in histological sections is less certain.

The characteristically lower level of CD45 expression in microglia as compared to all other differentiated hemopoetically derived cells is not merely a useful biomarker for differential isolation of microglia. Although the function of CD45 within microglia is as yet ill-defined, in peripheral macrophages, CD45 has been shown to function as both an activating signal and as a Janus kinase tyrosine phosphatase that negatively regulates cytokine-receptor signaling involved in the differentiation, proliferation, and antiviral immunity of haematopoietic cells *(82)*. The stable lower expression observed in microglia indicates that the set-point or homeostatic balance of intracellular signaling are fundamentally different in microglia as compared to other macrophage populations.

Using bone marrow chimeric animals and/or flow cytometric measures of CD45, several recent studies have begun to suggest that microglia and macrophages may be differentially recruited during CNS pathogenesis. For example, in response to transient middle cerebral artery occlusion (MCAO), both activated microglia and macrophages were recruited to the infarct site; however, microglia dominated the early response to the infarct (days 1–4 post-MCAO) *(79)*. Hematogenously derived macrophages were observed only in the CNS in significant numbers at days 4 and 7 post-MCAO, and even then, were the minority of the activated myeloid cells.

Similarly, in response to traumatic spinal cord injury, microglia and hematogenously derived macrophages were each recruited to different portions of the developing lesion, with hematogenous macrophage accumulation following microglial activation *(8,83)*. Hematogenously derived (CNS-infiltrating) macrophages accumulated within the regions with the most severe neurodegeneration and subsequent necrosis. In contrast, activated microglia were localized to the spared white-matter regions. Depletion of peripheral macrophages by C12MDP-liposome treatment dramatically decreased the numbers of hematogenously derived macrophages recruited to the injured spinal cord and dramatically decreased the area of spinal cord necrosis. In both the MCAO and spinal cord injury models, the putative cell-type specific morphologies (ramified and amoeboid) and cell-type specific markers (ED1,CD14) were displayed by both microglia and hematogenously derived macrophages.

Both of these studies clearly demonstrate the potential for microglia and macrophages to have significantly different roles in neurodegenerative disease. Since microglia and hematogenously derived macrophages and dendritic cells are likely to provide different types of targets for therapeutic intervention in MS, it is crucial to directly examine their differential ability to act as APCs in vivo.

4.4. Microglia Are a Central Nervous System-Specific Form of Antigen-Presenting Cell

Careful examinations of the potential for microglia to initiate and sustain antigen-specific T-cell responses suggest that their potential is dependent on their prior history and the status of their local environment *(see* Fig. 1). Microglia isolated from healthy adult rodent CNS were found to be relatively ineffective as compared to splenic or CNS-infiltrating macrophages at promoting CD4$^+$ T-cell proliferation when tested ex vivo, even when MHC expression was induced by IFN-γ treatment *(65,76,84)*. However, if microglia were activated by in vivo pathology (during EAE or by transgenic CNS overexpression of IL-3) to become not only MHC class II-positive but also CD45^{intermediate}, a slightly different picture was observed *(27,81,85)*. These microglia were still relatively poor at stimulating T-cell proliferation but were found to be very potent at promoting T-cell production of proinflammatory Th1 cytokines. Indeed, microglia were found to be much more potent at driving Th1 T-cell-effector function than the other macrophage populations examined in these studies because fewer T cells were producing greater levels of IFN-γ in the absence of antigen-induced T-cell proliferation *(27)*.

4.4.1. Microglial Antigen-Presenting Cell Function Is Regulated by Environmental Signals and Cellular Interactions

In the rodent models just described, microglia limit T-cell proliferation by at least two mechanisms: production of nitric oxide (NO) and prostaglandins *(27,85)*. Both NO and prostaglandin production not only directly inhibit T-cell proliferation but also these substances repress the ability of microglia, macrophages, and dendritic cells to present antigen by suppressing their expression of MHC class II and costimulatory molecules *(86,87)*. Therefore, the net effect of microglia antigen-presentation in vivo would be twofold: a strong brief burst of Th1 cytokine production coupled with the inhibition of antigen-presenting function of surrounding microglia, CNS-infiltrating macrophages, and/or dendritic cells. In an acute self-resolving form of CNS inflammation, this response would provide a robust defense against pathogens while simultaneously limiting exposure of CNS cells to activated immune cells. Consistent with this hypothesis, inhibition of NO production is sufficient to transform acute self-resolving EAE into a relapsing–remitting form of the disease *(86)*.

Analysis of cultured microglia further illustrates how strongly environmental factors can modify microglial-effector function. Cultured microglia, even if maintained in the presence of other CNS

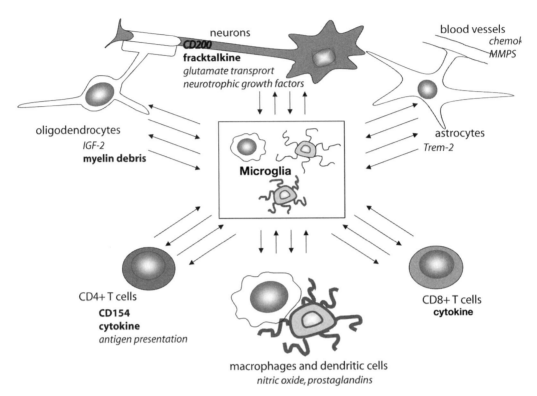

Fig. 1. Microglia are a heterogeneous class of resident central nervous system (CNS) macrophages. Capable of developing a broad array of effector functions and summating signals from a broad array of CNS and immune system cells, microglial phenotype can be precisely tailored to address the specific needs of each neuronal population. These same properties predispose microglia to amplify irrelevant or dysfunctional signals and thus inappropriately amplify or promote neurotoxic inflammation.

cells and in the absence of known stimulatory factors, already display a quasi-activated phenotype *(27,81,85)*. They express intermediate levels of CD45, and dependent on culture conditions, may be weakly positive for costimulatory factors and MHC class I and II. Using these cells, one set of studies has suggested that weakly activated microglia induce T-cell anergy or unresponsiveness, despite low-level expression of costimulatory molecules, CD40 and B7.2 *(88)*. If these microglia were treated with granulocyte-macrophage colony-stimulating factor (GM-CSF) and IFN-γ, molecules found in abundance in inflammatory infiltrates, these cells rapidly transformed into potent APCs *(88)*. Similar culture conditions also cause microglia to express high levels of the dendritic cell markers, CD11c and Dec-205 *(88)*. Even in the absence of stimulatory factors, a small percentage of cultured microglia spontaneously express the dendritic cell marker, Dec-205 *(27)*. This developmental plasticity is not only a feature of microglia derived from neonatal glial cultures but microglia isolated from adult murine CNS cultured with astrocytes and GM-CSF also begin to express dendritic cell antigens *(89)*.

4.4.2. Central Nervous System Viral Infections Cause Dramatic Changes in Microglial Antigen-Presenting Cell Function

Perhaps of greater pertinence to MS, Theiler's virus infection of the murine CNS results in a demyelinating encephalomyelitis (TMEV-IDD). TMEV-IDD is characterized by the activation of myelin-specific autoreactive CD4$^+$ T cells and mimics many of the clinical and histopathological features of the chronic progressive form of MS. In TMEV-IDD, microglia and macrophages are among the infected cells *(90)*. Early in the disease, microglia and macrophages were found to be equally effective at stimulating T-cell proliferation and IFN-γ production by myelin-specific T-cell lines *(84)*; however, as the disease progressed, hematogenous macrophages became much more effective presumably because of their much higher levels of MHC class II and costimulatory molecules. As it is not yet known whether the observed early increase in the antigen-presenting function of microglia was a consequence of direct viral infection or a signal provided by virally infected cells in the vicinity of the activated microglia.

Most of these studies examined the ability of microglia to present preprocessed peptide antigens. In vivo, it is more likely that antigens would be processed after phagocytosis of cellular debris. Although inactivated cultured microglia cannot efficiently process antigen, upon activation by IFN-γ or by viral infection, microglia can be stimulated to efficiently process and present endogenous (viral antigens) and exogenous myelin antigens *(91)*. Several studies also suggest that myelin phagocytosis itself can prime microglia to become APCs *(92,93)*. Having the ability to process antigen indicates that microglia have the potential to participate in the epitope switching that has been observed in viral models of CNS demyelination and that is presumed to occur in MS *(90)*. Here, an initial immune response is generated against viral antigens. As myelin damage occurs (as a consequence of oligodendrocyte infection and/or death or inflammatory products), macrophages and microglia phagocytose the debris. Presentation of the myelin epitopes causes the immune response to shift from a viral-specific response to a myelin-specific response.

4.5. Do Microglia Present Antigen In Vivo?

Because of the difficulty of separately measuring the relative abilities of microglia and macrophages to present antigen in vivo, most of the studies we have described examined these functions in vitro. To specifically examine the antigen-presenting function of microglia in vivo, some groups have selectively depleted the peripheral macrophage populations by treating animals with mannosylated liposome-encapsulated dichloromethyline diphophonate (Cl_2MDP) *(94,95)*. Without a peripheral myeloid population, an effective immune response cannot be generated after peripheral immunization of myelin proteins in adjuvant (the active immunization form of EAE). By contrast, depletion of peripheral macrophages by this method did not prevent T-cell extravasation or Th1 cytokine production following adoptive transfer of myelin-specific T cells, but it did inhibit demyelination, TNF-α production, T-cell infiltration into the CNS parenchyma, and induction of clinical EAE. These studies suggest the ability of microglia to present antigen is neither identical nor as potent as other APCs. These studies also show that parenchymal infiltration of T cells and/or activated macrophages are required for full-blown EAE; however, they do not distinguish between the roles of activated macrophages as initiators vs effectors of disease (APCs vs. phagocytes/producers of neurotoxic molecules). An additional complication is that the effects of Cl2MDP are not limited to peripheral macrophages and may alter microglial function.

Another method to separately examine the antigen-presenting functions of microglia vs. other myeloid populations in vivo is to use irradiation bone marrow chimeras. In these studies, rodents are generated in which only the APCs derived from the host (the radiation-resistant microglia) or only the APCs derived from the donor bone marrow (macrophages and dendritic cell populations) express the appropriate MHC to interact with MBP-specific T cells. Using this model, one set of studies has clearly shown that CNS-infiltration and activation of adoptively transferred MBP-specific T cells was not dependent on antigen-presentation by microglia in rats *(78)*. A separate study using mice confirmed that the radiation-insensitive component of the CNS (presumably microglia) was not required for induction of EAE *(96)*; however, it also demonstrated that the radiation-insensitive component was by itself sufficient to support induction of adoptively transferred EAE. Using bone marrow chimeric mice, microglial expression of CD40, IL-12, and/or IL-23 have been shown to be essential for the complete development of the clinical signs of EAE *(97,98)*. Interestingly, although clinical disease is greatly reduced when microglia fail to express these molecules, there is little change in the degree of immune cell infiltration into the CNS *(97,98)*.

4.6. Why Do Microglia Rapidly Acquire the Ability to Present Antigen in Response to Pathological Insults?

Recently several studies have demonstrated that not all forms of CNS inflammation are detrimental to CNS function. For example, less CNS regeneration is observed after mechanical trauma and more severe dysfunction results after cytokine-induced injury in mice deficient in T cells or APCs *(23,99,100)*. In vitro, antigen stimulation causes human lymphocytes to produce neurotrophic factors such as brain-derived neurotrophic factor (BDNF) and nerve growth factor (NGF) *(101)*. BDNF-positive cells morphologically resembling lymphoctyes have also been found within human MS lesions, indicating the potential for local antigen presentation within the CNS to promote growth factor production at the site of damage *(101)*.

A recent set of experiments has revealed that in at least one model, CD4+ T-cell-mediated neuroprotection is dependent on microglia acting as APCs *(102)*. Motoneuron degeneration following facial axotomy is associated with microglial activation and CNS infiltration of macrophages and T cells *(103)*. This inflammation was initially believed to be maladaptive and a contributing cause of motoneuron degeneration; however, in the absence of CD4+ T cells, motoneuron degeneration was much more rapid and severe than in their presence *(99)*. Using bone marrow chimeric mice, animals were generated in which either only microglia or only hematogenous immune cells could act as APCs *(102)*. Strikingly, microglia were not able to initiate the protective CD4+ T-cell response. Initiation of the T-cell response was entirely dependent on hematogenous macrophages. Although macrophages could initiate the response and did infiltrate the CNS, antigen presentation by hematogenous macrophages was insufficient to support CD4+ T-cell-mediated neuroprotection of motoneurons; however, once T-cell activation was initated by peripheral macrophages, protection of motoneurons following facial axotomy was absolutely dependent on antigen presentation by microglia activated by local neurodegenerative signals *(102)*.

The mechanisms underlying microglial-supported and T-cell-mediated neuroprotection are as yet undefined. To identify CNS-specific mechanisms regulating T-cell function, we recently compare the In-HA model of autoimmune diabetes (described in section 3.1.1) with our recently generated model of CNS autoimmunity. In these models, the target antigen (HA) and the responding T-cell population (HA-specific CD4+ T cells) were identical. In the Ins-HA mice, HA expression was restricted to the β cells of the pancreatic islets. In our recently generated CNS model, HA expression was restricted to CNS astrocytes (GFAP-HA). No expression was detected outside the CNS, such as in lymph nodes, enteric glia, or Schwann cells.

As described in Sections 3.1.1 and 3.1.3, when transferred into lymphopenic Ins-HA mice, HA-T cells underwent both antigen-independent (homeostatic) and antigen-induced proliferation *(47)*. Primed by homeostatic proliferation, the HA-T cells effectively triggered autoimmune destruction of HA-expression islets, as clearly evidenced by the rapid onset of clinical diabetes. In contrast, lymphopenic GFAP-HA mice receiving HA-T cells failed to develop any signs (clinical or histopathology) of autoimmune disease. This was not because HA-T cells failed to detect astrocyte-expressed HA. Rather, analysis of T-cell proliferation and activation revealed that the CNS-expressed HA was presented to the HA-T cells; however, presentation of HA within the CNS redirected T-cell activation and effector function, dramatically reducing both homeostatic and antigen-induced T-cell proliferation and activation. Further evidence of redirected T-cell-effector function by CNS antigen presentation was revealed by the incidence and type of disease induced in mice coexpressing HA in both the CNS and pancreas (GFAP-HA/Ins-HA). As compared to transfer into Ins-HA mice, HA-T cells induced diabetes in only 40% of the double GFAP-HA/Ins-HA transgenic mice. Protection from autoimmunity correlated with an increased ratio of IL-10/IFN-γ produced by antigen-triggered T cells. As described in Sections 3.1.2 and 3.1.3, homeostatic proliferation is a normal ongoing mechanism by which sufficient numbers of T cells are maintained in circulation. The protection provided by microglial presentation of antigen was overridden by treating mice with a strong adjuvant, such as PT. The proliferation and activation of HA-T cells transferred into PT-treated GFAP-HA mice was much more dramatic and accelerated than in lymphpenic Ins-HA mice. Not surprisingly, GFAP-HA mice receiving such treatment developed lethal but antigen-specific CNS inflammation. These data reveal that the CNS has evolved a mechanism to prevent the accidental proinflammatory activation of CNS-autoreactive T cells. In essence, these results indicate that CNS immune privilege is in part a consequence of continual presentation of CNS antigens to the immune system and that defects in these CNS intrinsic mechanisms are likely to contribute to destructive CNS autoimmunity.

These results confirm and extend the seminal findings by Streinlein and colleagues *(104,105)*. These authors previously demonstrated that injection of a foreign antigen into either the anterior chamber of the eye or the brain of rodents primes T cells to produce high levels of IL-10 and transforming growth factor-β if they subsequently encounter injected peptide outside the CNS (i.e., within the footpad). These phenomena have been termed *anterior-chamber induced immune deviation* and *brain-induced immune deviation* (BRAID), respectively.

These studies do not imply that molecular mimicry mechanisms are unable to operate in the CNS and cause demyelinating disease. Rather, these results indicate that autoimmunity is dependent on amplifying factors, such as PT or viral infection. For example, Olson et al. have generated a virus-induced molecular mimicry model by engineering a Theiler's murine encephalomyelitis (TMEV) to encode a myelin-protein epitope *(106)*. They find that the initial viral-specific immune response includes responses to the myelin protein that lead to early-onset CNS demyelination. In this TMEV model, many cells in the CNS, including the microglia, were actively infected. This infection caused robust production of inflammatory products and changes in neuronal and glial physiology. Thus, TMEV acted not only on the immune system but also within the CNS to change the local microenvironment.

Considered together, these four sets of results (facial axotomy, GFAP-HA, BRAID, TMEV studies) not only confirm the different functions of microglia and macrophages but also provide a clear explanation of why microglia rapidly express the molecular machinery to present antigen in response to almost any pathogenic signal. Appropriately activated, microglia are capable of redirecting and promoting neuroprotective T-cell responses; however, inappropriately activated microglia are just as likely to support maladaptive immune responses. In the context of MS, it is interesting to note that glatiramer acetate treatment is thought to act in part by promoting the generation of Th2 (IL-10) T-cell-effector function *(107)*.

4.7. How Does the Central Nervous System Regulate Microglial Function?

More recently, several groups have discovered multiple factors present in the healthy CNS capable of directly regulating microglial function *(108)*. For example, microglial expression of molecules required for antigen presentation is inhibited by electrically active neurons but is induced when electrical activity is suppressed *(108)*. Neuronal production of neurotrophins also suppresses the IFN-γ-induced MHC class II expression *(109)*. Many neuropepides have been shown in vitro to shape the innate immune responses of microglia *(110,111)*. Neuropeptides such as α-melanocyte-stimulating hormone (α-MSH) and vasoactive intestinal peptide (VIP) inhibit proinflammatory cytokine and NO production by lipopolysaccharide-activated microglia. Strikingly, studies using knock-out mice illustrate that CD200 expression by neurons actively prevents activation of myeloid cells expressing the CD200 receptor (e.g., microglia, macrophages, dendritic cells) *(112)*. Even in the CNS of healthy CD200 deficient mice, microglia display an activated phenotype (elevated expression of CD45, MHC class II, complement receptor 3). Furthermore, in CD200 deficient mice, microglial activation was accelerated in responses to axonal degeneration, and EAE occurred with a more rapid onset. Not all neuronal products inhibit microglia. Fractalkine released from injured neurons and the neuropeptide substance P augment microglial production of proinflammatory factors *(113,114)*.

4.8. All Microglia Are Not Created Equally

In this review, we have identified multiple potential microglial activation states and multiple levels of regulation, treating all microglia as equivalent; however, regional differences in cell morphology, antigenic markers, response to cytokines, and constitutive and inducible MHC expression have long been recognized as indicators of microglial heterogeneity in vivo *(114–116)*. Recent characterizations of microglial gene expression have revealed that a subset of microglia may also have a higher potential to differentiate into effective APCs. Triggering receptor expressed on myeloid cells-2 (TREM-2) has recently been implicated in mediating the differentiation of human monocyte-derived dendritic cells into APCs *(117,118)*. Although, TREM-2 is an orphan receptor, a TREM-2-binding activity is expressed by astocyte cell lines, implying that at least some forms of astrocytes may express the endogenous TREM-2 ligand *(117)*. Within the adult murine CNS, only a subset of microglia constitutively express TREM-2 *(119)*. Although TREM-2 expression is strongly downregulated by bacterial signals such as LPS, microglial expression of TREM-2 is dramatically upregulated in pathologies with abundant neurodegeneration and necrosis *(119)*. Strikingly, humans lacking this microglial-expressed molecule develop early-onset cognitive dementia, dying by their early 40s. Because TREM-2 is expressed by only microglia within the CNS, these data clearly demonstrate that microglia- and TREM-2-triggered functions are essential for normal function of CNS neurons. Considered with data presented in earlier sections of this chapter, it is tempting to speculate that microglial presentation to T cells is a necessary component to maintain optimal function of selected CNS neurons. If true, the induction of TREM-2 in degenerative diseases may not be in of itself maladaptive but an attempt to recruit T-cell-mediated neuroprotection.

Recent experiments indicate that the homeostatic function and balance of the different microglia populations within the CNS parenchyma may be altered by mechanical and ischemic damage not seen after an autoimmune or viral insult to the CNS. Using irradiation bone marrow chimeric mice, bone marrow-derived cells have been found to take up long-term residence near the site of injury in mice with facial axotomies or ischemic damage *(120,121)*. This response is in stark contrast to what occurs in healthy mice or in mice after EAE or virally-induced demyelinating disease *(76–78)*. In these situations, bone marrow-derived cells fail to contribute to the parenchymal microglial population. Although the bone marrow-derived parenchymal cells in the ischemia studies have been noted to reduce expression of CD45, additional studies are needed to explore whether these cells are phenotypically different than other parenchymal microglia. Specifically, do these cells display an activated CD45^{intermediate} phenotype or a CD45^{low} phenotype? Most macrophage populations are short lived in comparison to microglia. Therefore, does the CNS environment extend the lifespan of these cells? If reactivated, do these cells convert back to a full CD45^{high} macrophage phenotype? Upon activation or antigen capture, can these cells leave the CNS and travel to the draining lymph nodes? Answers to these questions could have important implications for the propensity to generate and regulate CNS-specific immune responses.

5. HOW DO WE DEFINE WHICH RESPONSES ARE INAPPROPRIATE?

It must be noted that many murine models of EAE are actually models of acute inflammation that successfully self-terminate. Indeed, in many murine models of EAE, CNS inflammation cannot be subsequently induced by the same antigen. By contrast relapsing–remitting EAE may represent an unbalanced immune response caused by either genetic or environmental predispositions. For example, the onset and relapse phases of EAE are associated with Th1 responses (IFN-γ) and the remitting phases with Th2 responses (IL-10, IL-5, IL-4) *(90)*. The toxic actions of Th1 responses have been well documented; however, Th2 responses by themselves are not protective and can even promote the production of pathogenic antibodies. Indeed, artificially inducing a pure Th2 myelin-specific T-cell response in RAG-/- mice leads to clinical EAE, and the addition of antibodies directed against the myelin protein, MOG, increases the severity of some forms of EAE *(122)*. Interestingly, some IgM antibodies reactive for oligodendrocyte surface antigens actually promote oligodendrocyte proliferation and myelin gene expression *(123)*. Thus, limited production of Th2 cytokines may limit the function of APCs and may even lead to the production of a therapeutic antibody response. An overly robust production of Th2 responses may promote pathogenic allergic responses (e.g., mast cell and neutrophil recruitment, IgG antibody production).

Proinflammatory Th1 responses and, in particular, IFN-γ production have been demonstrated to have causative roles in the acute destructive phase of EAE; however, knocking out IFN-γ production is by itself sufficient to transform EAE-resistant mouse strains, such as BALB/c and C57Bl/6, into EAE-susceptible strains *(94)*. The clinical disease that develops in the absence of IFN-γ is actually more rapid and severe than that triggered in traditional EAE-susceptible strains, such as the SJL mouse strain. In contrast to the perivascular inflammation and limited demyelination observed in most EAE models, demyelination was widespread and leukocytic infiltration was disseminated throughout the spinal cord in the absence of IFN-γ. The reasons for the increased severity of EAE in the absence of IFN-γ are not completely defined; however, although microglia are induced to produce TNF-α when treated with IFN-γ in vitro, they are also stimulated to produce insulin-like growth factor-2, which acts in part to counter the neurotoxic and glial toxic actions of TNF-α *(43)*.

6. MULTIPLE SCLEROSIS AS A DISEASE OF MISCOMMUNICATION BETWEEN THE CENTRAL NERVOUS SYSTEM AND IMMUNE SYSTEM

In the time frame immediately following Medwar's seminal experiments defining *immune privilege*, CNS function was thought to be dependent on successful isolation of the CNS from the immune system. Numerous in vivo and in vitro studies confirmed the neurotoxic potential of the products produced by activated immune cells (including nitric oxide, prostaglandins, cytokines). Furthermore, therapeutic interventions such as nonsteroidal anti-inflammatory drugs and steroids aimed at suppressing the immune system showed moderate, if incomplete success, at limiting the progression of secondary neurodegeneration in both humans and rodent models *(3)*. In this context, the very existence of a resident population of macrophages (microglia) stably distributed throughout the CNS appeared nonsensical at best and maladaptive at worst. Even more puzzling was the almost universal response of microglia to nearly all pathological insults (from the mildest to the most severe): the rapid induction of the molecular machinery required to present antigen to T cells (MHC and costimulatory molecules).

More recently, a very different concept of immune privilege has begun to evolve. In vivo and in vitro studies have revealed the potential for T cells, macrophages, and microglia to produce neurotrophins and other neuroprotective factors. Even more striking is the accumulating evidence that microglia are a unique class of tissue macrophage (*see* Fig. 2). Most notably, antigen presentation by microglia may serve substantially different functions in the healthy or modestly damaged CNS. Microglial activation and subsequent antigen presentation may actually serve to instruct the immune system that CNS antigens are immune-protected targets by diverting T-cell-effector function from proinflammatory to neuroprotective and T-cell-regulatory outcomes (Section 4.6). Failures in microglia to perform these homeostatic functions are likely to contribute toward either the predisposition or precipitation of CNS inflammation and autoimmunity.

In rodent models of CNS inflammation, the mere presence of lymphocytes within the CNS did not result in clinical disease and demyelination and/or irreversible neuronal damage. Rather, onset of severe clinical disease and damage were often dependent on the ability of microglia to directly and indirectly interact with T cells (CD40, IL-12-/IL-23-dependent responses). However, microglia always had maladaptive outcomes: T-cell interactions were always associated with the use of abnormally strong adjuvant treatments (such as CFA and PT).

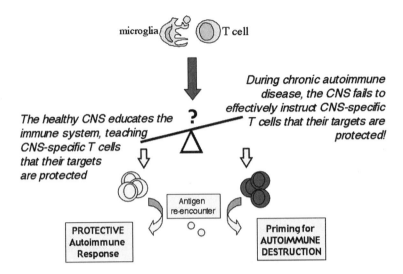

Fig. 2. In the healthy or modestly stressed microglial presentation of antigen directs T-cell-effector functions toward neuroprotective outcomes. Dysregulated activation of microglia could lead to inappropriate antigen presentation and triggering of neurotoxic T-cell-effector functions.

Microglial phenotype and function are due in large part to their interactions with other CNS cells (*see* Fig. 1). Treatments and/or environmental influences that alter CNS function will necessarily alter microglial function. Similarly, microglial phenotype and function are also a function of the nature of their interactions with T cells and other CNS-infiltrating immune cells. Thus, in MS, modest differences in neuronal, astrocytic, and oligodendrocyte physiology may result from normal human genetic polymorphisms. Small physiological differences, however, ultimately have the potential to lead to key differences in the basal and pathogen-triggered effector function of microglia. Subsequent encounters with pathogens and/or environmental toxins may serve to amplify or further polarize maladaptive forms of microglial activation either by direct modulation of the CNS or immune system.

This exquisite sensitivity of microglia to signals from the CNS and immune system allows microglial-effector function to be precisely tailored to support optimal CNS function, but the consequence of having so many adjustable toggle switches is the real possibility that microglia can amplify irrelevant and dysfunctional signals with severe consequences for CNS function. Consequently, although there is growing awareness of the necessary and beneficial in vivo functions of microglia, a dangerous presumption has become prevalent in the literature. Namely, it would be therapeutically advantageous to deactivate microglia. To date, many treatments aimed at suppressing microglial function have had limited success at ameliorating symptoms or histopathology of CNS inflammation; however, full and stable reversal of symptoms may ultimately depend not only on preventing the maladaptive responses of microglia but also on actively promoting (or artificially supplementing) their homeostatic and regenerative functions.

ACKNOWLEDGMENTS

The authors were supported by NIH grants NS045735 (MJC), NS39508 (MJC), and postdoctoral training grants from the NIH, NS41219 (CSA), and from the Fondation pour la Recherche Médicale and the Christopher Reeves Paralysis Foundation PBC1-0101-2 (CP).

REFERENCES

1. Bauer J, Rauschka H, Lassmann H. Inflammation in the nervous system: the human perspective. Glia 2001;36:235–243.
2. Carson MJ, Sutcliffe JG. Balancing function vs. self defense: the CNS as an active regulator of immune responses. J Neurosci Res 1999;55:1–8.
3. Stoll G, Jander S, Schroeter M. Detrimental and beneficial effects of injury-induced inflammation and cytokine expression in the nervous system. Adv Exp Med Biol 2002;513:87–113.
4. Owens T, Renno T, Taupin V, Krakowski M. Inflammatory cytokines in the brain: does the CNS shape immune responses? Immunol Today 1994;15:566–571.
5. Hickey WF. Leukocyte traffic in the central nervous system: the participants and their roles. Semin Immunol 1999;11:125–137.
6. Chabas D, Taheri S, Renier C, Mignot E. The genetics of narcolepsy. Annu Rev Genomics Hum Genet 2003;4:459–483.
7. Lagrange AH, Blaivas M, Gomez-Hassan D, Malow BA. Rasmussen's syndrome and new-onset narcolepsy, cataplexy, and epilepsy in an adult. Epilepsy Behav 2003;4:788–792.
8. Popovich PG, Hickey WF. Bone marrow chimeric rats reveal the unique distribution of resident and recruited macrophages in the contused rat spinal cord. J Neuropathol Exp Neurol 2001;60:676–685.
9. Matyszak MK. Inflammation in the CNS: balance between immunological privilege and immune responses. Prog Neurobiol 1998;56:19–35.
10. Stoll G, Jander S. The role of microglia and macrophages in the pathophysiology of the CNS. Prog Neurobiol 1999;58:233–247.
11. Wingerchuk DM, Weinshenker BG. Multiple sclerosis: epidemiology, genetics, classification, natural history, and clinical outcome measures. Neuroimaging Clin N Am 2000;10:611–624.
12. Noseworthy JH. Progress in determining the causes and treatment of multiple sclerosis. Nature 1999;399(Suppl. S):A40–A47.
13. Kreutzberg GW. Microglia: a sensor for pathological events in the CNS. Trends Neurosci 1996;19:312–318.
14. Medawar PB. Immunity to homologous grafted skin. III. The fate of skin homografts transplanted to the brain, to subcutaneous tissue, and to anterior chamber of the eye. Br J Exp Pathol 1948;29:58–69.
15. Perry VH. A revised view of the central nervous system microenvironment and major histocompatibility complex class II antigen presentation. J Neuroimmunol 1998;90:113–121.
16. Carson MJ, Sutcliffe JG. The role of microglia in CNS inflammatory disease: Friend or Foe? In: Bondy SC, Campbell A, eds. Inflammatory Events in Neurodegeneration. Scottsdale, AZ: Prominent Press; 2001:1–14.
17. Lo D, Feng LL, Li L, et al. Integrating innate and adaptive immunity in the whole animal. Immunol Rev 1999;169:225–239.
18. Medzhitov R, Janeway CA, Jr. Innate immune recognition and control of adaptive immune responses. Semin Immunol 1998;10:351–353.
19. Barker CF, Billingham RE. Immunologically privileged sites. Adv Immunol 1977;25:1–54.
20. Fujinami RS, Oldstone MB. Amino acid homology between the encephalitogenic site of myelin basic protein and virus: mechanism for autoimmunity. Science 1985;230:1043–1045.
21. Stohlman SA, Hinton DR. Viral induced demyelination. Brain Pathol 2001;11:92–106.
22. Kwidzinski E, Mutlu LK, Kovac AD, et al. Self-tolerance in the immune privileged CNS: lessons from the entorhinal cortex lesion model. J Neural Transm Suppl 2003;(65):29–49.
23. Schwartz M, Moalem G, Leibowitz-Amit R, Cohen IR. Innate and adaptive immune responses can be beneficial for CNS repair. Trends Neurosci 1999;22:295–299.
24. Streit WJ. Microglial response to brain injury: a brief synopsis. Toxicol Pathol 2000;28:28–30.
25. Irani DN. The susceptibility of mice to immune-mediated neurologic disease correlates with the degree to which their lymphocytes resist the effects of brain-derived gangliosides. J Immunol 1998;161:2746–2752.
26. Aloisi F. Immune function of microglia. Glia 2001;36:165–179.
27. Carson MJ, Sutcliffe JG, Campbell IL. Microglia stimulate naive T-cell differentiation without stimulating T-cell proliferation. J Neurosci Res 1999;55:127–134.
28. Scolding N. The differential diagnosis of multiple sclerosis. J Neurol Neurosurg Psychiatry 2001;71:9–15.
29. Leon SF, Arimura K, Osame M. Multiple sclerosis and HTLV-I associated myelopathy/tropical spastic paraparesis are two distinct clinical entities. Mult Scler 1996;2:88–90.
30. Howard AK, Li DK, Oger J. MRI contributes to the differentiation between MS and HTLV-I associated myelopathy in British Columbian coastal natives. Can J Neurol Sci 2003;30:41–48.
31. Hart BA, Amor S. The use of animal models to investigate the pathogenesis of neuroinflammatory disorders of the central nervous system. Curr Opin Neurol 2003;16:375–383.
32. Mix E, Pahnke J, Ibrahim SM. Gene-expression profiling of experimental autoimmune encephalomyelitis. Neurochem Res 2002;27:1157–1163.

33. Tsunoda I, Kuang LQ, Theil DJ, Fujinami RS. Antibody association with a novel model for primary progressive multiple sclerosis: induction of relapsing-remitting and progressive forms of EAE in H2s mouse strains. Brain Pathol 2000;10:402–418.

34. Lucchinetti C, Bruck W, Parisi J, Scheithauer B, Rodriguez M, Lassmann H. Heterogeneity of multiple sclerosis lesions: implications for the pathogenesis of demyelination. Ann Neurol 2000;47:707–717.

35. Trapp BD, Bo L, Mork S, Chang A. Pathogenesis of tissue injury in MS lesions. J Neuroimmunol 1999;98:49–56.

36. De Stefano N, Narayanan S, Francis GS, et al. Evidence of axonal damage in the early stages of multiple sclerosis and its relevance to disability. Arch Neurol 2001;58:65–70.

37. Brex PA, Ciccarelli O, O'Riordan JI, Sailer M, Thompson AJ, Miller DH. A longitudinal study of abnormalities on MRI and disability from multiple sclerosis. N Engl J Med 2002;346:158–164.

38. Bjartmar C, Wujek JR, Trapp BD. Axonal loss in the pathology of MS: consequences for understanding the progressive phase of the disease. J Neurol Sci 2003;206:165–171.

39. Prineas JW, Kwon EE, Cho ES, et al. Immunopathology of secondary-progressive multiple sclerosis. Ann Neurol 2001;50:646–657.

40. Bo L, Vedeler CA, Nyland H, Trapp BD, Mork SJ. Intracortical multiple sclerosis lesions are not associated with increased lymphocyte infiltration. Mult Scler 2003;9:323–331.

41. Banati RB, Newcombe J, Gunn RN, et al. The peripheral benzodiazepine binding site in the brain in multiple sclerosis: quantitative in vivo imaging of microglia as a measure of disease activity. Brain 2000;123(Pt 11): 2321–2337.

42. Gobin SJ, Montagne L, Van Zutphen M, Van Der Valk P, Van Den Elsen PJ, De Groot CJ. Upregulation of transcription factors controlling MHC expression in multiple sclerosis lesions. Glia 2001;36:68–77.

43. Nicholas RS, Stevens S, Wing MG, Compston DA. Microglia-derived IGF-2 prevents TNFalpha induced death of mature oligodendrocytes in vitro. J Neuroimmunol 2002;124:36–44.

44. Heese K, Hock C, Otten U. Inflammatory signals induce neurotrophin expression in human microglial cells. J Neurochem 1998;70:699–707.

45. Lo D, Reilly CR, Scott B, Liblau R, McDevitt HO, Burkly LC. Antigen-presenting cells in adoptively transferred and spontaneous autoimmune diabetes. Eur J Immunol 1993;23:1693–1698.

46. Lo D, Freedman J, Hesse S, Palmiter RD, Brinster RL, Sherman LA. Peripheral tolerance to an islet cell-specific hemagglutinin transgene affects both CD4+ and CD8+ T cells. Eur J Immunol 1992;22:1013–1022.

47. Ploix C, Lo D, Carson MJ. A ligand for the chemokine receptor CCR7 can influence the homeostatic proliferation of CD4 T cells and progression of autoimmunity. J Immunol 2001;167:6724–6730.

48. Surh CD, Sprent J. Homeostatic T cell proliferation: how far can T cells be activated to self-ligands? J Exp Med 2000;192:1–7.

49. Hug A, Korporal M, Schroder I, et al. Thymic export function and T cell homeostasis in patients with relapsing remitting multiple sclerosis. J Immunol 2003;171:432–437.

50. Koetz K, Bryl E, Spickschen K, O'Fallon WM, Goronzy JJ, Weyand CM. T cell homeostasis in patients with rheumatoid arthritis. Proc Natl Acad Sci USA 2000;97:9203–9208.

51. Ruddle NH. Lymphoid neo-organogenesis: lymphotoxin's role in inflammation and development. Immunol Res 1999;19:119–125.

52. Columba-Cabezas S, Serafini B, Ambrosini E, Aloisi F. Lymphoid chemokines CCL19 and CCL21 are expressed in the central nervous system during experimental autoimmune encephalomyelitis: implications for the maintenance of chronic neuroinflammation. Brain Pathol 2003;13:38–51.

53. Perry VH, Newman TA, Cunningham C. The impact of systemic infection on the progression of neurodegenerative disease. Nat Rev Neurosci 2003;4:103–112.

54. Brabb T, Goldrath AW, von Dassow P, Paez A, Liggitt HD, Goverman J. Triggers of autoimmune disease in a murine TCR-transgenic model for multiple sclerosis. J Immunol 1997;159:497–507.

55. Lo D. T-cell tolerance. Curr Opin Immunol 1992;4:711–715.

56. Lo D, Reilly C, Marconi LA, et al. Regulation of CD4 T cell reactivity to self and non-self. Int Rev Immunol 1995;13:147–160.

57. Boztug K, Carson MJ, Pham-Mitchell N, Asensio VC, DeMartino J, Campbell IL. Leukocyte infiltration, but not neurodegeneration, in the CNS of transgenic mice with astrocyte production of the CXC chemokine ligand 10. J Immunol 2002;169:1505–1515.

58. Lassmann S, Kincaid C, Asensio VC, Campbell IL. Induction of type 1 immune pathology in the brain following immunization without central nervous system autoantigen in transgenic mice with astrocyte-targeted expression of IL-12. J Immunol 2001;167:5485–5493.

59. Campbell IK, O'Donnell K, Lawlor KE, Wicks IP. Severe inflammatory arthritis and lymphadenopathy in the absence of TNF. J Clin Invest 2001;107:1519–1527.

60. Chen SC, Leach MW, Chen Y, et al. Central nervous system inflammation and neurological disease in transgenic mice expressing the CC chemokine CCL21 in oligodendrocytes. J Immunol 2002;168:1009–1017.

61. Winer S, Tsui H, Lau A, et al. Autoimmune islet destruction in spontaneous type 1 diabetes is not beta-cell exclusive. Nat Med 2003;9:198–205.

62. Baekkeskov S, Aanstoot HJ, Christgau S, et al. Identification of the 64K autoantigen in insulin-dependent diabetes as the GABA-synthesizing enzyme glutamic acid decarboxylase. Nature 1990;347:151–156.

63. Lohmann T, Hawa M, Leslie RD, Lane R, Picard J, Londei M. Immune reactivity to glutamic acid decarboxylase 65 in stiffman syndrome and type 1 diabetes mellitus. Lancet 2000;356:31–35.

64. Schulz RM, Hawa M, Leslie RD, et al. Proliferative responses to selected peptides of IA-2 in identical twins discordant for Type 1 diabetes. Diabetes Metab Res Rev 2000;16:150–156.

65. Carson MJ, Reilly CR, Sutcliffe JG, Lo D. Mature microglia resemble immature antigen-presenting cells. Glia 1998;22:72–85.

66. Becher B, Prat A, Antel JP. Brain-immune connection: immuno-regulatory properties of CNS-resident cells. Glia 2000;29:293–304.

67. Tan J, Town T, Saxe M, Paris D, Wu Y, Mullan M. Ligation of microglial CD40 results in p44/42 mitogen-activated protein kinase-dependent TNF-alpha production that is opposed by TGF-beta 1 and IL-10. J Immunol 1999; 163:6614–6621.

68. Nguyen VT, Benveniste EN. Critical role of TNF-alpha and NF-kB in IFN-gamma -induced CD40 expression in microglia/macrophages. J Biol Chem 2002;5:5.

69. Aloisi F, Penna G, Polazzi E, Minghetti L, Adorini L. CD40-CD154 interaction and IFN-gamma are required for IL-12 but not prostaglandin E2 secretion by microglia during antigen presentation to Th1 cells. J Immunol 1999;162:1384–1391.

70. Wolf SA, Gimsa U, Bechmann I, Nitsch R. Differential expression of costimulatory molecules B7-1 and B7-2 on microglial cells induced by Th1 and Th2 cells in organotypic brain tissue. Glia 2001;36:414–420.

71. Redwine JM, Buchmeier MJ, Evans CF. In vivo expression of major histocompatibility complex molecules on oligodendrocytes and neurons during viral infection. Am J Pathol 2001;159:1219–1224.

72. Hoftberger R, Aboul-Enein F, Brueck W, et al. Expression of major histocompatibility complex class I molecules on the different cell types in multiple sclerosis lesions. Brain Pathol 2004;14:43–50.

73. Hailer NP, Heppner FL, Haas D, Nitsch R. Fluorescent dye prelabelled microglial cells migrate into organotypic hippocampal slice cultures and ramify. Eur J Neurosci 1997;9:863–866.

74. Carson MJ, Reilly CR, Sutcliffe JG, Lo D. Disproportionate recruitment of CD8+ T cells into the central nervous system by professional antigen-presenting cells. Am J Pathol 1999;154:481–494.

75. Becher B, Fedorowicz V, Antel JP. Regulation of CD14 expression on human adult central nervous system-derived microglia. J Neurosci Res 1996;45:375–381.

76. Sedgwick JD, Schwender S, Imrich H, Dorries R, Butcher GW, ter Meulen V. Isolation and direct characterization of resident microglial cells from the normal and inflamed central nervous system. Proc Natl Acad Sci USA 1991;88:7438–7442.

77. Matsumoto Y, Fujiwara M. Absence of donor-type major histocompatibility complex class I antigen-bearing microglia in the rat central nervous system of radiation bone marrow chimeras. J Neuroimmunol 1987;17:71–82.

78. Hickey WF, Kimura H. Perivascular microglial cells of the CNS are bone marrow-derived and present antigen in vivo. Science 1988;239:290–292.

79. Schilling M, Besselmann M, Leonhard C, Mueller M, Ringelstein EB, Kiefer R. Microglial activation precedes and predominates over macrophage infiltration in transient focal cerebral ischemia: a study in green fluorescent protein transgenic bone marrow chimeric mice. Exp Neurol 2003;183:25–33.

80. Unger ER, Sung JH, Manivel JC, Chenggis ML, Blazar BR, Krivit W. Male donor-derived cells in the brains of female sex-mismatched bone marrow transplant recipients: a Y-chromosome specific in situ hybridization study. J Neuropathol Exp Neurol 1993;52:460–470.

81. Renno T, Krakowski M, Piccirillo C, Lin JY, Owens T. TNF-alpha expression by resident microglia and infiltrating leukocytes in the central nervous system of mice with experimental allergic encephalomyelitis. Regulation by Th1 cytokines. J Immunol 1995;154:944–953.

82. Irie-Sasaki J, Sasaki T, Penninger JM. CD45 regulated signaling pathways. Curr Top Med Chem 2003;3: 783–796.

83. Popovich PG, van Rooijen N, Hickey WF, Preidis G, McGaughy V. Hematogenous macrophages express CD8 and distribute to regions of lesion cavitation after spinal cord injury. Exp Neurol 2003;182:275–287.

84. Mack CL, Vanderlugt-Castaneda CL, Neville KL, Miller SD. Microglia are activated to become competent antigen presenting and effector cells in the inflammatory environment of the Theiler's virus model of multiple sclerosis. J Neuroimmunol 2003;144:68–79.

85. Juedes AE, Ruddle NH. Resident and infiltrating central nervous system APCs regulate the emergence and resolution of experimental autoimmune encephalomyelitis. J Immunol 2001;166:5168–5175.

86. Willenborg DO, Staykova MA, Cowden WB. Our shifting understanding of the role of nitric oxide in autoimmune encephalomyelitis: a review. J Neuroimmunol 1999;100:21–35.

87. Minghetti L, Polazzi E, Nicolini A, Greco A, Levi G. Possible role of microglial prostanoids and free radicals in neuroprotection and neurodegeneration. Adv Exp Med Biol 1999;468:109–119.

88. Matyszak MK, Denis-Donini S, Citterio S, Longhi R, Granucci F, Ricciardi-Castagnoli P. Microglia induce myelin basic protein-specific T cell anergy or T cell activation, according to their state of activation. Eur J Immunol 1999;29:3063–3076.

89. Santambrogio L, Belyanskaya SL, Fischer FR, et al. Developmental plasticity of CNS microglia. Proc Natl Acad Sci USA 2001;98:6295–6300.

90. Miller SD, Olson JK, Croxford JL. Multiple pathways to induction of virus-induced autoimmune demyelination: lessons from Theiler's virus infection. J Autoimmun 2001;16:219–227.

91. Olson JK, Girvin AM, Miller SD. Direct activation of innate and antigen-presenting functions of microglia following infection with Theiler's virus. J Virol 2001;75:9780–9789.

92. Cash E, Zhang Y, Rott O. Microglia present myelin antigens to T cells after phagocytosis of oligodendrocytes. Cell Immunol 1993;147:129–138.

93. Cash E, Rott O. Microglial cells qualify as the stimulators of unprimed CD4$^+$ and CD8$^+$ T lymphocytes in the central nervous system. Clin Exp Immunol 1994;98:313–318.

94. Tran EH, Hoekstra K, vanRooijen N, Dijkstra CD, Owens T. Immune invasion of the central nervous system parenchyma and experimental allergic encephalomyelitis, but not leukocyte extravasation from blood, are prevented in macrophage-depleted mice. J Immunol 1998;161:3767–3775.

95. Bauer J, Huitinga I, Zhao W, Lassmann H, Hickey WF, Dijkstra CD. The role of macrophages, perivascular cells, and microglial cells in the pathogenesis of experimental autoimmune encephalomyelitis. Glia 1995;15:437–446.

96. Myers KJ, Dougherty JP, Ron Y. In vivo antigen presentation by both brain parenchymal cells and hematopoietically derived cells during the induction of experimental autoimmune encephalomyelitis. J Immunol 1993;151:2252–2260.

97. Becher B, Durell BG, Miga AV, Hickey WF, Noelle RJ. The clinical course of experimental autoimmune encephalomyelitis and inflammation is controlled by the expression of CD40 within the central nervous system. J Exp Med 2001;193:967–974.

98. Becher B, Durell BG, Noelle RJ. IL-23 produced by CNS-resident cells controls T cell encephalitogenicity during the effector phase of experimental autoimmune encephalomyelitis. J Clin Invest 2003;112:1186–1191.

99. Serpe CJ, Kohm AP, Huppenbauer CB, Sanders VM, Jones KJ. Exacerbation of facial motoneuron loss after facial nerve transection in severe combined immunodeficient (scid) mice. J Neurosci 1999;19:RC7.

100. Stalder AK, Carson MJ, Pagenstecher A, et al. Late-onset chronic inflammatory encephalopathy in immune-competent and severe combined immune-deficient (SCID) mice with astrocyte-targeted expression of tumor necrosis factor. Am J Pathol 1998;153:767–783.

101. Kerschensteiner M, Gallmeier E, Behrens L, et al. Activated human T cells, B cells, and monocytes produce brain-derived neurotrophic factor in vitro and in inflammatory brain lesions: a neuroprotective role of inflammation? J Exp Med 1999;189:865–870.

102. Byram SC, Carson MJ, Deboy CA, Serpe CJ, Sanders VM, Jones KJ. CD4$^+$ T cell-mediated neuroprotection requires dual compartment antigen presentation. 2004;24:4333–4339.

103. Raivich G, Jones LL, Kloss CU, Werner A, Neumann H, Kreutzberg GW. Immune surveillance in the injured nervous system: T-lymphocytes invade the axotomized mouse facial motor nucleus and aggregate around sites of neuronal degeneration. J Neurosci 1998;18:5804–5816.

104. Stein-Streilein J, Streilein JW. Anterior chamber associated immune deviation (ACAID): regulation, biological relevance, and implications for therapy. International Reviews of Immunology 2002;21:123–152.

105. Wenkel H, Streilein JW, Young MJ. Systemic immune deviation in the brain that does not depend on the integrity of the blood-brain barrier. J Immunol 2000;164:5125–5131.

106. Olson JK, Croxford JL, Calenoff MA, Dal Canto MC, Miller SD. A virus-induced molecular mimicry model of multiple sclerosis. J Clin Invest 2001;108:311–318.

107. Chabot S, Yong FP, Le DM, Metz LM, Myles T, Yong VW. Cytokine production in T lymphocyte-microglia interaction is attenuated by glatiramer acetate: a mechanism for therapeutic efficacy in multiple sclerosis. Mult Scler 2002;8:299–306.

108. Neumann H. Control of glial immune function by neurons. Glia 2001;36:191–199.

109. Neumann H, Misgeld T, Matsumuro K, Wekerle H. Neurotrophins inhibit major histocompatibility class II inducibility of microglia: involvement of the p75 neurotrophin receptor. Proc Natl Acad Sci USA 1998;95:5779–5784.

110. Delgado R, Carlin A, Airaghi L, et al. Melanocortin peptides inhibit production of proinflammatory cytokines and nitric oxide by activated microglia. J Leukoc Biol 1998;63:740–745.

111. Kim WK, Kan Y, Ganea D, Hart RP, Gozes I, Jonakait GM. Vasoactive intestinal peptide and pituitary adenylyl cyclase-activating polypeptide inhibit tumor necrosis factor-alpha production in injured spinal cord and in activated microglia via a cAMP-dependent pathway. J Neurosci 2000;20:3622–3630.

112. Hoek RM, Ruuls SR, Murphy CA, et al. Down-regulation of the macrophage lineage through interaction with OX2 (CD200). Science 2000;290:1768–1771.

113. Sawynok J, Liu XJ. Adenosine in the spinal cord and periphery: release and regulation of pain. Prog Neurobiol 2003;69:313–340.

114. McCluskey LP, Lampson LA. Local immune regulation in the central nervous system by substance P vs. glutamate. J Neuroimmunol 2001;116:136–146.

115. Pedersen EB, McNulty JA, Castro AJ, Fox LM, Zimmer J, Finsen B. Enriched immune-environment of blood-brain barrier deficient areas of normal adult rats. J Neuroimmunol 1997;76:117–131.

116. Flaris NA, Densmore TL, Molleston MC, Hickey WF. Characterization of microglia and macrophages in the central nervous system of rats: definition of the differential expression of molecules using standard and novel monoclonal antibodies in normal CNS and in four models of parenchymal reaction. Glia 1993;7:34–40.

117. Daws MR, Sullam PM, Niemi EC, Chen TT, Tchao NK, Seaman WE. Pattern recognition by TREM-2: binding of anionic ligands. J Immunol 2003;171:594–599.

118. Cella M, Buonsanti C, Strader C, Kondo T, Salmaggi A, Colonna M. Impaired differentiation of osteoclasts in TREM-2-deficient individuals. J Exp Med 2003;198:645–651.

119. Schmid CD, Sautkulis LN, Danielson PE, et al. Heterogeneous expression of the triggering receptor expressed on myeloid cells-2 on adult murine microglia. J Neurochem 2002;83:1309–1320.

120. Flugel A, Bradl M, Kreutzberg GW, Graeber MB. Transformation of donor-derived bone marrow precursors into host microglia during autoimmune CNS inflammation and during the retrograde response to axotomy. J Neurosci Res 2001;66:74–82.

121. Priller J. Robert Feulgen Prize Lecture. Grenzganger: adult bone marrow cells populate the brain. Histochem Cell Biol 2003;120:85–91.

122. Laifaille JJ, Keere FV, Hsu AL, et al. Myelin basic protein-specific T helper 2 (Th2) cells cause EAE in immunodeficient hosts rather than protect them. J Exp Med 1997;186:307–312.

123. Rodriguez M, Miller BJ, Lennon VA. Immunoglobulin reactive with myelin promotes CNS remyelination. Neurology 1996;46:538–545.

CME QUESTIONS

1. Which statement about multiple sclerosis (MS) is correct?
   A. Axonal loss and neuronal dysfunction are major components of MS pathology.
   B. Axonal damage does not show any correlation with permanent disability in MS.
   C. Axonal transection does not occur in MS lesions.
   D. Neuronal loss occurs only in the late stages of MS.

2. In pathogenesis of MS, which cells act as antigen presenting cells?
   A. Central nervous system (CNS) astrocytes
   B. Cerebral endothelial cells
   C. Microglia
   D. All of the above

3. Based on Lucchinetti's classification of MS pathology, which types of MS lesions share features with experimentally induced autoimmune encephalomyelitis with predominance of myelin loss in perivenous locations?
   A. Type I
   B. Type II
   C. Type IV
   D. Types I and II

4. How is the CNS separated from the peripheral immune system?
   A. Absence of a lymphatic system in the CNS
   B. The presence of the blood brain barrier
   C. Absence of MHC class II molecules on resident cells within the CNS under normal conditions
   D. All of the above

3
Cytokines and Brain
Health and Disease

Tammy Kielian and Paul D. Drew

1. CYTOKINES IN THE NORMAL CENTRAL NERVOUS SYSTEM

The presence of proinflammatory cytokines in normal central nervous system (CNS) tissues remains an area of controversy (1). Several cytokines have been demonstrated in the normal CNS, and among them, tumor necrosis factor (TNF)-α, interleukin-1 (IL-1), transforming growth factor (TGF)-β, and macrophage migration inhibitory factor (MIF) have been studied in detail. The functions of TNF-α, IL-1, and TGF-β in the context of neuroinflammation have been described in detail elsewhere in this chapter; therefore, in this section, we will discuss only the potential roles these cytokines have in CNS development and physiological functions.

There have been conflicting reports regarding whether IL-1 is present in normal CNS tissues, suggesting that its expression is very low or undetectable (1). IL-1β mRNA and protein have been detected in the CNS of mice, rats, and humans, where expression was associated with specific brain regions, including the cortex, hippocampus, cerebellum, and spinal cord (2–9). Neurons and glial cells reportedly serve as the source of IL-1β in normal CNS (1). Interestingly, the levels of IL-1β mRNA have been shown to fluctuate with diurnal rhythm (10), which could account for the failure of some investigators to detect IL-1β in normal brain. In contrast to these reports, several groups have failed to detect IL-1β in the normal CNS, even when using sensitive techniques (11–14); however, the majority of evidence indicates that IL-1β mRNA and protein are expressed in normal CNS in a region-dependent manner in both neurons and glial cells (1).

The physiological role of endogenous IL-1β in the normal CNS has been linked to the regulation of sleep and feeding patterns, temperature, and synaptic plasticity (1). These outcomes are mediated by the type I IL-1 receptor (IL-1RI) expressed on numerous CNS cell types, including neurons and glia. Regarding sleep regulation, exogenous IL-1β has been shown to increase non-rapid eye movement in rodents, and IL-1RI knockout (KO) mice have been reported to sleep less compared to wild-type (WT) animals (15). The cyclic patterns of IL-1β expression observed in rodent brains correlates with many of these physiological pathways; however, the finding that IL-1 KO mice do not exhibit any developmental or neurological abnormalities suggests that other factors are capable of substituting for IL-1β in the normal CNS.

TNF-α is another cytokine that has been detected in normal CNS; however, similar to IL-1β, its expression is controversial (1,16). TNF-α and its receptors have been detected in discrete brain regions of normal mouse, rat, and human brain, including the hypothalamus, cortex, and cerebellum (17–20). In contrast, a few groups have been unable to demonstrate any TNF-α in the normal CNS

From: *Current Clinical Neurology: Inflammatory Disorders of the Nervous System: Pathogenesis, Immunology, and Clinical Management*
Edited by: A. Minagar and J. S. Alexander © Humana Press Inc., Totowa, NJ

(1), although the majority of available data indicate that TNF-α is expressed at very low levels in the brain. Similar to IL-1β, TNF-α expression is diurnally regulated, and a study demonstrating that TNF receptor (TNFR) KO mice sleep less compared to WT animals gave TNF-α a role in sleep–wake cycles *(15,18,21)*. In the developing rodent brain, TNF-α is transiently detected at high levels in neurons and astrocytes *(22)*, where its expression declines to low basal levels in the adult CNS. The finding that TNF-α KO mice do not display any overt CNS abnormalities suggests that the functional role of TNF-α in the developing CNS is either dispensable or is substituted for by alternative factors. Other physiological functions attributed to TNF-α include regulation of feeding and ion channel permeability in neurons *(1)*. Overall, the actions of IL-1β and TNF-α possess a large degree of overlap that may explain why single cytokine KO mice do not exhibit overt alterations in the majority of the physiological functions described above. It would be interesting to evaluate the consequences resulting from the loss of both TNF-α and IL-1β on these parameters by creating double KO mice.

TGF-β is a complex cytokine found in three isoforms: TGF-β1, TGF-β2, and TGF-β3. Each isoform is secreted from cells in a latent form that requires proteolytic processing extracellularly to become biologically active. TGF-β2 and TGF-β3, as well as their cognate receptors, are expressed in both the developing and adult CNS *(23,24)*. The functions of TGF-β2 and TGF-β3 in the normal CNS are not known, but in vitro and in vivo studies have demonstrated that astrocytes, microglia, neurons, and oligodendrocytes are targets for these cytokines *(25)*. TGF-β has been shown to inhibit the growth and motility of astrocytes *(26–28)* and influences ion channel activity, neurite outgrowth, and regeneration in neurons *(29–31)*. TGF-β also regulates the adhesion and migration of oligodendrocytes and inhibits microglial activation *(24,32,33)*. The functional importance of TGF-β2 and -β3 in the CNS is currently not known, since KO mice for each of these cytokines do not reveal any overt CNS abnormalities, which is likely caused by their redundant activities. The widespread expression of TGF-β during development and in the adult suggests it has a pivotal role in CNS homeostasis. It is possible that the absence of TGF-β2 and/or -β3 leads to subtle changes that are not yet understood.

We and others have detected MIF in the CNS *(34–38)*, where both neurons and glial cells are reportedly a source of this cytokine *(36,39,40)*. Paradoxically, MIF has been shown to have potent proinflammatory activities *(41)*; yet, the high levels of MIF expression in the CNS argue against a role for this cytokine in promoting cerebral inflammation. Although its precise function in the normal CNS is uncertain, MIF has been shown to convert toxic products derived from catecholamine neurotransmitters into inactive derivatives *(42)*, which suggests a protective role for MIF in neural tissues. Another potential function for MIF in normal CNS is suggested by recent studies demonstrating that MIF is a potent inhibitor of natural killer (NK) cells *(43,44)*. NK cells are activated upon recognizing cellular targets that lack major histocompatibility complex (MHC) class I expression. Because the majority of cells in the normal CNS do not express MHC class I, they theoretically could be susceptible to natural killer (NK)-mediated cell lysis. Speculatively, MIF could safeguard against this activity *(45,46)*.

In summary, evidence suggests that certain cytokines, including TNF-α, IL-1β, TGF-β2 and -β3, and MIF, are constitutively expressed in normal CNS. The inability to uniformly detect TNF-α and IL-1β in the brain suggest that these cytokines are present at very low and often undetectable levels. The discrepancies between reports evaluating the presence or absence of cytokines in the normal CNS may be related to the sensitivity of the assays used for detection, species differences, or the time of day at which cytokine levels are evaluated.

2. CYTOKINE EXPRESSION BY GLIA AND INFILTRATING IMMUNE CELLS IN THE CONTEXT OF CENTRAL NERVOUS SYSTEM INFLAMMATORY DISEASES

2.1. Glia

Microglia are the resident mononuclear phagocytes of the CNS parenchyma and participate in innate immune responses *(47,48)*. They constitute approx 10 to 15% of the total cell population in the parenchyma. Based on morphological and functional criteria in the normal and inflamed CNS, microglia have been categorized into various activation states. Resting microglia are highly ramified cells present in normal adult CNS tissue that display an immunologically quiescent phenotype characterized by the lack of phagocytic activity and expression of membrane receptors that are essential for normal macrophage functions. Subsequent to infection or trauma, ramified microglia transform into activated microglia that exhibit a rounded morphology and are highly phagocytic. At this stage, activated microglia have numerous functions in the CNS innate immune response, including the induction of neuroinflammation, phagocytosis, cytotoxicity, and regulation of T-lymphocyte responses through antigen presentation *(47)*.

Astrocytes influence neuronal activity and homeostasis in the CNS at several levels. Besides guiding neuronal development, astrocytes release neurotrophic factors, contribute to neurotransmitter metabolism, and regulate extracellular pH and K+ levels *(49,50)*. Astrocyte foot processes are intimately associated with the blood–brain barrier (BBB) *(51)*, and activated cells have been shown to express numerous adhesion molecules, including intercellular adhesion molecule (ICAM)-1 *(52–55)*. Because adhesion molecules have a pivotal role in the recruitment of peripheral immune cells into tissues, it appears likely that activated astrocytes are involved in regulating leukocyte trafficking into the CNS. It has also been shown that astrocytes increase the number of mature functional synapses on CNS neurons and are required for synaptic maintenance in vitro, suggesting that astrocytes may actively participate in synaptic plasticity *(56)*. Furthermore, astrocytes have an important function in initiating and regulating CNS immune responses through the release of proinflammatory cytokines *(46,57)*.

To achieve the effector functions mentioned above, numerous studies have demonstrated that microglia and astrocytes are capable of producing an array of proinflammatory mediators, including TNF-α, IL-1β, IL-10, and nitric oxide (NO), that initiate or regulate inflammatory processes in the CNS *(47,48,57)*. In addition to the beneficial effects that glia have in initiating protective immune responses in the CNS, these cells have been implicated in contributing to tissue damage when chronically and/or pathologically activated. For example, many reports demonstrate that activated microglia may exacerbate Alzheimer's disease (AD) and multiple sclerosis (MS), as described later in this chapter, through secreting a battery of inflammatory cytokines and cytotoxic agents, including TNF-α, IL-1β, and NO *(58–63)*. Although the array of cytokine mediators elaborated by activated astrocytes closely parallels those described for microglia, activated astrocytes have not been directly implicated as major contributors to neuronal toxicity in the CNS. This may be explained by the fact that their role in chronic neuroinflammatory disorders remains an understudied area. Therefore, the implications of glial activation in the context of CNS inflammation must be evaluated by recognizing the relative contributions of beneficial vs detrimental effector functions, which may have important implications in therapeutic approaches to disease. We describe the activities of TNF-α, IL-1β, IL-6, and TGF-β prior to explaining their involvement in CNS diseases to familiarize the reader with their biological functions in the context of neuroinflammation.

Activated microglia and astrocytes are a major source of TNF-α in the inflamed CNS *(46,47,57)*. TNF-α exerts numerous effects within CNS tissues, including modulation of BBB integrity, induction of adhesion molecule expression on cerebral microvascular endothelial cells, and subsequent activation of resident glia and infiltrating peripheral immune cells *(64–67)*. TNF-α is toxic to oligodendrocytes and oligodendrocyte-precursor cell lines, which has implications in demyelinating diseases, such as MS and its animal model experimental autoimmune encephalomyelitis (EAE) *(68–73,74)*. In addition, microglia-neuron co-culture studies have revealed that TNF-α produced by activated microglia is neurotoxic, which likely contributes to the significant neuronal loss associated with many CNS inflammatory diseases *(58,75)*; however, recent evidence has indicated that TNF-α has a beneficial role in demyelinating diseases by promoting the remyelination process *(76)*, as described later in this chapter. Therefore, the implications of TNF-α expression in various neuroinflammatory diseases may be complex and influenced by the nature of the CNS insult, the timing of its expression during disease, and/or the local concentration of TNF-α achieved within the CNS microenvironment.

Like TNF-α, IL-1 exerts a similar array of effects during CNS inflammation, including modulation of BBB integrity, induction of adhesion-molecule expression on cerebral microvascular endothelial cells, and subsequent activation of resident glia and infiltrating peripheral immune cells, resulting in the production of additional cytokines, such as IL-6 and TNF-α *(46,64–67)*. IL-1β is produced by both activated microglia and astrocytes in the CNS as an inactive proform that is enzymatically cleaved by caspase-1 (Casp-1) to produce the biologically active mature form of IL-1β. Similar to TNF-α, IL-1β has been shown to exert cytotoxic effects on numerous cell types in the CNS, including oligodendrocytes and neurons *(58,75,77)*, suggesting that IL-1β may contribute to neurodegeneration in the context of CNS inflammatory diseases; however, recent studies have demonstrated that IL-1β promotes remyelination in demyelinating disease *(78)*, revealing a dual role for this cytokine in the context of CNS inflammation. Like TNF-α, the beneficial vs detrimental effects of IL-1β in the CNS are probably influenced by a multitude of factors, including the concentrations of IL-1β achieved at the site of inflammation, the timing of cytokine induction during disease progression, and/or the nature of the inflammatory insult.

Astrocytes serve as the main source of IL-6 and TGF-β in the inflamed CNS *(46,57)*. IL-6 is a multifunctional cytokine with diverse actions, including regulation of acute phase reactions, immune responses, and cellular differentiation. In the CNS, IL-6 promotes astrocyte proliferation and neuronal survival *(57,79–81)*, suggesting that it may have a dual role in dictating beneficial vs detrimental responses in neuroinflammation. TGF-β is a complex cytokine found in three isoforms that have a function in mediating immune suppression during CNS inflammation. The majority of TGF-β-positive cells in the adult CNS are astrocytes; however, large neurons, microglia, and ependymal cells of the third ventricle of the hypothalamus have also been shown to produce TGF-β *(25,82,83)*. TGF-β is generally considered to possess anti-inflammatory properties and is capable of inhibiting macrophage as well as T- and B-lymphocyte activation, suggesting that it may have a role in downregulating CNS neuroinflammatory responses.

2.2. Peripheral Immune Cells

The neuroinflammatory diseases described in this chapter are associated with varying degrees and types of peripheral immune-cell infiltrates, including neutrophils, monocytes/macrophages, and T and B lymphocytes. In general, neutrophils are associated with acute immune responses, whereas lymphocytes are detected in chronic inflammation. Monocyte/macrophage infiltrates lie in between this continuum. Activated neutrophils and monocytes/macrophages produce many of the same proinflammatory cytokines as activated glia, including TNF-α and IL-1β *(84,85)*. In contrast, subsets of activated T cells secrete different mediators that dictate whether a cell-mediated or humoral immune response is elicited. A detailed discussion of the cytokine mediators released by activated T-cell subsets in the context of MS and EAE is provided later in this chapter.

3. CYTOKINES IN CNS INFECTIOUS DISEASES

3.1. Bacterial Meningitis

Despite advances made in vaccination and treatment strategies, bacterial meningitis remains associated with a high mortality rate and a high incidence of neurological sequelae, particularly in very young and elderly patients. Approximately 1.2 million cases of bacterial meningitis occur annually worldwide, with 135,000 deaths *(86)*. Long-term effects resulting from meningitis include hearing loss, hydrocephalus, and sequelae associated with parenchymal damage, including memory loss, cerebral palsy, learning disabilities, and seizures *(87)*. The majority of community-acquired meningitis cases are caused by organisms that colonize the mucosal membranes of the nasopharynx, including *Neisseria meningitidis*, *Streptococcus pneumoniae*, and *Haemophilus influenzae*;

however, the introduction of the *H. influenzae* conjugate vaccine in the United States and western Europe has greatly reduced the incidence of *H. influenzae* in these areas. The pathophysiology of bacterial meningitis begins with the colonization of the nasopharynx by the pathogen, microbial invasion into the bloodstream, and, finally, penetration of organisms into the subarachnoid space (SAS) *(88,89)*. Once the bacteria have entered the SAS, the initial response to infection is mediated by meningeal macrophages, ependymal cells, and choroid plexus epithelium, followed by responses from recruited peripheral blood leukocytes and resident glia *(89–94)*.

In addition to the direct damage induced by pathogens, the host antibacterial response elicited during bacterial meningitis can be detrimental to neurons and other glia in the CNS because of the toxic effects of cytokines, chemokines, proteolytic enzymes, and oxidants produced locally at the site of infection *(86,88,95)*. In addition, studies have shown that the inflammatory host response to bacterial products continues after organisms have been killed by antibiotics, revealing the challenging nature of the therapeutic manipulation of bacterial meningitis *(96)*. Proinflammatory cytokines, such as TNF-α, IL-1, and IL-6, and the antiinflammatory mediators IL-10 and TGF-β have been implicated in the pathophysiology of bacterial meningitis. Each of these mediators and their potential roles in the context of bacterial meningitis are discussed below.

TNF-α is one of the main proinflammatory cytokines detected in the cerebrospinal fluid (CSF) of patients with bacterial meningitis *(97–107)*. High levels of TNF-α in the CSF are associated with seizures, whereas elevated systemic levels correlate with a high mortality rate *(108,109)*. Interestingly, TNF-α is observed in the CSF following bacterial, but not viral meningitis *(100,103,104,107–109)*.

The role of TNF-α in bacterial meningitis has been investigated using experimental models in the mouse, rat, and rabbit. Similar to the findings obtained in human patients, elevated TNF-α levels have been detected in the CSF of animals infected with either *H. influenzae* type b or *S. pneumoniae* *(110–112)*. Using *in situ* hybridization, Bitsch et al. demonstrated that blood-derived monocytes were the major source of TNF-α production in the SAS during experimental *S. pneumoniae*-induced meningitis *(113)*. Collectively, these studies establish that TNF-α is a major constituent of the CSF inflammatory milieu in the context of bacterial meningitis.

To ascertain the functional consequences of TNF-α expression in bacterial meningitis, numerous studies have been performed in experimental animal models using TNF-α neutralizing antibodies, soluble receptors, and KO mice. In a rabbit model of experimental meningitis induced by an intracisternal (IC) inoculation of *H. influenzae* type b lipooligosaccharide, the simultaneous administration of a TNF-α-neutralizing antibody effectively attenuated meningeal inflammation *(94,114)*. However, in a separate study by the same group, IC delivery of soluble TNF receptor (sTNFR) had no effect on the meningeal inflammatory response *(115)*. The reason why these two independent approaches to neutralizing TNF-α expression did not yield similar results is not clear but may have resulted from insufficient neutralization of TNF-α levels in the CSF caused by suboptimal concentrations of sTNFR. Saukkonen et al. examined the role of TNF-α in rabbits in which meningitis was induced with an IC challenge of live *S. pneumoniae (116)*. The administration of a TNF-α-neutralizing antibody was capable of completely attenuating inflammation in this model. In contrast, researchers administering TNF-α monoclonal antibody to infant rats at the time of infection with group B Streptococcus type III revealed that the antibody had no effect on the degree of CSF inflammation or cortical injury, although hippocampal injury was significantly attenuated *(87)*. The inability of the TNF-α antibody to inhibit meningeal inflammation was observed regardless of the route of injection (i.e., both intraperitoneal [IP] and IC routes were ineffective). These findings contrasted those described above in similar models of bacterial meningitis, in which TNF-α appeared to have an important role in initiating CSF inflammation *(94,114,116)*. These discrepancies may be explained by examining the time points the various studies used to assess meningeal inflammation. For example, the beneficial effects of TNF-α-antibody treatment were observed during the acute stage of disease (i.e., time points up to 6 h following infection), whereas it had no impact at later time points (i.e., from 18 to 24 h postinfection) *(87)*. Collectively, these differences suggest that TNF-α has a critical pathophysiological role early in infection, although additional inflammatory mediators with redundant activities may compensate for its loss during the later stages of disease. Additional studies evaluating the role of TNF-α in *S. pneumoniae*-induced experimental meningitis were performed using TNF-α and TNFR KO mice *(117)*. Wellmer et al. found that leukocyte recruitment into the SAS and bacterial burdens were similar between TNF-α KO and WT mice *(117)*. In contrast, TNFR-deficient mice displayed decreased meningeal inflammation, suggesting that other TNFR ligands (such as lymphotoxin-α) contribute to the induction and/or maintenance of the inflammatory response during bacterial meningitis. The reasons for the reported discrepancies regarding the importance of TNF-α in the various bacterial meningitis models may have resulted from the different approaches used to evaluate TNF-α (i.e., TNF-α KO or TNFR KO mice vs administration of neutralizing antibodies or soluble TNF receptors), the strain of bacteria studied, or the route of pathogen infection. Nonetheless, the prevalence of TNF-α in the CSF of patients with meningitis coupled with findings from the majority of studies using experimental animal models of bacterial meningitis indicate that TNF-α plays a role in the pathophysiology of disease.

In patients with bacterial meningitis, IL-1 is present in the CSF, and elevated levels correlate with the development of neurological complications *(101,104,106,107,109,118–120)*. Several studies using experimental animal models of bacterial meningitis have also reported elevated levels of IL-1β in the CSF during the acute phase of disease *(110–112,121,122)*. Surprisingly, studies designed to directly examine the functional importance of IL-1 in the pathophysiology of bacterial meningitis are sparse. Only one group has investigated the role of IL-1 in *S. pneumoniae*-induced meningitis with IL-1R1 KO mice using an intranasal model of infection *(122)*. A role for endogenous IL-1 in host defense during pneumococcal meningitis was demonstrated by the finding that IL-1 RI KO mice displayed higher bacterial burdens and increased mortality compared to WT animals. Interestingly, leukocyte influx into the CSF was similar between IL-1 RI KO and WT animals, although the levels of the neutrophil-attracting chemokines macrophage inflammatory protein-2 (MIP-2/CXCL2) and KC/CXCL2 were lower in IL-1 RI KO compared to WT mice at later stages of disease (i.e., 72 h postinfection). This may be explained by the fact that bacterial products can serve as neutrophil chemoattractants that may compensate for the absence of these chemokines in IL-1 RI KO mice. Although this is the only study to date directly examining the role of IL-1 in the pathogenesis of bacterial meningitis, another report has indirectly examined its role in disease progression using both Casp-1 KO mice and pharmacological inhibition of Casp-1 activity *(86)*. Casp-1 is responsible for the proteolytic processing of the inactive proform of IL-1β into its mature active form. Casp-1 expression was increased in the brain during the course of experimental pneumococcal meningitis and correlated with increased IL-1β levels *(86)*. Evaluation of meningitis in Casp-1 KO mice and following the pharmacologic blockade of Casp-1 revealed a reduction in IL-1β levels, which was associated with a concomitant decrease in proinflammatory mediator expression (TNF-α, MIP-1α, and MIP-2) and leukocyte influx into the CSF *(86)*. In comparing the results of these two studies, the functional importance of IL-1 in bacterial meningitis remains unclear. Zwijenburg et al. reported that IL-1 was required to generate an effective host antibacterial immune response to contain the infection, whereas Koedel et al. found that indirect inhibition of IL-1β prevented the development of detrimental inflammatory responses implicated in the pathophysiology of bacterial meningitis *(86,122)*. These discrepancies may be explained by the fact that Casp-1 inactivation could affect additional pathways in the meningitis inflammatory cascade besides IL-1β, such as IL-18, which together act to prevent the pathophysiological changes typically associated with disease. Alternatively, IL-1β may be essential for generating an effective host antibacterial response during the early stages of meningitis, whereas the cytokine may exert toxic effects during the later phases of disease. In summary, further studies are required to definitively establish the role of IL-1β in bacterial meningitis.

IL-6 levels are elevated in the systemic circulation and CSF of patients with bacterial meningitis *(97,101,105,123,124)*. Likewise, IL-6 is also detected in various experimental models of bacterial meningitis *(101,110–112,125)*, confirming the results observed in human infection. Two studies that have yielded conflicting results have examined the functional importance of IL-6 in the pathogenesis of experimental bacterial meningitis using neutralizing antibodies and cytokine KO mice. Marby et al. demonstrated that the administration of an IL-6 antibody 1 h following an IC inoculation of heat-killed *S. pneumoniae* type 3 attenuated meningeal inflammation as measured by decreases in CSF leukocytosis and protein content, suggesting that IL-6 contributes to the pathophysiological response characteristic of bacterial meningitis *(126)*. In contrast, a separate study revealed that IL-6 inhibits meningeal inflammation, since IL-6 KO mice displayed significant elevations in CSF leukocyte counts and enhanced TNF-α, IL-1β, and MIP-2 levels *(127)*. Similar findings were obtained when rats were treated with IL-6-neutralizing antibodies *(127)*. The reasons for the reported discrepancies regarding the role of IL-6 in bacterial meningitis are not known but may be related to the methods used to evaluate IL-6 functional activity, the timing of antibody administration in neutralization studies, and/or the nature of the bacterial pathogen used in these model systems. Additional studies investigating the relative importance of IL-6 in bacterial meningitis are warranted to resolve these issues.

IL-10 is a prototypic anti-inflammatory cytokine produced by a variety of cells, including monocytes/macrophages, T and B lymphocytes, and resident CNS cells, such as microglia and neurons *(128,129)*. IL-10 is a potent inhibitor of proinflammatory cytokine production and has a role in attenuating immune responses *(130–132)*. Elevated levels of IL-10 have been detected in the CSF of patients with bacterial meningitis, suggesting that it may play a role in controlling ongoing pathological inflammation *(98,105,133–135)*. Likewise, IL-10 is increased in the CNS in several animal models of experimental meningitis *(110,111,136)*.

Numerous studies have directly examined the importance of IL-10 in experimental animal models of bacterial meningitis. Koedel et al. evaluated the effects of exogenously administered IL-10 on the course of experimental pneumococcal meningitis in a rat model *(125)*. In vehicle-treated rats, regional cerebral blood flow, brain water content, intracranial pressure, and leukocyte influx into the CSF were all elevated following pneumococcal infection. These parameters were significantly attenuated following the IP administration of IL-10. Interestingly, the inhibitory effects of IL-10 on meningeal inflammation were observed regardless of when the cytokine was administered *(125)*. IL-10 has also been shown to attenuate the production of IL-6 *(125)* and TNF-α *(137)* in experimental bacterial meningitis models, suggesting that IL-10 regulates the synthesis of proinflammatory mediators with purported pathophysiological roles in meningitis. Finally, a recent study using IL-10 KO mice has examined the functional importance of endogenous IL-10 on the course of bacterial meningitis *(136)*. Meningeal inflammation was more severe in IL-10 KO mice compared to WT animals, as revealed by elevated levels of IL-6, TNF-α, and leukocyte infiltrates 48 h postinfection *(136)*. Despite the ability of IL-10 to attenuate leukocyte entry into the CSF and proinflammatory mediator release, it appears to have little effect on dictating disease outcome, since the onset of meningitis and bacterial titers were similar between control animals, those receiving exogenous IL-10 *(137)*, and in IL-10 KO mice *(136)*. Thus, these studies suggest that although IL-10 is capable of attenuating certain inflammatory pathways during the evolution of bacterial meningitis, additional mediators are responsible for regulating bacterial burdens and disease severity. This is of critical importance when considering how to approach the therapeutic management of bacterial meningitis, since the available data indicate that disease outcome is dictated by a complex set of interactions, and targeting with a single anti-inflammatory agent (i.e., IL-10) likely will prove difficult.

Relatively little information is available regarding the expression and functional importance of IL-12 and IL-18 in the pathogenesis of bacterial meningitis. IL-12 is a heterodimeric cytokine composed of two covalently linked chains, p40 and p35, that form the biologically active form of IL-12 p70. During CNS inflammation, activated microglia, as well as infiltrating monocytes/macrophages, neutrophils, and dendritic cells, serve as the main source of IL-12, which is a potent inducer of interferon (IFN)-γ production by T and NK cells and promotes the differentiation of T helper (Th) 1 cells from naïve Th0 cells *(138,139)*. Two independent groups have been unable to demonstrate IL-12 p70 in the CSF of patients with bacterial meningitis *(140,141)*. Although Kornelisse et al. identified elevated levels of IL-12 p40 in the CSF of patients with bacterial meningitis *(140)*, IL-12 p40 is not the biologically active form of IL-12; therefore, its functional importance in disease pathology remains unknown. Further complicating the issue, IL-12 p40 is often secreted excessively over the p70 heterodimer and it can also associate with p19 to form IL-23 *(139)*. In light of these issues, it is difficult to speculate on the role of IL-12 p40 in disease, although it appears that IL-12 p70 may not have a pivotal role in the course of bacterial meningitis since T-lymphocyte and NK-cell infiltrates are not significant constituents of the CSF inflammatory infiltrate.

IL-18 is a member of the IL-1 cytokine superfamily and, like IL-1β, is produced as an inactive precursor (pro-IL-18) that is enzymatically cleaved by Casp-1 to generate the biologically active form of IL-18 *(142)*. IL-18 is produced by numerous cell types, including macrophages, dendritic cells, and microglia *(142,143)*. Biological functions of IL-18 include the enhancement of T- and NK-cell maturation, cytokine production, and toxicity; stimulation of cytokine production by macrophages; and neutrophil activation, reactive oxygen intermediate synthesis, cytokine release, and degranulation *(142)*. IL-18 has been detected in the CSF of patients with bacterial meningitis *(144)* and in a mouse model of *S. pneumoniae*-induced meningitis *(145)*, suggesting that this cytokine may be involved in the pathophysiological response to infection. A recent study examining bacterial meningitis in IL-18 KO mice supports a role of IL-18 in this disease *(145)*. In these studies, IL-18 KO mice were equally susceptible to meningitis as WT animals following the intranasal delivery of *S. pneumoniae*; however, IL-18 KO mice had fewer leukocytes in the meninges, reduced levels of proinflammatory mediators at the later stages of disease, and prolonged survival compared to WT animals *(145)*. Collectively, this suggests that IL-18 contributes to the pathological inflammatory response during the evolution of bacterial meningitis.

TGF-β is present in the CSF of patients with bacterial meningitis *(146–148)* and in experimental models of infection *(110,111)*. A beneficial role for this cytokine in bacterial meningitis was demonstrated using a rat model of pneumococcal meningitis *(149)*. A single IP inoculum of TGF-β2 was capable of reversing the deleterious changes in regional cerebral blood flow and intracranial pressure normally observed during acute meningitis. Because additional studies investigating the potential therapeutic benefits of TGF-β in bacterial meningitis are lacking, a more thorough analysis of the effects of TGF-β on the pathophysiology of bacterial meningitis is warranted to determine whether this cytokine may serve as an effective treatment modality for human disease.

In summary, bacterial meningitis is typified by the presence of both proinflammatory and anti-inflammatory cytokines in the CSF. The majority of proinflammatory cytokines, including TNF-α, IL-1β, and IL-6, have been implicated in mediating the pathophysiological changes associated with bacterial meningitis, whereas the anti-inflammatory mediators IL-10 and TGF-β may limit the extent of the ensuing host antibacterial immune response. Because it appears that the levels of anti-inflammatory cytokines produced during the acute phase of meningitis are not sufficient to offset the deleterious effects of the numerous proinflammatory mediators present in the CSF, the direct administration of anti-inflammatory cytokines or agents capable of shifting the ensuing response from inflammatory toward suppressive subsequent to effective bacterial neutralization may have therapeutic benefits in the clinical management of patients with bacterial meningitis. A large amount of experimental evidence from both animal models and clinical trials in humans shows that adjuvant therapy with corticosteroids provides protection against CNS tissue injury and improves disease outcome *(96)*, although corticosteroids, as broad-acting inflammatory inhibitors, may produce unwanted side effects. Therefore, combination therapies involving the use of antibiotics along with agents that skew the CNS inflammatory response toward neuroprotection may be more beneficial in regulating meningitis severity. Confirming the direct role of each specific cytokine in bacterial meningitis is difficult to demonstrate because of the redundant activities of many of the mediators released into the CSF. Models of experimental bacterial meningitis in cytokine KO or transgenic mice, when available, should add to our knowledge of the functional importance of individual cytokine mediators in disease pathology and host immunity. Finally, it will be important to evaluate and compare the responses of the major meningeal pathogens to determine whether differences exist in the nature of the ensuing host inflammatory response, as has been suggested by an earlier study *(110).*

3.2. Experimental Brain Abscess

Brain abscesses represent a significant medical problem—accounting for 1 in every 10,000 hospital admissions in the United States—and remain serious despite recent advances in detection and therapy *(150).* In addition, the emergence of multidrug-resistant strains of bacteria has become a confounding factor that is magnified by the inability of many antibiotics to reach high therapeutic levels in brain tissue. Besides infection containment, the immune response that is essential to abscess formation also destroys surrounding normal brain parenchyma, which can have detrimental consequences. Indeed, some long-term effects following brain abscess resolution include seizures, loss of mental acuity, and focal neurological defects. Our laboratory has developed an experimental brain abscess model in the mouse using *S. aureus,* one of the main etiological agents of brain abscess in humans *(35,151).* The mouse brain abscess model closely mimics human disease by progressing through a series of well-defined stages *(152,153).* The early stage, or early cerebritis, occurs from d 1 to 3 postinfection and is typified by neutrophil accumulation, tissue necrosis, and edema. Microglial and astrocyte activation are also hallmarks of this stage and persist throughout the evolution of the lesion. The intermediate, or late cerebritis stage, occurs from d 4 to 9 and is associated with a predominant macrophage and lymphocyte infiltrate. The final, or capsule stage, occurs from d 10 onward and is associated with the formation of a well-vascularized abscess wall, which, in effect, sequesters the lesion and protects the surrounding normal brain parenchyma.

We have established that *S. aureus* leads to the immediate induction of proinflammatory cytokine expression in the CNS parenchyma within 1 to 6 h following infection *(34,35).* Among the cytokines produced following *S. aureus* exposure include IL-1α, IL-1β, TNF-α, and IL-6 *(34,35).* The rapid kinetics of cytokine induction following *S. aureus* infection implicate resident CNS cells as the initial source, since peripheral immune cells do not begin to accumulate at significant levels until approximately 24 h following *S. aureus* exposure. In support of this hypothesis, we have recently demonstrated that both primary microglia and astrocytes are capable of recognizing both *S. aureus* and its cell wall product peptidoglycan and respond by elaborating a similar array of cytokines detected in brain abscesses in vivo, including IL-1β, TNF-α and IL-6, implicating these cells in the initial inflammatory response to bacteria in the brain parenchyma *(39,40).*

Although we have characterized the profile of cytokine gene expression during the course of experimental brain abscess development, relatively little is known regarding the functional importance of these mediators in disease pathogenesis. Recently, our laboratory has demonstrated that both IL-1 and TNF-α have a pivotal role during the acute phase of infection in the experimental brain abscess model using cytokine KO mice *(154).* This was demonstrated by significant increases in mortality rates and bacterial burdens in both IL-1 and TNF-α KO mice compared to WT animals. Interestingly, although there were no qualitative differences between IL-1 KO and WT animals in the nature of inflammatory infiltrates, brain abscesses appeared more severe in the former as revealed by enlarged abscess sizes and moderately increased neutrophil infiltrates. In contrast, there were no observable differences in the inflammatory cell profiles associated with brain abscesses from TNF-α KO and WT animals *(154).* Analysis of IL-6 KO mice revealed no significant differences in mortality rates, bacterial titers, or cellular infiltrates in brain abscesses, indicating that IL-6 is not a major contributor to the host antibacterial immune response in this model *(154).* These findings demonstrate that although IL-1 and TNF-α share many redundant activities, they are important for containing bacterial infection during the early stages of experimental brain abscess development.

Recently, we have expanded our analysis of cytokine mediators induced by *S. aureus* infection in the experimental brain abscess model by using a targeted microarray approach with samples from IL-1 KO and WT mice. Microarray analysis revealed several cytokines with significantly elevated expression in brain abscesses from IL-1 WT mice as compared to control animals, including IL-1β, IL-6, IL-7, TNFRSF1a, TNFRSF6, osteopontin, and erythropoietin *(154)*. A direct comparison of brain abscesses from *S. aureus*-infected IL-1 KO and WT animals on the same microarray revealed only three cytokine-related genes that were differentially expressed and statistically significant between the strains. As expected, IL-1β mRNA expression was significantly higher in IL-1 WT mice following *S. aureus* exposure as compared to KO animals. Similarly, the levels of IL-6 and IL-1 RII were significantly elevated in brain abscesses from IL-1 WT mice. The finding that IL-1 RII levels are increased in brain abscesses is intriguing since this receptor cannot transduce an activation signal and thus serves as a decoy receptor *(155)*. The host may be attempting to control the extent of inflammation in the brain parenchyma, although this remains speculative. Collectively, these findings suggest that the fundamental nature of the inflammatory response differs between IL-1 WT and KO animals either in its intensity or its dependence on IL-1 to induce the full array of proinflammatory mediators following infection.

In addition to the direct damage induced by pathogens, the host antibacterial response that ensues during the course of brain abscess development may be detrimental to neurons and other glia in the CNS because of the toxic effects of cytokines, chemokines, proteolytic enzymes, and oxidants produced locally at the site of infection. The finding that lesion sites are greatly exaggerated compared to the localized area of initial infection provides evidence of the establishment of an over-active immune response during the chronic stages of brain abscess development *(35,151)*, a phenomenon also observed in human brain abscess. Specifically, the continued release of proinflammatory mediators by activated glia and infiltrating peripheral immune cells may act through a positive feedback loop to potentiate the subsequent recruitment and activation of additional inflammatory cells and glia. This would effectively perpetuate the antibacterial inflammatory response via a vicious pathological cycle culminating in extensive collateral damage to normal brain tissue. Indeed, inappropriate immune responses have been implicated in mediating tissue damage in numerous CNS pathologies, including bacterial meningitis *(86,88,89)*, AD *(63,156,157)*, and EAE, the animal model for MS *(158)*. In contrast to their essential role during the acute phase of experimental brain abscess development, TNF-α and IL-1β, when released over a prolonged period, may exacerbate normal tissue damage, revealing a potential dual role for these cytokines in the context of brain abscess. Specifically, a potential detrimental role for IL-1β and TNF-α was suggested by the findings that cytokine expression persisted throughout the chronic stages of experimental brain abscess development in the context of relatively low bacterial burdens and was associated with continual disruption of the BBB *(159)*. These changes correlated with the continued presence of infiltrating neutrophils and macrophages/microglia. Notably, a dual role for proinflammatory cytokines in disease progression is a theme that we will revisit in our discussion of MS and EAE.

In summary, progress has been made toward dissecting the functional importance of proinflammatory cytokines in the pathogenesis of experimental brain abscess. Although the majority of studies demonstrate a pathological role for IL-1 and TNF-α in experimental bacterial meningitis, we have evidence to suggest that these cytokines have a dual role in the context of experimental brain abscess. Specifically, IL-1 and TNF-α are essential for the development of host antibacterial immune responses during the acute stages of infection, whereas the release of these mediators remains unchecked during the chronic phase of disease, which may effectively exacerbate damage to normal brain parenchyma via a bystander pathway. In general, these studies have revealed important differences regarding the roles of proinflammatory cytokines in two CNS infectious diseases, bacterial meningitis and experimental brain abscess, with distinct bacterial localization patterns.

3.3. *Human Immunodeficiency Virus-1 Encephalitis and Human Immunodeficiency Virus-Associated Dementia*

Human immunodeficiency virus (HIV)-1 is a neurotropic virus *(160,161)* linked to a variety of neurological disorders. CNS disease is usually a late complication of HIV-1 infection, although viral entry into the CNS is a relatively early phenomenon *(162–166)*, revealing a considerable lag between the initial establishment of CNS infection and the onset of clinically overt disease. HIV-1 strains have been categorized into two groups based upon their ability to infect cells of the mononuclear phagocyte lineage (M-tropic) vs. their ability to affect T lymphocytes (T-tropic). Generally, HIV-1 viruses that infect the CNS are M-tropic. The major pathway for HIV entry into the CNS is via infected monocytes/macrophages. Subsequent to penetrating the BBB, the principle targets of HIV-1 infection in the CNS are cells of the mononuclear phagocyte lineage in which viral RNA and antigens have been demonstrated in association with perivascular macrophages, microglia, multinucleated giant cells, and infiltrating monocytes/macrophages *(167–173)*. Subpopulations of HIV-1-infected persons develop cognitive, behavioral, and/or motor abnormalities commonly referred to as *HIV-1-associated dementia* (HAD). The frequency of HAD in HIV-infected individuals is reported to range from 20 to 40%, although its incidence has recently declined to approx 11% in developed countries because of the advent of highly active antiretroviral therapy (HAART) *(174,175)*. Although HAART reduces the incidence of HAD, a percentage of patients still present with symptoms caused by viral mutation, decreased penetration of antiretroviral drugs into the CNS, and HAART failure *(176–178)*. Another neurological sequelae associated with HIV-1 infection in the CNS is HIV encephalitis (HIVE), which is characterized histologically by monocyte/macrophage infiltration into the brain, microglial nodules, formation of macrophage-derived multinucleated giant cells, and myelin pallor *(179)*. It is important to note that HAD and HIVE are two distinct entities; HIVE refers to the histopathological changes in the brain that occur during HIV infection, whereas HAD describes the clinical syndrome. Patients could have HAD but not demonstrate pathological changes associated with HIVE. It is well established that the number of HIV-infected cells and the amount of viral antigen in the CNS do not correlate well with measures of cognitive deficits in HAD *(180–182)*. This phenomenon, along with the finding that the topographic distribution of apoptotic neurons in the CNS of HIV-infected individuals is closely associated with markers of macrophage/microglial activation, suggests that factors released from activated macrophages/microglia are the source of neurotoxic compounds leading to neuronal dysfunction *(183,184)*, as described in the following sections.

3.3.1. *Studies With Human Brain Tissue and Cerebral Spinal Fluid*

The majority of studies performed to date have suggested that the neuronal dysfunction associated with HIV infection in the CNS occurs by an indirect mechanism. One of the main pathogenic pathways leading to the destruction of CNS parenchyma is the continual release of proinflammatory cytokines produced by HIV-1-infected or activated macrophages/microglia *(185,186)*. Numerous studies on autopsy specimens from the brains of HIV-1-infected individuals, analysis of cytokines in the CSF, and in vitro studies evaluating the consequences of HIV-1 infection on cytokine release from macrophages/microglia support this theory.

Cytokine levels in autopsy-collected brain tissues of HIV-infected patients have provided insights into mediators that may have important roles in the pathogenesis of HIVE and HAD. One of the main cytokines detected in brain tissues from HIV-positive patients is TNF-α *(19,187–190)*, which is synthesized primarily by macrophages and microglia during infection *(191,192)*. Interestingly, a study by Nuovo and Alfieri demonstrated that the majority of TNF-α-producing cells in the CNS of HIV-positive patients were not productively infected with virus *(193)*. This suggests that other mechanisms, besides viral infection *per se*, are involved in stimulating TNF-α release during the course of HIV-1 infection in the brain. Possibilities include the autocrine/paracrine activation of neighboring macrophages/microglia via TNF receptors or stimulation by viral proteins (i.e., gp120, tat) secreted from infected cells or shed by the virus.

As mentioned previously, essentially all HIV-positive patients have CNS infection, but only 20–40% develop dementia. Therefore, attempts have been made to correlate cytokine expression in the brain with the development of HAD. The best pathological correlate for HAD is an increase in the number of activated macrophages in the white matter *(187,191,194)*. In addition, analysis of autopsy tissues from HIV-infected patients with and without dementia have revealed that TNF-α levels are elevated in the former *(19,191,192)*, suggesting that TNF-α has a pivotal role in dictating the onset of HAD. The mechanisms by which TNF-α could influence the onset of HAD are not known but may be related to the cytokine's neurotoxic effects or its ability to activate neighboring glia and infiltrating macrophages to release additional proinflammatory mediators that disturb neuronal homeostasis (i.e., glutamate uptake and release leading to neuronal cell death) *(195)*. In fact, activated macrophages/microglia in the CNS of patients with acquired immunodeficiency syndrome (AIDS) have been reported to upregulate both isoforms of the TNFR, providing a potential positive feedback loop to amplify pathological tissue damage and prolong cytokine release *(190)*.

In addition to TNF-α, other cytokines have been demonstrated in the brains of HIV-positive patients, including IL-1 *(19,187,190,196)*, IL-6 *(19,187,190)*, TGF-β *(19,197)*, and IFN-α *(198,199)*. Like TNF-α, the majority of these cytokines are produced by activated glia, which supports the concept that these cells are a significant source of neurotoxic compounds leading to neuronal dysfunction.

Elevated levels of numerous cytokines have also been reported in the CSF of HIV-infected individuals, including IL-1 *(200–203)*, IL-6 *(200–203)*, and IFN-α *(199,204)*. The source of these proinflammatory mediators is not known but likely includes activated macrophages/microglia. The presence of TNF-α in the CSF of patients with HIV is somewhat controversial. Several groups report detectable levels of TNF-α *(202,205–207)*, whereas others do not *(200,203,208)*. In studies that found TNF-α in the CSF, there was no correlation established between its concentrations and the incidence of HAD *(202,205)*. CSF cytokine levels are not used to establish a diagnosis of HIVE or HAD because they lack disease specificity. For example, it would be impossible to assess whether elevated proinflammatory cytokine levels in the CSF of a patient with AIDS resulted from the viral infection itself or from a subclinical CNS opportunistic infection. This becomes an issue when considering the heterogeneity of patient populations in many clinical studies. Therefore, the utility of assessing CSF cytokine concentrations in HIV-infected patients remains uncertain.

3.3.2. Cytokine Production From HIV-Infected Monocytes/Macrophages, Microglia, and Astrocytes

As previously mentioned, the primary reservoirs of HIV infection in the CNS are cells of the mononuclear phagocyte lineage, including perivascular macrophages, parenchymal microglia, infiltrating monocytes/macrophages, and multinucleated giant cells *(167–173)*. M-tropic strains of HIV-1 can productively infect microglia in vitro *(209–214)*, whereas HIV-1 has been shown to nonproductively infect astrocytes within the CNS *(173,189,215–218)*. Although viral replication is not sustained in HIV-1-infected astrocytes, studies have shown that treatment with cytokines that would be present in the inflammatory milieu during CNS infection, such as TNF-α and IL-1β, or co-culture with macrophages leads to the recovery of infectious virus from latently infected astrocytes *(218,219)*. These findings suggest that astrocytes may act as reservoirs of latent HIV-1 and, upon reactivation, may propagate the infection to neighboring macrophages/microglia.

Studies examining virus localization in the CNS have revealed that the topographic distribution of apoptotic neurons in HIV-infected individuals is closely associated with markers of macrophage/microglial activation, suggesting that factors released from activated macrophages/microglia are the source of neurotoxic compounds leading to neuronal dysfunction *(182–184)*. Indeed, studies with HIV-infected monocytes/macrophages have demonstrated the release of neurotoxic factors from infected cells in vitro *(220–222)*. In addition, soluble products released from HIV-infected macrophages have been shown to inhibit long-term potentiation and synaptic transmission *(223,224)*. Several cytokines are produced by HIV-infected macrophages/microglia, including IL-1, TNF-α, and IL-6 *(225–227)*. The numerous pathophysiological roles ascribed to TNF-α may contribute, in part, to the neuronal cell damage characteristic of HIVE and HAD. For example, TNF-α has been shown to inhibit glutamate uptake *(228–230)* and enhance viral replication in HIV-infected cells *(227,231–234)*. Differential expression and release of cytokines from activated macrophages/microglia and astrocytes in the context of HIV infection in the CNS may alter the normal balance of proinflammatory and anti-inflammatory cytokines, creating an environment in which the dysregulation of normal cytokine responses leads to a vicious cycle of cellular activation and toxicity *(185,235)*.

3.3.3. Animal Models of Immunodeficiency Virus Infection

Several studies using both simian and mouse systems to model the pathogenesis of HIV infection in humans support the hypothesis that macrophage/microglia infection leads to neuronal injury and dysfunction *(183,236)*. The simian immunodeficiency virus (SIV) animal model is an excellent system to investigate AIDS pathogenesis because SIV shares a high degree of homology with HIV strains and also infects cells of the mononuclear phagocyte lineage, including macrophages, microglia, and perivascular macrophages *(237–241)*. Although some studies of human patients have demonstrated that HIV invasion of the CNS was a relatively early event following infection *(164–166)*, these studies relied on the chance examination of HIV-positive patients who died of other causes, since death from AIDS normally occurs decades beyond initial infection. Therefore, studies in the SIV animal model allowed investigators to examine infected monkeys at time points early in the pathogenesis of disease to evaluate the extent of CNS involvement. As was observed in humans, CNS infection with SIV was found to be a frequent and early event in disease progression *(237,241–243)*. Similar to HAD, SIV encephalitis results in the loss of motor and cognitive functions that are not correlative with CNS viral burdens *(244)*. These deficits are likely the result of intense proinflammatory cytokine production from macrophages/microglia leading to neuronal toxicity. Indeed, SIV infection results in the induction of several proinflammatory cytokines in the brain, including TNF-α and IL-1β *(245,246)*. Activated microglia are one source of these mediators, since isolated cells from SIV-infected rhesus monkeys have been shown to produce elevated levels of IL-1β, TNF-α, and IL-6 *(247)*. Collectively, these studies support the concept that HIV-like infections of the CNS cause neuronal dysfunction that is mediated, in part, through the release of toxic mediators from activated macrophages/microglia.

Because of the strict viral host specificity of HIV, studies examining the pathogenesis of HIV infection in the mouse are limited; however, a mouse model has been developed that introduces HIV-infected human monocyte-derived macrophages (hMDM) into the brains of severe combined immunodeficiency (SCID) mice, providing a tool to examine the role of productively infected macrophages in the CNS *(248–250)*. The introduction of HIV-infected hMDM into the basal ganglia/cortex of SCID mice has been shown to recapitulate the pathological features associated with HIVE *(249,250)*. Studies in the SCID HIV-infected hMDM model revealed that the introduction of infected macrophages into the brain led to the local induction of endogenous mouse cytokines including TNF-α, IL-1β, and IL-6 *(249,250)*. These findings indicate that products released from virus-infected human macrophages are capable of activating resident CNS mouse cells to produce inflammatory cytokines, effectively amplifying the production of neurotoxic molecules that contribute to the pathogenesis of HIVE. This model is limited because SCID mice lack B and T lymphocytes, which may influence the nature of the observed inflammatory responses. Nonetheless, the HIV–SCID mouse model represents an important tool to dissect the role of the innate immune response to HIV infection in the CNS.

3.3.4. Immunostimulatory Effects of HIV-Encoded Proteins

In addition to HIV-1 infection triggering inflammatory-mediator release from macrophages/microglia, there is evidence to suggest that viral proteins either directly shed from the virus or released from infected cells are capable of inducing the activation of resident CNS glia and infiltrating monocytes/macrophages. Recombinant HIV-1 proteins, including Tat, Nef, and gp120, have been shown to induce cytokine production and neuropathology when directly injected into the brain, providing further support for the role of immune activation in the neurological dysfunction of HAD *(251–259)*. In addition, transgenic mice overexpressing HIV gp120 also demonstrate characteristics typical of HIVE, including microglial activation, astrocytosis, and alterations in neuronal morphology *(260)*. Importantly, both HIV Tat and gp120 have been detected within the CNS and the serum of HIV-positive patients *(261,262)*.

The HIV-1 Tat protein is a transcription factor that enhances viral gene transcription in infected cells. Several studies have demonstrated that Tat protein is released from HIV-infected cells and can be internalized by uninfected cells, where it is capable of stimulating gene expression *(222,263)*. Extracellular Tat is capable of inducing cytokine production in astrocytes *(264–266)*, microglia *(267,268)*, and monocytes *(269,270)*, providing a mechanism by which uninfected cells participate in the pathological amplification of inflammatory cytokines during HIV-1 infection of the CNS. This mechanism probably accounts for a significant portion of the cytokine levels observed in the CNS of HIV-infected individuals because, as alluded to earlier, the viral load in the CNS does not correlate with the degree of neurological impairment in HAD. In addition, TNF-α has been shown to synergize with Tat to promote neuronal cell death, which is thought to result from oxidative stress *(271)*.

Gp120 is an envelope glycoprotein of HIV-1 that mediates virus binding to CD4 and chemokine coreceptors on the surface of target cells. Some suggest that viral shedding of gp120 participates in the development of neurological dysfunction in HIV-infected individuals through its ability to stimulate cytokine release from resident glia and infiltrating immune cells. Indeed, HIV gp120 and its fragments are capable of stimulating IL-1, TNF-α, and IL-6 release from cultured CNS cells in vitro *(226,272–274)*. Similarly, gp120 has been shown to induce IL-1, TNF-α, and IL-6 release in monocytes *(275, 276)*. Again, these cytokines can indirectly lead to neuronal cell death and contribute to the pathological manifestations associated with HAD. Evidence for a role of astrocytes in gp120-mediated toxicity was suggested by a study demonstrating that treatment of primary rat and human astrocytes with gp120 led to alterations in ion transport and glutamate release *(277)*. The resultant dysfunctions in ion channels and glutamate regulation could lead to increases in neuron intracellular calcium levels and excititoxic cell death. Collectively, these studies suggest that extracellular HIV-1 proteins are capable of inducing cytokine production in both noninfected monocytes/macrophages and resident glia, providing potential mechanisms for not only augmenting HIV-1 replication in infected cells but also for amplifying CNS inflammatory responses following HIV-1 infection.

In summary, multiple mechanisms may exist for the large degree of neuronal dysfunction associated with HAD, all involving indirect damage mediated by activated macrophages/microglia and astrocytes within the CNS. First, direct infection of perivascular macrophages, microglia, and infiltrating macrophages in the CNS by HIV-1 leads to the elaboration of numerous cytokine mediators, including IL-1, TNF-α, and IL-6. The numerous effects that proinflammatory cytokines can have on the course of CNS infection include enhancing virus replication and release from infected cells, leading to new rounds of productive infection; toxic effects on neurons and oligodendrocytes, leading to demyelination; and activation of uninfected CNS cells in an autocrine/paracrine manner effectively augmenting local cytokine levels in the CNS parenchyma. In addition, HIV-1 infection induces in the CNS the expression of monocyte chemokines that have been implicated in the recruitment of new pools of peripheral blood mononuclear cells that can serve as additional targets for HIV-1 infection *(278,279)*. These facts, in combination with the finding that HIV proteins are capable of inducing cytokine expression in numerous CNS cell types, reveals the establishment of a vicious cycle of cytokine release that leads to the exacerbation of neuronal cell death.

4. CYTOKINES IN NONINFECTIOUS CENTRAL NERVOUS SYSTEM DISEASE

4.1. *Multiple Sclerosis*

MS is the most common neurological disorder of young adults. The majority of patients are diagnosed with MS during their third or fourth decade of life and thus suffer the effects of the disease for most of their adult life. Most patients with MS initially exhibit periods of disease exacerbations mixed with periods of disease remission (termed *relapsing–remitting MS*); however, over time, most patients enter a period of increased disability that is characterized by chronic inflammation without periods of significant disease remission (termed *secondary progressive MS*). Progressive disability in MS may be associated with axonal pathology that is likely initiated following acute inflammatory events during the early course of disease. It should be noted that approx 15% of MS patients exhibit a progressive course of disease without remissions from the onset. This is termed *primary progressive MS* and is generally characterized by less acute inflammation, as determined by MRI, and an escalated rate of development of disability *(280,281)*. The cause of MS is unknown although epidemiological studies, as well as studies examining identical twins, suggest that both genetics and environment, particularly viral infection, may have a role in pathogenesis *(282–284)*. T cells that are autoreactive to CNS antigens are believed to initiate MS. These autoreactive T cells may be activated in the periphery by microbial antigens exhibiting cross-reactivity to CNS antigens in a process termed *molecular mimicry (285,286)*. An autoimmune etiology of MS is further supported by the observation that MS is characterized by perivascular mononuclear cell inflammatory infiltrates and demyelination, features also characteristic of EAE, an established T-cell-mediated autoimmune disorder (described in detail in Section 4.1.1) *(282,287,288)*. Activated T cells are capable of extravasating through the BBB into the CNS. These activated T cells elicit a variety of cytokines and chemokines capable of activating resident brain microglia and astrocytes, as well as stimulating the migration of both CNS glia and peripheral macrophages to sites of CNS inflammation. Activated leukocytes, as well as resident glia, are believed to contribute to the demyelination characteristic of MS. The Food and Drug Administration has recently approved multiple drugs for use in the treatment of MS *(289,290)*. These drugs include IFN-β and glatiramer acetate that possess potent immunomodulatory activities and are preferable to previous MS therapies, including the immunosuppressive corticosteroids. IFN-β and glatiramer acetate likely modulate MS disease activity in part by modulating cytokine production by peripheral immune cells, as well as by resident CNS cells. It should be noted that because these new therapeutic agents do not cure disease, better treatment strategies for MS need development.

4.1.1 *Cytokine Modulation of T-Cell Phenotype*

EAE is an autoimmune disorder characterized by CNS inflammation, demyelination, and remittent paralysis, features consistent with MS *(282)*. During recent years, the understanding of immunologic mechanisms involved in demyelination has advanced greatly through the investigation of EAE, which can be induced either by active immunization of susceptible animals with components of myelin or by adoptive transfer of CD4$^+$ T cells specific for myelin antigens into syngeneic recipients *(291,292)*. The adoptive transfer experiments have clearly established that EAE is a T-cell-mediated autoimmune disease. CD4$^+$ T cells exhibit two distinct patterns of cytokine production and are designated Th1 and Th2 cells, both of which are believed to derive from a common precursor. Th1 cells produce IL-2, IFN-γ, TNF-α, and TNF-β/lymphotoxin. Th1 responses are associated with cell-mediated immunity and are responsible for delayed-type hypersensitivity. Th2 cells are characterized by the production of IL-4, -5, -6, -10, and -13. Th2 responses are associated with humoral immunity, enhanced antibody production by

B cells, and induction of the allergic response *(293)*. The cytokines IL-12 and IFN-γ are critical for the differentiation of Th1 cells, whereas IL-4 is pivotal for the differentiation of Th2 cells *(293)*. In EAE, Th1 cells are believed to be encephalitogenic, whereas Th2 cells may be protective *(294–297)*. In this section, we discuss the importance of four cytokines (IL-12, -18, -10, and -4) that have an important role in dictating Th1 vs Th2 responses in the context of MS and EAE.

IL-12 is an important mediator of EAE and MS. In the CNS, IL-12 is produced by microglia *(298–300)* and possibly at low levels in astrocytes *(301)*. The presence of IL-12 p40 RNA early in disease suggests a role for IL-12 in the initiation of MS *(302)*. In addition, IL-12 levels also appear to correlate with MS disease progression *(303,304)*. The functional importance of IL-12 in EAE was revealed by studies demonstrating that the administration of exogenous cytokine increases disease severity *(305)* and that IL-12 antibodies inhibit the development of EAE *(306)*. Similarly, EAE does not develop in IL-12-p40-deficient mice *(307)*. The role of IL-12 in the pathogenesis of EAE is likely to involve the generation of encephalogenic Th1 cells. Indeed, IL-12 triggers Th1 differentiation in vitro *(308,309)* and in vivo *(310)*. The cytokine also induces T-cell proliferation and IFN-γ production *(311,312)*. Several studies have revealed that IL-12 and IFN-γ cooperate in stimulating the development of Th1 cells. This likely represents an important mechanism for the generation of encephalogenic Th1 cells in MS and EAE, since both cytokines are present in the inflamed CNS. The importance of IL-12 in regulating IFN-γ production is supported by studies in mice lacking IL-12 or signal transducers and activators of transcription (STAT-4) (which is responsible for IL-12 signaling) that exhibit impaired IFN-γ production *(313-315)*. IFN-γ stimulates monocytes to produce IL-12 *(316,317)* and T cells to express IL-12R *(318)*. Therefore, the interplay between IL-12 and IFN-γ in regulating Th1 development suggests that these cytokines are pivotal in dictating the pathogenesis of MS and EAE. It should be noted that some of the actions attributed to IL-12 in modulating MS and EAE may actually be due to IL-23 because these cytokines both function as heterodimers and share a common p40 subunit. IL-12 consists of a p40/p35 heterodimer, whereas IL-23 exists as a heterodimer containing p40 and p19. The observation that p35-deficient mice are susceptible to EAE, whereas p40-deficient mice are not susceptible may suggest that IL-23 plays a more important role than IL-12 in modulating EAE (reviewed in ref. *318a*).

Another cytokine that has been implicated in the development of EAE and MS is IL-18. In the CNS, IL-18 is produced by microglia and possibly by astrocytes *(143,319)*. Increased levels of IL-18 RNA were observed in the brains of rodents with EAE *(320)*, and IL-18 protein is expressed in demyelinating brain lesions in MS *(321)*. Furthermore, the level of Casp-1, the protein responsible for the activational cleavage of IL-18, correlates with the severity of EAE *(322)* and MS *(323)*. In EAE, IL-18-neutralizing antibodies blocked the disorder, suggesting that this occurred because of a shift in the Th1/Th2 balance toward Th2 cells *(324)*. The effects of IL-18 in MS and EAE are likely mediated by its ability to influence Th1 development. For example, IL-18 alone does not induce the formation of Th1 cells, but it greatly potentiates Th1 development in response to IL-12 *(325)*. Similar to the cooperative effects of IL-12 and IFN-γ, IL-18 has also been shown to associate with these cytokines to influence T-cell activation. For example, IL-18, together with IL-12, synergistically induces T cells to produce IFN-γ *(326–328)*. In addition, IL-12 induces the expression of IL-18R on Th1 cells, whereas IL-18 stimulates IL-12R expression *(329,330)*. Thus, the synergistic induction of IFN-γ by Th1 cells in response to IL-12 and IL-18 may result in part from this reciprocal induction of their corresponding receptors, although the synergistic induction of IFN-γ by IL-12 and IL-18 may occur through alternative mechanisms. For example, IL-12 signals are transduced by STAT-4 *(331)*, and IL-18 activates NF-κB *(332)*. The IFN-γ-gene promoter contains binding elements for these transcription factors *(333)*, suggesting that these proteins may synergistically induce transcription of the IFN-γ gene. The complex interactions between IL-18, IL-12, and IFN-γ likely dictate the nature and extent of encephalogenic Th1 development in MS and EAE.

IL-10 is a cytokine that may function to limit the extent of inflammation in MS and EAE. IL-10 is principally produced by Th2 cells that are considered protective in these diseases. Other cells, including antigen-presenting macrophages and B cells, also produce this cytokine *(334,335)*. In the CNS, microglia and astrocytes are both capable of producing IL-10 *(336–341)*. Because IL-10 levels appear to inversely correlate with symptoms in patients with MS, the cytokine may have a protective role in disease *(342–344)*. Numerous studies indicating that IL-10 suppresses disease directly support its protective role in EAE *(345–348)*. IL-10 may regulate the extent of neuroinflammation in MS and EAE through its ability to repress IFN-γ production by Th1 cells, which favors Th2 differentiation *(349)*. In turn, IFN-γ can also inhibit monocytes from expressing IL-10 *(350,351)*, which favors development of Th1 cells. Thus, IFN-γ and IL-10 cross-regulate each other's expression in monocytes and differentially affect T-cell phenotype. Based on IL-10's reported ability to attenuate disease severity in EAE, therapies designed to augment its expression in the CNS may have beneficial effects on the progression of MS.

IL-4 is a cytokine produced by Th2 cells that also has a critical role in their differentiation. This cytokine is also produced by eosinophils, mast cells, and NK cells. Administration of IL-4 has been demonstrated to suppress EAE *(352,353)*. Although some reports have indicated that IL-4 KO mice are more susceptible than WT controls to the development of EAE *(354)*, other studies indicate that IL-4-deficient mice do not develop more severe disease *(346,355,356)*. Thus, the role of IL-4 in the pathogenesis of EAE is somewhat controversial. Relevant to its reported protective effects in EAE, one of the principle functions of IL-4 involves the polarization of CD4+ T cells toward a Th2 phenotype. IL-4 also skews T cells toward a Th2 phenotype by suppressing the production of IFN-γ-producing Th1 cells *(357)*. IL-4 likely stimulates Th2 differentiation through activation of STAT-6 following receptor binding, which is supported by studies indicating that STAT-6 knockout mice have impaired Th2-cell differentiation and that activation of STAT-6 is sufficient to trigger Th2 differentiation *(358,359)*. In response to IL-4, STAT-6 mediates the induction of the transcription factor GATA-3 *(359,360)*. GATA-3 has a critical role in Th2 differentiation, and the expression of this protein is elevated during Th2 differentiation and decreased during Th1 differentiation *(361,362)*. GATA-3 stimulates Th2 differentiation, at least in part, by inhibiting IFN-γ *(363)*. Future studies are needed to clarify the exact role of IL-4 in modulating the course of EAE.

4.1.2. Role of Innate Immune Cytokines in MS and EAE

In addition to autoreactive T cells, activated glia participate in the pathology associated with MS that is thought to result in part from the excessive production of TNF-α, IL-1β, and NO *(58,364)*. NO is a gaseous molecule that performs a variety of cellular functions. It is produced by a series of enzymes termed *NO synthases*. Inducible NOS (iNOS) was first demonstrated in monocytes but is now known to be expressed in a variety of cells, including microglia and astrocytes. Expression of iNOS is stimulated by a variety of inflammatory cytokines (e.g, IFN-γ, TNF-α, and IL-1β, which are elevated in patients with MS) and bacterial products, including lipopolysaccharide (LPS) *(365)*. Although molecules including NO, TNF-α, and IL-1β may be toxic to pathogens, these agents can also be toxic to CNS cells, including myelin-producing oligodendrocytes *(58)*, which are compromised in MS *(366)*. These molecules may also be toxic to neurons and thus may contribute to axonal degeneration characteristic of MS *(75)*, although there is also compelling evidence that NO, TNF-α, and IL-1β may contribute to the resolution of CNS inflammatory conditions, particularly in vivo *(22,367)*. These issues are discussed in detail in the following paragraphs.

In vitro, activated glia can produce molecules, including NO, TNF-α, and IL-1β. The vast majority of studies indicate that these molecules are toxic to oligodendrocytes in vitro, suggesting that they may contribute to the pathogenesis of MS. Specifically, TNF-α and IL-1β are reportedly toxic to oligodendrocytes and oligodendrocyte-precursor cell lines *(68–74,77)*. Likewise, NO has also been demonstrated to be toxic to these cells *(368–370)*. Interestingly, a few studies indicate that NO can exert either toxic or protective effects on oligodendrocytes, depending on the intracellular redox state of the cells *(371,372)*.

In vivo studies have suggested that NO and proinflammatory cytokines may suppress or alternatively contribute to CNS inflammation and degeneration. A potential dual role for numerous proinflammatory mediators in the context of CNS inflammatory diseases is a theme that is just beginning to be appreciated. For example, inhibition of NO synthesis has been reported to block development of EAE *(373–375)*. Furthermore, NO reacts with superoxide to form peroxynitrite, which is a strong lipid-peroxidizing agent capable of altering myelin integrity *(376)*. Peroxynitrite has been detected in the CNS in both EAE and MS *(377,378)*, suggesting it may contribute to NO-stimulated oligodendrocyte death. These findings indicate that agents that inhibit NO synthesis may be effective in the treatment of MS. Contrary to these studies, mice genetically deficient in iNOS are susceptible to the development of EAE. In fact, these animals exhibit earlier onset of disease and increased disability than do WT mice *(379,380)*. Increased severity of EAE in iNOS KO mice may be explained in part by studies indicating that NO has a critical role in the resolution of EAE by inhibiting T-cell proliferation in established disease *(381)*. A dual role for NO in the inductive vs resolution phases of EAE is supported by studies in Lewis rats that generally exhibit monophasic disease on active immunization with myelin basic protein (MBP) in the presence of CFA. For example, treatment of recovered rats with the NO-synthase inhibitor *N*-methyl-L-arginine acetate precipitated a second episode of disease *(382)*. Administration of the selective iNOS inhibitor aminoguanidine indicated that NO is a pathogenic factor in the inductive phase and has an inhibitory role in the progressive phase of EAE *(383)*. Inhibition of iNOS production using antisense oligonucleotides immediately following the transfer of myelin-specific T cells further supports the conclusion that NO is pathogenic in the inductive phase of EAE *(375)*. Collectively, these studies indicate that the role of NO in EAE and MS is complex and is likely dictated by the timing of its expression during disease and/or the local concentrations achieved within the CNS microenvironment.

The role of TNF-α in vivo in modulating EAE is also controversial. Many studies indicate that genetic deficiency of TNF-α results in the development of EAE that is not significantly different or is less severe than in WT animals *(384–386)*. Neutralization of TNF-α activity also reportedly results in less severe EAE *(387,388)*. This reduction in disease severity may result primarily from decreased movement of leukocytes into the CNS parenchyma *(389)*. Studies demonstrating that MBP-specific T-cells retrovirally transduced to express TNF-α increased the severity of EAE, support the idea that this cytokine has a pathogenic role in the disease *(390)*. Conversely, other studies demonstrate that TNF-α-deficient mice develop more severe EAE and that TNF-α treatment reduces the severity of their disease *(391,392)*. Elucidation of the role of TNF-α in EAE has been complicated by the fact that both lymphotoxin and TNF receptors can also influence the initiation and clinical course of EAE *(393–397)*.

IL-1 likely contributes to pathogenesis in EAE, as reflected by studies demonstrating that IL-1 administration increases disease severity *(398)*. In addition, targeted disruption of the IL-1RI gene and IL-1-receptor antagonist studies indicate that IL-1 receptors are critical for the development of EAE *(399–401)*; however, priming with IL-1β can suppress the development of EAE, likely through effects on the hypothalamus-pituitary-adrenal axis *(402)*. Therefore, further studies must be conducted to clarify the role of IL-1 and IL-1 receptors in EAE and MS.

Recent studies have begun to clarify the apparently disparate roles of NO, TNF-α, and IL-1β in demyelinating disorders using a cuprizone model of demyelination. Although it is acknowledged that the mechanisms of remyelination in the cuprizone model may be distinct from EAE, the cuprizone system offers advantages, such as the ability to control remyelination temporally, which is very difficult to achieve in the EAE model. In the cuprizone model, the genetic deficiency of either TNF-α and IL-1β resulted in the failure to remyelinate, likely the result of the inability of oligodendrocyte precursors to differentiate into mature oligodendrocytes *(76,78)*. Inducible NOS KO mice also exhibited an inability to remyelinate following cuprizone administration that was coincident with the depletion of mature oligodendrocytes *(403)*. Additional studies indicated that TNFR2, and not TNFR1, is critical to oligodendrocyte regeneration *(403)*. Interestingly, previous studies in the EAE model suggested that TNFR1, and not TNFR2, may contribute to the initial exacerbation of disease because of increased demyelination *(70,391,399)*. Collectively, these studies suggest that NO, TNF-α, and IL-1β likely contribute to the inductive phase of EAE but also are critical for remyelination and resolution of existing disease. The studies also suggest that the efficacy of therapies designed to alter the expression or function of NO, TNF-α, and IL-1β may depend on the timing of drug administration.

In summary, cytokines are critical mediators of MS and EAE. IFN-γ and IL-12 have a pivotal role in Th1 differentiation, which is associated with the development of these disorders, whereas IL-4 is critical in Th2-cell differentiation, which protects against the diseases. Cytokines elicited by T cells also control the responses of innate immune cells, including peripheral macrophages and CNS-derived microglia and astrocytes. On activation, these cells produce cytokines, including TNF-α and IL-1β, as well as NO. These molecules are required for the resolution of microbial infections; however, in the context of noninfectious neuroinflammatory disorders, such as MS and EAE, these mediators may also be toxic to oligodendrocytes and neurons. Interestingly, these same molecules appear to facilitate remyelination and thus may facilitate recovery from disease. Therefore, future therapies designed to regulate the expression of these molecules must consider their dual role in exacerbating and resolving disease. Experimentally, it is difficult to assess the role of specific cytokines in modulating EAE because of the redundant activities of these mediators. Future studies involving the conditional knock-in and knock-out of genes encoding these cytokines will be useful in determining the role of the cytokines in modulating disease.

4.2. Alzheimer's Disease

AD is the most common form of dementia. The disease is characterized by progressive neurodegeneration associated with impairment of memory, deterioration of language skills, altered judgment, confusion, and restlessness. The incidence of AD increases with age, and the probability of developing the disease approximately doubles every 5 yr beyond the age of 65. Concerns exist that the personal and societal costs of AD may become staggering as life expectancy increases in developing countries. The causes of AD are not completely understood. Approximately 5 to 10% of AD cases are familial and linked to gene mutations, whereas the majority of cases are sporadic in nature. AD is characterized by brain atrophy resulting from loss of neurons and the presence of neurofibrillary tangles as well as amyloid plaques containing β-amyloid peptide (β-AP). This peptide has a tendency to aggregate and is highly insoluble *(404,405)*.

Several lines of evidence suggest that inflammation contributes to the neuropathology associated with AD. For example, many clinical studies have indicated that anti-inflammatory drugs, including nonsteroidal anti-inflammatory drugs, protect against the development of AD *(406–408)*. In addition, large numbers of activated microglia and astrocytes are observed in the brains of patients with AD *(409–411)*. Activated microglia (and possibly astrocytes) may contribute to AD pathology, likely through the production of neurotoxic molecules, including inflammatory cytokines. In addition to CNS parenchymal cells, a limited number of T cells can be observed near postcapillary venules in areas of severe inflammation in the brains of patients with AD *(412)*, although cell-mediated immunity is not believed to take place in AD. It is possible however, that these limited T cells may contribute to AD pathology through the production of IFN-γ, which potently stimulates the production of inflammatory cytokines by microglia and astrocytes. The localization of activated glia near amyloid plaques supports the hypothesis that these cells contribute to neurodegeneration. For example, active amyloid plaques that contain degenerating neuritic processes (designated *neuritic plaques*) are associated with activated microglia. Activated astrocytes are also observed at the periphery of these neuritic plaques; however, end stage *burnt out* plaques are devoid of injured neuritic processes as well as activated glia

(413,414). Finally, a tremendous variety of proinflammatory mediators are observed in the brains of patients with AD. These include cytokines, chemokines, complement proteins, acute phase reactants, and oxidative stress molecules *(415)*. As mentioned previously, AD is characterized by the presence of neurofibrillary tangles and plaques associated with the highly insoluble β-AP. Although inflammation is not likely to initiate disease, it is highly probable that inflammation perpetuates neurodegeneration through the production of proinflammatory and neurotoxic molecules by activated glia in response to insoluble β-AP. The following sections focus on the role of cytokines in mediating AD pathogenesis.

A variety of cytokines are associated with AD plaques, including IL-1α, IL-1β, IL-6, TNF-α, and TGF-β *(413,415–422)*. These cytokines are produced by activated glia and some (IL-1β and TNF-α) are capable of perpetuating glial activation, leading to a cycle of overproduction of these potentially neurotoxic molecules. It should be noted, however, that these same cytokines at low concentrations may be neuroprotective. Microglia isolated post-mortem from AD patients have been shown to either constitutively express cytokines, including IL-1β, IL-6, and TNF-α, or produce these cytokines in response to β-AP *(423)*. Likewise, β-AP and other amyloid-associated proteins are capable of stimulating the production of these same cytokines by rodent glia *(415,423–425)*. Polymorphisms in the regulatory regions of the genes that encode these cytokines have been demonstrated to affect the risk of developing AD *(426–433)*. The probability of developing AD is increased in individuals who exhibit more than one of these high-risk cytokine alleles.

As mentioned previously, a variety of cytokines, including IL-1, IL-6, TNF-α, and TGF-β, are expressed in the brains of AD patients. Each of these cytokines may contribute to or alternatively protect against neuropathology associated with neuroinflammatory disorders, including AD. The strongest evidence for cytokine involvement in the pathology of AD originates from studies of IL-1. Griffin et al. *(416)* first described IL-1 overexpression in AD. IL-1 is primarily associated with microglia surrounding AD plaques *(434)*. Importantly, microglial expression of IL-1 correlates with the transformation of AD plaques. For example, diffuse non-neuritic *pre-amyloid* deposits contain microglia expressing relatively low levels of IL-1, whereas neuritic plaques are associated with microglia expressing high levels of this cytokine. Finally, end-stage burnt out plaques devoid of neuritic structures also lack IL-1-expressing microglia *(413)*. These studies suggest that IL-1 contributes to neuron loss in AD *(435)*.

IL-1 may stimulate neuron death in AD through a number of mechanisms. First, IL-1 stimulates the synthesis *(436,437)* and processing of β-amyloid precursor protein (βAPP), thus promoting the release of amyloid proteins. Furthermore, IL-1 activates glia *(438–440)*, which perpetuates the continued release of neurotoxic molecules by these cells. IL-1 also stimulates the release of S-100B by astrocytes *(420)*. This molecule contributes to the pathology associated with AD by promoting neuritic growth *(441)* and stimulating increased intracellular calcium levels in neurons, which may lead to cell death *(442)*. Additional support for the role of IL-1 in AD pathogenesis comes from studies indicating that polymorphisms in the genes encoding IL-1α and IL-1β can increase the risk of developing disease *(428,429)*. These polymorphisms are associated with increased production of IL-1α and IL-1β, which supports the role of these cytokines in the pathogenesis of disease *(443,444)*.

In summary, additional studies demonstrating the functional involvement of cytokines in the pathogenesis of AD are needed to begin to understand the role of these mediators in dementia; however, these types of studies have been limited to date by the lack of available animal models of AD in cytokine KO mice. The generation of cytokine transgenic or KO mice in Alzheimer's-susceptible strains would facilitate the establishment of the role of individual mediators in disease pathogenesis.

4.3. Parkinson's Disease

Parkinson's disease (PD) is a common progressive neurodegenerative disorder characterized by motor system dysfunction. Patients commonly exhibit tremor, rigidity, bradykinesia or slowness of movement, and postural instability or impaired balance and coordination. PD is distinguished neuropathologically by the selective loss of dopaminergic neurons of the substantia nigra and in related brainstem nuclei. Loss of the neurotransmitter dopamine results in uncontrolled firing of spared neurons, resulting in movement disorders in patients. The causes of PD as well as the mechanisms that result in neurodegeneration are largely unknown. Inheritance contributes to the development of familial forms of the disease, which represent only about 10% of all cases of PD. Most forms of PD are sporadic in nature and are not inherited. Oxidative stress and mitochondrial dysfunction have been suggested to have roles in PD *(445)*. Metabolism of dopamine results in increased production of free radicals that may be toxic to dopaminergic neurons. Increased lipid peroxidation and iron levels and decreased glutathione transferase observed in the substantia nigra of patients with PD supports a hypothesis that reactive oxygen formation may contribute to pathology *(446)*. The finding that complex I of the mitochondrial respiratory chain is defective in some patients with PD, in addition to the identification of missense mutations in mitochondrial complex I genes *(447)*, supports mitochondrial dysfunction as a contributor to the development of disease *(448,449)*.

There are several lines of evidence to suggest that neuroinflammation plays a role in the degeneration of dopaminergic neurons in PD. Seminal studies by McGeer demonstrated elevated levels of human leukocyte antigen-DR positive microglial cells in the substantia nigra of patients with PD *(450)*. These findings are supported by studies of a cohort of patients who developed parkinsonian syndrome following 1-methyl-4-phenyl-1,2,3,6-tetrahydropyridine (MPTP) intoxication during drug use *(451)*. Postmortem neuropathology studies of these individuals demonstrated that years following MPTP intoxication, reactive gliosis and activated microglia clustered around dopaminergic neurons were still evident in the CNS. These studies suggest that following an initiating event, reactive glia may perpetuate neurodegeneration in parkinsonian syndromes. Although the initiating event in these studies was MPTP intoxication, the initiating event in the development of most cases of PD is unknown. Animal models of PD support the hypothesis that activated glia contribute to neurodegeneration. In vitro studies demonstrate that LPS, a potent activator of glia, is capable of killing dopaminergic neurons in culture and that loss of neurons is more profound in neuron–glial mixed cultures. This suggests that products of activated glia contribute to neuron death *(452)*. Furthermore, agents including methylphenylpyridinium or 6-hydroxydopamine were shown to be directly toxic to dopaminergic neurons, which was enhanced when the cells were co-cultured with activated astrocytes *(453)*. In vivo studies demonstrated that LPS injected into rats damaged dopaminergic neurons in the substantia nigra without damaging GABAergic and serotoninergic neurons *(454,455)*. Interestingly, dexamethasone, a potent immunosuppressive agent, inhibited microglial/ macrophage activation and protected dopaminergic neurons in this in vivo model *(456)*. Collectively, these studies suggest that activated glia contribute to the loss of dopaminergic neurons observed in PD.

A variety of cytokines are expressed at higher levels in the substantia nigra, striatum, and/or CSF of patients with PD relative to control subjects. These include TNF-α, IL-1β, IL-6, and TGF-β that are known to be produced by glia, and IL-2, IL-4, and IFN-γ produced primarily by T and/or NK cells *(457)*. The potential role of these cytokines in mediating PD has not been elucidated; however, as previously mentioned, TNF-α and IL-1β elicited by activated glia may be directly toxic to neurons. TGF-β is an anti-inflammatory cytokine capable of suppressing glial activation and thus may aid in the resolution of inflammation associated with PD. CD4$^+$ and CD8$^+$ T cells have been shown to infiltrate the CNS of MPTP-intoxicated rodents *(458)*. In addition, CD8$^+$ T cells have been identified in the substantia nigra of patients with PD, although the abundance of T cells in the CNS in these disorders is relatively low and their potential role in modulating PD has not been defined. It is possible that the limited number of T cells present in the CNS in parkinsonian disorders may affect the viability of dopaminergic neurons by eliciting cytokines, such as IFN-γ and IL-4 that control the activation state of glia. This possibility is supported by the fact that both IL-4 and IFN-γ have been detected in the brain tissue and CSF of patients with PD.

Hunet et al. *(459)* present two hypotheses that may explain how cytokines could cause neurodegeneration in PD. They suggest that proinflammatory cytokines, including IFN-γ, TNF-α, and IL-1β, may stimulate production of NO by glial cells. Although NO can protect neurons under some circumstances, in profound inflammatory conditions, NO likely contributes to neuron cell death, possibly through lipid peroxidation. In support of this hypothesis, glia expressing iNOS have been identified in the substantia nigra of patients with PD *(460)* and NO has been observed in the CSF of these patients *(461)*. Hunet et al. further hypothesize that TNF-α produced by activated glia may stimulate the death of TNFR1-expressing dopaminergic neurons by activating the TNFR1 signaling pathway, which, under certain conditions, is capable of inducing apoptosis.

Studies demonstrating that anti-inflammatory drugs are capable of suppressing neurodegeneration in animal models of PD support the notion that inflammation contributes to disease. These anti-inflammatory drugs likely suppress disease, at least in part, by modulating the expression of both pro- and anti-inflammatory cytokines. In general, modification of a single inflammatory pathway has not proved effective in protecting dopaminergic neurons in these model systems *(462)*. Inhibition of apoptotic pathways using Casp inhibitors have also proved largely ineffective in preventing neurodegeneration *(463)*. Agents with a broader spectrum of anti-inflammatory actions have been more effective in protecting dopaminergic neurons in these models. For example, the peroxisome proliferator-activated receptor-γ agonist pioglitazone blocked glial activation and protected dopaminergic neurons in the substantia nigra of MPTP-treated mice *(464)*, although pioglitazone neither suppressed glial activation nor protected neurons in the striatum. These and other studies suggest that the mechanisms that regulate glial cell activation and neuron viability may be different in the terminals relative to cell bodies of dopaminergic neurons. Minocycline, a tetracycline derivative, has been demonstrated to block glial cell activation and protect neurons in the entire stratonigral system in MPTP and in 6-hydroxydopamine-treated rats *(465–467)*. This suggests the intriguing possibility that minocycline or other broad-spectrum anti-inflammatory agents may be effective in delaying the progression of PD.

5. CONCLUSIONS AND PERSPECTIVES

In this work, we have attempted to provide detailed discussions regarding the roles of cytokines in the context of the healthy CNS, in addition to a wide variety of infectious and noninfectious inflammatory diseases of this tissue. Although the overexpression of numerous proinflammatory cytokines likely contributes in part to the neurodegeneration associated with these inflammatory diseases, many of these same mediators have also been shown to contribute to the resolution of disease. Therefore, the functional role of cytokines in various neuroinflammatory disorders is likely dictated by a complex interplay between the nature of the CNS insult, the timing of cytokine expression during disease, the balance of pro- vs anti-inflammatory mediators, and/or the local concentration of cytokines within the CNS microenvironment. It is interesting to note that many cytokines, such as TNF-α and IL-1β, are detected in a wide range of both infectious and non-infectious neuroinflammatory diseases, suggesting that the fundamental response of the CNS to inflammatory insults is conserved at some level. The development of new animal models to evaluate the functional importance of cytokines in neuroinflammatory diseases should provide important insights into the role of these mediators in CNS pathology and recovery. Specifically, the generation of conditional cytokine-inducible and KO mice along with double-cytokine KO animals would greatly add to our knowledge base regarding the roles of these mediators in both the normal and diseased CNS.

ACKNOWLEDGMENTS

The authors would like to thank Jean Chaunsumlit for excellent administrative assistance. This work was supported by grants from the National Institutes of Health (NS40730 and MH65297 to TK and NS42860 to PDD) and the National Multiple Sclerosis Society (RG 3198A1 to PDD).

REFERENCES

1. Vitkovic L, Bockaert J, Jacque C. "Inflammatory" cytokines: neuromodulators in normal brain? J Neurochem 2000;74:457–471.
2. Breder CD, Dinarello CA, Saper CB. Interleukin-1 immunoreactive innervation of the human hypothalamus. Science 1988;240:321–324.
3. Lechan RM, Toni R, Clark BD, et al. Immunoreactive interleukin-1 beta localization in the rat forebrain. Brain Res 1990;514:135–140.
4. Bandtlow CE, Meyer M, Lindholm D, Spranger M, Heumann R, Thoenen H. Regional and cellular codistribution of interleukin 1 beta and nerve growth factor mRNA in the adult rat brain: possible relationship to the regulation of nerve growth factor synthesis. J Cell Biol 1990;111:1701–1711.
5. da Cunha A, Jefferson JJ, Tyor WR, Glass JD, Jannotta FS, Vitkovic L. Control of astrocytosis by interleukin-1 and transforming growth factor-beta 1 in human brain. Brain Res 1993;631:39–45.
6. Quan N, Zhang Z, Emery M, et al. In vivo induction of interleukin-1 bioactivity in brain tissue after intracerebral infusion of native gp 120 and gp 160. Neuroimmunomodulation 1996;3:56–61.
7. Ilyin SE, Plata-Salaman CR. HIV-1 gp120 modulates hypothalamic cytokine mRNAs in vivo: implications to cytokine feedback systems. Biochem Biophys Res Commun 1997;231:514–518.
8. Streit WJ, Semple-Rowland SL, Hurley SD, Miller RC, Popovich PG, Stokes BT. Cytokine mRNA profiles in contused spinal cord and axotomized facial nucleus suggest a beneficial role for inflammation and gliosis. Exp Neurol 1998;152:74–87.
9. Yu AC, Lau LT. Expression of interleukin-1 alpha, tumor necrosis factor alpha and interleukin-6 genes in astrocytes under ischemic injury. Neurochem Int 2000;36:369–377.
10. Taishi P, Bredow S, Guha-Thakurta N, Obal F Jr, Krueger JM. Diurnal variations of interleukin-1 beta mRNA and beta-actin mRNA in rat brain. J Neuroimmunol 1997;75:69–74.
11. Meltzer JC, Sanders V, Grimm PC, et al. Production of digoxigenin-labeled RNA probes and the detection of cytokine mRNA in rat spleen and brain by in situ hybridization. Brain Res Brain Res Protoc 1998;2:339–351.
12. Higgins GA, Olschowka JA. Induction of interleukin-1 beta mRNA in adult rat brain. Brain Res Mol Brain Res 1991;9:143–148.
13. Pousset F. Developmental expression of cytokine genes in the cortex and hippocampus of the rat central nervous system. Brain Res Dev Brain Res 1994;81:143–146.
14. Fontana A, Weber E, Dayer JM. Synthesis of interleukin 1/endogenous pyrogen in the brain of endotoxin-treated mice: a step in fever induction? J Immunol 1984;133:1696–1698.
15. Krueger JM, Fang J, Taishi P, Chen Z, Kushikata T, Gardi J. Sleep. A physiologic role for IL-1 beta and TNF-alpha. Ann N Y Acad Sci 1998;856:148–159.
16. Perry SW, Dewhurst S, Bellizzi MJ, Gelbard HA. Tumor necrosis factor-alpha in normal and diseased brain: conflicting effects via intraneuronal receptor crosstalk? J Neurovirol 2002;8:611–624.
17. Hunt JS, Chen HL, Hu XL, Chen TY, Morrison DC. Tumor necrosis factor-alpha gene expression in the tissues of normal mice. Cytokine 1992;4:340–346.
18. Bredow S, Guha-Thakurta N, Taishi P, Obal F Jr, Krueger JM. Diurnal variations of tumor necrosis factor alpha mRNA and alpha-tubulin mRNA in rat brain. Neuroimmunomodulation 1997;4:84–90.
19. Wesselingh SL, Power C, Glass JD, et al. Intracerebral cytokine messenger RNA expression in acquired immunodeficiency syndrome dementia. Ann Neurol 1993;33:576–582.
20. Breder CD, Tsujimoto M, Terano Y, Scott DW, Saper CB. Distribution and characterization of tumor necrosis factor-alpha-like immunoreactivity in the murine central nervous system. J Comp Neurol 1993;337:543–567.
21. Floyd RA, Krueger JM. Diurnal variation of TNF alpha in the rat brain. Neuroreport 1997;8:915–918.
22. Munoz-Fernandez MA, Fresno M. The role of tumour necrosis factor, interleukin 6, interferon-gamma and inducible nitric oxide synthase in the development and pathology of the nervous system. Prog Neurobiol 1998;56:307–340.
23. Krieglstein K, Unsicker K. Bovine chromaffin cells release a transforming growth factor-beta-like molecule contained within chromaffin granules. J Neurochem 1995;65:1423–1426.
24. Bottner M, Krieglstein K, Unsicker K. The transforming growth factor-betas: structure, signaling, and roles in nervous system development and functions. J Neurochem 2000;75:2227–2240.
25. Unsicker K, Strelau J. Functions of transforming growth factor-beta isoforms in the nervous system. Cues based on localization and experimental in vitro and in vivo evidence. Eur J Biochem 2000;267:6972–6975.

26. Flanders KC, Ludecke G, Engels S, et al. Localization and actions of transforming growth factor-betas in the embryonic nervous system. Development 1991;113:183–191.

27. Hunter KE, Sporn MB, Davies AM. Transforming growth factor-betas inhibit mitogen-stimulated proliferation of astrocytes. Glia 1993; 7:203-211.

28. Toru-Delbauffe D, Baghdassarian-Chalaye D, Gavaret JM, Courtin F, Pomerance M, Pierre M. Effects of transforming growth factor beta 1 on astroglial cells in culture. J Neurochem 1990;54:1056–1061.

29. Cameron JS, Lhuillier L, Subramony P, Dryer SE. Developmental regulation of neuronal K^+ channels by target-derived TGF beta in vivo and in vitro. Neuron 1998;21:1045–1053.

30. Ishihara A, Saito H, Abe K. Transforming growth factor-beta 1 and -beta 2 promote neurite sprouting and elongation of cultured rat hippocampal neurons. Brain Res 1994;639:21–25.

31. Abe K, Chu PJ, Ishihara A, Saito H. Transforming growth factor-beta 1 promotes re-elongation of injured axons of cultured rat hippocampal neurons. Brain Res 1996;723:206–209.

32. Fok-Seang J, Mathews GA, French-Constant C, Trotter J, Fawcett JW. Migration of oligodendrocyte precursors on astrocytes and meningeal cells. Dev Biol 1995;171:1–15.

33. Schnadelbach O, Mandl C, Faissner A. Expression of DSD-1-PG in primary neural and glial-derived cell line cultures, upregulation by TGF-beta, and implications for cell-substrate interactions of the glial cell line Oli-neu. Glia 1998;23:99–119.

34. Kielian T, Hickey WF. Proinflammatory cytokine, chemokine, and cellular adhesion molecule expression during the acute phase of experimental brain abscess development. Am J Pathol 2000;157:647–658.

35. Kielian T, Cheung A, Hickey WF. Diminished virulence of an alpha-toxin mutant of *Staphylococcus aureus* in experimental brain abscesses. Infect Immun 2001;69:6902–6911.

36. Bacher M, Meinhardt A, Lan HY, et al. MIF expression in the rat brain: implications for neuronal function. Mol Med 1998;4:217–230.

37. Nishibori M, Nakaya N, Mori S, Saeki K. Immunohistochemical localization of macrophage migration inhibitory factor (MIF) in tanycytes, subcommissural organ and choroid plexus in the rat brain. Brain Res 1997;758:259–262.

38. Busche S, Gallinat S, Fleegal MA, Raizada MK, Sumners C. Novel role of macrophage migration inhibitory factor in angiotensin II regulation of neuromodulation in rat brain. Endocrinology 2001;142:4623–4630.

39. Kielian T, Mayes, P, Kielian M. Characterization of microglial responses to *Staphylococcus aureus:* effects on cytokine, costimulatory molecule, and Toll-like receptor expression. J Neuroimmunol. 2002;130:86–99.

40. Esen N, Tanga FY, DeLeo JA, Kielian T. Toll-like receptor 2 (TLR2) mediates astrocyte activation in response to the Gram-positive bacterium *Staphylococcus aureus.* J Neurochem 2004;88:746–758.

41. Fingerle-Rowson GR, Bucala R. Neuroendocrine properties of macrophage migration inhibitory factor (MIF). Immunol Cell Biol 2001;79:368–375.

42. Matsunaga J, Sinha D, Pannell L, et al. Enzyme activity of macrophage migration inhibitory factor toward oxidized catecholamines. J Biol Chem 1999;274:3268–3271.

43. Repp AC, Mayhew ES, Apte S, Niederkorn JY. Human uveal melanoma cells produce macrophage migration-inhibitory factor to prevent lysis by NK cells. J Immunol 2000;165:710–715.

44. Apte RS, Sinha D, Mayhew E, Wistow GJ, Niederkorn JY. Cutting edge: role of macrophage migration inhibitory factor in inhibiting NK cell activity and preserving immune privilege. J Immunol 1998;160:5693–5696.

45. Streilein JW, Stein-Streilein J. Does innate immune privilege exist? J Leukoc Biol 2000;67:479–487.

46. John GR, Lee SC, Brosnan CF. Cytokines: powerful regulators of glial cell activation. Neuroscientist 2003;9:10–22.

47. Aloisi F. Immune function of microglia. Glia 2001;36:165–179.

48. Hanisch UK. Microglia as a source and target of cytokines. Glia 2002;40:140–155.

49. Walz W, Hertz L. Functional interactions between neurons and astrocytes. II. Potassium homeostasis at the cellular level. Prog Neurobiol 1983;20:133–183.

50. Chen Y, Swanson RA. Astrocytes and brain injury. J Cereb Blood Flow Metab 2003;23:137–149.

51. Wolburg H, Risau W. Formation of the blood brain barrier. In: Ransom BR KH, ed. Neuroglia. New York: Oxford University Press, 1995: 763–776.

52. Frohman EM, Frohman TC, Dustin ML, et al. The induction of intercellular adhesion molecule 1 (ICAM-1) expression on human fetal astrocytes by interferon-gamma, tumor necrosis factor alpha, lymphotoxin, and interleukin-1: relevance to intracerebral antigen presentation. J Neuroimmunol 1989;23:117–124.

53. Hurwitz AA, Lyman WD, Guida MP, Calderon TM, Berman JW. Tumor necrosis factor alpha induces adhesion molecule expression on human fetal astrocytes. J Exp Med 1992;176:1631–1636.

54. Aloisi F, Borsellino G, Samoggia P, et al. Astrocyte cultures from human embryonic brain: characterization and modulation of surface molecules by inflammatory cytokines. J Neurosci Res 1992;32:494–506.

55. Lee SJ, Benveniste EN. Adhesion molecule expression and regulation on cells of the central nervous system. J Neuroimmunol 1999;98:77–88.

56. Ullian EM, Sapperstein SK, Christopherson KS, Barres BA. Control of synapse number by glia. Science 2001; 291:657–661.

57. Dong Y, Benveniste EN. Immune function of astrocytes. Glia 2001;36:180–190.
58. Benveniste EN. Role of macrophages/microglia in multiple sclerosis and experimental allergic encephalomyelitis. J Mol Med 1997;75:165–173.
59. Combs CK, Karlo JC, Kao SC, Landreth GE. beta-Amyloid stimulation of microglia and monocytes results in TNFalpha-dependent expression of inducible nitric oxide synthase and neuronal apoptosis. J Neurosci 2001; 21:1179–1188.
60. Meda L, Cassatella MA, Szendrei GI, et al. Activation of microglial cells by beta-amyloid protein and interferon-gamma. Nature 1995;374:647–650.
61. Renno T, Krakowski M, Piccirillo C, Lin JY, Owens T. TNF-alpha expression by resident microglia and infiltrating leukocytes in the central nervous system of mice with experimental allergic encephalomyelitis. Regulation by Th1 cytokines. J Immunol 1995;154:944–953.
62. Tran EH, Hardin-Pouzet H, Verge G, Owens T. Astrocytes and microglia express inducible nitric oxide synthase in mice with experimental allergic encephalomyelitis. J Neuroimmunol 1997;74:121–129.
63. Griffin WS, Mrak RE. Interleukin-1 in the genesis and progression of and risk for development of neuronal degeneration in Alzheimer's disease. J Leukoc Biol 2002;72:233–238.
64. Claudio L, Martiney JA, Brosnan CF. Ultrastructural studies of the blood-retina barrier after exposure to interleukin-1 beta or tumor necrosis factor-alpha. Lab Invest 1994;70:850–861.
65. Quagliarello VJ, Wispelwey B, Long WJ Jr, Scheld WM. Recombinant human interleukin-1 induces meningitis and blood-brain barrier injury in the rat. Characterization and comparison with tumor necrosis factor. J Clin Invest 1991;87:1360–1366.
66. Wong D, Dorovini-Zis K. Upregulation of intercellular adhesion molecule-1 (ICAM-1) expression in primary cultures of human brain microvessel endothelial cells by cytokines and lipopolysaccharide. J Neuroimmunol 1992;39:11–21.
67. Wong D, Dorovini-Zis K. Regulation by cytokines and lipopolysaccharide of E-selectin expression by human brain microvessel endothelial cells in primary culture. J Neuropathol Exp Neurol 1996;55:225–235.
68. Selmaj KW, Raine CS. Tumor necrosis factor mediates myelin and oligodendrocyte damage in vitro. Ann Neurol 1988;23:339–246.
69. Hisahara S, Shoji S, Okano H, Miura M. ICE/CED-3 family executes oligodendrocyte apoptosis by tumor necrosis factor. J Neurochem 1997;69:10–20.
70. Akassoglou K, Bauer J, Kassiotis G, et al. Oligodendrocyte apoptosis and primary demyelination induced by local TNF/p55TNF receptor signaling in the central nervous system of transgenic mice: models for multiple sclerosis with primary oligodendrogliopathy. Am J Pathol 1998;153:801–813.
71. Andrews T, Zhang P, Bhat NR. TNFalpha potentiates IFNgamma-induced cell death in oligodendrocyte progenitors. J Neurosci Res 1998;54:574–583.
72. Ladiwala U, Li H, Antel JP, Nalbantoglu J. p53 induction by tumor necrosis factor-alpha and involvement of p53 in cell death of human oligodendrocytes. J Neurochem 1999;73:605–611.
73. Ye P, D'Ercole AJ. Insulin-like growth factor I protects oligodendrocytes from tumor necrosis factor-alpha-induced injury. Endocrinology 1999;140:3063–3072.
74. Merrill JE. Effects of interleukin-1 and tumor necrosis factor-alpha on astrocytes, microglia, oligodendrocytes, and glial precursors in vitro. Dev Neurosci 1991;13:130–137.
75. Trapp BD, Peterson J, Ransohoff RM, Rudick R, Mork S, Bo L. Axonal transection in the lesions of multiple sclerosis. N Engl J Med 1998;338:278–285.
76. Arnett HA, Mason J, Marino M, Suzuki K, Matsushima GK, Ting JP. TNF alpha promotes proliferation of oligodendrocyte progenitors and remyelination. Nat Neurosci 2001;4:1116–1122.
77. Brogi A, Strazza M, Melli M, Costantino-Ceccarini E. Induction of intracellular ceramide by interleukin-1 beta in oligodendrocytes. J Cell Biochem 1997;66:532–541.
78. Mason JL, Suzuki K, Chaplin DD, Matsushima GK. Interleukin-1beta promotes repair of the CNS. J Neurosci 2001;21:7046–7052.
79. Gruol DL, Nelson TE. Physiological and pathological roles of interleukin-6 in the central nervous system. Mol Neurobiol 1997;15:307–339.
80. Van Wagoner NJ, Benveniste EN. Interleukin-6 expression and regulation in astrocytes. J Neuroimmunol 1999;100:124–139.
81. Selmaj KW, Farooq M, Norton WT, Raine CS, Brosnan CF. Proliferation of astrocytes in vitro in response to cytokines. A primary role for tumor necrosis factor. J Immunol 1990;144:129–135.
82. Constam DB, Schmid P, Aguzzi A, Schachner M, Fontana A. Transient production of TGF-beta 2 by postnatal cerebellar neurons and its effect on neuroblast proliferation. Eur J Neurosci 1994;6:766–778.
83. Lindholm D, Castren E, Kiefer R, Zafra F, Thoenen H. Transforming growth factor-beta 1 in the rat brain: increase after injury and inhibition of astrocyte proliferation. J Cell Biol 1992;117:395–400.
84. Cassatella MA. The production of cytokines by polymorphonuclear neutrophils. Immunol Today 1995;16:21–26.
85. Cassatella MA. Neutrophil-derived proteins: selling cytokines by the pound. Adv Immunol 1999;73:369–509.

86. Koedel U, Scheld WM, Pfister HW. Pathogenesis and pathophysiology of pneumococcal meningitis. Lancet Infect Dis 2002;2:721–736.

87. Bogdan I, Leib SL, Bergeron M, Chow L, Tauber MG. Tumor necrosis factor-alpha contributes to apoptosis in hippocampal neurons during experimental group B streptococcal meningitis. J Infect Dis 1997;176:693–697.

88. Scheld WM, Koedel U, Nathan B, Pfister HW. Pathophysiology of bacterial meningitis: mechanism(s) of neuronal injury. J Infect Dis 2002;186(Suppl 2):S225–233.

89. Nau R, Bruck W. Neuronal injury in bacterial meningitis: mechanisms and implications for therapy. Trends Neurosci 2002;25:38–45.

90. van Furth AM, Roord JJ, van Furth R. Roles of proinflammatory and anti-inflammatory cytokines in pathophysiology of bacterial meningitis and effect of adjunctive therapy. Infect Immun 1996;64:4883–4890.

91. Zysk G, Bruck W, Huitinga I, et al. Elimination of blood-derived macrophages inhibits the release of interleukin-1 and the entry of leukocytes into the cerebrospinal fluid in experimental pneumococcal meningitis. J Neuroimmunol 1997;73:77–80.

92. Trostdorf F, Bruck W, Schmitz-Salue M, et al. Reduction of meningeal macrophages does not decrease migration of granulocytes into the CSF and brain parenchyma in experimental pneumococcal meningitis. J Neuroimmunol 1999;99:205–210.

93. Tauber MG, Moser B. Cytokines and chemokines in meningeal inflammation: biology and clinical implications. Clin Infect Dis 1999;28:1–11; quiz 12.

94. Ramilo O, Saez-Llorens X, Mertsola J, et al. Tumor necrosis factor alpha/cachectin and interleukin 1 beta initiate meningeal inflammation. J Exp Med 1990;172:497–507.

95. Pfister HW, Scheld WM. Brain injury in bacterial meningitis: therapeutic implications. Curr Opin Neurol 1997;10:254–259.

96. van der Flier M, Geelen SP, Kimpen JL, Hoepelman IM, Tuomanen EI. Reprogramming the host response in bacterial meningitis: how best to improve outcome? Clin Microbiol Rev 2003;16:415–429.

97. Dulkerian SJ, Kilpatrick L, Costarino AT Jr, et al. Cytokine elevations in infants with bacterial and aseptic meningitis. J Pediatr 1995;126:872–876.

98. van Furth AM, Seijmonsbergen EM, Langermans JA, Groeneveld PH, de Bel CE, van Furth R. High levels of interleukin 10 and tumor necrosis factor alpha in cerebrospinal fluid during the onset of bacterial meningitis. Clin Infect Dis 1995;21:220–222.

99. van Deuren M, van der Ven-Jongekrijg J, Bartelink AK, van Dalen R, Sauerwein RW, van der Meer JW. Correlation between proinflammatory cytokines and antiinflammatory mediators and the severity of disease in meningococcal infections. J Infect Dis 1995;172:433–439.

100. Leist TP, Frei K, Kam-Hansen S, Zinkernagel RM, Fontana A. Tumor necrosis factor alpha in cerebrospinal fluid during bacterial, but not viral, meningitis. Evaluation in murine model infections and in patients. J Exp Med 1988;167:1743–1748.

101. Waage A, Halstensen A, Shalaby R, Brandtzaeg P, Kierulf P, Espevik T. Local production of tumor necrosis factor alpha, interleukin 1, and interleukin 6 in meningococcal meningitis. Relation to the inflammatory response. J Exp Med 1989;170:1859–1867.

102. Nadal D, Leppert D, Frei K, Gallo P, Lamche H, Fontana A. Tumour necrosis factor-alpha in infectious meningitis. Arch Dis Child 1989;64:1274–1279.

103. Glimaker M, Kragsbjerg P, Forsgren M, Olcen P. Tumor necrosis factor-alpha (TNF alpha) in cerebrospinal fluid from patients with meningitis of different etiologies: high levels of TNF alpha indicate bacterial meningitis. J Infect Dis 1993;167:882–889.

104. Ohga S, Aoki T, Okada K, et al. Cerebrospinal fluid concentrations of interleukin-1 beta, tumour necrosis factor-alpha, and interferon gamma in bacterial meningitis. Arch Dis Child 1994;70:123–125.

105. Kornelisse RF, Savelkoul HF, Mulder PH, et al. Interleukin-10 and soluble tumor necrosis factor receptors in cerebrospinal fluid of children with bacterial meningitis. J Infect Dis 1996;173:1498–1502.

106. Sharief MK, Ciardi M, Thompson EJ. Blood-brain barrier damage in patients with bacterial meningitis: association with tumor necrosis factor-alpha but not interleukin-1 beta. J Infect Dis 1992;166:350–358.

107. Akalin H, Akdis AC, Mistik R, Helvaci S, Kilicturgay K. Cerebrospinal fluid interleukin-1 beta/interleukin-1 receptor antagonist balance and tumor necrosis factor-alpha concentrations in tuberculous, viral and acute bacterial meningitis. Scand J Infect Dis 1994;26:667–674.

108. Arditi M, Manogue KR, Caplan M, Yogev R. Cerebrospinal fluid cachectin/tumor necrosis factor-alpha and platelet-activating factor concentrations and severity of bacterial meningitis in children. J Infect Dis 1990;162:139–147.

109. Lopez-Cortes LF, Cruz-Ruiz M, Gomez-Mateos J, Jimenez-Hernandez D, Palomino J, Jimenez E. Measurement of levels of tumor necrosis factor-alpha and interleukin-1 beta in the CSF of patients with meningitis of different etiologies: utility in the differential diagnosis. Clin Infect Dis 1993;16:534–539.

110. Diab A, Zhu J, Lindquist L, Wretlind B, Bakhiet M, Link H. *Haemophilus influenzae* and *Streptococcus pneumoniae* induce different intracerebral mRNA cytokine patterns during the course of experimental bacterial meningitis. Clin Exp Immunol 1997;109:233–241.

111. Diab A, Zhu J, Lindquist L, Wretlind B, Link H, Bakhiet M. Cytokine mRNA profiles during the course of experimental *Haemophilus influenzae* bacterial meningitis. Clin Immunol Immunopathol 1997;85:236–245.

112. Winkler F, Koedel U, Kastenbauer S, Pfister HW. Differential expression of nitric oxide synthases in bacterial meningitis: role of the inducible isoform for blood-brain barrier breakdown. J Infect Dis 2001;183:1749–1759.

113. Bitsch A, Trostdorf F, Bruck W, Schmidt H, Fischer FR, Nau R. Central nervous system TNFalpha-mRNA expression during rabbit experimental pneumococcal meningitis. Neurosci Lett 1997;237:105–108.

114. Mustafa MM, Ramilo O, Olsen KD, et al. Tumor necrosis factor in mediating experimental *Haemophilus influenzae* type B meningitis. J Clin Invest 1989;84:1253–1259.

115. Paris MM, Friedland IR, Ehrett S, et al. Effect of interleukin-1 receptor antagonist and soluble tumor necrosis factor receptor in animal models of infection. J Infect Dis 1995;171:161–169.

116. Saukkonen K, Sande S, Cioffe C, et al. The role of cytokines in the generation of inflammation and tissue damage in experimental gram-positive meningitis. J Exp Med 1990;171:439–448.

117. Wellmer A, Gerber J, Ragheb J, et al. Effect of deficiency of tumor necrosis factor alpha or both of its receptors on *Streptococcus pneumoniae* central nervous system infection and peritonitis. Infect Immun 2001;69:6881–6886.

118. Mustafa MM, Lebel MH, Ramilo O, et al. Correlation of interleukin-1 beta and cachectin concentrations in cerebrospinal fluid and outcome from bacterial meningitis. J Pediatr 1989;115:208–213.

119. Mustafa MM, Ramilo O, Saez-Llorens X, Mertsola J, Magness RR, McCracken GH Jr. Prostaglandins E2 and I2, interleukin 1-beta, and tumor necrosis factor in cerebrospinal fluid in infants and children with bacterial meningitis. Pediatr Infect Dis J 1989;8:921–922.

120. van Deuren M, van der Ven-Jongekrijg J, Vannier E, et al. The pattern of interleukin-1beta (IL-1beta) and its modulating agents IL-1 receptor antagonist and IL-1 soluble receptor type II in acute meningococcal infections. Blood 1997;90:1101–1108.

121. Zwijnenburg PJ, van der Poll T, Florquin S, van Deventer SJ, Roord JJ, van Furth AM. Experimental pneumococcal meningitis in mice: a model of intranasal infection. J Infect Dis 2001;183:1143–1146.

122. Zwijnenburg PJ, van der Poll T, Florquin S, Roord JJ, Van Furth AM. IL-1 receptor type 1 gene-deficient mice demonstrate an impaired host defense against pneumococcal meningitis. J Immunol 2003;170:4724–4730.

123. Chavanet P, Bonnotte B, Guiguet M, et al. High concentrations of intrathecal interleukin-6 in human bacterial and nonbacterial meningitis. J Infect Dis 1992;166:428–431.

124. Matsuzono Y, Narita M, Akutsu Y, Togashi T. Interleukin-6 in cerebrospinal fluid of patients with central nervous system infections. Acta Paediatr 1995;84:879–883.

125. Koedel U, Bernatowicz A, Frei K, Fontana A, Pfister HW. Systemically (but not intrathecally) administered IL-10 attenuates pathophysiologic alterations in experimental pneumococcal meningitis. J Immunol 1996;157:5185–5191.

126. Marby D, Lockhart GR, Raymond R, Linakis JG. Anti-interleukin-6 antibodies attenuate inflammation in a rat meningitis model. Acad Emerg Med 2001;8:946–949.

127. Paul R, Koedel U, Winkler F, et al. Lack of IL-6 augments inflammatory response but decreases vascular permeability in bacterial meningitis. Brain 2003;126:1873–1882.

128. Howard M, O'Garra A, Ishida H, de Waal Malefyt R, de Vries J. Biological properties of interleukin 10. J Clin Immunol 1992;12:239–247.

129. Strle K, Zhou JH, Shen WH, et al. Interleukin-10 in the brain. Crit Rev Immunol 2001;21:427–449.

130. Molina-Holgado F, Grencis R, Rothwell NJ. Actions of exogenous and endogenous IL-10 on glial responses to bacterial LPS/cytokines. Glia 2001;33:97–106.

131. Opal SM, Wherry JC, Grint P. Interleukin-10: potential benefits and possible risks in clinical infectious diseases. Clin Infect Dis 1998;27:1497–1507.

132. Pajkrt D, Camoglio L, Tiel-van Buul MC, et al. Attenuation of proinflammatory response by recombinant human IL-10 in human endotoxemia: effect of timing of recombinant human IL-10 administration. J Immunol 1997;158:3971–3977.

133. Frei K, Nadal D, Pfister HW, Fontana A. Listeria meningitis: identification of a cerebrospinal fluid inhibitor of macrophage listericidal function as interleukin 10. J Exp Med 1993;178:1255–1261.

134. Torre D, Zeroli C, Martegani R, Speranza F. Levels of interleukin-10 and tumor necrosis factor alpha in patients with bacterial meningitis. Clin Infect Dis 1996;22:883–885.

135. Lehmann AK, Halstensen A, Sornes S, Rokke O, Waage A. High levels of interleukin 10 in serum are associated with fatality in meningococcal disease. Infect Immun 1995;63:2109–2112.

136. Zwijnenburg PJ, van der Poll T, Florquin S, Roord JJ, van Furth AM. Interleukin-10 negatively regulates local cytokine and chemokine production but does not influence antibacterial host defense during murine pneumococcal meningitis. Infect Immun 2003;71:2276–2279.

137. Paris MM, Hickey SM, Trujillo M, Ahmed A, Olsen K, McCracken GH Jr. The effect of interleukin-10 on meningeal inflammation in experimental bacterial meningitis. J Infect Dis 1997;176:1239–1246.

138. Adorini L. Interleukin-12, a key cytokine in Th1-mediated autoimmune diseases. Cell Mol Life Sci 1999;55:1610–1625.

139. Trinchieri G, Pflanz S, Kastelein RA. The IL-12 family of heterodimeric cytokines: new players in the regulation of T cell responses. Immunity 2003;19:641–644.

140. Kornelisse RF, Hack CE, Savelkoul HF, et al. Intrathecal production of interleukin-12 and gamma interferon in patients with bacterial meningitis. Infect Immun 1997;65:877–881.
141. Mastroianni CM, Paoletti F, Lichtner M, D'Agostino C, Vullo V, Delia S. Cerebrospinal fluid cytokines in patients with tuberculous meningitis. Clin Immunol Immunopathol 1997;84:171–176.
142. Gracie JA, Robertson SE, McInnes IB. Interleukin-18. J Leukoc Biol 2003;73:213–224.
143. Prinz M, Hanisch UK. Murine microglial cells produce and respond to interleukin-18. J Neurochem 1999;72:2215–2218.
144. Fassbender K, Mielke O, Bertsch T, et al. Interferon-gamma-inducing factor (IL-18) and interferon-gamma in inflammatory CNS diseases. Neurology 1999;53:1104–1106.
145. Zwijnenburg PJ, van der Poll T, Florquin S, et al. Interleukin-18 gene-deficient mice show enhanced defense and reduced inflammation during pneumococcal meningitis. J Neuroimmunol 2003;138:31–37.
146. Huang CC, Chang YC, Chow NH, Wang ST. Level of transforming growth factor beta 1 is elevated in cerebrospinal fluid of children with acute bacterial meningitis. J Neurol 1997;244:634–638.
147. Ossege LM, Voss B, Wiethege T, Sindern E, Malin JP. Detection of transforming growth factor beta 1 mRNA in cerebrospinal fluid cells of patients with meningitis by non-radioactive in situ hybridization. J Neurol 1994;242:14–19.
148. Ossege LM, Sindern E, Voss B, Malin JP. Expression of tumor necrosis factor-alpha and transforming growth factor-beta 1 in cerebrospinal fluid cells in meningitis. J Neurol Sci 1996;144:1–13.
149. Pfister HW, Frei K, Ottnad B, Koedel U, Tomasz A, Fontana A. Transforming growth factor beta 2 inhibits cerebrovascular changes and brain edema formation in the tumor necrosis factor alpha-independent early phase of experimental pneumococcal meningitis. J Exp Med 1992;176:265–268.
150. Townsend GC, Scheld WM. Infections of the central nervous system. Adv Intern Med 1998;43:403–447.
151. Kielian T, Barry B, Hickey WF. CXC chemokine receptor-2 ligands are required for neutrophil-mediated host defense in experimental brain abscesses. J Immunol 2001;166:4634–4643.
152. Flaris NA, Hickey WF. Development and characterization of an experimental model of brain abscess in the rat. Am J Pathol 1992;141:1299–1307.
153. Kielian T, Hickey, W.F. Chemokines and neural inflammation in experimental brain abscesses. In: Ransohoff RM, Suzuki K, Proudfoot AEI, Hickey WF, Harrison JK, ed. Universes in Delicate Balance: Chemokines and the Nervous System. Amsterdam: Elsevier Science B.V., 2002: 217–224.
154. Kielian T, Bearden ED, Baldwin AC, Esen N. IL-1 and TNF-α play a pivotal role in the host immune response in a mouse model of *Staphylococcus aureus*-induced experimental brain abscess. J Neuropathol Exp Neurol. 2004; 63:381–396.
155. Re F, Sironi M, Muzio M, et al. Inhibition of interleukin-1 responsiveness by type II receptor gene transfer: a surface "receptor" with anti-interleukin-1 function. J Exp Med 1996;183:1841–1850.
156. Eikelenboom P, Bate C, Van Gool WA, et al. Neuroinflammation in Alzheimer's disease and prion disease. Glia 2002;40:232–239.
157. McGeer PL, McGeer EG. Local neuroinflammation and the progression of Alzheimer's disease. J Neurovirol 2002;8:529–538.
158. Hemmer B, Cepok S, Nessler S, Sommer N. Pathogenesis of multiple sclerosis: an update on immunology. Curr Opin Neurol 2002;15:227–231.
159. Baldwin A, Kielian T. Persistent immune activation associated with a mouse model of *Staphylococcus aureus*-induced experimental brain abscess. J Neuroimmunol. 2004; 151:24–32.
160. Ho DD, Rota TR, Schooley RT, et al. Isolation of HTLV-III from cerebrospinal fluid and neural tissues of patients with neurologic syndromes related to the acquired immunodeficiency syndrome. N Engl J Med 1985;313:1493–1497.
161. Gabuzda DH, Ho DD, de la Monte SM, Hirsch MS, Rota TR, Sobel RA. Immunohistochemical identification of HTLV-III antigen in brains of patients with AIDS. Ann Neurol 1986;20:289–295.
162. Davis LE, Hjelle BL, Miller VE, et al. Early viral brain invasion in iatrogenic human immunodeficiency virus infection. Neurology 1992;42:1736–1739.
163. Gray F, Scaravilli F, Everall I, et al. Neuropathology of early HIV-1 infection. Brain Pathol 1996;6:1–15.
164. Goudsmit J, de Wolf F, Paul DA, et al. Expression of human immunodeficiency virus antigen (HIV-Ag) in serum and cerebrospinal fluid during acute and chronic infection. Lancet 1986;2:177–180.
165. Resnick L, Berger JR, Shapshak P, Tourtellotte WW. Early penetration of the blood-brain-barrier by HIV. Neurology 1988;38:9–14.
166. Achim CL, Wiley CA. Inflammation in AIDS and the role of the macrophage in brain pathology. Curr Opin Neurol 1996;9:221–225.
167. Koenig S, Gendelman HE, Orenstein JM, et al. Detection of AIDS virus in macrophages in brain tissue from AIDS patients with encephalopathy. Science 1986;233:1089–1093.
168. Stoler MH, Eskin TA, Benn S, Angerer RC, Angerer LM. Human T-cell lymphotropic virus type III infection of the central nervous system. A preliminary *in situ* analysis. JAMA 1986;256:2360–2364.

169. Michaels J, Price RW, Rosenblum MK. Microglia in the giant cell encephalitis of acquired immune deficiency syndrome: proliferation, infection and fusion. Acta Neuropathol (Berl) 1988;76:373–379.

170. Kure K, Lyman WD, Weidenheim KM, Dickson DW. Cellular localization of an HIV-1 antigen in subacute AIDS encephalitis using an improved double-labeling immunohistochemical method. Am J Pathol 1990;136:1085–1092.

171. Peudenier S, Hery C, Montagnier L, Tardieu M. Human microglial cells: characterization in cerebral tissue and in primary culture, and study of their susceptibility to HIV-1 infection. Ann Neurol 1991;29:152–161.

172. An SF, Groves M, Giometto B, Beckett AA, Scaravilli F. Detection and localisation of HIV-1 DNA and RNA in fixed adult AIDS brain by polymerase chain reaction/*in situ* hybridisation technique. Acta Neuropathol (Berl) 1999;98:481–487.

173. Takahashi K, Wesselingh SL, Griffin DE, McArthur JC, Johnson RT, Glass JD. Localization of HIV-1 in human brain using polymerase chain reaction/*in situ* hybridization and immunocytochemistry. Ann Neurol 1996;39:705–711.

174. McArthur JC, Hoover DR, Bacellar H, et al. Dementia in AIDS patients: incidence and risk factors. Multicenter AIDS Cohort Study. Neurology 1993;43:2245–2252.

175. Maschke M, Kastrup O, Esser S, Ross B, Hengge U, Hufnagel A. Incidence and prevalence of neurological disorders associated with HIV since the introduction of highly active antiretroviral therapy (HAART). J Neurol Neurosurg Psychiatry 2000;69:376–380.

176. Sacktor N, Lyles RH, Skolasky R, et al. HIV-associated neurologic disease incidence changes: Multicenter AIDS Cohort Study, 1990–1998. Neurology 2001;56:257–260.

177. Sacktor N, McDermott MP, Marder K, et al. HIV-associated cognitive impairment before and after the advent of combination therapy. J Neurovirol 2002;8:136–142.

178. Sacktor N. The epidemiology of human immunodeficiency virus-associated neurological disease in the era of highly active antiretroviral therapy. J Neurovirol 2002;8(Suppl 2):115–121.

179. Lipton SA, Gendelman HE. Seminars in medicine of the Beth Israel Hospital, Boston. Dementia associated with the acquired immunodeficiency syndrome. N Engl J Med 1995;332:934–940.

180. Glass JD, Fedor H, Wesselingh SL, McArthur JC. Immunocytochemical quantitation of human immunodeficiency virus in the brain: correlations with dementia. Ann Neurol 1995;38:755–762.

181. Masliah E, Heaton RK, Marcotte TD, et al. Dendritic injury is a pathological substrate for human immunodeficiency virus-related cognitive disorders. HNRC Group. The HIV Neurobehavioral Research Center. Ann Neurol 1997;42:963–972.

182. Adle-Biassette H, Chretien F, Wingertsmann L, et al. Neuronal apoptosis does not correlate with dementia in HIV infection but is related to microglial activation and axonal damage. Neuropathol Appl Neurobiol 1999;25:123–133.

183. Garden GA. Microglia in human immunodeficiency virus-associated neurodegeneration. Glia 2002;40:240–251.

184. Kaul M, Garden GA, Lipton SA. Pathways to neuronal injury and apoptosis in HIV-associated dementia. Nature 2001;410:988–994.

185. Glass JD, Wesselingh SL. Microglia in HIV-associated neurological diseases. Microsc Res Tech 2001;54:95–105.

186. Persidsky Y, Gendelman HE. Mononuclear phagocyte immunity and the neuropathogenesis of HIV-1 infection. J Leukoc Biol 2003;74:691–701.

187. Tyor WR, Glass JD, Griffin JW, et al. Cytokine expression in the brain during the acquired immunodeficiency syndrome. Ann Neurol 1992;31:349–360.

188. Achim CL, Heyes MP, Wiley CA. Quantitation of human immunodeficiency virus, immune activation factors, and quinolinic acid in AIDS brains. J Clin Invest 1993;91:2769–2775.

189. Nuovo GJ, Gallery F, MacConnell P, Braun A. *In situ* detection of polymerase chain reaction-amplified HIV-1 nucleic acids and tumor necrosis factor-alpha RNA in the central nervous system. Am J Pathol 1994;144:659–666.

190. Sippy BD, Hofman FM, Wallach D, Hinton DR. Increased expression of tumor necrosis factor-alpha receptors in the brains of patients with AIDS. J Acquir Immune Defic Syndr Hum Retrovirol 1995;10:511–521.

191. Wesselingh SL, Takahashi K, Glass JD, McArthur JC, Griffin JW, Griffin DE. Cellular localization of tumor necrosis factor mRNA in neurological tissue from HIV-infected patients by combined reverse transcriptase/polymerase chain reaction *in situ* hybridization and immunohistochemistry. J Neuroimmunol 1997;74:1–8.

192. Seilhean D, Kobayashi K, He Y, et al. Tumor necrosis factor-alpha, microglia and astrocytes in AIDS dementia complex. Acta Neuropathol (Berl) 1997;93:508–517.

193. Nuovo GJ, Alfieri ML. AIDS dementia is associated with massive, activated HIV-1 infection and concomitant expression of several cytokines. Mol Med 1996;2:358–366.

194. Griffin DE. Cytokines in the brain during viral infection: clues to HIV-associated dementia. J Clin Invest 1997;100:2948–2951.

195. Saha RN, Pahan K. Tumor necrosis factor-alpha at the crossroads of neuronal life and death during HIV-associated dementia. J Neurochem 2003;86:1057–1071.

196. Stanley LC, Mrak RE, Woody RC, et al. Glial cytokines as neuropathogenic factors in HIV infection: pathogenic similarities to Alzheimer's disease. J Neuropathol Exp Neurol 1994;53:231–238.

197. Wahl SM, Allen JB, McCartney-Francis N, et al. Macrophage- and astrocyte-derived transforming growth factor beta as a mediator of central nervous system dysfunction in acquired immune deficiency syndrome. J Exp Med 1991;173:981–991.
198. Perrella O, Carreiri PB, Perrella A, et al. Transforming growth factor beta-1 and interferon-alpha in the AIDS dementia complex (ADC): possible relationship with cerebral viral load? Eur Cytokine Netw 2001;12:51–55.
199. Rho MB, Wesselingh S, Glass JD, et al. A potential role for interferon-alpha in the pathogenesis of HIV-associated dementia. Brain Behav Immun 1995;9:366–377.
200. Gallo P, Frei K, Rordorf C, Lazdins J, Tavolato B, Fontana A. Human immunodeficiency virus type 1 (HIV-1) infection of the central nervous system: an evaluation of cytokines in cerebrospinal fluid. J Neuroimmunol 1989;23:109–116.
201. Gallo P, Laverda AM, De Rossi A, et al. Immunological markers in the cerebrospinal fluid of HIV-1-infected children. Acta Paediatr Scand 1991;80:659–666.
202. Perrella O, Carrieri PB, Guarnaccia D, Soscia M. Cerebrospinal fluid cytokines in AIDS dementia complex. J Neurol 1992;239:387–388.
203. Laverda AM, Gallo P, De Rossi A, et al. Cerebrospinal fluid analysis in HIV-1-infected children: immunological and virological findings before and after AZT therapy. Acta Paediatr 1994;83:1038–1042.
204. Krivine A, Force G, Servan J, et al. Measuring HIV-1 RNA and interferon-alpha in the cerebrospinal fluid of AIDS patients: insights into the pathogenesis of AIDS Dementia Complex. J Neurovirol 1999;5:500–506.
205. Mastroianni CM, Paoletti F, Massetti AP, Falciano M, Vullo V. Elevated levels of tumor necrosis factor (TNF) in the cerebrospinal fluid from patients with HIV-associated neurological disorders. Acta Neurol (Napoli) 1990;12:66–67.
206. Grimaldi LM, Martino GV, Franciotta DM, et al. Elevated alpha-tumor necrosis factor levels in spinal fluid from HIV-1-infected patients with central nervous system involvement. Ann Neurol 1991;29:21–25.
207. Franciotta DM, Melzi d'Eril GL, Bono G, Brustia R, Ruberto G, Pagani I. Tumor necrosis factor alpha levels in serum and cerebrospinal fluid of patients with AIDS. Funct Neurol 1992;7:35–38.
208. Shaskan EG, Thompson RM, Price RW. Undetectable tumor necrosis factor-alpha in spinal fluid from HIV-1-infected patients. Ann Neurol 1992;31:687–689.
209. Watkins BA, Dorn HH, Kelly WB, et al. Specific tropism of HIV-1 for microglial cells in primary human brain cultures. Science 1990;249:549–553.
210. Jordan CA, Watkins BA, Kufta C, Dubois-Dalcq M. Infection of brain microglial cells by human immunodeficiency virus type 1 is CD4 dependent. J Virol 1991;65:736–742.
211. Strizki JM, Albright AV, Sheng H, O'Connor M, Perrin L, Gonzalez-Scarano F. Infection of primary human microglia and monocyte-derived macrophages with human immunodeficiency virus type 1 isolates: evidence of differential tropism. J Virol 1996;70:7654–7662.
212. Albright AV, Shieh JT, O'Connor MJ, Gonzalez-Scarano F. Characterization of cultured microglia that can be infected by HIV-1. J Neurovirol 2000;6(Suppl 1):S53–60.
213. Lee SC, Hatch WC, Liu W, Kress Y, Lyman WD, Dickson DW. Productive infection of human fetal microglia by HIV-1. Am J Pathol 1993;143:1032–1039.
214. Ioannidis JP, Reichlin S, Skolnik PR. Long-term productive human immunodeficiency virus-1 infection in human infant microglia. Am J Pathol 1995;147:1200–1206.
215. Ranki A, Nyberg M, Ovod V, et al. Abundant expression of HIV Nef and Rev proteins in brain astrocytes in vivo is associated with dementia. Aids 1995;9:1001–1008.
216. Bagasra O, Lavi E, Bobroski L, et al. Cellular reservoirs of HIV-1 in the central nervous system of infected individuals: identification by the combination of *in situ* polymerase chain reaction and immunohistochemistry. Aids 1996;10:573–585.
217. Fiala M, Rhodes RH, Shapshak P, et al. Regulation of HIV-1 infection in astrocytes: expression of Nef, TNF-alpha and IL-6 is enhanced in coculture of astrocytes with macrophages. J Neurovirol 1996;2:158–166.
218. Sabri F, Tresoldi E, Di Stefano M, et al. Nonproductive human immunodeficiency virus type 1 infection of human fetal astrocytes: independence from CD4 and major chemokine receptors. Virology 1999;264:370–384.
219. Janabi N, Di Stefano M, Wallon C, Hery C, Chiodi F, Tardieu M. Induction of human immunodeficiency virus type 1 replication in human glial cells after proinflammatory cytokines stimulation: effect of IFNgamma, IL1beta, and TNFalpha on differentiation and chemokine production in glial cells. Glia 1998;23:304–315.
220. Giulian D, Vaca K, Noonan CA. Secretion of neurotoxins by mononuclear phagocytes infected with HIV-1. Science 1990;250:1593–1596.
221. Pulliam L, Herndier BG, Tang NM, McGrath MS. Human immunodeficiency virus-infected macrophages produce soluble factors that cause histological and neurochemical alterations in cultured human brains. J Clin Invest 1991; 87:503–512.
222. Tardieu M, Hery C, Peudenier S, Boespflug O, Montagnier L. Human immunodeficiency virus type 1-infected monocytic cells can destroy human neural cells after cell-to-cell adhesion. Ann Neurol 1992;32:11–17.
223. Xiong H, Zheng J, Thylin M, Gendelman HE. Unraveling the mechanisms of neurotoxicity in HIV type 1-associated dementia: inhibition of neuronal synaptic transmission by macrophage secretory products. AIDS Res Hum Retroviruses 1999;15:57–63.

224. Xiong H, Zeng YC, Zheng J, Thylin M, Gendelman HE. Soluble HIV-1 infected macrophage secretory products mediate blockade of long-term potentiation: a mechanism for cognitive dysfunction in HIV-1-associated dementia. J Neurovirol 1999;5:519–528.

225. Genis P, Jett M, Bernton EW, et al. Cytokines and arachidonic metabolites produced during human immunodeficiency virus (HIV)-infected macrophage-astroglia interactions: implications for the neuropathogenesis of HIV disease. J Exp Med 1992;176:1703–1718.

226. Merrill JE, Koyanagi Y, Zack J, Thomas L, Martin F, Chen IS. Induction of interleukin-1 and tumor necrosis factor alpha in brain cultures by human immunodeficiency virus type 1. J Virol 1992;66:2217–2225.

227. Wilt SG, Milward E, Zhou JM, et al. In vitro evidence for a dual role of tumor necrosis factor-alpha in human immunodeficiency virus type 1 encephalopathy. Ann Neurol 1995;37:381–394.

228. Chao CC, Hu S. Tumor necrosis factor-alpha potentiates glutamate neurotoxicity in human fetal brain cell cultures. Dev Neurosci 1994;16:172–179.

229. Gelbard HA, Dzenko KA, DiLoreto D, del Cerro C, del Cerro M, Epstein LG. Neurotoxic effects of tumor necrosis factor alpha in primary human neuronal cultures are mediated by activation of the glutamate AMPA receptor subtype: implications for AIDS neuropathogenesis. Dev Neurosci 1993;15:417–422.

230. Fine SM, Angel RA, Perry SW, et al. Tumor necrosis factor alpha inhibits glutamate uptake by primary human astrocytes. Implications for pathogenesis of HIV-1 dementia. J Biol Chem 1996;271:15,303–15,306.

231. Griffin GE, Leung K, Folks TM, Kunkel S, Nabel GJ. Induction of NF-kappa B during monocyte differentiation is associated with activation of HIV-gene expression. Res Virol 1991;142:233–238.

232. Khanna KV, Yu XF, Ford DH, Ratner L, Hildreth JK, Markham RB. Differences among HIV-1 variants in their ability to elicit secretion of TNF-alpha. J Immunol 2000;164:1408–1415.

233. Mellors JW, Griffith BP, Ortiz MA, Landry ML, Ryan JL. Tumor necrosis factor-alpha/cachectin enhances human immunodeficiency virus type 1 replication in primary macrophages. J Infect Dis 1991;163:78–82.

234. Tadmori W, Mondal D, Tadmori I, Prakash O. Transactivation of human immunodeficiency virus type 1 long terminal repeats by cell surface tumor necrosis factor alpha. J Virol 1991;65:6425–6429.

235. Chao CC, Hu S, Peterson PK. Glia: the not so innocent bystanders. J Neurovirol 1996;2:234–239.

236. Williams KC, Hickey WF. Central nervous system damage, monocytes and macrophages, and neurological disorders in AIDS. Annu Rev Neurosci 2002;25:537–562.

237. Hurtrel B, Chakrabarti L, Hurtrel M, Montagnier L. Target cells during early SIV encephalopathy. Res Virol 1993; 144:41–46.

238. Watry D, Lane TE, Streb M, Fox HS. Transfer of neuropathogenic simian immunodeficiency virus with naturally infected microglia. Am J Pathol 1995;146:914–923.

239. Czub S, Muller JG, Czub M, Muller-Hermelink HK. Impact of various simian immunodeficiency virus variants on induction and nature of neuropathology in macaques. Res Virol 1996;147:165–170.

240. Lane JH, Sasseville VG, Smith MO, et al. Neuroinvasion by simian immunodeficiency virus coincides with increased numbers of perivascular macrophages/microglia and intrathecal immune activation. J Neurovirol 1996;2:423–432.

241. Williams KC, Corey S, Westmoreland SV, et al. Perivascular macrophages are the primary cell type productively infected by simian immunodeficiency virus in the brains of macaques: implications for the neuropathogenesis of AIDS. J Exp Med 2001;193:905–915.

242. Chakrabarti L, Hurtrel M, Maire MA, et al. Early viral replication in the brain of SIV-infected rhesus monkeys. Am J Pathol 1991;139:1273–1280.

243. Gonzalez RG, Cheng LL, Westmoreland SV, et al. Early brain injury in the SIV-macaque model of AIDS. Aids 2000;14:2841–2849.

244. Rausch DM, Heyes MP, Murray EA, et al. Cytopathologic and neurochemical correlates of progression to motor/cognitive impairment in SIV-infected rhesus monkeys. J Neuropathol Exp Neurol 1994;53:165–175.

245. Lane TE, Buchmeier MJ, Watry DD, Fox HS. Expression of inflammatory cytokines and inducible nitric oxide synthase in brains of SIV-infected rhesus monkeys: applications to HIV-induced central nervous system disease. Mol Med 1996;2:27–37.

246. Orandle MS, MacLean AG, Sasseville VG, Alvarez X, Lackner AA. Enhanced expression of proinflammatory cytokines in the central nervous system is associated with neuroinvasion by simian immunodeficiency virus and the development of encephalitis. J Virol 2002;76:5797–5802.

247. Sopper S, Demuth M, Stahl-Hennig C, et al. The effect of simian immunodeficiency virus infection in vitro and in vivo on the cytokine production of isolated microglia and peripheral macrophages from rhesus monkey. Virology 1996;220:320–329.

248. Tyor WR, Power C, Gendelman HE, Markham RB. A model of human immunodeficiency virus encephalitis in SCID mice. Proc Natl Acad Sci U S A 1993;90:8658–8662.

249. Persidsky Y, Limoges J, McComb R, et al. Human immunodeficiency virus encephalitis in SCID mice. Am J Pathol 1996;149:1027–1053.

250. Persidsky Y, Buttini M, Limoges J, Bock P, Gendelman HE. An analysis of HIV-1-associated inflammatory products in brain tissue of humans and SCID mice with HIV-1 encephalitis. J Neurovirol 1997;3:401–416.

251. Philippon V, Vellutini C, Gambarelli D, et al. The basic domain of the lentiviral Tat protein is responsible for damages in mouse brain: involvement of cytokines. Virology 1994;205:519–529.

252. Wang P, Barks JD, Silverstein FS. Tat, a human immunodeficiency virus-1-derived protein, augments excitotoxic hippocampal injury in neonatal rats. Neuroscience 1999;88:585–597.

253. Bagetta G, Corasaniti MT, Berliocchi L, et al. Involvement of interleukin-1beta in the mechanism of human immunodeficiency virus type 1 (HIV-1) recombinant protein gp120-induced apoptosis in the neocortex of rat. Neuroscience 1999;89:1051–1066.

254. Bansal AK, Mactutus CF, Nath A, Maragos W, Hauser KF, Booze RM. Neurotoxicity of HIV-1 proteins gp120 and Tat in the rat striatum. Brain Res 2000;879:42–49.

255. Sporer B, Koedel U, Paul R, et al. Human immunodeficiency virus type-1 Nef protein induces blood-brain barrier disruption in the rat: role of matrix metalloproteinase-9. J Neuroimmunol 2000;102:125–130.

256. Corasaniti MT, Piccirilli S, Paoletti A, et al. Evidence that the HIV-1 coat protein gp120 causes neuronal apoptosis in the neocortex of rat via a mechanism involving CXCR4 chemokine receptor. Neurosci Lett 2001;312:67–70.

257. Corasaniti MT, Maccarrone M, Nistico R, Malorni W, Rotiroti D, Bagetta G. Exploitation of the HIV-1 coat glycoprotein, gp120, in neurodegenerative studies in vivo. J Neurochem 2001;79:1–8.

258. Barak O, Goshen I, Ben-Hur T, Weidenfeld J, Taylor AN, Yirmiya R. Involvement of brain cytokines in the neurobehavioral disturbances induced by HIV-1 glycoprotein120. Brain Res 2002;933:98–108.

259. Pu H, Tian J, Flora G, et al. HIV-1 Tat protein upregulates inflammatory mediators and induces monocyte invasion into the brain. Mol Cell Neurosci 2003;24:224–237.

260. Toggas SM, Masliah E, Rockenstein EM, Rall GF, Abraham CR, Mucke L. Central nervous system damage produced by expression of the HIV-1 coat protein gp120 in transgenic mice. Nature 1994;367:188–193.

261. Wiley CA, Baldwin M, Achim CL. Expression of HIV regulatory and structural mRNA in the central nervous system. Aids 1996;10:843–847.

262. Hudson L, Liu J, Nath A, et al. Detection of the human immunodeficiency virus regulatory protein tat in CNS tissues. J Neurovirol 2000;6:145–155.

263. Ensoli B, Buonaguro L, Barillari G, et al. Release, uptake, and effects of extracellular human immunodeficiency virus type 1 Tat protein on cell growth and viral transactivation. J Virol 1993;67:277–287.

264. Cupp C, Taylor JP, Khalili K, Amini S. Evidence for stimulation of the transforming growth factor beta 1 promoter by HIV-1 Tat in cells derived from CNS. Oncogene 1993;8:2231–2236.

265. Chen P, Mayne M, Power C, Nath A. The Tat protein of HIV-1 induces tumor necrosis factor-alpha production. Implications for HIV-1-associated neurological diseases. J Biol Chem 1997;272:22,385–22,388.

266. Sawaya BE, Thatikunta P, Denisova L, Brady J, Khalili K, Amini S. Regulation of TNFalpha and TGFbeta-1 gene transcription by HIV-1 Tat in CNS cells. J Neuroimmunol 1998;87:33–42.

267. Sheng WS, Hu S, Hegg CC, Thayer SA, Peterson PK. Activation of human microglial cells by HIV-1 gp41 and Tat proteins. Clin Immunol 2000;96:243–251.

268. Bruce-Keller AJ, Barger SW, Moss NI, Pham JT, Keller JN, Nath A. Pro-inflammatory and pro-oxidant properties of the HIV protein Tat in a microglial cell line: attenuation by 17 beta-estradiol. J Neurochem 2001;78:1315–1324.

269. Gibellini D, Zauli G, Re MC, et al. Recombinant human immunodeficiency virus type-1 (HIV-1) Tat protein sequentially up-regulates IL-6 and TGF-beta 1 mRNA expression and protein synthesis in peripheral blood monocytes. Br J Haematol 1994;88:261–267.

270. Scala G, Ruocco MR, Ambrosino C, et al. The expression of the interleukin 6 gene is induced by the human immunodeficiency virus 1 TAT protein. J Exp Med 1994;179:961–971.

271. Shi B, Raina J, Lorenzo A, Busciglio J, Gabuzda D. Neuronal apoptosis induced by HIV-1 Tat protein and TNF-alpha: potentiation of neurotoxicity mediated by oxidative stress and implications for HIV-1 dementia. J Neurovirol 1998;4:281–290.

272. Koka P, He K, Zack JA, et al. Human immunodeficiency virus 1 envelope proteins induce interleukin 1, tumor necrosis factor alpha, and nitric oxide in glial cultures derived from fetal, neonatal, and adult human brain. J Exp Med 1995;182:941–951.

273. Yeung MC, Pulliam L, Lau AS. The HIV envelope protein gp120 is toxic to human brain-cell cultures through the induction of interleukin-6 and tumor necrosis factor-alpha. Aids 1995;9:137–143.

274. Kong LY, Wilson BC, McMillian MK, Bing G, Hudson PM, Hong JS. The effects of the HIV-1 envelope protein gp120 on the production of nitric oxide and proinflammatory cytokines in mixed glial cell cultures. Cell Immunol 1996;172:77–83.

275. Wahl LM, Corcoran ML, Pyle SW, Arthur LO, Harel-Bellan A, Farrar WL. Human immunodeficiency virus glycoprotein (gp120) induction of monocyte arachidonic acid metabolites and interleukin 1. Proc Natl Acad Sci USA 1989;86:621–625.

276. Clouse KA, Cosentino LM, Weih KA, et al. The HIV-1 gp120 envelope protein has the intrinsic capacity to stimulate monokine secretion. J Immunol 1991;147:2892–2901.

277. Benos DJ, Hahn BH, Bubien JK, et al. Envelope glycoprotein gp120 of human immunodeficiency virus type 1 alters ion transport in astrocytes: implications for AIDS dementia complex. Proc Natl Acad Sci USA 1994;91:494–498.

278. Reinhart TA. Chemokine induction by HIV-1: recruitment to the cause. Trends Immunol 2003;24:351–353.

279. Kielian T. Microglia and chemokines in infectious diseases of the nervous system: views and reviews. Front Biosci 2004;9:732–750.

280. Keegan BM, Noseworthy JH. Multiple sclerosis. Annu Rev Med 2002;53:285–302.

281. Owens T. The enigma of multiple sclerosis: inflammation and neurodegeneration cause heterogeneous dysfunction and damage. Curr Opin Neurol 2003;16:259–265.

282. Martin R, McFarland HF, McFarlin DE. Immunological aspects of demyelinating diseases. Annu Rev Immunol 1992;10:153–187.

283. Sadovnick AD, Ebers GC. Epidemiology of multiple sclerosis: a critical overview. Can J Neurol Sci 1993;20:17–29.

284. Martyn C. The epidemiology of multiple sclerosis. In: WB M, ed. McAlpine's Multiple Sclerosis. New York: Churchill Livingstone, 1991.

285. Croxford JL, Olson JK, Miller SD. Epitope spreading and molecular mimicry as triggers of autoimmunity in the Theiler's virus-induced demyelinating disease model of multiple sclerosis. Autoimmun Rev 2002;1:251–260.

286. Wekerle H, Hohlfeld R. Molecular mimicry in multiple sclerosis. N Engl J Med 2003;349:185–186.

287. Arnason BG. Relevance of experimental allergic encephalomyelitis to multiple sclerosis. Neurol Clin 1983;1:765–782.

288. Raine CS. Biology of disease. Analysis of autoimmune demyelination: its impact upon multiple sclerosis. Lab Invest 1984;50:608–635.

289. Johnson KP, Brooks BR, Cohen JA, et al. Copolymer 1 reduces relapse rate and improves disability in relapsing-remitting multiple sclerosis: results of a phase III multicenter, double-blind placebo-controlled trial. The Copolymer 1 Multiple Sclerosis Study Group. Neurology 1995;45:1268–1276.

290. Jacobs LD, Cookfair DL, Rudick RA, et al. Intramuscular interferon beta-1a for disease progression in relapsing multiple sclerosis. The Multiple Sclerosis Collaborative Research Group (MSCRG). Ann Neurol 1996;39:285–294.

291. Panitch HS, McFarlin DE. Experimental allergic encephalomyelitis: enhancement of cell-mediated transfer by con-canavalin A. J Immunol 1977;119:1134–1137.

292. Pettinelli CB, McFarlin DE. Adoptive transfer of experimental allergic encephalomyelitis in SJL/J mice after in vitro activation of lymph node cells by myelin basic protein: requirement for Lyt 1+ 2- T lymphocytes. J Immunol 1981;127:1420–1423.

293. Seder R, Mosmann TM. Differentiation of effectos phenotypes of CD4$^+$ and CD8$^+$ T cells. In: Paul W, ed. Fundamental Immunology. Philadelphia: Lippencott-Raven, 1999: 1879–1908.

294. Ando DG, Clayton J, Kono D, Urban JL, Sercarz EE. Encephalitogenic T cells in the B10.PL model of experimental allergic encephalomyelitis (EAE) are of the Th-1 lymphokine subtype. Cell Immunol 1989;124:132–143.

295. Powell MB, Mitchell D, Lederman J, et al. Lymphotoxin and tumor necrosis factor-alpha production by myelin basic protein-specific T cell clones correlates with encephalitogenicity. Int Immunol 1990;2:539–544.

296. Liblau RS, Singer SM, McDevitt HO. Th1 and Th2 CD4$^+$ T cells in the pathogenesis of organ-specific autoimmune diseases. Immunol Today 1995;16:34–38.

297. Olsson T. Critical influences of the cytokine orchestration on the outcome of myelin antigen-specific T-cell autoimmunity in experimental autoimmune encephalomyelitis and multiple sclerosis. Immunol Rev 1995;144:245–268.

298. Becher B, Dodelet V, Fedorowicz V, Antel JP. Soluble tumor necrosis factor receptor inhibits interleukin 12 production by stimulated human adult microglial cells in vitro. J Clin Invest 1996;98:1539–1543.

299. Lodge PA, Sriram S. Regulation of microglial activation by TGF-beta, IL-10, and CSF-1. J Leukoc Biol 1996;60:502–508.

300. Suzumura A, Sawada M, Takayanagi T. Production of interleukin-12 and expression of its receptors by murine microglia. Brain Res 1998;787:139–142.

301. Stalder AK, Pagenstecher A, Yu NC, et al. Lipopolysaccharide-induced IL-12 expression in the central nervous system and cultured astrocytes and microglia. J Immunol 1997;159:1344–1351.

302. Windhagen A, Newcombe J, Dangond F, et al. Expression of costimulatory molecules B7-1 (CD80), B7-2 (CD86), and interleukin 12 cytokine in multiple sclerosis lesions. J Exp Med 1995;182:1985–1996.

303. Balashov KE, Smith DR, Khoury SJ, Hafler DA, Weiner HL. Increased interleukin 12 production in progressive multiple sclerosis: induction by activated CD4$^+$ T cells via CD40 ligand. Proc Natl Acad Sci USA 1997;94:599–603.

304. Comabella M, Balashov K, Issazadeh S, Smith D, Weiner HL, Khoury SJ. Elevated interleukin-12 in progressive multiple sclerosis correlates with disease activity and is normalized by pulse cyclophosphamide therapy. J Clin Invest 1998;102:671–678.

305. Santambrogio L, Crisi GM, Leu J, Hochwald GM, Ryan T, Thorbecke GJ. Tolerogenic forms of auto-antigens and cytokines in the induction of resistance to experimental allergic encephalomyelitis. J Neuroimmunol 1995;58:211–22.

306. Leonard JP, Waldburger KE, Goldman SJ. Prevention of experimental autoimmune encephalomyelitis by antibodies against interleukin 12. J Exp Med 1995;181:381–386.

307. Segal BM, Dwyer BK, Shevach EM. An interleukin (IL)-10/IL-12 immunoregulatory circuit controls susceptibility to autoimmune disease. J Exp Med 1998;187:537–546.

308. Hsieh CS, Macatonia SE, Tripp CS, Wolf SF, O'Garra A, Murphy KM. Development of TH1 CD4⁺ T cells through IL-12 produced by Listeria-induced macrophages. Science 1993;260:547–549.

309. Manetti R, Parronchi P, Giudizi MG, et al. Natural killer cell stimulatory factor (interleukin 12 [IL-12]) induces T helper type 1 (Th1)-specific immune responses and inhibits the development of IL-4-producing Th cells. J Exp Med 1993;177:1199–1204.

310. Afonso LC, Scharton TM, Vieira LQ, Wysocka M, Trinchieri G, Scott P. The adjuvant effect of interleukin-12 in a vaccine against Leishmania major. Science 1994;263:235–237.

311. Seder RA, Gazzinelli R, Sher A, Paul WE. Interleukin 12 acts directly on CD4+ T cells to enhance priming for interferon gamma production and diminishes interleukin 4 inhibition of such priming. Proc Natl Acad Sci USA 1993;90:10,188–10,192.

312. Trinchieri G. Interleukin-12: a cytokine produced by antigen-presenting cells with immunoregulatory functions in the generation of T-helper cells type 1 and cytotoxic lymphocytes. Blood 1994;84:4008–4027.

313. Kaplan MH, Sun YL, Hoey T, Grusby MJ. Impaired IL-12 responses and enhanced development of Th2 cells in Stat4-deficient mice. Nature 1996;382:174–177.

314. Magram J, Sfarra J, Connaughton S, et al. IL-12-deficient mice are defective but not devoid of type 1 cytokine responses. Ann N Y Acad Sci 1996;795:60–70.

315. Thierfelder WE, van Deursen JM, Yamamoto K, et al. Requirement for Stat4 in interleukin-12-mediated responses of natural killer and T cells. Nature 1996;382:171–174.

316. Hayes MP, Wang J, Norcross MA. Regulation of interleukin-12 expression in human monocytes: selective priming by interferon-gamma of lipopolysaccharide-inducible p35 and p40 genes. Blood 1995;86:646–650.

317. Ma X, Chow JM, Gri G, et al. The interleukin 12 p40 gene promoter is primed by interferon gamma in monocytic cells. J Exp Med 1996;183:147–157.

318. Szabo SJ, Dighe AS, Gubler U, Murphy KM. Regulation of the interleukin (IL)-12R beta 2 subunit expression in developing T helper 1 (Th1) and Th2 cells. J Exp Med 1997;185:817–824.

318a.Gran, B, Zhang G-X, Rostami A. Role of the IL-12/IL-23 system in the regulation of T-cell responses in central nervous system inflammatory demyelination. Critical Rev Immunol 2004; 24:87–110.

319. Conti B, Park LC, Calingasan NY, et al. Cultures of astrocytes and microglia express interleukin 18. Brain Res Mol Brain Res 1999;67:46–52.

320. Jander S, Stoll G. Differential induction of interleukin-12, interleukin-18, and interleukin-1beta converting enzyme mRNA in experimental autoimmune encephalomyelitis of the Lewis rat. J Neuroimmunol 1998;91:93–99.

321. Balashov KE, Rottman JB, Weiner HL, Hancock WW. CCR5(+) and CXCR3(+) T cells are increased in multiple sclerosis and their ligands MIP-1alpha and IP-10 are expressed in demyelinating brain lesions. Proc Natl Acad Sci USA 1999;96:6873–6878.

322. Furlan R, Martino G, Galbiati F, et al. Caspase-1 regulates the inflammatory process leading to autoimmune demyelination. J Immunol 1999;163:2403–2409.

323. Furlan R, Filippi M, Bergami A, et al. Peripheral levels of caspase-1 mRNA correlate with disease activity in patients with multiple sclerosis; a preliminary study. J Neurol Neurosurg Psychiatry 1999;67:785–788.

324. Wildbaum G, Youssef S, Grabie N, Karin N. Neutralizing antibodies to IFN-gamma-inducing factor prevent experimental autoimmune encephalomyelitis. J Immunol 1998;161:6368–6374.

325. Robinson D, Shibuya K, Mui A, et al. IGIF does not drive Th1 development but synergizes with IL-12 for interferon-gamma production and activates IRAK and NFkappaB. Immunity 1997;7:571–581.

326. Micallef MJ, Ohtsuki T, Kohno K, et al. Interferon-gamma-inducing factor enhances T helper 1 cytokine production by stimulated human T cells: synergism with interleukin-12 for interferon-gamma production. Eur J Immunol 1996;26:1647–1651.

327. Ahn HJ, Maruo S, Tomura M, et al. A mechanism underlying synergy between IL-12 and IFN-gamma-inducing factor in enhanced production of IFN-gamma. J Immunol 1997;159:2125–2131.

328. Kohno K, Kataoka J, Ohtsuki T, et al. IFN-gamma-inducing factor (IGIF) is a costimulatory factor on the activation of Th1 but not Th2 cells and exerts its effect independently of IL-12. J Immunol 1997;158:1541–1550.

329. Xu D, Chan WL, Leung BP, et al. Selective expression and functions of interleukin 18 receptor on T helper (Th) type 1 but not Th2 cells. J Exp Med 1998;188:1485–1492.

330. Yoshimoto T, Takeda K, Tanaka T, et al. IL-12 up-regulates IL-18 receptor expression on T cells, Th1 cells, and B cells: synergism with IL-18 for IFN-gamma production. J Immunol 1998;161:3400–3407.

331. Kaplan MH, Grusby MJ. Regulation of T helper cell differentiation by STAT molecules. J Leukoc Biol 1998;64:2–5.

332. Dinarello CA, Novick D, Puren AJ, et al. Overview of interleukin-18: more than an interferon-gamma inducing factor. J Leukoc Biol 1998;63:658–664.

333. Young HA. Regulation of interferon-gamma gene expression. J Interferon Cytokine Res 1996;16:563–568.

334. O'Garra A, Stapleton G, Dhar V, et al. Production of cytokines by mouse B cells: B lymphomas and normal B cells produce interleukin 10. Int Immunol 1990;2:821–832.

335. de Waal Malefyt R, Abrams J, Bennett B, Figdor CG, de Vries JE. Interleukin 10 (IL-10) inhibits cytokine synthesis by human monocytes: an autoregulatory role of IL-10 produced by monocytes. J Exp Med 1991;174:1209–1220.

336. Mizuno T, Sawada M, Marunouchi T, Suzumura A. Production of interleukin-10 by mouse glial cells in culture. Biochem Biophys Res Commun 1994;205:1907–1915.

337. Sheng WS, Hu S, Kravitz FH, Peterson PK, Chao CC. Tumor necrosis factor alpha upregulates human microglial cell production of interleukin-10 in vitro. Clin Diagn Lab Immunol 1995;2:604–608.

338. Williams K, Dooley N, Ulvestad E, Becher B, Antel JP. IL-10 production by adult human derived microglial cells. Neurochem Int 1996;29:55–64.

339. Jander S, Pohl J, D'Urso D, Gillen C, Stoll G. Time course and cellular localization of interleukin-10 mRNA and protein expression in autoimmune inflammation of the rat central nervous system. Am J Pathol 1998;152:975–982.

340. Aloisi F, De Simone R, Columba-Cabezas S, Levi G. Opposite effects of interferon-gamma and prostaglandin E2 on tumor necrosis factor and interleukin-10 production in microglia: a regulatory loop controlling microglia pro- and anti-inflammatory activities. J Neurosci Res 1999;56:571–580.

341. Yoshikawa M, Suzumura A, Tamaru T, Takayanagi T, Sawada M. Effects of phosphodiesterase inhibitors on cytokine production by microglia. Mult Scler 1999;5:126–133.

342. Calabresi PA, Tranquill LR, McFarland HF, Cowan EP. Cytokine gene expression in cells derived from CSF of multiple sclerosis patients. J Neuroimmunol 1998;89:198–205.

343. Link H. The cytokine storm in multiple sclerosis. Mult Scler 1998;4:12–15.

344. van Boxel-Dezaire AH, Hoff SC, van Oosten BW, et al. Decreased interleukin-10 and increased interleukin-12p40 mRNA are associated with disease activity and characterize different disease stages in multiple sclerosis. Ann Neurol 1999;45:695–703.

345. Rott O, Fleischer B, Cash E. Interleukin-10 prevents experimental allergic encephalomyelitis in rats. Eur J Immunol 1994;24:1434–1440.

346. Bettelli E, Das MP, Howard ED, Weiner HL, Sobel RA, Kuchroo VK. IL-10 is critical in the regulation of autoimmune encephalomyelitis as demonstrated by studies of IL-10- and IL-4-deficient and transgenic mice. J Immunol 1998;161:3299–3306.

347. Xiao BG, Bai XF, Zhang GX, Link H. Suppression of acute and protracted-relapsing experimental allergic encephalomyelitis by nasal administration of low-dose IL-10 in rats. J Neuroimmunol 1998;84:230–237.

348. Cua DJ, Groux H, Hinton DR, Stohlman SA, Coffman RL. Transgenic interleukin 10 prevents induction of experimental autoimmune encephalomyelitis. J Exp Med 1999;189:1005–1010.

349. Fiorentino DF, Bond MW, Mosmann TR. Two types of mouse T helper cell. IV. Th2 clones secrete a factor that inhibits cytokine production by Th1 clones. J Exp Med 1989;170:2081–2095.

350. Chomarat P, Rissoan MC, Banchereau J, Miossec P. Interferon gamma inhibits interleukin 10 production by monocytes. J Exp Med 1993;177:523–527.

351. Libraty DH, Airan LE, Uyemura K, et al. Interferon-gamma differentially regulates interleukin-12 and interleukin-10 production in leprosy. J Clin Invest 1997;99:336–341.

352. Shaw MK, Lorens JB, Dhawan A, et al. Local delivery of interleukin 4 by retrovirus-transduced T lymphocytes ameliorates experimental autoimmune encephalomyelitis. J Exp Med 1997;185:1711–1714.

353. Inobe J, Slavin AJ, Komagata Y, Chen Y, Liu L, Weiner HL. IL-4 is a differentiation factor for transforming growth factor-beta secreting Th3 cells and oral administration of IL-4 enhances oral tolerance in experimental allergic encephalomyelitis. Eur J Immunol 1998;28:2780–2790.

354. Falcone M, Rajan AJ, Bloom BR, Brosnan CF. A critical role for IL-4 in regulating disease severity in experimental allergic encephalomyelitis as demonstrated in IL-4-deficient C57BL/6 mice and BALB/c mice. J Immunol 1998; 160:4822–4830.

355. Liblau R, Steinman L, Brocke S. Experimental autoimmune encephalomyelitis in IL-4-deficient mice. Int Immunol 1997;9:799–803.

356. Samoilova EB, Horton JL, Chen Y. Acceleration of experimental autoimmune encephalomyelitis in interleukin-10-deficient mice: roles of interleukin-10 in disease progression and recovery. Cell Immunol 1998;188:118–124.

357. Agnello D, Lankford CS, Bream J, et al. Cytokines and transcription factors that regulate T helper cell differentiation: new players and new insights. J Clin Immunol 2003;23:147–161.

358. Kurata H, Lee HJ, O'Garra A, Arai N. Ectopic expression of activated Stat6 induces the expression of Th2-specific cytokines and transcription factors in developing Th1 cells. Immunity 1999;11:677–688.

359. Zhu J, Guo L, Watson CJ, Hu-Li J, Paul WE. Stat6 is necessary and sufficient for IL-4's role in Th2 differentiation and cell expansion. J Immunol 2001;166:7276–7281.

360. Lawless VA, Zhang S, Ozes ON, et al. Stat4 regulates multiple components of IFN-gamma-inducing signaling pathways. J Immunol 2000;165:6803–6308.

361. Zhang DH, Cohn L, Ray P, Bottomly K, Ray A. Transcription factor GATA-3 is differentially expressed in murine Th1 and Th2 cells and controls Th2-specific expression of the interleukin-5 gene. J Biol Chem 1997;272:21,597–21,603.

362. Zheng W, Flavell RA. The transcription factor GATA-3 is necessary and sufficient for Th2 cytokine gene expression in CD4 T cells. Cell 1997;89:587–596.

363. Ferber IA, Lee HJ, Zonin F, et al. GATA-3 significantly downregulates IFN-gamma production from developing Th1 cells in addition to inducing IL-4 and IL-5 levels. Clin Immunol 1999;91:134–144.

364. Sriram S, Rodriguez M. Indictment of the microglia as the villain in multiple sclerosis. Neurology 1997;48:464–470.

365. MacMicking J, Xie QW, Nathan C. Nitric oxide and macrophage function. Annu Rev Immunol 1997;15:323–350.

366. Raine CS. The Norton Lecture: a review of the oligodendrocyte in the multiple sclerosis lesion. J Neuroimmunol 1997;77:135–152.

367. Mattson MP, Barger SW, Furukawa K, et al. Cellular signaling roles of TGF beta, TNF alpha and beta APP in brain injury responses and Alzheimer's disease. Brain Res Brain Res Rev 1997;23:47–61.

368. Merrill JE, Ignarro LJ, Sherman MP, Melinek J, Lane TE. Microglial cell cytotoxicity of oligodendrocytes is mediated through nitric oxide. J Immunol 1993;151:2132–2141.

369. Mitrovic B, Ignarro LJ, Montestruque S, Smoll A, Merrill JE. Nitric oxide as a potential pathological mechanism in demyelination: its differential effects on primary glial cells in vitro. Neuroscience 1994;61:575–585.

370. Mitrovic B, Parkinson J, Merrill JE. An in vitro model of o ligodendrocyte destruction by nitric oxide and its relevance to multiple sclerosis. Methods 1996;10:501–513.

371. Boullerne AI, Nedelkoska L, Benjamins JA. Synergism of nitric oxide and iron in killing the transformed murine oligodendrocyte cell line N20.1. J Neurochem 1999;72:1050–1060.

372. Rosenberg PA, Li Y, Ali S, Altiok N, Back SA, Volpe JJ. Intracellular redox state determines whether nitric oxide is toxic or protective to rat oligodendrocytes in culture. J Neurochem 1999;73:476–484.

373. Zhao W, Tilton RG, Corbett JA, et al. Experimental allergic encephalomyelitis in the rat is inhibited by aminoguanidine, an inhibitor of nitric oxide synthase. J Neuroimmunol 1996;64:123–133.

374. Hooper DC, Bagasra O, Marini JC, et al. Prevention of experimental allergic encephalomyelitis by targeting nitric oxide and peroxynitrite: implications for the treatment of multiple sclerosis. Proc Natl Acad Sci USA 1997; 94:2528–2533.

375. Ding M, Zhang M, Wong JL, Rogers NE, Ignarro LJ, Voskuhl RR. Antisense knockdown of inducible nitric oxide synthase inhibits induction of experimental autoimmune encephalomyelitis in SJL/J mice. J Immunol 1998; 160:2560–2564.

376. van der Veen RC, Roberts LJ. Contrasting roles for nitric oxide and peroxynitrite in the peroxidation of myelin lipids. J Neuroimmunol 1999;95:1–7.

377. Cross AH, Manning PT, Stern MK, Misko TP. Evidence for the production of peroxynitrite in inflammatory CNS demyelination. J Neuroimmunol 1997;80:121–130.

378. Cross AH, Manning PT, Keeling RM, Schmidt RE, Misko TP. Peroxynitrite formation within the central nervous system in active multiple sclerosis. J Neuroimmunol 1998;88:45–56.

379. Fenyk-Melody JE, Garrison AE, Brunnert SR, et al. Experimental autoimmune encephalomyelitis is exacerbated in mice lacking the NOS2 gene. J Immunol 1998;160:2940–2946.

380. Sahrbacher UC, Lechner F, Eugster HP, Frei K, Lassmann H, Fontana A. Mice with an inactivation of the inducible nitric oxide synthase gene are susceptible to experimental autoimmune encephalomyelitis. Eur J Immunol 1998;28:1332–1338.

381. Juedes AE, Ruddle NH. Resident and infiltrating central nervous system APCs regulate the emergence and resolution of experimental autoimmune encephalomyelitis. J Immunol 2001;166:5168–5175.

382. O'Brien NC, Charlton B, Cowden WB, Willenborg DO. Inhibition of nitric oxide synthase initiates relapsing remitting experimental autoimmune encephalomyelitis in rats, yet nitric oxide appears to be essential for clinical expression of disease. J Immunol 2001;167:5904–5912.

383. Okuda Y, Sakoda S, Fujimura H, Yanagihara T. Aminoguanidine, a selective inhibitor of the inducible nitric oxide synthase, has different effects on experimental allergic encephalomyelitis in the induction and progression phase. J Neuroimmunol 1998;81:201–210.

384. Korner H, Riminton DS, Strickland DH, Lemckert FA, Pollard JD, Sedgwick JD. Critical points of tumor necrosis factor action in central nervous system autoimmune inflammation defined by gene targeting. J Exp Med 1997; 186:1585–1590.

385. Riminton DS, Korner H, Strickland DH, Lemckert FA, Pollard JD, Sedgwick JD. Challenging cytokine redundancy: inflammatory cell movement and clinical course of experimental autoimmune encephalomyelitis are normal in lymphotoxin-deficient, but not tumor necrosis factor-deficient, mice. J Exp Med 1998;187:1517–1528.

386. Kassiotis G, Pasparakis M, Kollias G, Probert L. TNF accelerates the onset but does not alter the incidence and severity of myelin basic protein-induced experimental autoimmune encephalomyelitis. Eur J Immunol 1999;29:774–780.

387. Ruddle NH, Bergman CM, McGrath KM, et al. An antibody to lymphotoxin and tumor necrosis factor prevents transfer of experimental allergic encephalomyelitis. J Exp Med 1990;172:1193–1200.

388. Selmaj K, Raine CS, Farooq M, Norton WT, Brosnan CF. Cytokine cytotoxicity against oligodendrocytes. Apoptosis induced by lymphotoxin. J Immunol 1991;147:1522–1529.

389. Sedgwick JD, Riminton DS, Cyster JG, Korner H. Tumor necrosis factor: a master-regulator of leukocyte movement. Immunol Today 2000;21:110–113.

390. Dal Canto RA, Shaw MK, Nolan GP, Steinman L, Fathman CG. Local delivery of TNF by retrovirus-transduced T lymphocytes exacerbates experimental autoimmune encephalomyelitis. Clin Immunol 1999;90:10–14.

391. Liu J, Marino MW, Wong G, et al. TNF is a potent anti-inflammatory cytokine in autoimmune-mediated demyelination. Nat Med 1998;4:78–83.

392. Kassiotis G, Kollias G. Uncoupling the proinflammatory from the immunosuppressive properties of tumor necrosis factor (TNF) at the p55 TNF receptor level: implications for pathogenesis and therapy of autoimmune demyelination. J Exp Med 2001;193:427–434.

393. Suen WE, Bergman CM, Hjelmstrom P, Ruddle NH. A critical role for lymphotoxin in experimental allergic encephalomyelitis. J Exp Med 1997;186:1233–1240.

394. Bachmann R, Eugster HP, Frei K, Fontana A, Lassmann H. Impairment of TNF-receptor-1 signaling but not fas signaling diminishes T-cell apoptosis in myelin oligodendrocyte glycoprotein peptide-induced chronic demyelinating autoimmune encephalomyelitis in mice. Am J Pathol 1999;154:1417–1422.

395. Eugster HP, Frei K, Bachmann R, Bluethmann H, Lassmann H, Fontana A. Severity of symptoms and demyelination in MOG-induced EAE depends on TNFR1. Eur J Immunol 1999;29:626–632.

396. Probert L, Eugster HP, Akassoglou K, et al. TNFR1 signalling is critical for the development of demyelination and the limitation of T-cell responses during immune-mediated CNS disease. Brain 2000;123(Pt 10):2005–2019.

397. Suvannavejh GC, Lee HO, Padilla J, Dal Canto MC, Barrett TA, Miller SD. Divergent roles for p55 and p75 tumor necrosis factor receptors in the pathogenesis of MOG(35–55)-induced experimental autoimmune encephalomyelitis. Cell Immunol 2000;205:24–33.

398. Mannie MD, Dinarello CA, Paterson PY. Interleukin 1 and myelin basic protein synergistically augment adoptive transfer activity of lymphocytes mediating experimental autoimmune encephalomyelitis in Lewis rats. J Immunol 1987;138:4229–4235.

399. Schiffenbauer J, Streit WJ, Butfiloski E, LaBow M, Edwards C, 3rd, Moldawer LL. The induction of EAE is only partially dependent on TNF receptor signaling but requires the IL-1 type I receptor. Clin Immunol 2000; 95:117–123.

400. Martin D, Near SL. Protective effect of the interleukin-1 receptor antagonist (IL-1ra) on experimental allergic encephalomyelitis in rats. J Neuroimmunol 1995;61:241–245.

401. Badovinac V, Mostarica-Stojkovic M, Dinarello CA, Stosic-Grujicic S. Interleukin-1 receptor antagonist suppresses experimental autoimmune encephalomyelitis (EAE) in rats by influencing the activation and proliferation of encephalitogenic cells. J Neuroimmunol 1998;85:87–95.

402. Huitinga I, Schmidt ED, van der Cammen MJ, Binnekade R, Tilders FJ. Priming with interleukin-1beta suppresses experimental allergic encephalomyelitis in the Lewis rat. J Neuroendocrinol 2000;12:1186–1193.

403. Arnett HA, Hellendall RP, Matsushima GK, et al. The protective role of nitric oxide in a neurotoxicant-induced demyelinating model. J Immunol 2002;168:427–433.

404. Morishima-Kawashima M, Ihara Y. Alzheimer's disease: beta-Amyloid protein and tau. J Neurosci Res 2002; 70:392–401.

405. Ritchie K, Lovestone S. The dementias. Lancet 2002;360:1759–1766.

406. Stewart WF, Kawas C, Corrada M, Metter EJ. Risk of Alzheimer's disease and duration of NSAID use. Neurology 1997;48:626–632.

407. Broe GA, Grayson DA, Creasey HM, et al. Anti-inflammatory drugs protect against Alzheimer disease at low doses. Arch Neurol 2000;57:1586–1591.

408. Zandi PP, Anthony JC, Hayden KM, Mehta K, Mayer L, Breitner JC. Reduced incidence of AD with NSAID but not H2 receptor antagonists: the Cache County Study. Neurology 2002;59:880–886.

409. McGeer PL, Itagaki S, Tago H, McGeer EG. Reactive microglia in patients with senile dementia of the Alzheimer type are positive for the histocompatibility glycoprotein HLA-DR. Neurosci Lett 1987;79:195–200.

410. McGeer EG, McGeer PL. Inflammatory processes in Alzheimer's disease. Prog Neuropsychopharmacol Biol Psychiatry 2003;27:741–749.

411. Rogers J, Luber-Narod J, Styren SD, Civin WH. Expression of immune system-associated antigens by cells of the human central nervous system: relationship to the pathology of Alzheimer's disease. Neurobiol Aging 1988;9:339–349.

412. Togo T, Akiyama H, Iseki E, et al. Occurrence of T cells in the brain of Alzheimer's disease and other neurological diseases. J Neuroimmunol 2002;124:83–92.

413. Griffin WS, Sheng JG, Roberts GW, Mrak RE. Interleukin-1 expression in different plaque types in Alzheimer's disease: significance in plaque evolution. J Neuropathol Exp Neurol 1995;54:276–281.

414. Fukumoto H, Asami-Odaka A, Suzuki N, Iwatsubo T. Association of A beta 40-positive senile plaques with microglial cells in the brains of patients with Alzheimer's disease and in non-demented aged individuals. Neurodegeneration 1996;5:13–17.

415. Akiyama H, Barger S, Barnum S, et al. Inflammation and Alzheimer's disease. Neurobiol Aging 2000;21:383–421.

416. Griffin WS, Stanley LC, Ling C, et al. Brain interleukin 1 and S-100 immunoreactivity are elevated in Down syndrome and Alzheimer disease. Proc Natl Acad Sci U S A 1989;86:7611–7615.

417. van der Wal EA, Gomez-Pinilla F, Cotman CW. Transforming growth factor-beta 1 is in plaques in Alzheimer and Down pathologies. Neuroreport 1993;4:69–72.

418. Wood JA, Wood PL, Ryan R, et al. Cytokine indices in Alzheimer's temporal cortex: no changes in mature IL-1 beta or IL-1RA but increases in the associated acute phase proteins IL-6, alpha 2-macroglobulin and C-reactive protein. Brain Res 1993;629:245–252.

419. Cacabelos R, Alvarez XA, Fernandez-Novoa L, et al. Brain interleukin-1 beta in Alzheimer's disease and vascular dementia. Methods Find Exp Clin Pharmacol 1994;16:141–151.

420. Sheng JG, Ito K, Skinner RD, et al. In vivo and in vitro evidence supporting a role for the inflammatory cytokine interleukin-1 as a driving force in Alzheimer pathogenesis. Neurobiol Aging 1996;17:761–766.

421. Griffin WS, Sheng JG, Royston MC, et al. Glial-neuronal interactions in Alzheimer's disease: the potential role of a 'cytokine cycle' in disease progression. Brain Pathol 1998;8:65–72.

422. Tarkowski E, Blennow K, Wallin A, Tarkowski A. Intracerebral production of tumor necrosis factor-alpha, a local neuroprotective agent, in Alzheimer disease and vascular dementia. J Clin Immunol 1999;19:223–230.

423. Lue LF, Walker DG, Rogers J. Modeling microglial activation in Alzheimer's disease with human postmortem microglial cultures. Neurobiol Aging 2001;22:945–956.

424. Barger SW, Harmon AD. Microglial activation by Alzheimer amyloid precursor protein and modulation by apolipoprotein E. Nature 1997;388:878–881.

425. Chong Y. Effect of a carboxy-terminal fragment of the Alzheimer's amyloid precursor protein on expression of proinflammatory cytokines in rat glial cells. Life Sci 1997;61:2323–2333.

426. Collins JS, Perry RT, Watson B Jr, et al. Association of a haplotype for tumor necrosis factor in siblings with late-onset Alzheimer disease: the NIMH Alzheimer Disease Genetics Initiative. Am J Med Genet 2000;96:823–830.

427. Du Y, Dodel RC, Eastwood BJ, et al. Association of an interleukin 1 alpha polymorphism with Alzheimer's disease. Neurology 2000;55:480–483.

428. Grimaldi LM, Casadei VM, Ferri C, et al. Association of early-onset Alzheimer's disease with an interleukin-1alpha gene polymorphism. Ann Neurol 2000;47:361–365.

429. Nicoll JA, Mrak RE, Graham DI, et al. Association of interleukin-1 gene polymorphisms with Alzheimer's disease. Ann Neurol 2000;47:365–368.

430. Papassotiropoulos A, Bagli M, Jessen F, et al. A genetic variation of the inflammatory cytokine interleukin-6 delays the initial onset and reduces the risk for sporadic Alzheimer's disease. Ann Neurol 1999;45:666–668.

431. Rebeck GW. Confirmation of the genetic association of interleukin-1A with early onset sporadic Alzheimer's disease. Neurosci Lett 2000;293:75–77.

432. McCusker SM, Curran MD, Dynan KB, et al. Association between polymorphism in regulatory region of gene encoding tumour necrosis factor alpha and risk of Alzheimer's disease and vascular dementia: a case-control study. Lancet 2001;357:436–439.

433. Hedley R, Hallmayer J, Groth DM, Brooks WS, Gandy SE, Martins RN. Association of interleukin-1 polymorphisms with Alzheimer's disease in Australia. Ann Neurol 2002;51:795–797.

434. Sheng JG, Mrak RE, Griffin WS. Microglial interleukin-1 alpha expression in brain regions in Alzheimer's disease: correlation with neuritic plaque distribution. Neuropathol Appl Neurobiol 1995;21:290–301.

435. Sheng JG, Zhou XQ, Mrak RE, Griffin WS. Progressive neuronal injury associated with amyloid plaque formation in Alzheimer disease. J Neuropathol Exp Neurol 1998;57:714–717.

436. Goldgaber D, Harris HW, Hla T, et al. Interleukin 1 regulates synthesis of amyloid beta-protein precursor mRNA in human endothelial cells. Proc Natl Acad Sci USA 1989;86:7606–7610.

437. Forloni G, Demicheli F, Giorgi S, Bendotti C, Angeretti N. Expression of amyloid precursor protein mRNAs in endothelial, neuronal and glial cells: modulation by interleukin-1. Brain Res Mol Brain Res 1992;16:128–134.

438. Lee SC, Liu W, Dickson DW, Brosnan CF, Berman JW. Cytokine production by human fetal microglia and astrocytes. Differential induction by lipopolysaccharide and IL-1 beta. J Immunol 1993;150:2659–2667.

439. Sebire G, Emilie D, Wallon C, et al. In vitro production of IL-6, IL-1 beta, and tumor necrosis factor-alpha by human embryonic microglial and neural cells. J Immunol 1993;150:1517–1523.

440. Das S, Potter H. Expression of the Alzheimer amyloid-promoting factor antichymotrypsin is induced in human astrocytes by IL-1. Neuron 1995;14:447–456.

441. Marshak DR. S100 beta as a neurotrophic factor. Prog Brain Res 1990;86:169–181.

442. Barger SW, Van Eldik LJ. S100 beta stimulates calcium fluxes in glial and neuronal cells. J Biol Chem 1992;267:9689–9694.

443. Pociot F, Molvig J, Wogensen L, Worsaae H, Nerup J. A TaqI polymorphism in the human interleukin-1 beta (IL-1 beta) gene correlates with IL-1 beta secretion in vitro. Eur J Clin Invest 1992;22:396–402.

444. Shirodaria S, Smith J, McKay IJ, Kennett CN, Hughes FJ. Polymorphisms in the IL-1A gene are correlated with levels of interleukin-1alpha protein in gingival crevicular fluid of teeth with severe periodontal disease. J Dent Res 2000;79:1864–1869.

445. McGeer PL, Yasojima K, McGeer EG. Inflammation in Parkinson's disease. Adv Neurol 2001;86:83–89.

446. Jenner P, Olanow CW. Understanding cell death in Parkinson's disease. Ann Neurol 1998;44:S72–84.

447. Kosel S, Grasbon-Frodl EM, Mautsch U, et al. Novel mutations of mitochondrial complex I in pathologically proven Parkinson disease. Neurogenetics 1998;1:197–204.

448. Mann VM, Cooper JM, Krige D, Daniel SE, Schapira AH, Marsden CD. Brain, skeletal muscle and platelet homogenate mitochondrial function in Parkinson's disease. Brain 1992;115(Pt 2):333–342.

449. Ebadi M, Govitrapong P, Sharma S, et al. Ubiquinone (coenzyme q10) and mitochondria in oxidative stress of parkinson's disease. Biol Signals Recept 2001;10:224–253.

450. McGeer PL, Itagaki S, Boyes BE, McGeer EG. Reactive microglia are positive for HLA-DR in the substantia nigra of Parkinson's and Alzheimer's disease brains. Neurology 1988;38:1285–1291.

451. Langston JW, Ballard P, Tetrud JW, Irwin I. Chronic Parkinsonism in humans due to a product of meperidine-analog synthesis. Science 1983;219:979–980.

452. Bronstein DM, Perez-Otano I, Sun V, et al. Glia-dependent neurotoxicity and neuroprotection in mesencephalic cultures. Brain Res 1995;704:112–116.

453. McNaught KS, Jenner P. Altered glial function causes neuronal death and increases neuronal susceptibility to 1-methyl-4-phenylpyridinium- and 6-hydroxydopamine-induced toxicity in astrocytic/ventral mesencephalic co-cultures. J Neurochem 1999;73:2469–2476.

454. Herrera AJ, Castano A, Venero JL, Cano J, Machado A. The single intranigral injection of LPS as a new model for studying the selective effects of inflammatory reactions on dopaminergic system. Neurobiol Dis 2000;7:429–447.

455. Gao HM, Jiang J, Wilson B, Zhang W, Hong JS, Liu B. Microglial activation-mediated delayed and progressive degeneration of rat nigral dopaminergic neurons: relevance to Parkinson's disease. J Neurochem 2002;81:1285–1297.

456. Castano A, Herrera AJ, Cano J, Machado A. The degenerative effect of a single intranigral injection of LPS on the dopaminergic system is prevented by dexamethasone, and not mimicked by rh-TNF-alpha, IL-1beta and IFN-gamma. J Neurochem 2002;81:150–157.

457. Nagatsu T, Mogi M, Ichinose H, Togari A. Changes in cytokines and neurotrophins in Parkinson's disease. J Neural Transm Suppl 2000:277–290.

458. Kurkowska-Jastrzebska I, Wronska A, Kohutnicka M, Czlonkowski A, Czlonkowska A. MHC class II positive microglia and lymphocytic infiltration are present in the substantia nigra and striatum in mouse model of Parkinson's disease. Acta Neurobiol Exp (Wars) 1999;59:1–8.

459. Hunot S, Hirsch EC. Neuroinflammatory processes in Parkinson's disease. Ann Neurol 2003;53(Suppl 3):S49–58; discussion S58–60.

460. Hunot S, Dugas N, Faucheux B, et al. FcepsilonRII/CD23 is expressed in Parkinson's disease and induces, in vitro, production of nitric oxide and tumor necrosis factor-alpha in glial cells. J Neurosci 1999;19:3440-3447.

461. Qureshi GA, Baig S, Bednar I, Sodersten P, Forsberg G, Siden A. Increased cerebrospinal fluid concentration of nitrite in Parkinson's disease. Neuroreport 1995;6:1642–1644.

462. Rousselet E, Callebert J, Parain K, et al. Role of TNF-alpha receptors in mice intoxicated with the parkinsonian toxin MPTP. Exp Neurol 2002;177:183–192.

463. Hartmann A, Troadec JD, Hunot S, et al. Caspase-8 is an effector in apoptotic death of dopaminergic neurons in Parkinson's disease, but pathway inhibition results in neuronal necrosis. J Neurosci 2001;21:2247–2255.

464. Breidert T, Callebert J, Heneka MT, Landreth G, Launay JM, Hirsch EC. Protective action of the peroxisome proliferator-activated receptor-gamma agonist pioglitazone in a mouse model of Parkinson's disease. J Neurochem 2002;82:615–624.

465. Du Y, Ma Z, Lin S, et al. Minocycline prevents nigrostriatal dopaminergic neurodegeneration in the MPTP model of Parkinson's disease. Proc Natl Acad Sci U S A 2001;98:14,669–14,674.

466. He Y, Appel S, Le W. Minocycline inhibits microglial activation and protects nigral cells after 6-hydroxydopamine injection into mouse striatum. Brain Res 2001;909:187–193.

467. Wu DC, Jackson-Lewis V, Vila M, et al. Blockade of microglial activation is neuroprotective in the 1-methyl-4-phenyl-1,2,3,6-tetrahydropyridine mouse model of Parkinson disease. J Neurosci 2002;22:1763–1771.

CME QUESTIONS

1. Which of the following statements is *not* correct?
   A. The majority of neuronal cell death in the central nervous system of human immunodeficiency virus (HIV)-infected individuals is believed to occur via an indirect mechanism through the release of neurotoxic products from activated macrophages/microglia.
   B. The levels of cerebrospinal fluid cytokines are routinely used to establish a diagnosis of HIV encephalitis or HIV-associated dementia.
   C. The HIV-1 viral proteins Tat and gp120 can directly stimulate proinflammatory cytokine production by microglia.
   D. The number of HIV-1 infected cells and the amount of viral antigen in the CNS do not correlate well with measures of cognitive deficits in HAD.

2. Which of the following statements is *false*?
   A. The initial response to infection in bacterial meningitis is mediated by meningeal macrophages, ependymal cells, and choroid plexus epithelium.
   B. The incidence of *Haemophilus influenzae* meningitis has decreased in developed countries because of the introduction of the *H. influenzae* conjugate vaccine.
   C. The cytokines induced during the course of bacterial meningitis are always considered to be beneficial to the host.
   D. TNF-α is unequivocally detected in the CSF of patients with bacterial meningitis.

3. Which of the following statements is *not* correct?
   A. T helper 1 (Th1) cells are believed to protect against experimental autoimmune encephalomyelitis (EAE).
   B. Interleukin (IL)-4 is critical in the development of Th2 cells.
   C. Tumor necrosis factor-α has been proposed to both contribute to and alternatively protect against EAE.
   D. IL-12 is critical in the development of Th1 cells.

4. Which of the following statements is *not* correct?
   A. Polymorphisms in the genes encoding cytokines may contribute to the development of Alzheimer's disease (AD)
   B. Glia likely contribute to neurodegeneration in AD.
   C. AD is believed to be an autoimmune disease.
   D. IL-1 likely contributes to the development of Alzheimer's disease.

Chemokines and Central Nervous System Disorders

William J. Karpus

1. CHEMOKINES AND CHEMOKINE RECEPTORS

Chemokines are small molecular-weight chemotactic cytokines that can be classified into four subfamilies based on the position of the amino-terminal cysteines (1,2). The CXC chemokines can be further categorized based on the presence or absence of a glutamate-leucine-arginine (ELR) motif in the amino terminus. Chemokines that possess the ELR motif are generally chemotactic for neutrophils and are angiogenic, whereas the non-ELR CxC chemokines are chemotactic for activated T cells and are angiostatic (3). The CC family of chemokines are chemoattractant for a variety of cell types, including monocytes/macrophages, T lymphocytes, basophils, eosinophils, and dendritic cells (4–6). The C family, lymphotactin, is chemotactic for T cells and natural killer (NK) cells (7) and the CX3C chemokine contains a chemokine domain attached to a membrane-bound mucin chain that produces a soluble chemoattractant after proteolysis or mRNA processing (8). This chemokine is a chemoattractant for T cells, NK cells, and neutrophils (2). Chemokines and chemokine receptor-like molecules are also encoded by viruses and used in a variety of strategies to subvert the immune response (9).

Chemokines induce a variety of downstream cellular-signaling cascades through specific seven-transmembrane spanning, G protein-coupled receptors (10,11). The most well-studied response is cellular chemotaxis, although other cellular outcomes, such as cytokine expression, cellular differentiation, and cellular survival, have been described (11). Chemokine receptors can also be subdivided into four families based on the chemokine family members that are specific ligands for particular receptors. The working hypothesis in the field of neuroimmunology has been that chemokines induce leukocyte accumulation in the central nervous system (CNS) through interaction with specific receptors on the cell surface of T cells, monocytes, and neutrophils (12). The induction of chemokine expression in the CNS is a result of few constitutively expressed chemokines (13–15), as well as a number of transcriptionally upregulated chemokines (16,17). The precise regulation of CNS-specific chemokine regulatory events is not well understood.

2. EXPERIMENTAL AUTOIMMUNE ENCEPHALOMYELITIS

Experimental autoimmune encephalomyelitis (EAE) is a CD4$^+$ T cell-mediated, CNS demyelinating disease that serves as a model for the study of multiple sclerosis (MS) and its underlying pathophysiologic mechanisms (18). Several reports have demonstrated an association between chemokine mRNA or protein expression and appearance of clinical disease (16,19,20). Hulkower et al. (21) were the first to demonstrate the correlation between chemokine expression and development of EAE in

From: *Current Clinical Neurology: Inflammatory Disorders of the Nervous System:*
Pathogenesis, Immunology, and Clinical Management
Edited by: A. Minagar and J. S. Alexander © Humana Press Inc., Totowa, NJ

the Lewis rat model. Subsequently, Ransohoff et al. *(22)* described expression of chemokine mRNA in the CNS of SJL/J mice with relapsing EAE. Using semiquantitative reverse transcription polymerase chain reactionand in situ hybridization, they demonstrated that CXCL10 and CCL2 were expressed in the spinal cord. Additional studies of relapsing EAE demonstrated upregulation of mRNA chemokine expression for CCL5, CCL4, CCL3, CCL1, CXCL10, CCL2, CXCL1, and CCL7 just prior to the first appearance of clinical symptoms in a mouse model of EAE and elevated chemokine levels throughout the course of the disease *(16)*. Additionally, CCL6 expression has also been associated with EAE *(23)*. As evidence that chemokines are tightly associated with disease induction, CNS chemokine mRNA expression correlates with histological signs of inflammation, whereas expression is not detected in the absence of leukocyte infiltration *(19,24)*. Colocalization experiments have shown that CCL3 and CCL5 were expressed by infiltrating leukocytes, although CXCL10 and CCL2 were expressed only by astrocytes *(17)*. In addition to the link between CNS mRNA levels and tissue-specific inflammation, CNS chemokine protein levels have been associated with differential phases of relapsing disease. Elevated CCL3 and CXCL10 protein levels have been demonstrated in the CNS following adoptive transfer of activated neuroantigen-specific T cells *(25–27)* and correlate with acute disease development, whereas CCL2 levels increase with the development of the relapsing phase of disease *(20)*. It should be emphasized that emerging data suggests different chemokine-expression patterns in different EAE models and also in different mouse strains *(12)*. The biological importance of CNS chemokine expression in EAE as been demonstrated using in vivo anti-chemokine antibody treatments and chemokine knockout mice. Anti-CCL3 *(25)* and anti-CXCL10 *(26,27)* treatment prevented acute clinical EAE, whereas anti-CCL2 treatment prevented relapsing disease *(20)*. In addition to CCL2's role in relapsing EAE, it has also been shown to be important for CNS monocyte accumulation during acute clinical disease through the use of knockout mice *(28)*. Notably, in vivo neutralization studies have shown that although a variety of chemokines may be expressed during inflammatory autoimmune disease, only a subset of chemokines actually has a significant biological role in disease pathogenesis. In addition to regulating the migration/accumulation of leukocytes in the CNS during disease development and progression, chemokines also appear to regulate the trafficking of antigen-presenting cells that are necessary to prime the autoreactive T-cell response *(29)*.

Similar to the relationship between chemokines and EAE development, chemokine-receptor mRNA analysis has also shown a link between development of inflammation and accumulation of inflammatory cells bearing chemokine receptors *(30–33)*. Correspondingly, a reduction in CNS inflammation results in less chemokine-receptor mRNA expression. A number of recent studies using genetically deficient mice have shown that CCR1 *(34)* and CCR2 *(35)* expression are biologically important for the development of acute EAE. In the CCR1-knockout mice, there was about a 50% decrease in clinical disease severity; however, the mechanism behind disease attenuation is unknown. Since both T cells and monocytes have been shown to express CCR1 *(36)*, it is possible that CCR1 expression by either lymphocytes or monocytes, or perhaps both, is required for EAE development. In the CCR2-knockout mice, there was an almost total absence of disease caused by failure of monocytes, and not T cells, to traffic to the CNS *(35)*. These two examples contrast EAE induction in CCR5-knockout mice, in which the same level of disease severity was also seen in wild-type control animals *(37)*. An advance that has come from both the chemokine and chemokine-receptor studies in EAE is development of small-molecular-weight antagonists to chemokine receptors. Indeed, a small-molecular-weight antagonist of CCR1 has shown efficacy in the inhibition of clinical EAE *(38,39)*.

3. VIRUS-INDUCED DEMYELINATING DISEASE MODELS

A number of virus-induced CNS demyelinating disease models for MS exist, and two of these, murine hepatitis virus (MHV) *(40)* and Theiler's murine encephalomyelitis virus (TMEV) *(41,42)*, are well studied with respect to pathogenetic mechanisms of disease induction and progression. CXCL10-, CXCL9-, CCL5-, CCL2-, CCL7-, CCL4-, and CXCL1-mRNA expression have been shown to correlate with viral encephalitis in the brains of MHV-infected mice *(40,43)*. Furthermore, CXCL10-, CCL5-, and CCL4-mRNA expression were related to the demyelinating phase of this disease. In vivo neutralization experiments using the anti-chemokine treatment approach revealed that CXCL9 *(43)* and CXCL10 *(44)* were functionally important for early CNS viral clearance, whereas CCL5 was shown to be a pivotal chemokine in the recruitment of inflammatory cells during the demyelinating phase of disease *(45,46)*.

Chemokine expression has also been linked to clinical disease development in TMEV-induced demyelinating disease *(47)*. CXCL10-, CCL5-, and CCL2-mRNA expression were found in the CNS of both susceptible and resistant mouse strains following viral infection *(48)*. This same study demonstrated re-expression of CXCL10, CCL5, and CCL2 in the CNS of susceptible, but not resistant, mouse strains following viral clearance and coinciding with development of demyelination. CCL2- and CCL3-protein expression in the spinal cords of the susceptible SJL mouse strain also correlated with development of clinical disease symptoms *(49)*, with CCL2, and not CXCL10, being biologically important for clinical disease development, since CCL2 overexpression in a transgenic mouse line resulted in exacerbated, early disease development *(50)*. These examples demonstrate the correlation of chemokine presence with development of histological and clinical CNS demyelinating disease, as well as the functional contribution of chemokines to the demyelinating disease process.

4. MULTIPLE SCLEROSIS

Although chemokines have been demonstrated in the CNS of MS patients and alterations of chemokine receptor-bearing leukocytes in the peripheral blood of MS patients, the role of chemokines in the pathogenesis of MS has not been well established. An early study demonstrated elevated CCL3 expression in the cerebrospinal fluid (CSF) of MS patients compared to control patients with other neurological diseases and that the increased levels correlated with CSF leukocyte counts *(51)*. Bennetts et al. *(52)* analyzed a population of MS and control patients for a correlation between the absence of one of the CCL3 receptors, CCR5, and clinical disease presentation. Although they found that the absence of functional CCR5 had a significant protective effect against HIV infection, it did not have a protective effect against development of MS. However, the CCR5Δ32 mutation has been reported to confer a lower risk of recurrent disease activity *(53)*. A number of investigators have demonstrated the expression of chemokines in CNS tissue of MS patients *(54–60)*. Recent studies of the expression of chemokines in the CSF of MS patients undergoing clinical episodes of disease have shown that CXCL10 and CCL5 production were elevated in MS patients as compared to controls and that the levels of CXCL10 correlated with increased CSF leukocyte counts *(61)*. Because both CXCL10 and CCL5 are potent T-cell chemoattractants, it is reasonable to postulate that the elevated levels of these chemokines during active episodes of MS induced migration of T cells into the CNS. CXCL10 has also been demonstrated in MS lesions *(60)*. An increase in CXCR3[+] and CCR5[+] T cells in the peripheral blood of MS patients has been recently reported *(56)*; however, the significance of this finding with respect to disease progression is not known. Interferon (IFN)-β is a common treatment modality for MS, and a recent study has shown that in vitro exposure of T cells to IFN-β selectively inhibited mRNA expression for CCL5 and CCL3 *(62)*. Collectively, these results demonstrate the emerging significance of chemokine expression in the CNS during human demyelinating disease, as well as the increase in chemokine-receptor-bearing cells, and suggest a critical role for these molecules in the pathogenesis of disease development and progression. In fact, it has been postulated that a chemokine-receptor-antagonist approach could be feasible as a new therapeutic strategy for MS *(63)*.

5. ALZHEIMER'S DISEASE

It is becoming increasingly evident that Alzheimer's disease (AD) has an inflammatory component and that chemokine expression may contribute to its development and/or its progression *(64)*. Immunohistochemical analysis of the human brain for CCL4, CCL3, CCL5, CCL11, and CCL7 indicated that CCL4 was predominantly expressed in a subpopulation of reactive astrocytes that were more widespread in AD than in control brains, whereas CCL3 was predominantly expressed in neurons and weakly in some microglia in both AD and controls *(65)*. In this same study, the investigators noted that many of the CCR3[+]- or CCR5[+]-reactive microglia and CCL4-reactive astrocytes were linked to amyloid deposits. Additional evidence for chemokine-involvement in AD suggests that Aβ can activate both astrocytes and oligodendrocytes to express CCL2 and CCL5 *(66)*. Moreover, Aβ1-42 has been shown to induce the in vitro CCL2-, CCL3-, CCL4-, and CXCL8-dependent migration of monocytes *(67)*. Aβ 25–35 was also shown to induce CCL3 and CXCL10 expression by cultured human monocytes and mouse microglial cells *(68)*. Finally, neurons in AD tissue have been shown to express CXCR3, with the corresponding ligand expressed by reactive astrocytes *(69)*, suggesting a relationship between chemokines and the disease process. Collectively, these studies do not explicitly demonstrate a causal role for chemokines and pathogenesis, but they are the first steps toward understanding the role of chemokines and inflammation in AD.

6. HIV-ASSOCIATED DEMENTIA

CNS dysfunction has been described in HIV-infected individuals and most likely results from viral infection of cells through the use of chemokine receptors as coreceptors (reviewed in ref. *70)*. Chemokine receptors, most notably CCR5, CXCR4, and CX3CR1, have been described as coreceptors for HIV, and a number of studies have shown chemokine receptor expression on neurons *(71)*, astrocytes *(72,73)*, endothelia *(74)*, and microglia *(75,76)*. Neuronal damage following HIV infection could result from either an infiltration of inflammatory leukocytes *(77)* resulting in cellular death, direct neuronal apoptosis *(78)*, or indirect stimulation of glia-derived neurotoxic factors *(79)*. The role of chemokines in HIV-associated dementia (HAD) is not well understood. For instance, in patients with HAD, the levels of CCL3, CCL4, and CCL5 in the CSF positively correlate with dementia, although low levels of CCL3 may be neuroprotective *(80)*. This result suggests that chemokine-mediated induction of CNS leukocyte accumulation may result in disease by attracting virus-containing cells. CCL3, CCL4, and CCL5 also have been shown to protect neurons from gp120-induced cell death *(79,81)*. It is clear that chemokines and chemokine receptors are involved in the pathogenesis of HAD, although the mechanisms are not clearly understood.

7. CNS BACTERIAL INFECTIONS

The role of chemokines in the control of CNS bacterial infections is also not well understood; however, there has been significant progress toward understanding the functions of these molecules in both experimental models and in patients. In experimental bacterial meningitis induced by *Listeria monocytogenes*, both CXC and CC chemokines (namely CCL3, CCL4, and CXCL1) are produced intrathecally by meningeal macrophages and leukocytes that infiltrate the CNS. In comparison, patients with bacterial meningitis demonstrate CXCL8, CXCL1, CCL2, CCL3, and CCL4 expression in the CSF *(82)*. In experimental CNS infections using *Haemophilus influenzae* type b, mRNA for CXCL1, CCL3, CCL2, and CCL5 was detected in the brains of neonatal rats *(83)*. In vivo neutralization of CXCL1 or CCL3 resulted in a reduction of neutrophil accumulation, whereas anti-CCL2 treatment resulted in reduction of monocyte accumulation in the CNS *(83)*. The study of a bacterial-induced brain abscess model has increased the understanding of chemokine function in CNS infections. When mouse brains were infected with *Staphylococcus aureus*, a number of chemokines were expressed locally. These included CCL3, CCL4, CXCL1, CCL2, and CCL1 *(84)*. Control of bacterial clearance and disease development appeared to be a function of CXCL1 expression as mice without CXCR2 expression failed to clear the infection because of reduced neutrophil accumulation *(84)*. These examples point to the requirement of CXC chemokines for the control of CNS bacterial infections and the subsequent development of bystander tissue destruction that results in CNS inflammatory disease.

8. CHEMOKINE TRANSGENIC MODELS

Transgenic mice have been constructed in which CNS-specific promoters have driven various chemokines of interest to restrict expression to that particular compartment. One of the earliest models was the MBP-CCL2 transgenic mouse created by Lira and colleagues *(85)*. In these mice, over-expression of CCL2 in the CNS by oligodendrocytes resulted in a higher number of organ-specific infiltrating mononuclear cells than in control littermates. The vast majority of the recruited cells in the brain were monocytes and macrophages, as defined by light microscopy and ultrastructural and immunohistochemical criteria. The cells were found in a perivascular orientation with minimal parenchymal infiltration, with the authors suggesting the possibility of CCL2 accumulation in the vessels. The mononuclear cell infiltrate in the brain was significantly amplified by lipopolysaccharide treatment of transgenic but not littermate controls, suggesting that the recruitment properties of CCL2 can be potentiated by additional factors. It should be noted that despite the enhanced mononuclear cell recruitment in the brain, there was little, if any, pathologic change. This model provided some of the first evidence that forced expression of a chemokine in the CNS can result in specific local cellular accumulation.

We constructed a similar transgenic mouse using the glial fibrillary acidic protein (GFAP) promoter to drive CCL2 and limit its expression to CNS astrocytes *(50)*. In this study, we demonstrated that transgenic expression of CCL2 in the CNS resulted in diffuse CNS monocyte infiltration and accumulation compared to littermate controls. Transgenic CCL2 expression did not alter normal development, differentiation, or function of peripheral T cells. Importantly, there was no evidence of overt CNS disease or other pathologic phenotype when mice were left unchallenged with antigen or unchallenged with bacteria or virus. However, when CCL2 transgenic mice were given a peripheral challenge of lipopolysaccharide, an inflammatory infiltrate with organized perivascular lesions developed. Infection of the transgenic mice with TMEV resulted in accelerated onset and increased severity of clinical and histological disease. These results suggested that CCL2 expression in the CNS has the potential to be a major pathogenic factor that drives macrophage accumulation in the development of CNS inflammatory disease. Moreover, these results support the idea that organ-restricted chemokine expression alone is incapable of inducing tissue-specific disease and that additional activation signals are necessary.

Ransohoff and colleagues constructed a GFAP-CCL2 transgenic mouse that demonstrated very high levels of chemokine expression in the CNS *(86)*. In this model, they described pertussis toxin-induced reversible encephalopathy dependent on monocyte chemoattractant protein-1 (CCL2) overexpression. This is a novel animal model that exhibits features of human encephalopathic complications of inflammatory disorders such as viral meningoencephalitis and *Lyme neuroborreliosis*, as well as the mild toxic encephalopathy that commonly precedes MS relapses. The transgenic mouse line that overexpressed CCL2 at a high level manifested transient, severe encephalopathy with high mortality after peripheral injections of pertussis toxin (PTx), along with complete Freund's adjuvant (CFA), despite being relatively normal when unchallenged. Surviving mice showed markedly improved function and did not relapse during a prolonged period of observation. This study characterized a novel model of reversible inflammatory encephalopathy that is dependent on both genetic and environmental factors.

Similar experiments were designed using a chemokine primarily responsible for T-cell accumulation. It is well known that CXCL10 is expressed in the CNS following inflammatory disease induction *(26)*; therefore, Campbell and colleagues examined the biological outcome in transgenic mice with astrocyte-directed production of this chemokine *(87)*. The GFAP-CXCL10 transgenic mice spontaneously developed transgene dose- and age-related leukocyte infiltrates in the perivascular, meningeal, and ventricular regions of the brain that were composed of neutrophils and T cells. As with the CNS CCL2 transgenic models, no other overt pathological or physical changes were evident. The extent of leukocyte recruitment to the brain was enhanced by peripheral immunization of GFAP-CXCL10 mice with CFA and PTx. This was paralleled by a modest, transient increase in the expression of some cytokine and chemokine genes. The biological function of forced CNS CXCL10 expression was demonstrated by observing enrichment for CXCR3-expressing leukocytes from CNS of immunized GFAP-CXCL10 transgenic mice. It is again important to note that although astrocyte production of CXCL10 can promote and potentiate spontaneous immune-induced recruitment of leukocytes to the CNS, this ability is not associated with activation of a degenerative immune pathology. These models have been instructive in developing new hypotheses that additional, perhaps Toll-like receptor, stimulation is needed to elevate chemokine-regulated leukocyte accumulation to a pathologic state.

9. SUMMARY

Chemokines and their receptors are a growing family of inflammatory molecules that are associated with many tissue-specific inflammatory events, and the CNS is no exception. One current view of chemokines is that they regulate the migration to and/or accumulation of leukocytes at a particular tissue site to clear infection and repair tissue. However, aberrant accumulation of leukocytes, including antigen-specific T cells and monocytes, can induce pathology and result in tissue-specific autoimmune and/or inflammatory disease. Our greatest understanding of the role of chemokines in CNS disorders comes from the EAE model, in which the temporal and spatial chemokine expression patterns appear to regulate mononuclear cell accumulation and subsequent disease development *(12)*. In the case of autoimmune disease or bystander inflammatory disease, it would be beneficial to limit the biological effect of chemokine expression, thus limiting the extent of self-tissue damage. To this end, small-molecular-weight chemokine-receptor antagonists have been developed and are being evaluated for efficacy in disease models as well as human disease *(63)*. In the case of CNS bacterial infections, it would be deleterious to generally inhibit the function of chemokines as a subset, as these molecules are required for the accumulation of neutrophils and the resulting clearance of infection. In this particular instance, it might be beneficial to use selective antagonists for monocytes and T cells to inhibit self-tissue destruction while allowing accumulation of neutrophils. Nevertheless, understanding the role of this superfamily of inflammatory molecules in diseases of the CNS will shed light on specific pathogenetic mechanisms as well as provide targets for therapeutic intervention.

ACKNOWLEDGMENTS

The author's work is supported in part by National Institutes of Health grants AI35934, NS34510, and NS023349.

REFERENCES

1. Zlotnik A, Yoshie O. Chemokines: a new classification system and their role in immunity. Immunity 2000;12:121–127.
2. Murphy PM, Baggiolini M, Charo IF, et al. International Union of Pharmacology. XXII. Nomenclature for chemokine receptors. Pharmacol Rev 2000;52:145–176.
3. Strieter RM, Polverini PJ, Kunkel SL, et al. The functional role of the ELR motif in CXC chemokine-mediated angiogenesis. J Biol Chem 1995;270:27348–27357.
4. Davatelis G, Tekamp-Olson P, Wolpe SD, et al. Cloning and characterization of a cDNA for murine macrophage inflammatory protein (MIP), a novel monokine with inflammatory and chemokine properties. J Exp Med 1988;167:1939–1944.
5. Schall TJ. Biology of the RANTES/SIS cytokine family. Cytokine 1991;3:165–183.
6. Taub DD, Conlon K, Lloyd AR, Oppenheim JJ, Kelvin DJ. Preferential migration of activated CD4$^+$ and CD8$^+$ T cells in response to MIP-1α and MIP-1β. Science 1993;260:355–358.
7. Hedrick JA, Saylor V, Figueroa D, et al. Lymphotactin is produced by NK cells and attracts both NK cells and T cells in vivo. J Immunol 1997;158:1533–1540.
8. Bazan JF, Bacon KB, Hardiman G, et al. A new class of membrane-bound chemokine with a CX3C motif. Nature 1997;385:640–644.
9. Lindow M, Luttichau HR, Schwartz TW. Viral leads for chemokine-modulatory drugs. Trends Pharmacol Sci 2003;24:126–130.
10. Horuk R. Chemokine receptors. Cytokine Growth Factor Rev 2001;12:313–335.

11. Ward SG, Westwick J. Chemokines: understanding their role in T-lymphocyte biology. Biochem J 1998;333 (Pt 3):457–470.

12. Karpus WJ, Ransohoff RM. Chemokine regulation of experimental autoimmune encephalomyelitis: temporal and spatial expression patterns govern disease pathogenesis. J Immunol 1998;161:2667–2671.

13. Hesselgesser J, Taub D, Baskar P, et al. Neuronal apoptosis induced by HIV-1 gp120 and the chemokine SDF-1 alpha is mediated by the chemokine receptor CXCR4. Curr Biol 1998;8:595–598.

14. Pan Y, Lloyd C, Zhou H, et al. Neurotactin, a membrane-anchored chemokine upregulated in brain inflammation. Nature 1997;387:611–617.

15. Alt C, Laschinger M, Engelhardt B. Functional expression of the lymphoid chemokines CCL19 (ELC) and CCL 21 (SLC) at the blood-brain barrier suggests their involvement in G-protein-dependent lymphocyte recruitment into the central nervous system during experimental autoimmune encephalomyelitis. Eur J Immunol 2002;32: 2133–2144.

16. Godiska R, Chantry D, Dietsch GN, Gray PW. Chemokine expression in murine experimental allergic encephalomyelitis. J Neuroimmunol 1995;58:167-176.

17. Glabinski AR, Tani M, Strieter RM, Tuohy VK, Ransohoff RM. Synchronous synthesis of α- and β-chemokines by cells of diverse lineage in the central nervous system of mice with relapses of chronic experimental autoimmune encephalomyelitis. Am J Pathol 1997;150:617–630.

18. Segal BM. Experimental autoimmune encephalomyelitis: cytokines, effector T Cells, and antigen-presenting cells in a prototypical Th1-mediated autoimmune disease. Curr Allergy Asthma Rep 2003;3:86–93.

19. Glabinski AR, Tani M, Tuohy VK, Tuthill RJ, Ransohoff RM. Central nervous system chemokine mRNA accumulation follows initial leukocyte entry at the onset of acute murine experimental autoimmune encephalomyelitis. Brain Behav Immun 1995;9:315–330.

20. Kennedy KJ, Strieter RM, Kunkel SL, Lukacs NW, Karpus WJ. Acute and relapsing experimental autoimmune encephalomyelitis are regulated by differential expression of the CC chemokines macrophage inflammatory protein-1α and monocyte chemotactic protein-1. J Neuroimmunol 1998;92:98–108.

21. Hulkower K, Brosnan CF, Aquino DA, et al. Expression of CSF-1, c-fms, and MCP-1 in the central nervous system of rats with experimental allergic encephalomyelitis. J Immunol 1993;150:2525–2533.

22. Ransohoff RM, Hamilton TA, Tani M, et al. Astrocyte expression of mRNA encoding cytokines IP-10 and JE/MCP-1 in experimental autoimmune encephalomyelitis. FASEB J 1993;7:592–600.

23. Asensio VC, Lassmann S, Pagenstecher A, Steffensen SC, Henriksen SJ, Campbell IL. C10 is a novel chemokine expressed in experimental inflammatory demyelinating disorders that promotes recruitment of macrophages to the central nervous system. Am J Pathol 1999;154:1181–1191.

24. Glabinski AR, Tuohy VK, Ransohoff RM. Expression of chemokines RANTES, MIP-1alpha and GRO-alpha correlates with inflammation in acute experimental autoimmune encephalomyelitis. Neuroimmunomodulation 1998;5:166–171.

25. Karpus WJ, Lukacs NW, McRae BL, Strieter RM, Kunkel SL, Miller SD. An important role for the chemokine macrophage inflammatory protein-1α in the pathogenesis of the T cell-mediated autoimmune disease, experimental autoimmune encephalomyelitis. J Immunol 1995;155:5003–5010.

26. Fife BT, Kennedy KJ, Paniagua MC, et al. CXCL10 (IFN-gamma-inducible protein-10) control of encephalitogenic CD4+ T cell accumulation in the central nervous system during experimental autoimmune encephalomyelitis. J Immunol 2001;166:7617–7624.

27. Karpus WJ, Fife BT, Kennedy KJ. Immunoneutralization of chemokines for the prevention and treatment of central nervous system autoimmune disease. Methods 2003;29:362–368.

28. Huang DR, Wang J, Kivisakk P, Rollins BJ, Ransohoff RM. Absence of monocyte chemoattractant protein 1 in mice leads to decreased local macrophage recruitment and antigen-specific T helper cell type 1 immune response in experimental autoimmune encephalomyelitis. J Exp Med 2001;193:713–726.

29. Kohler RE, Caon AC, Willenborg DO, Clark-Lewis I, McColl SR. A role for macrophage inflammatory protein-3 alpha/CC chemokine ligand 20 in immune priming during T cell-mediated inflammation of the central nervous system. J Immunol 2003;170:6298.

30. Jiang Y, Salafranca MN, Adhikari S, et al. Chemokine receptor expression in cultured glia and rat experimental allergic encephalomyelitis. J Neuroimmunol 1998;86:1–12.

31. Charles PC, Weber KS, Cipriani B, Brosnan CF. Cytokine, chemokine and chemokine receptor mRNA expression in different strains of normal mice: implications for establishment of a Th1/Th2 bias. J Neuroimmunol 1999;100:64–73.

32. Rajan AJ, Asensio VC, Campbell IL, Brosnan CF. Experimental autoimmune encephalomyelitis on the SJL mouse: effect of gamma delta T cell depletion on chemokine and chemokine receptor expression in the central nervous system. J Immunol 2000;164:2120–2130.

33. Matejuk A, Vandenbark AA, Burrows GG, Bebo BF Jr, Offner H. Reduced chemokine and chemokine receptor expression in spinal cords of TCR BV8S2 transgenic mice protected against experimental autoimmune encephalomyelitis with BV8S2 protein. J Immunol 2000;164:3924–3931.

34. Rottman JB, Slavin AJ, Silva R, Weiner HL, Gerard CG, Hancock WW. Leukocyte recruitment during onset of experimental allergic encephalomyelitis is CCR1 dependent. Eur J Immunol 2000;30:2372–2377.

35. Fife BT, Huffnagle GB, Kuziel WA, Karpus WJ. CC chemokine receptor 2 is critical for induction of experimental autoimmune encephalomyelitis. J Exp Med 2000;192:899–906.

36. Gao JL, Wynn TA, Chang Y, et al. Impaired host defense, hematopoiesis, granulomatous inflammation and type 1-type 2 cytokine balance in mice lacking CC chemokine receptor 1. J Exp Med 1997;185:1959–1968.

37. Tran EH, Kuziel WA, Owens T. Induction of experimental autoimmune encephalomyelitis in C57BL/6 mice deficient in either the chemokine macrophage inflammatory protein-1alpha or its CCR5 receptor. Eur J Immunol 2000;30:1410–1415.

38. Hesselgesser J, Ng HP, Liang M, et al. Identification and characterization of small molecule functional antagonists of the CCR1 chemokine receptor. J Biol Chem 1998;273:15687–15692.

39. Liang M, Mallari C, Rosser M, et al. Identification and characterization of a potent, selective, and orally active antagonist of the CC chemokine receptor-1. J Biol Chem 2000;275:19000–19008.

40. Lane TE, Asensio VC, Yu N, Paoletti AD, Campbell IL, Buchmeier MJ. Dynamic regulation of alpha- and beta-chemokine expression in the central nervous system during mouse hepatitis virus-induced demyelinating disease. J Immunol 1998;160:970–978.

41. Jakob J, Roos RP. Molecular determinants of Theiler's murine encephalomyelitis-induced disease. J Neurovirol 1996;2:70–77.

42. Kim BS, Lyman MA, Kang BS, et al. Pathogenesis of virus-induced immune-mediated demyelination. Immunol Res 2001;24:121–130.

43. Liu MT, Armstrong D, Hamilton TA, Lane TE. Expression of Mig (monokine induced by interferon-gamma) is important in T lymphocyte recruitment and host defense following viral infection of the central nervous system. J Immunol 2001;166:1790–1795.

44. Liu MT, Chen BP, Oertel P, et al. The T cell chemoattractant IFN-inducible protein 10 is essential in host defense against viral-induced neurologic disease. J Immunol 2000;165:2327–2330.

45. Lane TE, Liu MT, Chen BP, et al. A central role for CD4(+) T cells and RANTES in virus-induced central nervous system inflammation and demyelination. J Virol 2000;74:1415–1424.

46. Glass WG, Hickey MJ, Hardison JL, Liu MT, Manning JE, Lane TE. Antibody targeting of the CC chemokine ligand 5 results in diminished leukocyte infiltration into the central nervous system and reduced neurologic disease in a viral model of multiple sclerosis. J Immunol 2004;172:4018–4025.

47. Hoffman LM, Karpus WJ. Chemokine regulation of CNS T-cell infiltration in experimental autoimmune encephalomyelitis. Res Immunol 1998;149:790–794.

48. Murray PD, Krivacic K, Chernosky A, Wei T, Ransohoff RM, Rodriguez M. Biphasic and regionally-restricted chemokine expression in the central nervous system in the Theiler's virus model of multiple sclerosis. J Neurovirol 2000;6 (Suppl 1):S44-52.

49. Hoffman LM, Fife BT, Begolka WS, Miller SD, Karpus WJ. Central nervous system chemokine expression during Theiler's virus-induced demyelinating disease. J Neurovirol 1999;5:635–642.

50. Bennett JL, Elhofy A, Canto MCD, Tani M, Ransohoff RM, Karpus WJ. CCL2 transgene expression in the central nervous system directs diffuse infiltration of CD45^{high}CD11b$^+$ monocytes and enhanced Theiler's murine encephalomyelitis virus-induced demyelinating disease. J Neurovirol 2003;9:623–636.

51. Miyagishi R, Kikuchi S, Fukazawa T, Tashiro K. Macrophage inflammatory protein-1 alpha in the cerebrospinal fluid of patients with multiple sclerosis and other inflammatory neurological diseases. J Neurol Sci 1995;129:223–227.

52. Bennetts BH, Teutsch SM, Buhler MM, Heard RN, Stewart GJ. The CCR5 deletion mutation fails to protect against multiple sclerosis. Hum Immunol 1997;58:52–59.

53. Sellebjerg F, Madsen HO, Jensen CV, Jensen J, Garred P. CCR5 delta32, matrix metalloproteinase-9 and disease activity in multiple sclerosis. J Neuroimmunol 2000;102:98–106.

54. Hvas J, McLean C, Justesen J, et al. Perivascular T cells express the pro-inflammatory chemokine RANTES mRNA in multiple sclerosis lesions. Scand J Immunol 1997;46:195–203.

55. Van DV, Tekstra J, Beelen RH, Tensen CP, Van DV, De GC. Expression of MCP-1 by reactive astrocytes in demyelinating multiple sclerosis lesions. Am J Pathol 1999;154:45–51.

56. Balashov KE, Rottman JB, Weiner HL, Hancock WW. CCR5$^+$ and CXCR3$^+$ T cells are increased in multiple sclerosis and their ligands MIP-1alpha and IP-10 are expressed in demyelinating brain lesions. Proc Natl Acad Sci USA 1999;96:6873–6878.

57. McManus C, Berman JW, Brett FM, Staunton H, Farrell M, Brosnan CF. MCP-1, MCP-2 and MCP-3 expression in multiple sclerosis lesions: an immunohistochemical and *in situ* hybridization study. J Neuroimmunol 1998;86:20–29.

58. Simpson JE, Newcombe J, Cuzner ML, Woodroofe MN. Expression of monocyte chemoattractant protein-1 and other beta-chemokines by resident glia and inflammatory cells in multiple sclerosis lesions. J Neuroimmunol 1998;84:238–249.

59. Simpson J, Rezaie P, Newcombe J, Cuzner ML, Male D, Woodroofe MN. Expression of the beta-chemokine receptors CCR2, CCR3 and CCR5 in multiple sclerosis central nervous system tissue. J Neuroimmunol 2000;108:192–200.

60. Simpson JE, Newcombe J, Cuzner ML, Woodroofe MN. Expression of the interferon-gamma-inducible chemokines IP-10 and Mig and their receptor, CXCR3, in multiple sclerosis lesions. Neuropathol Appl Neurobiol 2000;26: 133–142.

61. Sorensen TL, Tani M, Jensen J, et al. Expression of specific chemokines and chemokine receptors in the central nervous system of multiple sclerosis patients. J Clin Invest 1999;103:807–815.

62. Zang YC, Halder JB, Samanta AK, Hong J, Rivera VM, Zhang JZ. Regulation of chemokine receptor CCR5 and production of RANTES and MIP-1alpha by interferon-beta. J Neuroimmunol 2001;112:174–180.

63. Ransohoff RM, Bacon KB. Chemokine receptor antagonism as a new therapy for multiple sclerosis. Expert Opin Investig Drugs 2000;9:1079–1097.

64. Xia MQ, Hyman BT. Chemokines/chemokine receptors in the central nervous system and Alzheimer's disease. J Neurovirol 1999;5:32–41.

65. Xia MQ, Qin SX, Wu LJ, Mackay CR, Hyman BT. Immunohistochemical study of the beta-chemokine receptors CCR3 and CCR5 and their ligands in normal and Alzheimer's disease brains. Am J Pathol 1998;153:31–37.

66. Johnstone M, Gearing AJ, Miller KM. A central role for astrocytes in the inflammatory response to beta-amyloid; chemokines, cytokines and reactive oxygen species are produced. J Neuroimmunol 1999;93:182–193.

67. Fiala M, Zhang L, Gan X, et al. Amyloid-beta induces chemokine secretion and monocyte migration across a human blood–brain barrier model. Mol Med 1998;4:480–489.

68. Meda L, Baron P, Prat E, et al. Proinflammatory profile of cytokine production by human monocytes and murine microglia stimulated with beta-amyloid[25-35]. J Neuroimmunol 1999;93:45–52.

69. Xia MQ, Bacskai BJ, Knowles RB, Qin SX, Hyman BT. Expression of the chemokine receptor CXCR3 on neurons and the elevated expression of its ligand IP-10 in reactive astrocytes: in vitro ERK1/2 activation and role in Alzheimer's disease. J Neuroimmunol 2000;108:227–235.

70. Kaul M, Garden GA, Lipton SA. Pathways to neuronal injury and apoptosis in HIV-associated dementia. Nature 2001;410:988–994.

71. Horuk R, Martin AW, Wang Z, et al. Expression of chemokine receptors by subsets of neurons in the central nervous system. J Immunol 1997;158:2882–2890.

72. Tanabe S, Heesen M, Yoshizawa I, et al. Functional expression of the CXC-chemokine receptor-4/fusin on mouse microglial cells and astrocytes. J Immunol 1997;159:905–911.

73. Cota M, Kleinschmidt A, Ceccherini-Silberstein F, et al. Upregulated expression of interleukin-8, RANTES and chemokine receptors in human astrocytic cells infected with HIV-1. J Neurovirol 2000;6:75–83.

74. Molino M, Woolkalis MJ, Prevost N, et al. CXCR4 on human endothelial cells can serve as both a mediator of biological responses and as a receptor for HIV-2. Biochim Biophys Acta 2000;1500:227–240.

75. He JL, Chen YZ, Farzan M, et al. CCR3 and CCR5 are co-receptors for HIV-1 infection of microglia. Nature 1997;385:645–649.

76. Ghorpade A, Xia MQ, Hyman BT, et al. Role of the beta-chemokine receptors CCR3 and CCR5 in human immunodeficiency virus type 1 infection of monocytes and microglia. J Virol 1998;72:3351–3361.

77. Persidsky Y, Ghorpade A, Rasmussen J, et al. Microglial and astrocyte chemokines regulate monocyte migration through the blood–brain barrier in human immunodeficiency virus-1 encephalitis. Am J Pathol 1999;155:1599–1611.

78. Zheng J, Thylin MR, Ghorpade A, et al. Intracellular CXCR4 signaling, neuronal apoptosis and neuropathogenic mechanisms of HIV-1-associated dementia. J Neuroimmunol 1999;98:185–200.

79. Kaul M, Lipton SA. Chemokines and activated macrophages in HIV gp120-induced neuronal apoptosis. Proc Natl Acad Sci USA 1999;96:8212–8216.

80. Letendre SL, Lanier ER, McCutchan JA. Cerebrospinal fluid beta chemokine concentrations in neurocognitively impaired individuals infected with human immunodeficiency virus type 1. J Infect Dis 1999;180:310–319.

81. Meucci O, Fatatis A, Simen AA, Bushell TJ, Gray PW, Miller RJ. Chemokines regulate hippocampal neuronal signaling and gp120 neurotoxicity. Proc Natl Acad Sci USA 1998;95:14500–14505.

82. Lahrtz F, Piali L, Spanaus KS, Seebach J, Fontana A. Chemokines and chemotaxis of leukocytes in infectious meningitis. J Neuroimmunol 1998;85:33–43.

83. Diab A, Abdalla H, Li HL, et al. Neutralization of macrophage inflammatory protein 2 (MIP-2) and MIP-1alpha attenuates neutrophil recruitment in the central nervous system during experimental bacterial meningitis. Infect Immun 1999;67:2590–2601.

84. Kielian T, Barry B, Hickey WF. CXC chemokine receptor-2 ligands are required for neutrophil-mediated host defense in experimental brain abscesses. J Immunol 2001;166:4634–4643.

85. Fuentes ME, Durham SK, Swerdel MR, et al. Controlled recruitment of monocytes and macrophages to specific organs through transgenic expression of monocyte chemoattractant protein-1. J Immunol 1995;155:5769–5776.

86. Huang D, Tani M, Wang J, et al. Pertussis toxin-induced reversible encephalopathy dependent on monocyte chemoattractant protein-1 overexpression in mice. J Neurosci 2002;22:10633–10642.

87. Boztug K, Carson MJ, Pham-Mitchell N, Asensio VC, DeMartino J, Campbell IL. Leukocyte Infiltration, But Not Neurodegeneration, in the CNS of Transgenic Mice with Astrocyte Production of the CXC Chemokine Ligand 10. J Immunol 2002;169:1505–1515.

CME QUESTIONS

1. Which statement about chemokines is correct?
   A. Chemokines are small-molecular-weight chemotactic cytokines that can be classified into four sub-families based on the position of the amino-terminal cysteines.
   B. The CXC chemokines can be further categorized based on the presence or absence of a glutamate-leucine-arginine (ELR) motif in the amino terminus. Those chemokines that possess the ELR motif are generally chemotactic for neutrophils and are argiogenic, although the non-ELR CXC chemokines are chemotactic for activated T cells and are angiostatic.
   C. The CC family of chemokines are chemoattractant for a wide variety of cell types, including monocytes/macrophages, T lymphocytes, basophils, eosinophils, and dendritic cells.
   D. All of the above are correct.

2. Which statement about Alzheimer's disease and chemokines is incorrect?
   A. Chemokines do not have any role in pathogenesis of Alzheimer's disease.
   B. Immunohistochemical analysis of human brains for CCL4, CCL3, CCL5, CCL11, and CCL7 indicated that CCL4 has been predominantly expressed in a subpopulation of reactive astrocytes that were more widespread in AD than control brains, although CCL3 was predominantly expressed in neurons and weakly in some microglia in both AD and controls.
   C. CCR3+ or CCR5+ reactive microglia and CCL4-reactive astrocytes have been associated with amyloid deposits.
   D. Aβ can activate both astrocytes and oligodendrocytes to express CCL2 and CCL5.

3. Which statement is correct about the role of chemokines in pathogenesis of HIV-associated dementia?
   A. HIV-associated dementia is a degenerative process without any involvement of chemokines.
   B. Of Chemokine receptors, most notably CCR5, CXCR4, and CX3CR1 have been described as core-ceptors for HIV, and a number of studies have shown chemokine-receptor expression on neurons, astrocytes, endothelia, and microglia.
   C. Chemokines have only a destructive role in pathogenesis of HIV-associated dementia.
   D. Chemokines have only a marginal neuro-protective role in pathogenesis of HIV-associated dementia.

4. Which statement about chemokines is incorrect?
   A. Chemokines and their receptors are a growing family of inflammatory molecules that are associated with many tissue-specific inflammatory events, and the CNS is no exception.
   B. One current view of chemokines is that they regulate the migration and/or accumulation of leukocytes at a particular tissue site for the general function of infection clearance and tissue repair.
   C. Our greatest understanding of the role of chemokines in CNS disorders comes from the EAE model, in which the temporal and spatial chemokine expression patterns appear to regulate mononuclear cell accumulation and subsequent disease development.
   D. Chemokines and their receptors are not potential therapeutic targets.

5

Circulating Cell-Derived Microparticles in Thrombotic and Inflammatory Disorders

Wenche Jy, Lawrence L. Horstman, Joaquin J. Jimenez, Alireza Minagar, and Yeon S. Ahn

1. BACKGROUND

1.1. Introduction

It is now recognized that all circulating blood cells, as well as endothelial cells (EC), continuously shed small membranous vesicles (*microparticles* [MPs]), which are approximately less than 1 μm, and that levels of circulating MPs are sensitive indicators of disease activity. The first type extensively studied in patients was platelet MP (PMPs) *(1)*. Currently, endothelial-derived MP (EMPs) have risen to the fore as sensitive markers of EC perturbation, recently reviewed *(2)* and further considered in this article. Although other reviews may differ in viewpoint and emphasis *(3,4)*, it is generally agreed that circulating MPs comprise different subspecies of membrane vesicles released from endothelium and blood cells, such as platelets, leukocytes, and red blood cells (RBCs). MPs containing negatively charged phospatidylserine (PS) and/or tissue factor are highly procoagulant. MPs that express specific adhesion molecules are capable of interacting with leukocytes and endothelia to initiate inflammatory responses.

Leukocyte MPs (LMPs) are less commonly studied, even though they are potentially of great interest. Because erythrocyte MPs (RBCMPs) are rarest in blood and are studied mainly in relation to disorders involving RBCs, such as hemolytic anemias, sickle-cell disease, and thallasemias, they are not considered in this chapter.

The focus of this review is on MPs as markers of inflammation and thrombosis. Additionally, their potential role in pathophysiology is also a major topic. Accordingly, we develop some novel hypotheses implied by experimental findings concerning the pathophysiology of certain disease conditions.

1.2. Methodologies

At present, results from different laboratories on the same type of patient may differ radically because of differences in methodological procedures. This situation led us to write a recent forum article in which principals of six laboratories active in MP studies presented their methods side by side *(5)*. Although most employ flow-cytometric techniques based on addition of fluorescent-labeled antihuman monoclonal antibodies to the MPs in plasma (or resuspended after centrifugation), it is evident *(5)* that different results will be found by different laboratories from the same sample owing to differences in methods. We will not attempt to discuss methodological details, but this situation must be noted when examining findings from different laboratories. Future workshops are planned to improve agreement on measurement methods.

From: *Current Clinical Neurology: Inflammatory Disorders of the Nervous System: Pathogenesis, Immunology, and Clinical Management*
Edited by: A. Minagar and J. S. Alexander © Humana Press Inc., Totowa, NJ

1.3. Soluble Inflammatory Markers

Several studies of inflammatory disorders have relied on measurement of so-called *soluble markers* of endothelial perturbation. For example, CD31 (platelet-endothelial cell adhesion molecule-1 [PECAM-1]) has been used to assess disease activity in multiple sclerosis (MS) *(6)*. However, we have demonstrated that the majority of CD31 can be removed by filtration through 0.1 μm filter and that it is clearly associated with PMP and EMP *(7–10)*; thus, it is not a true soluble species. (A minimum of several hundred fluorescent molecules is needed to trigger a signal in clinical flow cytometers; therefore, they cannot detect true soluble molecules.) Similarly, E-selectin (CD62E) is widely measured as a soluble marker of endothelial stress *(11–14)*, but we routinely use it to identify EMP *(15–17)*, demonstrating that it is actually at least partially MP-bound.

Similar considerations apply to many other markers now regarded as soluble, including intercellular adhesion molecule-1 (ICAM-1), vascular cell adhesion molecule-1 (VCAM-1), P-selectin, tissue factor (TF), von Willebrand factor (vWF; partly bound to EMP *[18]* and PMP), thrombomodulin *(19)*, and CD40L *(20)*. As our recent review further details *(2)*, these observations lead to the conclusion that many or most so-called soluble markers of EC disturbance are in reality not soluble, but are at least partially bound to MPs.

It is well established that some of these markers do exist in true soluble form, usually owing to enzymatic cleavage from the membrane or by posttranslational editing *(21)*, but it is equally well established by our lab and others that a significant fraction, up to 80 to 90%, of these markers occur on cell-derived MPs, presumably with their transmembrane domains intact and normally adjacent proteins present.

The practical importance of this lies in the fact that release of true soluble species occurs by mechanisms entirely different from membrane vesiculation and hence reflect different pathophysiologies. Additionally, true soluble species often have properties functionally different from their MP-bound forms, as we have shown for vWF *(18)*. In view of these considerations, it is expected that when the MP-bound markers are clearly distinguished by independent measurement from the true soluble species, better-defined relations will emerge between disease states and the marker in question.

In summary, many so-called soluble species are in reality MPs. Accordingly, to the extent that they are recognized as valuable clinical and research tools, MP analysis deserves at least equal recognition.

1.4. Generation of MPs

MPs can be released under many different conditions, such as (a) activation or apoptosis induced by numerous agents; (b) partial or complete lysis, such as by complement; (c) oxidative injury; or (d) other insults, such as high-shearing stress *(22)*. The detailed mechanisms for MP release remain obscure. However, a rise in cytosolic calcium concentration, either from internal stores or from plasma membrane, appears to be a necessary triggering event or common pathway for vesicle release. Elevated cytoplasmic calcium has been shown to activate several cytoplasmic enzymes involving MP shedding. First, elevated calcium can induce cytoskeletal contraction, which is thought to be the driving force for the formation of membrane blebs *(23)*. To allow the membrane blebs to be shed from plasma membrane, the membrane cytoskeleton must be broken down. It has been demonstrated that calcium-dependent proteases, such as calpain *(24)* and caspases *(25)* are capable of breaking down cytoskeleton and facilitating MP releases.

1.5. Composition of MPs

MPs consist mainly of phospholipids and proteins. Their composition depends on the cell origin and the cellular processes inducing their release. Inside the vesicles, MPs may carry some cytoplasmic materials. The redistributed lipid bilayers of plasma membrane have been shown to be disturbed prior to the release of MPs *(26)*, leading to the expression of negatively charged PS on the MP. The expression of PS on MP has been shown to play an important role in blood coagulation *(26)*.

Weerheim et al. *(27)* have analyzed the phospholipid composition of cell-derived microparticles in normal blood and found that the composition comprises 60% phosphatidylcholine (PC), with remainder in sphingomyelin, phosphatidylethanolamine (PE), and phosphatidylserine (PS). In contrast, Fourcade et al. have reported that MPs from synovial fluids from inflamed joints of arthritis patients contained evenly distributed PC, PE, sphingomyelin, and lysophospholipids *(28)*. MPs in the synovial fluids are mainly derived from leukocytes. However, MPs in blood are mainly released from platelets *(29,30)*. These studies indicate that the difference in MP lipid composition may be caused by differences in cell origin and types of stimulation.

The surface antigens on MPs are a unique indicator of parent cell status. We have found that EMPs derived from activated ECs are enriched with CD62E and CD54 antigens. In contrast, EMPs derived from apoptotic ECs are enriched with CD31 antigen *(15)*. However, not all the surface antigens on the parent cells are expressed on MPs. For example, T cell-derived MPs lack CD28 and CD45 antigens, which are among the most abundant antigens on the parent T cells *(31)*. We have also observed that CD51 antigens are highly expressed on ECs but seldom on EMPs. Together, it is very likely that MP shedding is a well-controlled process. It may involve membrane antigen clustering/capping and the formation of lipid raft *(32,33)*.

2. CIRCULATING MPS IN THROMBOTIC AND INFLAMMATORY DISEASES

Berckmans et al. have assayed the number, cellular origin, and thrombin-generation properties of MPs in healthy individuals *(29)*. They found that normal blood contains the highest number of PMPs (237×10^6/L), as compared to EMP (64×10^6/L), granulocyte MPs (46×10^6/L), or red cell MPs (28×10^6/L). In this chapter, we review only MPs originating from platelets, endothelia, and leukocytes.

2.1. Platelet Microparticles

Among all cell-derived MPs, PMPs were the first discovered *(34)* and are the most widely studied. Glycoprotein (GP) IIb/IIIa (CD41), GP Ib/IX (CD42), and CD62P are the most frequently used markers to label and quantitate PMPs. In addition, they also carry other factors including vascular endothelial growth factor (VEGF) *(35)*, thrombospondin *(36)*, platelet-activating factor (PAF) *(37)*, β-amyloid protein precursor *(38)*, anticoagulant protein C/S *(39)*, and complement components *(40)*. These factors carried by PMP can further amplify PMP's role in thrombosis and inflammation.

Abnormal PMP have been reported in many thrombotic and inflammatory disorders including immune thrombocytopenic purpura (ITP), transient ischemic attacks (TIAs), acute coronary syndrome (ACS), thrombosis, antiphospholipid antibodies, lupus anticoagulant, thrombotic thrombocytopenic purpura (TTP), heparin-induced thrombocytopenia/heparin-induced thrombocytopenia with thrombosis (HIT/HITT), paroxysmal nocturnal hemoglobinuria (PNH), and multiple sclerosis (MS). For detailed information, please refer to our previous review of this subject *(1)*. In contrast, low-PMP generation was reported in Scott's syndrome, a rare bleeding disorder *(41)*. Most of these studies focus quantitatively on the EMP levels and do not follow up longitudinally on the studied patients. The value of PMP as a predictive marker in prethrombotic state remained mostly unknown.

In addition to assaying the PMP counts, some studies tried to identify the functionality of PMP by examining special antigens or proteins on PMP. For example, Tans et al. found that some PMPs contain anticoagulant factor protein C/S; therefore, they concluded that some PMP are anticoagulant *(39)*.

2.2. Endothelial Microparticles

EMPs have been investigated intensively in the past several years. Cumulative studies have shown that EMPs comprise subsets of membrane vesicles with different surface antigens. There is no consensus on which markers or methodologies are best for evaluating EMPs in disease activities. Sometimes, conflicting results arise from different research groups owing to their different methodologies.

2.2.1. Lupus Anticoagulant

The first report of clinical application of EMP assay was by Combes et al. in lupus anticoagulant *(42)*. Using CD31/CD51 markers, they found that patients with lupus anticoagulant had significantly higher EMPs (by twofold) than normal controls. Interestingly, the levels of EMPs were not reduced in those treated for thrombosis with anticoagulant.

2.2.2. Thrombotic Thrombocytopenic Purpura

Jimenez et al. reported elevated EMPs in patients with TTP by measuring CD31+/CD42b- EMP species and observed that EMP levels rose in acute stages, returned to normal in remission, and correlated with disease activity *(7)*. In a more recent study, CD62E rather CD31 was used as the main marker, yielding higher EMP counts and better correlation with other markers *(16)*.

2.2.3. Multiple Sclerosis

Minagar et al. reported an elevation of CD31$^+$ EMPs during MS exacerbations in contrast to remission. However, CD51$^+$ EMPs do not distinguish exacerbation from remission *(8)*. Elevated CD31$^+$ EMPs were well correlated with the presence of gadolinium-enhancing lesions in brain magnetic resonance imagings. Jy et al. used a simple in vitro model of transendothelial migration (TEM) to study the role of EMPs in the transmigration of the monocytic cell U937 *(5)*. The most recent work demonstrated that (a) plasma from MS patients sharply increase TEM; (b) pretreatment of the leukocytes with EMPs further facilitated TEM; (c) leukocytes exhibited bound EMPs after passing through the monolayer; and (d) drugs, such as interferon-β-1b and danazol, inhibited TEM *(17)*.

2.2.4. Acute Coronary Syndrome

Mallat et al. *(43)* measured MPs in ACS by first capturing MP with immobilized Annexin V (ANV), quantitating them by prothrombinase activity, then identifying cell origins using an ELISA method with anti-CD3, -CD11a, -CD31, -CD146, or -GPIb. Their main finding was that EMP, but not other MP, were elevated by 2.5-fold in acute myocardial infarction (MI). In this study, neither EMP nor other MP levels differentiated between stable angina (SA) and normal controls, between unstable angina (UA) and MI, or between UA and controls.

At the same time, Bernal-Mizrachi et al. *(9)* similarly found elevated EMP in ACS when they studied a larger number of patients ($N = 84$) using flow cytometry. A number of Bernal-Mizrachi's findings are notable. First, they found distinctly different EMP results when they used two markers, CD31$^+$ and CD51$^+$. For example, CD51$^+$ EMP, although clearly elevated in ACS relative to controls, did not distinguish new ACS from recurring disease, as CD31$^+$ EMP did. The authors concluded that CD31$^+$ EMP mainly acts as a marker of acute events, whereas CD51$^+$ EMP reflects chronic endothelial stress, which has also been observed in MS *(8)*.

2.2.5. Hypertension

Preston et al. *(44)* investigated a possible relationship between hypertension (HTN) and endothelial injury, as measured primarily by EMPs. They studied patients with untreated severe (diastolic blood pressure [BP] ≥120) or mild (BP > 95 <100) HTN compared to normal controls. They observed that EMP was highest in severe HTN ($p = 0.002$) and showed a significant correlation with systolic and diastolic BP. Interestingly, they found no correlation between BP and soluble markers of endothelial activation, such as sVCAM-1, and thus concluded that EMP assay appears to be the most sensitive method for assessing BP-induced effects on the endothelium and subsequent risk of impending hypertensive vascular and organ damage.

2.2.6. Preeclampsia

Gonzalez-Qintero et al. *(10)* applied EMP analysis to a prospective, case-controlled study of 20 patients with preeclampsia (PE) and 20 healthly pregnant controls. They demonstrated that a significant elevation of CD31+/CD42- EMP in PE *(10)*. In a more recent follow-up that also employed CD62E, results were clearer and more dramatic. Additionally, EMP correlated with proteinuria in patients with PE. They also observed a correlation between EMP and mean arterial BP, as in the work by Preston et al. cited earlier (*see* Section 2.2.5.). VanWijk et al. *(4)* also investigated MP in patients with PE. They failed to demonstrated significant differences in EMP levels between patients and controls. We suggest that the discrepancy may have been caused by the use of different methodologies.

2.2.7. Diabetes Mellitus

Sabatier et al. *(45)* compared MP numbers in controls vs patients with diabetes mellitus types 1 and 2, finding that patients with type 1 had elevated PMP, EMP, and total MP. Patients with diabetes mellitus type 2 showed elevation only in total MP, not in PMP or EMP. The authors suggested that these findings may be related to vascular complications in diabetes mellitus.

2.2.8. Paroxysmal Nocturnal Hemoglobinuria and Sickle Cell Crisis

Simak et al. *(46)* studied circulating EMP in PNH, aplastic anaemia (AA), and sickle cell disease (SCD). They found that both $CD54^+$ and $CD144^+$ EMP were significantly elevated in PNH and SCD but not in AA or healthy controls. Their findings indicate an involvement of endothelial injury in the acute phase of PNH and SC crisis.

2.3. Leukocyte Microparticles

The role of LMP as a maker of disease activities recently has received increasing attention. Several laboratories have reported that LMPs were elevated in thrombotic or inflammatory disorders. Biro et al. *(47)* have shown that MP originated from granulocyte-expressed TF, indicating that they may promote thrombus formation in a tissue factor-dependent manner.

2.3.1. Preeclampsia

VanWijk et al. *(4)* have investigated the cellular origin and numbers of circulating MP in normal pregnancy and PE. They found that the number of circulating MPs was unaltered in pregnancy and PE; however, numbers of T-cell and granulocyte MPs are increased in PE. Whether these altered MP levels cause vascular dysfunction in PE or are a consequence of the disease remains to be established.

2.3.2. Sepsis

Nieuwland et al. *(48)* have studied circulating MPs in meningococcal sepsis. They found that on admission, all patients had increased levels of MPs originating from platelets or granulocytes when compared to controls. In addition, they reported that these MPs supported thrombin generation more strongly in vitro than controls did. Plasma from the patient with the most fulminant disease course and severe disseminated intravascular coagulation contained MPs that expressed both CD14 and TF, and these microparticles demonstrated extreme thrombin generation in vitro.

2.3.3. Antiphospholipid Syndrome

Nagahama et al. *(49)* have reported that the concentration of monocyte-derived and platelet-derived MP in patients with antiphospholipid syndrome (APS) was significantly higher than that in normal subjects and patients with systemic lupus erythematosus. Twenty one of the 37 APS patients (56.8%) had elevated levels of anti-oxLDL antibody. In addition, the patients with elevated monocyte-derived MPs were frequently associated with positive anti-oxLDL antibody *(49)*.

2.3.4. Sickle Cell Disease

Shet et al. *(50)* found total MPs were elevated in crisis and steady state in subjects with SCD, compared to those without it. These MP were derived from erythrocytes, platelets, monocytes, and EC. Total TF-positive MPs were elevated in SCD crisis vs steady-state and control subjects and were derived from both monocytes and EC. Their data support the concept that SCD is an inflammatory state with monocyte and endothelial activation and abnormal TF activity.

2.3.5. Trauma

Fujimi et al. *(51)* have evaluated the production of polymorphonuclear leukocyte (PMNL)-derived MPs in severely injured patients at three time points: days 0 to 1, days 2 to 5, and days 6 to 12 after the trauma event. They found that production of PMNL-derived MPs increased along with adhesion-molecule expression on days 2 to 5 after severe trauma. CD62L expression was enhanced on MPs at all three time points, and CD11b expression was enhanced on MPs less than 1.0 μm in diameter at all three time points. However, soluble E2-selectin and thrombomodulin in blood did not change significantly between time points, indicating no significant endothelial injury.

2.3.6. Venous Thrombosis

Myers et al. *(52)* have studied P-selectin and leukocyte MPs in thrombogenesis in mice. The evaluation of MP revealed that mice with the highest thrombus mass showed a high amount of mean channel fluorescence for MAC-1 (phycoerythrin) antibody, indicative of leukocyte MPs. An antibody directed against PSGL-1 was more effective than rPSGL-Ig in decreasing TM and limiting leukocyte-derived MP fluorescence. These data suggest that leukocyte MPs are associated with venous thrombus formation.

3. FUNCTIONS OF MICROPARTICLES

3.1. Coagulation

Exposing TF usually triggersblood coagulation. Completing the coagulation cascade, not only requires coagulation factors and calcium ions but also a membrane surface exposing negatively charged phospholipids, such as PS, to facilitate the formation of tenase and prothrombinase complex. MPs have been shown to carry anionic phospholipids, especially PS and TF. Both of these procoagulant activities are known to occur on EMP, LMP, and PMP *(7,43,47,53,54)*; however, it is not yet possible to ascertain the relative importance of these activities on EMP vs PMP and LMP or on whole cell surfaces (such as PF3 activity of activated platelets or TF expression on leukocytes or activated EC).

TF activity in particular has been difficult to quantify; conflicting reports may be caused by variable expression of "cryptic" TF and masking by tissue factor pathway inhibitor *(55,56)* and partly to sensitivity to sulfhydryl redox state *(57)*. Although more work is needed, much evidence suggests that EMP likely have important roles in coagulation, especially at local sites of injury, not only by virtue of PF3 and TF activities but also by possibly modulating the protein C/S-thrombomodulin anticoagulant system.

Although the majority of MP are procoagulant, some reports also demonstrate that MP may be anticoagulant under certain conditions. Tans et al. suggested that PMP could serve an anticoagulant function by supporting the protein C/S/TM pathway *(39)*. Gris et al. *(58)* demonstrated that a large part of protein S is MP-associated and that clinical assays using PEG precipitation cause underestimation of protein S because much of it is precipitated with MP. More recently but in a similar spirit, Berckmans et al. have shown that low levels of thrombin generation by MP in normal controls occurs via the contact pathway (independent of TF) and may serve an anticoagulant function because protein C could be activated by the trace of thrombin *(29)*.

3.2. Inflammation

Jy et al. *(59)* first demonstrated the interaction of PMPs and leukocytes. They showed that PMPs can bind to leukocytes via a P-selectin-dependent pathway. The binding of PMPs to leukocytes leads to leukocyte activation and aggregation. Barry et al. *(60)* showed that PMPs interact

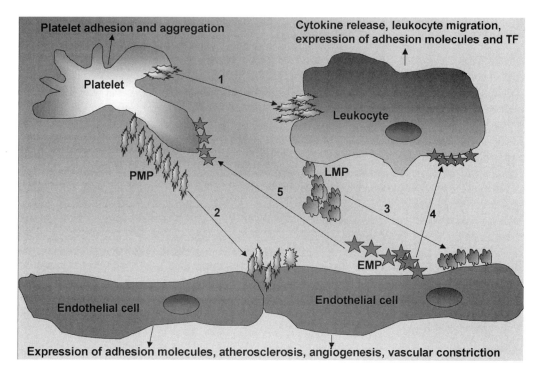

Fig. 1. Current findings on interactions among MPs species and cells.

with ECs, which results in upregulation of CD54 and the subsequent adhesion of monocytes. Mesri and his coworker also showed that leukocyte microparticles can interact with endothelium to induce interleukin-6 release *(61)*.

Recently, Sabattier et al. *(62)* demonstrated that EMPs can bind to and activate cultured monocytes, as judged by induced expression of TF antigen and that this effect could be largely inhibited by anti-CD54. Building on previous work on PMP–leukocyte interactions, Jy et al. *(59)* had independently found similar results (including selective inhibition of the interaction by anti-CD54) but used a different approach: studying leukocytes in whole blood and measuring leukocyte activation in response to added EMP by expression of CD11b *(5)*. Their findings also indicated that EMPs interacted only weakly with PMNs relative to monocytes and hardly at all with lymphocytes.

Of particular interest was the finding that EMPs generated by apoptosis in ECs were weak compared to equal concentration of EMPs from ECs activated by tumor necrosis factor (TNF)-α *(5)*. This may be the result of higher levels of CD54$^+$ EMP induced by TNF-α compared to apoptotic ECs. In a binding study using U937 cells exposed to EMP labeled with various markers, the EMPs labeled with ICAM-1 (CD54) exhibited the greatest apparent binding, followed by EMPs labeled with PECAM-1 (CD31), E-selectin (CD62E), and vitronectin receptor (CD51). Accordingly, the CD54- labeled EMP was largely depleted in the cell-free supernatant, consistent with the majority binding to the U937 cells *(5)*. Those authors also proposed that the relatively low concentration of CD54$^+$ EMP found in blood in various disease states is explained by the finding that these EMPs preferentially and strongly bind to leukocytes, reducing their free concentration. Finally, they demonstrated that monocytes with adhering EMPs were facilitated in their passage through an endothelial monolayer *(5)*. Taken together, these findings suggest that at least one function of EMPs may be to modulate inflammation via leukocyte activation and transendothelial migration. The complete interaction between MPs and platelets, leukocytes and endothelium was summarized in Fig. 1.

3.3. Vascular Function

It has been reported that MPs released from platelets or leukocytes can influence endothelial function. Boulanger et al. *(63)* reported that MPs from patients with acute MI impaired endothelium-dependent relaxation in isolated arteries. In contrast, MPs isolated from patients with non-ischemic chest pain had no such effect. High concentrations of microparticles from patients with MI affected neither endothelium-independent relaxation to sodium nitroprusside nor expression of the endothelial nitric oxide (NO) synthase. The origin of the MP isolated from patients with MI has not been identified. Their data indicate that circulating MPs from patients with MI selectively impair the endothelial NO transduction pathway. VanWijk et al. also demonstrated that MPs isolated from patients with PE impaired endothelium-dependent relaxation in isolated myometrial arteries *(64)*. It is suggested that these MPs may contain oxidized phospholipids, which are a potent inhibitor of endothelial function *(65)*. Some MPs, however, may have a beneficial effect on endothelium. Barry et al. showed that PMPs can transfer arachidonic acid to ECs, which results in prostacyclin production and will induce vascular relaxation *(66)*. It has been reported recently that PMPs promote proliferation, survival, migration, and tube formation in human umbilical vein endothelial cells *(67)*. In addition, PMPs were also shown to augment endothelial progenitor cell differentiation in peripheral blood mononuclear cells. Their results suggest that lipid components of the PMP may be major active factors and that protein components may be minor contributors.

4. CONCLUSION

Cell-derived MPs have received increasing attention in recent years, both as a diagnostic aid and investigative tool. Because they carry markers of the parent cell, including those induced by activation or apoptosis, EMPs can provide valuable information on the status of the parent cell, which can be obtained no other way. In addition, there is a growing belief that MPs can function as important diffusible vectors of specific adhesins and cytokines promoting cellular interactions and signal transmission.

Thus, MP analysis constitutes a new avenue for investigation of pathologies in various diseases. Although still considered investigational, recent results from several laboratories suggest that MP analysis may be poised to enter the mainstream of clinical testing. In summary, it appears that MP analysis is emerging as the method of choice for assessing cell involvement in disease states. Although few studies have yet undertaken direct comparison of results using EMP compared to soluble markers, our EMP results for TTP, coronary artery disease, and MS appear to offer superior discrimination of clinical states as compared to other published studies employing soluble markers of endothelial disturbance.

REFERENCES

1. Horstman LL, Ahn YS. Platelet microparticles: a wide-angle perspective. Crit Rev Oncol Hematol 1999;30:111–142.
2. Horstman LL, Jy W, Jimenez JJ, Ahn YS. Endothelial microparticles as markers of endothelial dysfunction. Front Biosci 2004;9:1118–1135.
3. Freyssinet JM. Cellular microparticles: what are they bad or good for? J Thromb Haemost 2003;1:1655–1662.
4. VanWijk MJ, Nieuwland R, Boer K, van der Post JA, VanBavel E, Sturk A. Microparticle subpopulations are increased in preeclampsia: possible involvement in vascular dysfunction? Am J Obstet Gynecol 2002;187:4506.
5. Jy W, Minagar A, Jimenez JJ, et al. Endothelial microparticles (EMP) bind and activate monocytes: elevated EMP-monocyte conjugates in multiple sclerosis. Front Biosci 2004;9:3137–3144.
6. Losy J, Niezgoda A, Wender M. Increased serum levels of soluble PECAM-1 in multiple sclerosis patients with brain gadolinum-enhancing lesions. J Neuroimmunol 1999;99:169–172.
7. Jimenez J, Jy W, Mauro L, Horstman L, Ahn YS. Elevated endothelial microparticles in thrombotic thrombocytopenic purpura (TTP): findings from brain and renal microvascular cell culture and patients with active disease. Br J Haematol 2001;112:81–90.
8. Minagar A, Jy W, Jimenez JJ, Mauro LM, Horstman LL, Ahn YS, Sheremata WA. Elevated plasma endothelial microparticles in multiple sclerosis. Neurology 2001;56:1319–1324.

9. Bernal-Mizrachi L, Jy W, Jimenez JJ, et al. High levels of circulating endothelial microparticles in patients with acute coronary syndromes. Am Heart J 2003;145:962–970.

10. Gonzalez-Quintero V, Jimenez JJ, Jy W, Mauro LM, Horstman L, O'Sullivan M, Ahn YS. Elevated plasma endothelial microparticles in preeclampsia. Am J Obstet Gynecol 2003;189:589–593.

11. Roldan V, Marin F, Lip GYH, Blann AD. Soluble E-selectin in cardiovascular disease and its risk factors. Thromb Haemost 2003;90:1007–1020.

12. Seeman HB, Gurbel PA, Anderson JL, Muhlestein JB, Carlquist JF, Horne BD, Serebruany VL. Soluble VCAM-1 and E-selectin, but not ICAM-1, discriminate endothelial injury in patients with documented coronary artery disease. Cardiology 2000;93:7–10.

13. Hwang SJ, Ballantyne CM, Sharrett R, Smith LC, Davis CE, Gotto AM, Boerwinkle E. Circulating adhesion molecules VCAM-1, ICAM-1, and E-selectin in carotid atherosclerosis and incident coronary heart disease cases. Circulation 1997;96:4219–4225.

14. Lieuw-a-Fa M, Schalkwijk C, vanHinsbergh VWM. Distinct accumulation patterns of soluble forms of E-selectin, VCAM-1 and ICAM-1 upon infusion of TNF-alpha in tumor patients. Thromb Haemost 2003;89:1052–1057.

15. Jimenez JJ, Jy W, Mauro L, Soderland C, Horstman LL, Ahn YS. Endothelial cells release phenotypically and quantitatively distinct microparticles in activation and apoptosis. Thromb Res 2003;109:175–180.

16. Jimenez JJ, Jy W, Mauro LM, Horstman LL, Soderland C, Ahn YS. Endothelial microparticles released in thrombotic thrombocytopenic purpura express von Willebrand factor and markers of endothelial activation. Br J Haematol 2003;12:896–902.

17. Jimenez JJ, Jy W, Mauro LM, Minagar A, Solderland C, Horstman LL, Ahn YS. Transendothelial migration (TEM) in multiple sclerosis (MS): induction by patient plasma and its augmentation by leukocyte endothelial microparticles (L-EMP) complexes. Blood 2003;102:72b Ab 9.

18. Jy W, Jimenez JJ, Mauro LM, et al. Endothelial microparticles (EMP) interact with platelets via a vWF dependent pathway to form platelet aggregates, more resistant to dissociation than those induced by soluble vWF. Blood 2003;102:783a Ab 2896.

19. Satta N, Freyssinet JM, Toti F. The significance of human monocyte thrombomodulin during membrane vesiculation and after stimulation by lipopolysaccharide. Brit J Haematol 1997;96:534–542.

20. Amirkhosravi A, Meyer T, Sackel D, Desai H, Biddinger R, Amaya M, Francis JL. Platelet microparticles upregulate TF and VEGF in endothelial and melanoma cells in a CD40 ligand-dependent manner: Possible role in angiogenesis and metastasis. Blood 2002;100(11, Part II):63b Ab 3721.

21. Heaney ML, Golde DW. Soluble cytokine receptors. Blood 1996;87:847–857.

22. Miyazaki Y, Nomura S, Miyake T, et al. High shear stress can initiate both platelet aggregation and shedding of procoagulant containing microparticles. Blood 1996;88:3456–3464.

23. Mills JC, Stone NL, Erhardt J, Pittman RN. Apoptotic membrane blebbing is regulated by myosin light chain phosphorylation. J Cell Biol 1998;140:627–636.

24. Fox JE, Austin CD, Boyles JK, Steffen PK. Role of the membrane skeleton in preventing the shedding of procoagulant-rich microvesicles from the platelet plasma membrane. J Cell Biol 1990;111:483–493.

25. Rohn TT, Cusack SM, Kessinger SR, Oxford JT. Caspase activation independent of cell death is required for proper cell dispersal and correct morphology in PC12 cells. Exp Cell Res 2004;295:215–225.

26. Zwaal RF, Schroit AJ. Pathophysiologic implications of membrane phospholipid asymmetry in blood cells. Blood 1997;89:1121–1132.

27. Weerheim AM, Kolb AM, Sturk A, Nieuwland R. Phospholipid composition of cell-derived microparticles determined by one-dimensional high-performance thin-layer chromatography. Anal Biochem 2002;302:191–198.

28. Fourcade O, Simon MF, Viode C, et al. Secretory phospholipase A2 generates the novel lipid mediator lysophosphatidic acid in membrane microvesicles shed from activated cells. Cell 1995;80:919–927.

29. Berckmans RJ, Neiuwland R, Boing AN, Romijn FP, Hack CE, Sturk A. Cell-derived microparticles circulate in healthy humans and support low grade thrombin generation. Thromb Haemost 2001;85:639–646.

30. Berckmans RJ, Nieuwland R, Tak PP, et al. Cell-derived microparticles in synovial fluid from inflamed arthritic joints support coagulation exclusively via a factor VII-dependent mechanism. Arthritis Rheum 2002; 46:2857–2866.

31. Blanchard N, Lankar D, Faure F, Regnault A, Dumont C, Raposo G, Hivroz C. TCR activation of human T cells induces the production of exosomes bearing the TCR/CD3/zeta complex. J Immunol 2002;168:3235–3241.

32. Jy W, Jimenez JJ, Mauro LM, et al. Agonist-induced capping of adhesion proteins and microparticle shedding in cultures of human renal microvascular endothelial cells. Endothelium 2002;9:179–189.

33. Salzer U, Hinterdorfer P, Hunger U, Borken C, Prohaska R. Ca(++)-dependent vesicle release from erythrocytes involves stomatin-specific lipid rafts, synexin (annexin VII), and sorcin. Blood 2002;99:2569–2577.

34. Wolf P. The nature and significanc of platelet product in human plasma Br J Haematol 1967;13:269–288.

35. Wartiovaara U, Salven P, Mikkola H, et al. Peripheral blood platelets express VEGF-C and VEGF which are released during platelet activation. Thromb Haemost 1998;80:171–175.

36. George JN, Pickett EB, Saucerman S, McEver RP, Kunicki TJ, Kieffer N, Newman PJ. Platelet surface glycoproteins. Studies on resting and activated platelets and platelet membrane microparticles in normal subjects, and observations in patients during adult respiratory distress syndrome and cardiac surgery. J Clin Invest 1986;78:340–348.

37. Iwamoto S, Kawasaki T, Kambayashi J, Ariyoshi H, Monden M. Platelet microparticles: a carrier of platelet-activating factor? Biochem Biophys Res Commun 1996;218:940–944.

38. Nomura S, Komiyama Y, Miyake T, et al. Amyloid beta-protein precursor-rich platelet microparticles in thrombotic disease. Thromb Haemost 1994;72:519–522.

39. Tans G, Rosing J, Thomassen MC, Heeb MJ, Zwaal RF, Griffin JH. Comparison of anticoagulant and procoagulant activities of stimulated platelets and platelet-derived microparticles. Blood 1991;77:2641–2648.

40. Sims PJ, Faioni EM, Wiedmer T, Shattil SJ. Complement proteins C5b-9 cause release of membrane vesicles from the platelet surface that are enriched in the membrane receptor for coagulation factor Va and express prothrombinase activity. J Biol Chem 1988;263:18205–18212.

41. Sims PJ, Wiedmer T, Esmon CT, Weiss HJ, Shattil SJ. Assembly of the platelet prothrombinase complex is linked to vesiculation of the platelet plasma membrane. Studies in Scott syndrome: an isolated defect in platelet procoagulant activity. J Biol Chem 1989;264:17,049–17,057.

42. Combes V, Simon AC, Grau GE, et al. In vitro generation of endothelial microparticles and possible prothrombotic activity in patients with lupus anticoagulant. J Clin Invest 1999;104:93–102.

43. Mallat Z, Hugel B, Ohan J, Leseche G, Freyssinet JM, Tedgui A. Shed membrane microparticles with procoagulant potential in human atherosclerotic plaques: a role for apoptosis in plaque thrombogenicity. Circulation 1999;99:348–353.

44. Preston RA, Jy W, Jimenez JJ, et al. Effects of severe hypertension on endothelial and platelet microparticles. Hypertension 2003;41:211–217.

45. Sabatier F, Darmon P, Hugel B, et al. Type 1 and type 2 diabetic patients display different patterns of cellular microparticles. Diabetes 2002;51:2840–2845.

46. Simak J, Holada K, Risitano AM, Zivny JH, Young NS, Vostal JG. Elevated circulating endothelial membrane microparticles in paroxysmal nocturnal haemoglobinuria. Br J Haematol 2004;125:804–813.

47. Biro E, Sturk-Maquelin KN, Vogel GM, et al. Human cell-derived microparticles promote thrombus formation in vivo in a tissue factor-dependent manner. J Thromb Haemost 2003;1:2561–2568.

48. Nieuwland R, Berckmans RJ, McGregor S, et al. Cellular origin and procoagulant properties of microparticles in meningococcal sepsis. Blood 2000;95:930–935.

49. Nagahama M, Nomura S, Kanazawa S, Ozaki Y, Kagawa H, Fukuhara S. Significance of anti-oxidized LDL antibody and monocyte-derived microparticles in anti-phospholipid antibody syndrome. Autoimmunity 2003;36:125–131.

50. Shet AS, Aras O, Gupta K, et al. Sickle blood contains tissue factor-positive microparticles derived from endothelial cells and monocytes. Blood 2003;102:2678–2683.

51. Fujimi S, Ogura H, Tanaka H, et al. Increased production of leukocyte microparticles with enhanced expression of adhesion molecules from activated polymorphonuclear leukocytes in severely injured patients. J Trauma 2003;54:114–119.

52. Myers DD, Hawley AE, Farris DM, et al. P-selectin and leukocyte microparticles are associated with venous thrombogenesis. J Vasc Surg 2003;38:1075–1089.

53. Kagawa H, Komiyama Y, Nakamura S, et al. Expression of functional tissue factor on small vesicles of lipopolysaccharide-stimulated human vascular endothelial cells. Thromb Res 1998;91:297–304.

54. Mallat Z, Benamer H, Hugel B, Benessiano J, Steg PG, Freyssinet JM, Tedgui A. Elevated levels of shed membrane microparticles with procoagulant potential in the peripheral circulating blood of patients with acute coronary syndromes. Circulation 2000;101:841–843.

55. Bajaj MS, Birktoft JJ, Steer SA, Bajaj SP. Structure and biology of tissue factor pathway inhibitor. Thromb Haemost 2001;86:959–972.

56. Camerer E, Kolsto AB, Prydz H. Cell biology of tissue factor, the principal initiator of blood coagulation. Thromb Res 1996;81:1–41.

57. Horstman LL, Cast L, Jy W, Jimenez JJ, Ahn YS. Tissue factor activity is controlled by its inhibitor and redox state: findings in endothelial microparticles, monocytes and a porcine trauma model. Presented at the 19th Annual ISTH Congress, Birmingham, U.K. July 12–18, 2003.

58. Gris JC, Toulon P, Brun S, Maugard C, Sarlat C, Schved JF, Berlan J. The relationship between plasma microparticles, protein S and anticardiolipin antibodies in patients with human immunodeficiency virus infection. Thromb Haemost 1996;76:38–45.

59. Jy W, Mao WW, Horstman L, Tao J, Ahn YS. Platelet microparticles bind, activate and aggregate neutrophils in vitro. Blood Cells Mol Dis 1995;21:217–231.

60. Barry OP, Pratico D, Savani RC, FitzGerald GA. Modulation of monocyte-endothelial cell interactions by platelet microparticles. J Clin Invest 1998;102:136–144.

61. Mesri M, Altieri DC. Endothelial cell activation by leukocyte microparticles. J Immunol 1998;161:4382–4387.

62. Sabatier F, Roux V, Anfosso F, Camoin L, Sampol J, Dignat-George F. Interaction of endothelial microparticles with monocytic cells in vitro induces tissue factor-dependent procoagulant activity. Blood 2002;99:3962–3970.

63. Boulanger CM, Scoazec A, Ebrahimian T, Henry P, Mathieu E, Tedgui A, Mallat Z. Circulating microparticles from patients with myocardial infarction cause endothelial dysfunction. Circulation 2001;104:2649–2652.

64. VanWijk MJ, Svedas E, Boer K, Nieuwland R, Vanbavel E, Kublickiene KR. Isolated microparticles, but not whole plasma, from women with preeclampsia impaired endothelium-dependent relaxation in isolated myometrial arteries from healthy pregnant women. Am J Obstet Gynecol 2002;187:1686–1693.

65. Rikitake Y, Hirata K, Kawashima S, et al. Inhibition of endothelium-dependent arterial relaxation by oxidized phosphatidylcholine. Atherosclerosis 2000;152:79–87.

66. Barry OP, Pratico D, Lawson JA, FitzGerald GA. Transcellular activation of platelets and endothelial cells by bioactive lipids in platelet microparticles. J Clin Invest 1997;99:2118–2127.

67. Kim HK, Song KS, Chung JH, Lee KR, Lee SN. Platelet microparticles induce angiogenesis in vitro. Br J Haematol 2004;124:376–384.

CME QUESTIONS

1. Which statement is correct?
   A. It is now recognized that all circulating blood cells, as well as endothelial cells, continuously shed small membranous vesicles (*microparticles*), which are approximately less than 1.0 μm.
   B. Plasma levels of circulating microparticles may be sensitive indicators of disease activity.
   C. Endothelial microparticles have been reported as markers of endothelial disturbance.
   D. All of the above are correct.

2. Which statement about microparticles is correct?
   A. Microparticles consist mainly of phospholipids and proteins.
   B. Composition of microparticles depends on the cell origin and the cellular processes inducing their release. Inside the vesicles, microparticles may carry some cytoplasmic materials.
   C. Microparticles carry one or multiple adhesion molecules from their parent cells.
   D. All of the above are correct.

3. Which statement is incorrect?
   A. Elevated endothelial microparticles plasma levels have been reported in multiple sclerosis.
   B. Microparticles probably have a role in coagulation.
   C. Microparticles interact with leukocytes and participate in the cascade of inflammation.
   D. Microparticles have no known function in endothelial biology.

6
Multiple Sclerosis
Clinical Features, Immunopathogenesis, and Clinical Management

William A. Sheremata

1. INTRODUCTION

1.1. History

Multiple sclerosis (MS) was first described by Charcot in mid-19th century Paris. Charcot, however, attributed the original recognition of this disorder to Cruveillier, the famed professor of anatomy. Although others also described the pathological anatomy of the disease in remarkable detail, it was Charcot who characterized the clinical illness and correlated the illness with its unique neuropathology *(1)*. From the outset, researchers recognized that the illness differed from one patient to another, with the majority of patients experiencing a relapsing–remitting disease (relapsing–remitting MS) *(1,2)*. Charcot recognized that a minority of patients had a fundamentally different illness, which he described as an "incomplete" form of the disease *(1,2)*. From their first symptoms, these patients showed signs of a progressive spinal cord disease without relapses. These patients are now designated as having *primary progressive MS* (PPMS) *(2)*.

Remarkably, the first person documented to have suffered clearly from MS was a grandson of King George III of England, Sir August D'Este *(3)*. He recorded the course of his illness in his diary, which was edited by Firth and published in 1947. Although MS is an illness that is more common in the higher socioeconomic strata of society, it is not limited to the well-to-do *(2,4,5)*. The disease occurs predominantly in persons of European descent *(2,4,5)* and is diagnosed in African-Americans at approximately half the rate of Caucasians in the United States *(4,5)*.

1.2. Clinical Features of Multiple Sclerosis

MS is characterized by relapses of neurological deficits followed by remissions, with varying degrees of recovery *(1–6)*. The occurrence and severity of the exacerbations are unpredictable, although several factors are recognized as increasing the risk of attacks. Patients experiencing their initial attacks are more likely to recover fully, but an experienced neurologist can virtually always find evidence of the previous neurological deficit, no matter how complete the recovery seems to have been. For example, retrobulbar (ocular) neuritis heralds the onset of disease in 10 to 15% of MS patients. The severity of the visual impairment varies greatly, with a very small percentage of patients suffering complete loss of light perception. Most patients recover their vision, but occasionally, especially if complete loss of vision occurs, there may be little or no recovery. The

From: *Current Clinical Neurology: Inflammatory Disorders of the Nervous System: Pathogenesis, Immunology, and Clinical Management*
Edited by: A. Minagar and J. S. Alexander © Humana Press Inc., Totowa, NJ

skilled examiner can usually find an afferent papillary defect (Marcus Gunn pupil) and impaired color saturation (color desaturation) in the vast majority of patients with retrobulbar neuritis who seem to have recovered normal visual acuity.

MS typically involves recurrent acute onset of neurological difficulties, reflecting damage to multiple areas of the brain and spinal cord, defined clinically as *attacks* or *relapses (1,2,4)*. Symptoms associated with these events typically remit, but subsequent relapses occur unpredictably and may become associated with residual disability *(1,3,4)*. This dissemination in time and space characterizes MS and is its principal diagnostic feature *(6,8–10)*. Interval progression between attacks signifies the onset of secondary progressive MS *(2)*. About 10 to 15% of the overall patient population develops a progressive form of illness, usually appearing in midlife, termed *PPMS (2,11)*. This form of illness is slightly more common in men and is approximately three times more common in Irish and Ashkenazi Jewish populations *(2,11)*. Should one or more exacerbations occur after onset of primary progressive illness at outset, patients are designated as having *relapsing progressive MS (2)*, although there is no universal agreement that secondary progressive and relapsing progressive patients differ in any fundamental way. The majority of the MS population will experience relapsing–remitting illness, but residual persistent disability may follow despite remission *(7,12,13)*, although the presence of residual disability following exacerbations *does not* signify the onset of secondary progressive illness.

Illness or increases in body temperature may result in the transient reappearance of neurological MS symptoms (*Uhthoff phenomenon*), despite a previous remission of those same symptoms *(2)*. Although Uhthoff's phenomenon is not an exacerbation, it is commonly misinterpreted as such. Occasionally, heat exposure appears to acutely worsen the severity of an exacerbation, and in other circumstances, worsens a minimal or subclinical event, making it more clearly apparent clinically *(14)*. These events probably reflect the ability of heat to impair the blood–brain barrier (BBB), allowing activated lymphocytes and immunoglobulins to enter the brain and spinal cord *(14)*.

The most common initial symptoms of MS are sensory disturbances and fatigue, which are often ignored by both patients and physicians. Perceptions of numbness and tingling may not be accompanied by obvious abnormalities on initial examination, especially a neurologist does not examine a patient at the onset of his or her symptoms. Almost half of initially recognized exacerbations principally affect ambulation. Acute paraparesis varies greatly in the degree and symmetry of the weakness. During examination, many MS patients who have motor weakness describe their difficulty as "heaviness" in their legs or stumbling when their feet seem to catch uneven areas on the sidewalk. Sometimes, the difficulty during ambulation is recognized only by a family member or a friend. Gait problems may be caused by motor difficulties and/or ataxia. Ataxia may occur as a result of vestibular, cerebellar, or sensory impairments. Thus, gait difficult may reflect motor deficits or ataxia caused by one or more problems.

Up to one out of five or six patients with MS will have unilateral retrobulbar neuritis as their initial clinical difficulty *(2,7)*. Other common symptoms at onset include diplopia, facial weakness and/or facial myokymia, vertigo, and bladder and bowel symptoms. Seizures will eventually occur in 10% during the clinical illness but rarely (about 1%) are a presenting sign of illness *(2)*. Some symptoms, such as hearing loss and impaired night vision, are less obviously related to MS. Other less commonly recognized symptoms include extrapyramidal symptoms and a family of paroxysmal manifestations *(15)*.

Recurrent brief stereotyped manifestations in MS include paroxysmal dystonias (tonic seizures), paroxysmal dysarthria, paroxysmal akinesis (paroxysmal falling), and pains (e.g., trigeminal neuralgia, glossopharyngeal neuralgia) *(2)*. Lhermitte's sign is precipitated by neck flexion and consists of transient shock-like sensations radiating down the neck and back and often into the limbs. It is commonly recognized as a sign of MS, especially when it occurs in the young, although it may occur with compressive cervical disc disease or spinal tumors. Except for Lhermitte's sign, these paroxysmal symptoms seem to occur in a minority of patients and are often not recognized as part of the spectrum of illness, although these paroxysmal phenomena are of great diagnostic value because they are rarely associated with other illnesses. When viewed in a cross-section of a patient population, they are evident in only about 3% of patients; however, we have found that paroxysmal phenomena will eventually occur in up to one-fourth of patients with MS. Occasionally paroxysmal dystonia involves all four limbs and the trunkal muscles and may be accompanied by severe pain. Fortunately, there is usually a prompt and complete response to 400 mg of carbamazepine per day, but a course of parenteral corticotrophin may be needed. Unfortunately, many of these patients are incorrectly diagnosed as having an acute psychiatric problem.

These paroxysmal symptoms are commonly attributed to ephaptic transmission (cross talk between damaged/demyelinated axons), but we suspect that they may be caused by inflammatory mediators, such as macrophage-produced leukotriene C, which is an extremely potent depolarizing agent. Often, the time course of these paroxysmal events approximates that of an exacerbation.

Although fatigue and fatigability become more prominent with time, especially during periods of disease activity, they may be prominent presenting signs of MS. Additionally, anxiety, depression, and cognitive issues may dominate the presentation of illness and delay disease recognition. In our experience, cognitive problems and accompanying emotional reaction occurring early in the course of illness are more important than physical disability as reasons for social dislocation and for leaving studies or the workplace.

A bewildering variety of manifestations may occur in MS, alone or in combination with other difficulties. These include limb weakness, useless-limb syndrome caused by severe proprioceptive loss, memory impairment, word-finding difficulty, acalculia, tremor, unusual nonphysiological patterns of sensory loss, and sexual impotence *(2,7)*.

1.3. Diagnosis of Multiple Sclerosis

The diagnosis of MS depends on the recognition of symptoms and neurological findings that typically accompany disease exacerbations *and* affect different parts of the nervous system over time *(8–10)*.

1.3.1. Diagnostic Criteria

In the past, experienced neurologists could easily recognize MS, but long delays in diagnosis and misdiagnosis were common in many patients. The need for standardized criteria led to the formation of a National Institutes of Health (NIH) committee led by Dr. George Schumacher. Diagnostic criteria have evolved from the 1965 Schumacher criteria *(8)*, which were established primarily for the selection of subjects for MS studies, to the 1983 Poser criteria *(9)*, which for the first time included laboratory support (magnetic resonance imaging [MRI], evoked-response testing, as well as cerebrospinal fluid [CSF] examination). The 2001 McDonald criteria are based on the original criteria but include validated specific MRI features as well as visual evoked and new CSF criteria *(10)*. These new criteria (*see* Table 1) allow the identification of clinically isolated syndromes (optic neuritis, and brainstem or acute myelitis) with very high (80%) probability of MS. Imaging provides the additional evidence required to establish the presence of dissemination of lesions both in time and space. Early diagnosis of MS and earlier introduction of treatment portends a better outcome, at least for interferon (IFN)-β-1a (Avonex®, Biogen Idec) *(20)*.

Another issue impacting early diagnosis of MS is the quality of spinal fluid examination. Importantly, a new Food and Drug Administration (FDA) laboratory standard for oligoclonal banding testing prevents technically inadequate studies, which have been common. Accurate CSF immunoglobulin and albumen quantitation are often difficult to obtain and results are limited by the quality of the reagents and technology used for testing. Evoked-response testing is relied on less but can be helpful, especially visual evoked responses *(10)*.

Table 1
McDonald Diagnostic Criteria

Clinical attacks	Objective lesions	Additional requirements for diagnosis
≥2	≥2	Clinical evidence is enough
≥2	1	Disseminated in space by MRI or positive CSF and =2 MRI lesions consistent with MS or additional clinical attack in different site
1	2 or more	Disseminated in time by MRI or second clinical attack
1 Monosymptomatic	1	Disseminated in space by MRI or positive CSF and ≥2 MRI lesions consistent with MS and disseminated in time by MRI or second attack
0 Progressive from start	1	Positive CSF and disseminated in space by MRI evidence of three or more T2 brain lesions or two or more cord lesions or —four to eight brain lesions and one cord lesions or positive VEP and —four to eight MS lesions or positive VEP and four brain lesions and one cord lesion and disseminated in time by MRI or continued progression for 1 yr.

MRI, magnetic resonance imaging; CSF, cerebrospinal fluid; MS, multiple sclerosis; VEP, visual evoked potentials.

1.3.2. Differential Diagnosis

There is a large differential diagnosis (*see* Table 2). In the past, meningovascular syphilis topped the list of imitators. Today, a variety of granulomatous diseases and other diseases are considered in the differential diagnosis, but sarcoidosis and systemic lupus erythematosis are the major differential diagnoses considered. The retroviruses human immunodeficiency virus (HIV) and human T-cell lymphotropic virus (HTLV)-I/II rarely can present as a granulomatous disease or mimic MS.

Central nervous system (CNS) lymphoma may require brain biopsy to establish a diagnosis, but a positive test for HIV rules out the diagnosis of MS. Biopsy is ordinarily required to make a diagnosis of primary CNS vasculitis, which is rare, and like progressive multifocal leukoencephalopathy (PML), is associated with MS-like attacks and increasing neurological deficit progressing in a stepwise fashion. Unlike PML, there may be temporary partial resolution of neurological deficit with high-dose steroids or pulse cytoxan therapy in patients with CNS vasculitis. Despite its rarity, diagnosis of CNS vasculitis is important because it is typically fatal if not aggressively treated with chronic systemic immunosuppression.

MS may occasionally present with prominent sensory complaints and marked, symmetrical weakness of the lower extremities and be mistakenly diagnosed as an acute demyelinative polyneuropathy (Guillain-Barre syndrome), although albumino-cytological dissociation is rarely found in MS.

Symptoms of MS must last at least 24 h. To be considered a new relapse, a new symptom or a relapse of a prior symptom must occur at least 1 mo after the previous exacerbation. The symptoms and findings should be associated with MS. Only a neurologist can diagnose MS (8–10).

PPMS is more difficult than other forms of MS to diagnosis. This form of MS presents most commonly in midlife (about 40 ± 5 yr on average) and distinguishing it from other potentially

Table 2
Differential Diagnosis of Multiple Sclerosis

Acquired Diseases

1. ADEM vs CIS (MS)
2. Infectious disease
     Syphilis
     Retroviral infection
       HIV
       HTLV–I/II
3. CNS vasculitis
     Granulomatous vasculitis (e.g., sarcoid, HIV)
     Primary CNS vasculitis
4. Autoimmune diseases (e.g., SLE)
5. Tumors of the CNS
6. Trauma to CNS
7. Psychiatric illness

Hereditary Diseases

1. Leukodystrophies
2. Spinocerebellar diseases
3. Hereditary spastic paraparesis

ADEM, acute disseminated encephalomyelitis; CIS, clinically isolated syndrome; MS, multiple sclerosis; HIV, human immunodeficiency virus; HTLV, human T-cell lymphotropic virus; CNS, central nervous system; SLE, systemic lupus erythematosus.

treatable illnesses may be extremely difficult *(7,16)*. Symptoms should be present for 6 mo before accepted as evidence of PPMS. Several other disorders must be ruled out of the differential diagnosis. Syphilis, vitamin B_{12} deficiency (subacute combined myelopathy) and retrovirus-associated myelopathy (HIV–associated myelopathy and human T-cell-leukemia-associated myelopathy) *(2,7,17)* can be easily ruled out by laboratory testing. Antibody testing by Western blot for HTLV-I/II, if negative, may not be insufficient. Genetic (polymerase chain reaction) testing in a reliable laboratory is the most sensitive and specific test for this purpose and is positive in up to 20% of antibody-negative patients infected with either HTLV-I/II virus, in our experience *(18)*. Radiation myelopathy continues to be an important differential diagnosis in patients with a history of radiation therapy to the head and neck.

Importantly, neuroimaging should be carried out to rule out spinal cord compression, congenital abnormalities, and intraparenchymal tumors. At times, imaging will not reveal the presence of one or more intraparenchymal spinal cord lesions discovered in clinical examination. The finding of hypothyroidism is common in MS, and myelopathy should not be attributed to thyroid disease alone. Adrenocortical leukodystrophy and hereditary spastic paraplegia are easily distinguished from PPMS by infantile age of presentation and presence of a family history *(2,19)*.

Repeated clinical visits and examinations, as well as repeated imaging, may clarify the nature of the illness in difficult cases. This is particularly important when cognitive and emotional issues dominate and obscure the presentation *(3,7)*. The McDonald criteria greatly assist early diagnosis and justify the institution of treatment. For the first time, the criteria now also include guidelines for establishing a diagnosis of PPMS. When using the criteria for patients with clinically isolated syndromes, the majority will be correctly diagnosed as having MS, but about 20% of patients may never meet criteria for a definite diagnosis. On the other hand, we regularly document relapses within weeks to months in many patients with clinically isolated syndromes who initially had no evidence of brain lesions in their MRI scans at clinical presentation. MS remains a clinical diagnosis *(10)*.

1.4. Prognosis

Exacerbation rates in patients with MS vary greatly but tend to diminish with increasing duration of illness *(12,13,20)*. When a patient has established disability, exacerbations do not appear to correlate with increasing disability *(12)*. Pregnancy has long been thought to decrease the risk of relapse, but this has only recently been proven in a large prospective French study *(22)*. The study also confirmed a long-recognized phenomenon of markedly increased risk of MS exacerbation for 3 mo postpartum. This study also showed that this risk continued at a somewhat lower level for the 33 mo of follow-up in the study. The importance of infection as a precipitating factor for exacerbations has long been recognized, and recent studies have provided further evidence *(23)*.

Emotional stress and its impact on MS has been the subject of a number of excellent studies *(24–27)*, which have consistently shown a correlation between major life stress and a significantly increased risk of exacerbation. In a remarkable recent study, Mohr et al. have demonstrated a correlation between stress, including "hassles," and the appearance of new active gadolinium-enhancing brain lesions *(27)*. The perception of stress, rather than a particular life event, is related to an increased risk of exacerbation *(24–27)*. Although other factors are thought to influence prognosis in MS patients, no similar studies have addressed them adequately.

Several neurologists at academic centers in the United States and elsewhere have concluded that the majority of patients with MS develop secondary progressive disease and then progress rapidly to disability. Confavreux et al. have published their studies of the natural history of a large population of French patients *(12)*. The French researchers have concluded that there is no relationship between relapses and progression, once disability is established. They have further concluded that only 30% of their relapsing–remitting patients had secondary progressive MS. Pittock et al. at Mayo Clinic recently published important observations of a 10-yr follow-up of the MS population from Olmsted County, Minnesota *(13)*. They also found that disability in the majority of their patients did not progress measurably during the observation period. Only 30% of their patients progressed to needing a cane or a wheelchair, and most patients remained stable despite the fact that only 15% had received immunomodulatory therapy. Thus, it is obvious that the perception that the vast majority of MS patients develop secondary progressive disease with rapid progression to serious disability is incorrect. The French group also found that longer periods of follow-up show that patients thought to have "benign MS" do develop some neurological impairment during 20 to 30 yr of follow-up.

1.5. Neuroimaging in Multiple Sclerosis

Computed tomography (CT) neuroimaging for the first time revealed areas of decreased radio density in the brain, as well as occasional enhancing brain and spinal cord lesions, in MS. Interestingly, the MS community largely ignored increasing brain atrophy, although it was reported early *(28–30)*. Comparative studies of CT and MRI revealed the relative strength of the latter test in MS *(32,33)*. In contrast to the limitations encountered with CT, MRI has had an important impact on both the diagnosis and subsequent management of MS because of the relative ease with which it can detect white-matter lesions in the brain and spinal cord.

Investigators have sought brain MRI correlations with clinical symptoms of MS, prognosis of the illness, other laboratory findings, as well as with CNS pathology. Increased T2-weighted signals, reflecting increases in water content of white-matter lesions, were emphasized in earlier studies, but their presence correlates poorly with symptoms and neurological findings (Fig. 1A). Very early in the course of clinical disease, we found that only half of patients with clinically definite MS had cerebral white-matter lesions *(32,34)*, although almost half of those who did not have plaques in their brains exhibited spinal cord lesions that were clearly evident *(35)*. Even though not all CSF had diagnostic abnormalities, only 5% of patients did not have either brain MRI abnormality or significant CSF abnormality. In part, the difficulty with the MRI findings was related to technical issues, such as image slice thickness and noncontiguous sections.

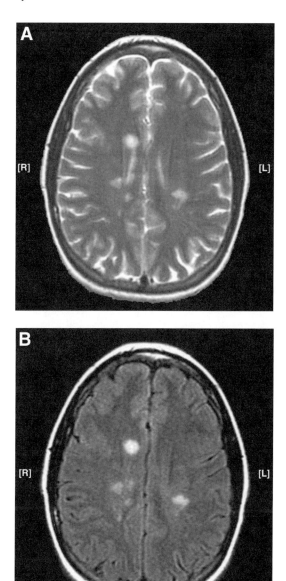

Fig. 1. MRI scans of the brain of a 19-yr-old woman with relapsing–remitting multiple sclerosis. Axial T2-weighted (**A**) and fluid-attenuated inversion recovery (**B**) views show hyperintense lesions in subcortical white matter. Axial T1-weighted postcontrast (**C**) of the same patient reveals an enhancing lesion, indicating the breakdown of the blood–brain barrier.

Advances in hardware and software have made practicable the use of fluid attenuated inversion recovery) sequences, which are easier to visualize (Fig. 1B). Newer acquisition paradigms and the use of gadolinium to identify active inflammatory lesions, in particular, as well as continued hardware improvements, have remarkably improved the quality and utility of MRI.

Because all patients with MS, particularly those with primary progressive disease, do not exhibit white-matter lesions in their cerebral hemispheres, the absence of MRI abnormality does

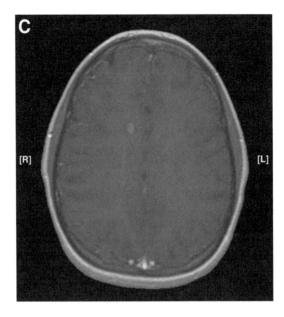

Fig. 1. *(Continued).*

not negate the diagnosis of MS *(10)*. We have found that after 9 to 12 yr the same proportion of MS patients will have white-matter lesions evidenced by MRI and pathology *(32,34)*.

A strong correlation between increased volume of cerebral MRI T2-weighted signals and long-term disability in MS has been reported in patients followed for 5 yr after the onset of a clinically isolated syndrome, although further follow-up of this cohort has shown only a moderate correlation at 10 yr *(35)*. A number of short-term correlations have been shown between stabilization or reduction of T2-weighted volumes and clinical stabilization in patients treated with each of the approved immunomodulatory drugs (*see* Section 3.). General experience follows these observations. After the initial 5 yr of illness, with some notable exceptions, changes from one year to the next are difficult to see in brain MRI scans. Clearly, there must be some reservation about the use of T2-weighted lesion volumes for assessment of any form of long-term treatment.

Gadolinium enhancement of white-matter lesions is an accepted indicator of active disease, but enhancing lesions are seen several times more often than acute exacerbations of illness in MS (Fig. 1C). This surrogate measure of disease activity has been used effectively in preliminary drug efficacy studies to detect a treatment effect. Despite the earlier negative reports, Leist et al. reported a correlation between gadolinium-enhancing lesions and the subsequent appearance of cerebral atrophy *(36)*. Unlike the earlier studies that found no correlation, this NIH study was based on frequent (monthly) gadolinium-enhanced brain MRI studies.

Although T1-weighted hypointensities have been a focus of interest more recently and have been reported to correlate with cerebral atrophy, other studies have shown that this type MRI lesion does not correlate well with either the amount of demyelination or gliosis in tissue lesions. This lack of correlation with tissue changes makes it difficult to understand and accept these observations at face value *(37)*. Importantly, De Stefano et al. have reported data supporting a role between evidence of early axonal damage and the subsequent development of disability in MS *(38)*. The value of MR spectroscopy remains under investigation. Although there have been many conflicting claims, it is obvious that MRI is especially helpful in the evaluation of patients early in the course of their illness. Unfortunately, the usefulness of MRI or other surrogate measures to evaluate the long-term response to treatment remains essentially unanswered. Thus, cerebral atrophy may be the most valuable measure.

1.6. Other Laboratory Measures

1.6.1. Cerebrospinal Fluid

CSF analysis can be helpful if performed in a specialty laboratory. Increased intrathecal immunoglobulin-G (IgG) synthesis, measurement of the increase in the proportion of γ-globulin by CSF electrophoresis, and the presence of CSF oligoclonal bands increases the likelihood of a diagnosis of MS *(7–10)*.

1.6.2. Evoked-Response Testing

Visual evoked responses carried out in an established laboratory also can be helpful in making a diagnosis *(10)*. Other evoked responses, brainstem and somatosensory, can be abnormal in MS, as well as in other diseases, and the studies are technically more difficult. For example, spinocerebellar degenerations often had marked abnormal auditory evoked potentials.

1.7. Epidemiology

To yield useful data, epidemiological studies must be performed by trained personnel in large populations with good access to good medical care. Several good studies have been performed, and there is evidence indicating that incidence rates for MS may be increasing.

1.7.1. Age and Sex Distribution

Relapsing–remitting MS is more common in women than men. About 70% of all patients in most recently studied populations, including our large southern population, had this variation, with onset of illness in both sexes occurring by the age of 30 in two-thirds of patients *(7)*. PPMS is slightly more common in men than women and typically begins in midlife.

1.7.2. Incidence of Multiple Sclerosis

Incidence is the rate of occurrence of newly diagnosed cases (i.e., MS) per unit of population (usually described per million) per time period and is usually reported on an annual basis. The incidence of MS is relatively low (1–5 per million) but seems to have increased during the last century *(7)*. In the United States, the most useful current data comes from Olmsted County, Minnesota, where the incidence rate has increased during the last century from two per million to three times that figure *(7)*.

A number of confounding factors influence incidence figures. Over the last half century, there has been a dramatic increase in the number of trained neurologists. With the advent of effective therapies, more neurologists are interested in MS and are trained in this subspecialty. Consistent, easily interpreted diagnostic criteria and improved diagnostic testing (especially MRI) have greatly facilitated MS diagnosis. Undoubtedly, these factors partly account for the apparent increased incidence of MS. Additionally, neuropathologists have found that 1 to 2% of postmortem examinations reveal tissue evidence of demyelinating disease in the absence of a clinical history *(40)*. It is possible that with the increasing availability of neurologists, the increasing awareness of MS, and the improved diagnostic facilities available, many cases that were undiagnosed in the past would now be labeled as MS.

Despite the low incidence of MS, this illness is the most common cause of chronic disability in young adults because of its currently minimal impact on longevity. The observations in Olmsted County clearly indicate a real increase in the incidence, as well as prevalence, of MS *(10)*.

It is often stated that there are 250,000 to 350,000 patients in the United States *(7)*, although these figures are not based on any current national epidemiological studies. When prevalence figures were reported to be low in the southern United States, there were not any neurologists in the area, for practical purposes. In Florida, for example, the first neurologist established a practice in 1953 but then entered military service. The appearance of neurologists in the south, as in virtually all under-serviced communities in the United States, is bound to have had a dramatic impact on the recognition and diagnosis of nervous system diseases, especially MS.

The impact of MRI on the recognition of neurological disease, especially MS, has been dramatic. Considering the increased availability of neurological consultation, improved diagnostic criteria, and the availability to MRI and improved CSF examination, it is likely that more patients will be recognized with MS later in life. Thus, prevalence rates of MS may be unrealistically low.

1.8. Pathology of Multiple Sclerosis

Charcot recognized as the cardinal features of MS *multiple* areas of discoloration and hardness (*sclerosis*) scattered throughout the brain and spinal cord, which he termed *plaques* (plate-like); hence, the he diagnosed *sclerose en plaque*, or multiple sclerosis (1). By microscopy, Charcot found that plaques exhibited loss of myelin with relative sparing of axons and varying amounts of gliotic scarring. He also described the presence of inflammatory cells, including large numbers of fat-laden cells. The demyelinated plaque remains the pathological hallmark of this disease (41).

Early in the disease, small plaques are prominent in subcortical white matter (42), but, in the usual necropsy material obtained after many years of disease, large coalesced plaques are predominantly periventricular (41–45). No regular association between MS plaques and blood vessels was observed by Adams and Kubik (43) or Zimmerman and Netsky (44). Subsequently, however, Lampert (45) and others performed whole-brain serial sections of a number of cases, including those previously studied, and reported that brain plaques were invariably perivenular (45). Although oligodendrocyte loss had earlier been reported as a major feature of MS (43,44), study of whole-brain serial sections did not reveal this as a consistent feature (45). Another important finding is that so-called *shadow plaques* seen at the white-matter cortical junction are actually areas of remyelination rather than areas of incomplete demyelination, as had been previously thought (41).

Recently, the neuropathology of MS has been revisited (46–48), and a new view of the histopathology of MS has emerged based on a study of 51 biopsies and 37 autopsies. A central role for CD4$^+$ T cells and macrophages in the immunopathogenesis of MS lesions seemed to have been well established (Fig. 2A) (47); however, Luchinetti et al. suggested four different types of neuropathology in MS, pointing to a predominant role for CD3$^+$ cells and macrophages in type 1, with antibody-mediated demyelination added in type 2, and to loss of oligodendrocytes in types 3 and 4 (49).

In type 1, in patients from whom tissue samples were obtained very early, prominent perivascular infiltrates composed of CD3$^+$ cells and macrophages were present without antibody (IgG) or complement. In type 2, a similar perivascular picture was seen, except that IgG and complement, without cells, were seen at the edges of active demyelination. Although prominent loss of myelin basic protein (MBP) and myelin-associated glycoprotein was found, remyelination was reported to be prominent in types 1 and 2. In types 3 and 4, oligodendrocyte loss was prominent, raising the question of primary oligodendrocyte pathology. Plaques were poorly defined and not related to vessels. Additionally, the authors reported that CD3$^+$ (T) cells and macrophages were present in all four types of MS pathology included in their classification, a finding consistent with other recent analysis of lesions (49). Luchinetti et al.'s findings that tissue obtained from a small number of patients studied shortly after onset of illness revealed prominent CD3$^+$ and macrophage cellular infiltrates but lacked antibody (type 1) are reminiscent of Lumsden's findings of patients who died early in the course of their illness (42). Type 2, in which antibody is present in lesions, is seen at necropsy with some frequency and resembles changes seen in chronic relapsing forms of experimental autoimmune encephalomyelitis (EAE). In EAE, the initial cellular infiltrate initially is composed primarily of CD4$^+$ cells, but eventually much larger numbers of macrophages, which induce the damage to myelin and oligodendrocytes, begin to appear (50).

Despite the impressive amount of research Lunichetti et al.'s research encompasses (49), the observations that the pathology of MS in a proportion of cases may consist of oligodendrocyte loss, with pathology not associated with blood vessels, raises questions. The numbers of cases were relatively small and many were biopsy specimens, in which sampling necessarily was limited and, most

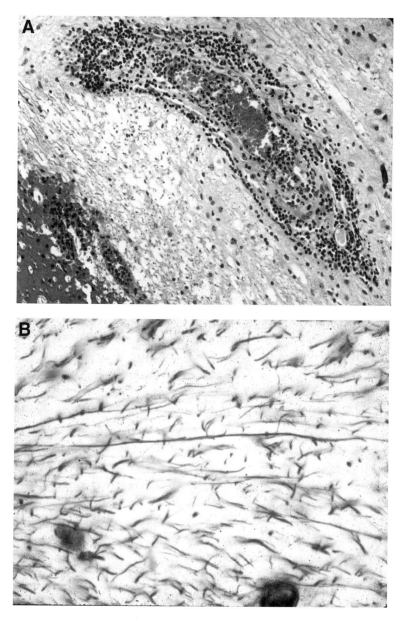

Fig. 2. Biopsy of a large left frontal lobe plaque from a 29-yr-old woman with new onset multiple sclerosis with recurrent right hemiparesis during 3 mo and new mild speech difficulty. **(A)** Specimen is stained with luxol fast blue and counterstained with eosin. Visible is a new active plaque, which is not sharply demarcated but exhibits prominent perivascular cellularity with varying myelin damage and relative sparing of axons. The inflammatory infiltrate is composed of lymphocytes (predominantly CD4+ Th1 cells) and a large number of macrophages. These cells are predominantly of hematogenous origin and are considered the perpetrators of tissue damage. These features are in contrast to chronic or inactive plaques, which exhibit relatively few or no inflammatory cells but contain prominent myelin damage and gliosis. Axonal loss may be prominent. **(B)** Specimen is stained with luxol fast blue and counterstained with eosin. Higher power view shows loss of axons and more prominent myelin loss. Note that preserved axons exhibit variable loss of myelin.

importantly, was not based on study of whole-brain serial sections. Considering the past contributions of Lampert *(45)*, these conclusions should be considered preliminary. Poser has raised other questions about type I pathology *(51)*.

2. PATHOGENESIS OF MULTIPLE SCLEROSIS

2.1. Genetics

A large MS database in Vancouver, Canada and our large database reveal a 20% familial incidence. The Canadian twin study shows a concordance of more than 31%, similar to findings in other twin studies *(52)*. Mothers confer a 20- to 40-times increased risk to their children, and the risk is greater for girls than boys. Other first-degree relatives also have a much increased risk of MS *(53)*.

Several genes are more common in MS than in population controls, principally at the major histocompatibility (MHC) gene locus located on chromosome 6. Jersild et al. found that the alleles A3, B7, and DR2 (15) occurred twice as commonly in patients with MS, compared to the unaffected population. They observed that patients who possessed both human leukocyte antigen (HLA)-B7 and DR2 had particularly severe disease *(54)*. Many genes important in normal immune function and immune-mediated tissue damage, such as tumor necrosis factor (TNF), are located in the region between HLA-B7 and the DR locus. Several mutations of genes residing in this area are under investigation. An important study looking for single nucleotide polymorphisms, modeled on a Crohn's disease study, is currently under way as part of the human genome project. As yet there is no single gene, or combination of genes, implicated in the risk of MS.

Population migration studies have suggested the presence of an environmental factor. Although viral infection is generally implicated as the factor, no evidence of a specific virus's role in MS has been produced *(7)*.

2.2. Myelin Biochemistry

The genetic basis of a number of leukodystrophies has been firmly established. Of these disorders, the most common are adrenocortical leukodystrophy and metachromatic leukodystrophy. At one time, both were considered to have some relationship to MS *(2,7)*. Of some importance is Marburg's disease, sometimes referred to as *acute MS*, which has been attributed to a defect in MBP synthesis and structure *(55)*. Work on alterations of the three-dimensional structure of MBP and its relationship to various demyelinating disease is continuing. Interestingly, several mutations of myelin's proteolipid are causative of Pelizaeus-Merzbacher disease, as well as several types of hereditary spastic paraparesis. These leukodystrophies ordinarily should not be confused with MS because of their early age of presentation, their inexorably progressive course, and their familial setting.

2.3. Immunology

MS is now generally accepted as an immune-mediated illness, although its pathogenesis is incompletely understood. The occurrence of MS following about one-third of acute disseminated encephalomyelitis-complicating infections *(56–58)*, as well as after immunizations (including Semple vaccine, which contains spinal cord and killed virus), suggested an autoimmune origin. Although EAE has been studied in animal models for decades as a means of understanding the nature of the immune response *(59)*, these studies have also provided insight into the pathogenesis of MS. Transfer of EAE from immunized to naive animals was first successfully accomplished using lymph node cells, thus pointing to a central role for lymphocytes *(59)*. Nevertheless, antibody from immunized animals and patients with MS can induce demyelination in vitro *(60,61)*.

More recently, attention has centered on the primary role of T cells in the pathogenesis of EAE, regardless of the nervous system antigen used to induce disease *(62,63)*. There is a consensus that

T cells are the primary effectors both in MS and EAE *(63)*, although B cells, plasma cells, and antibody can be found both in EAE pathology and MS plaques *(48,49)*. Despite emphasizing other findings, these recent studies of MS pathology show that the predominant cells in active lesions are lymphocytes, particularly CD3$^+$ T cells, and macrophages *(49)*.

In early studies, multiple injections of whole spinal cord were used to induce EAE, but single immunizations of equivalent amounts of purified myelin or MBP combined with adjuvants were shown to be very effective in disease induction *(63)*. Myelin proteins other than MBP have also been investigated, notably proteolipid and myelin-oligodendrocyte glycoprotein (MOG). Proteolipid protein can induce forms of experimental disease in animal models and, although antibody as well as T cells reactive to this antigen may be present in plaques, no role for sensitization to this antigen has been established *(63)*. An interesting model using MOG to induce EAE in marmosets indicates that antibody may mediate demyelination *(64,65)*. Passive transfer of the disease by serum from sensitized animals has also been accomplished *(65)*. T cells (CD4$^+$ T helper [Th]2, rather than CD4$^+$ Th1 cells) may be the primary mediators of myelin damage in MOG-sensitized marmosets *(65)*. The situation is complicated by the fact that MBP-reactive CD4$^+$ cells capable of inducing EAE are present in naive animals, as well as in immunized animals, coincidently with anti-MOG antibody *(65)*. Anti-MOG antibody has been reported at the outset of MS and is common in relapsing MS *(66,67)*. Whereas anti-MOG antibody are limited to MS relapse, MOG-reactive CD4$^+$ cells are ubiquitous *(68)*.

When antigen is presented to T cells by MHC class I- or MHC class II antigen-presenting cells (APC), an immune response is initiated; either antibody production or a cellular immune response occurs. Activated CD4$^+$ cells fall into two functionally distinct classes, Th1 and Th2, each with distinctive lymphokine-production profiles. Following antigenic stimulation, Th1 cells, which are also called CD4$^+$ Th1 cells, produce interleukin (IL)-1, IL-2, interferon (IFN)-γ, and TNF-α and mediate inflammatory pathological processes in immune-mediated tissue damage seen in MS and EAE *(69)*. In contrast, Th2 cells produce IL-4, IL-5, IL-6, and IL-10 and induce upregulation of antibody production and downregulation of Th1 cellular responses (Fig. 3) *(69)*.

Macrophages are the principal sources of IL-1, IL-12 and TNF-α and are driven by IL-2 production from antigen-activated CD4$^+$ cells. Importantly, IL-12 production is IFN-γ dependant and TNF-α production is IL-12 dependent *(70)*. Not only are macrophages the principal APC but also they are central effector cells in cell-mediated immunity. After antigen presentation, CD4$^+$ cells undergo clonal proliferation and recruit other CD4$^+$ cells to participate in the initiation of cellular immune responses. Cytotoxic CD8$^+$ cells driven by IL-12 may exert their effect directly or target antigen-complexed antibody on target tissue (i.e., antibody-dependent cytotoxicity) *(63,71)*. Macrophages may also target these complexes. The spectrum of CD4$^+$ Th2 responses includes regulating the switch from CD8$^+$ cell cytotoxic function to active suppression of CD4$^+$ Th1 responses, creating *suppressor T cells*. In the CNS, microglial cells can function as APC and exhibit certain other macrophage behaviors.

The BBB is a physical barrier that prevents intravascular cellular elements, antibodies, and other proteins from having free access to the brain and spinal cord *(72)*. The endothelial cells in the brain and spinal cord possess tight junctions that are impervious to intravascular fluids, as well as to nonactivated cells. These endothelial cells are also surrounded by astrocytic foot processes, which further support and maintain the integrity of the BBB. Although activated CD4$^+$ cells do cross the BBB *(72–78)*, the BBB is an actual physical barrier that may be breached only in an organized and well–orchestrated fashion *(72,77,78)*. The mechanisms of cellular transmigration across the BBB are now well understood *(72–78)*.

2.4. Adhesion Molecules

Venules control CD4$^+$ and other cell migration from blood into the nervous system. Attachment requires cellular adhesion molecules and endothelial counterreceptors to overcome the considerable

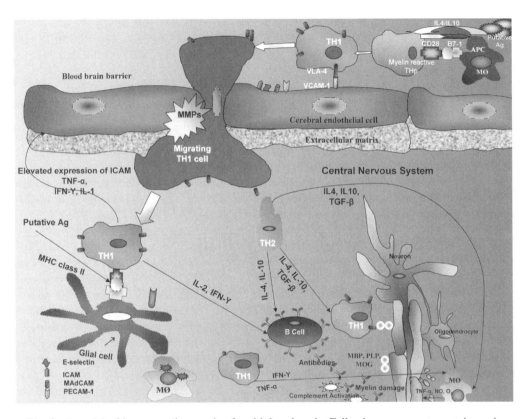

Fig. 3. A model of immunopathogenesis of multiple sclerosis. Following exposure to certain environmental antigen(s) in genetically susceptible individuals, myelin-reactive T cells migrate from peripheral circulation to the central nervous system. Interaction between activated T cell and cerebral endothelial cells leads to upregulation of the adhesion molecules (E-selectin, vascular cell adhesion molecule, intercellular adhesion molecule, mucosal addressin cell adhesion molecule, and platelet endothelial cells adhesion molecule. Transendothelial migration of reactive T cells is heralded by the disruption of the blood–brain barrier, which is in part mediated by the activities of the matrix metalloproteinases (MMPs). MMPs digest extracellular matrix and facilitate migration of the activated T cells. Proinflammatory cytokines released by the activated T cells (such as tumor necrosis factor-α and interferon-γ) upregulate the expression of cell-surface molecules on antigen-presenting cells (in this figure, glial cell). Binding of putative multiple sclerosis antigen (e.g., myelin basic protein and myelin oligodendrocyte glycoprotein by the trimolecular complex T cell receptor and class II major histocompatibility molecules on the antigen presenting cells precipitates a massive inflammatory cascade, which leads to production of both pro- and anti-inflammatory cytokines. This inflammatory reaction ultimately results in loss of myelin-oligodendrocyte complexes.

shear stresses produced by blood flow. Adhesion molecules on CD4+ cells and macrophages are functional anchors that form stable bonds with their ligands on the vascular wall. In addition to functioning as mechanical anchors, adhesion molecules are tissue-specific recognition molecules *(72–78)*.

Entry of CD4+ cells and macrophages into the CNS is accomplished by a series of steps, including tethering or rolling, adhesion (binding), and finally transendothelial migration across the BBB *(73–78)*. Subsequent to their egress, they migrate through the extracellular matrix in the CNS. Selectins mediate the initial step of tethering, which leads to rolling *(78–80)*, but selectin-mediated bonds are reversible. To arrest these cells on the endothelium, these low-affinity interactions must be supplemented by high-affinity adhesion molecules, the integrins *(80,81)*. The integrins, including α4β1-integrin (VLA-4), are members of the endothelial immunoglobulin superfamily *(81,82)*. The predominant function of the β2- integrin leukocyte function antigen (LFA)-1 and α4 integrins (integrin-α4β1/VLA-4) is to bind the cells to their ligands' intercellular adhesion molecule (ICAM)-1 and vascular cell adhesion molecule (VCAM)-1 *(80–82)*

Selectins expressed on leukocytes (P-selectin and L-selectin) and endothelium (E-selectin) results in rolling and slowing of the cells. P-selectin and its ligand PECAM-1 appear to have a special role in EAE and MS *(83,84)*. In contrast, L-selectin has a primary role in lymphocyte recruitment for lymphoid tissues. As cells roll and are slowed by the interaction of selectins and their ligands, they respond to endothelial cell chemokines.

Specific chemokines are fixed on the endothelial surface and are molecular signals that direct cells to tissues and confer organ specificity with specific adhesion molecules *(77)*. Chemokines are divided into four families, which are specific for different T-cell subgroups *(77)*. Distinctive chemokine receptors on Th1 cells include CCR5 and CXCR3. In MS and rheumatoid arthritis, all of the infiltrating Th1 cells express these chemokine receptors *(85)*. They have a central role in the egress of specific lymphocyte subgroups into specific target organs. Selectin binding to ligand is an activating signal that induces rapid activation of α4 integrins and β2 integrins *(80–82)*.

Integrins are a large family of cell-surface glycoproteins that mediate intercellular interactions and interactions with matrix protein *(75–78)*. They possess high affinity for their ligands, ICAM-1 and VCAM-1 *(79,80)*. Under inflammatory conditions, the integrin heterodimers adopt a high-affinity open molecular conformation and can mediate activation-independent rolling interactions, as well as arrest rolling leukocytes. In MS, the integrins responsible for leukocyte binding are LFA-1, also referred to as *CD11aCD18* and α4β1 *integrins* (VLA-4). In the CNS, α4β1 is of primary importance because VCAM-1 is expressed on CNS at low levels on nonactivated endothelium and at high levels on activated endothelium *(73,86,87)*.

2.4.1. Adhesion Molecules in EAE

Yednock established that the α4β1-integrin molecule has a key role in antigen-specific CD4[+] cell entry into the CNS in EAE *(73)*. A murine monoclonal antibody (MAb) to α4β1 integrin prevented migration of CD4[+] cells into the CNS in the guinea pig EAE model. This anti-α4 integrin MAb also suppressed and reversed inflammatory demyelination in EAE *(86)*. These studies established that the development of demyelinating lesions in EAE is entirely α4β1-integrin dependent *(73,86,87)*.

More recently, a number of small molecules have been studied with demonstrated efficacy in blocking integrins LFA-1 and VLA-4 from binding with their ligands ICAM-1 and VCAM-1 in vitro and in vivo *(88–90)*. Canella et al. investigated a synthetic small, nonpeptide molecule antagonist of integrin $\alpha_4\beta_1$, (TBC 3486) in the SJL mouse relapsing EAE model *(90)*. TBC 3486 had previously been shown to inhibit binding of integrin $\alpha_4\beta_1$ to the connecting segment-1 (CS-1) of fibronectin. CS-1 binds to both VLA-4 and VCAM-1 *(91)*. Clinical benefit has been documented in models of arthritis and pulmonary inflammation *(92)*. Daily administration of TBC 3486 in EAE for 14 d markedly delayed onset of acute EAE. In the chronic relapsing EAE disease model, it prevented relapse *(92)*. A reduction in the clinical severity of disease was seen, and severity of demyelination in the lesions reduced. Immunocytochemistry and Western blot assays of CNS tissue showed that acutely treated animals demonstrated a shift from a Th1-type proinflammatory cytokine profile toward a Th2-type cytokine profile.

Evidence shows that the $\alpha_4\beta_1$-integrin molecule may have a pivotal role in the pathogenesis of EAE and MS because of its crucial function in transendothelial migration of myelin-specific CD4[+] T lymphocytes into the CNS *(77,78)*. The molecule has also been implicated in the interactions between MBP-primed T lymphocytes and microglial cells *(93,94)*. Studies have examined the following:

1. The role of MBP-primed T lymphocytes.
2. The release of nitric oxide (NO).
3. The expression of the inducible form of NO synthase (iNOS) protein.
4. mRNA in mouse BV-2 microglial cells *(93)*.

The investigators reported that an anti-α_4 chain MAb of the of $\alpha_4\beta_1$ integrin blocked expression of the $\alpha_4\beta_1$ integrin adhesion molecule on the surface of the MBP-primed T lymphocytes. MAb treatment also blocked microglial NO production. Within the context of the experimental paradigm, $\alpha_4\beta_1$ integrin appeared to function as a regulator of cell–cell contact-mediated induction of iNOS. The investigators' subsequent research provided evidence that MBP-primed T lymphocytes modulate expression of proinflammatory cytokines in microglial cells *(95)*. These MBP-primed T lymphocytes express $\alpha_4\beta_1$-integrin on their surface. Functional blocking of these adhesion molecules by the same anti-α_4 chain MAb inhibited T-lymphocyte induction of microglial proinflammatory cytokines.

There has been great interest in lovastatin, a commercially available cholesterol-lowering statin that has the ability to modulate LFA-1 expression in animals and humans *(96,97)*. The investigators researched TNF-α and NO expression in EAE, studying expression in macrophages and brain. Treatment with lovastatin resulted in a lymphokine shift with treatment, indicating a switch from Th1 to Th2 cellular function. A preliminary study using lovasatin in MS recently been reported a reduction in the number of gadolinium-enhancing lesions in MRI scans after 6 mo of treatment, as compared to pretreatment *(98)*.

A new intervention involves in vivo blockade of the lymphokine macrophage migration inhibitory factor (MIF) by anti-MIF MAb in an EAE model employing sensitization to PL in SJL mice. Treatment with the anti-MIF MAb decreased the size of the clone of Th1 cells and impaired homing of neuroreactive Th1 cells to the CNS by blocking the expression of VCAM. Treatment also reduced the severity of acute EAE and accelerated recovery *(99)*.

We studied MIF intensively in MS several years ago and showed production of this lymphokine after peripheral blood lymphocytes were stimulated with MBP. Production of MIF correlated well with acute exacerbations of disease *(100,101)*. Indeed, production of MIF in serially studied patients was increased up to 3 wk prior to and during clinically identified exacerbations *(102)*. In contrast, serum antibody to MBP correlated inversely with the appearance of MIF production. Antibody to MBP was not seen at the onset of exacerbations but only during convalescence and disappeared with full recovery, suggesting the presence of antibody correlated with a Th2 response *(103,104)*. Although in unpublished studies we found antibody to proteolipid protein (PLP) of myelin in MS, we did not discover a correlation with clinical activity, and the same low frequency of antibody in MS was seen in other neurological diseases. Perhaps we can anticipate future clinical trials of a humanized version of the anti-MIF MAb in MS.

2.4.2. Adhesion Molecules in Multiple Sclerosis

The central role of $\alpha_4\beta_1$-integrin found in EAE *(73,86,87)* led to an intense interest in the importance of adhesion molecules in human autoimmune disease, including MS. A decrease in $\alpha_4\beta_1$-integrin expression on CD3$^+$ lymphocytes after INF-β1b (Betaseron®) treatment was reported in MS patients *(105)*. Another study implemented monthly contrast-enhanced MRI 2 mo prior to initiation of treatment and through 3 mo of IFN-β1b treatment. Results showed a reduction of MRI activity with IFN-β1b treatment in MS patients that correlated with decreased integrin expression on lymphocytes *(106)*. The MRI results correlated closely with laboratory evidence of downregulation of $\alpha_4\beta_1$-integrin expression on CD4$^+$ and CD8$^+$/CD54RO$^+$ "memory" cells. Expression of $\alpha4\beta1$-integrin appeared to modulate differentially the proportion of CD4$^+$, CD8$^+$, and CD27$^+$ T lymphocytes *(106)*. The observed effect of IFN-β1b on MRI activity was not unexpected because of IFN-β1b's demonstrated ability to downregulate of metalloproteinases *(107)*.

Commonly used to treat acute exacerbations of MS, intravenous methylprednisolone reportedly reduces upregulation of soluble VLA-4, LFA-1, VCAM-1, and ICAM-1 adhesion molecules in blood and CSF in relapsing–remitting and secondary progressive MS *(108)*. An in vitro study also showed that methylprednisolone decreased transmigration of peripheral blood mononuclear cells through a cerebral endothelial cell layer *(109)*. Sustained downregulation of in vitro soluble adhesion molecules and clinical benefits from steroid administration, comparable to that of IFN-β1b in MS, has not been reported. Should chronic use of intravenous high-dose methylprednisolone produce sustained downregulation of adhesion molecules in MS, apart from existing concerns, caution should be exercised since methylprednisolone has recently been reported to induce neuronal apoptosis *(110)*. Stated otherwise, methylprednisolone does not have any neuroprotective effect; rather, it appears to have neurotoxic properties.

2.5. MS Treatment Trials With Adhesion Molecule Modulators

2.5.1. Natalizumab Clinical Trials

Natalizumab (Antegren®) is converted from murine MAb to human $\alpha_4\beta_1$-integrin humanized by grafting the complementary determining portion of the hypervariable region of the murine antibody-encoding gene onto a human immunoglobulin G4 framework *(73)*. As mentioned above, treatment of guinea pig EAE with either the murine parent AN100226m or natalizumab, the humanized molecule, results in a dose-dependent reversal of clinical manifestations and leukocyte infiltration of the nervous system *(73,86)*.

Also previously mentioned, in EAE and, by inference, in inflammatory human nervous system diseases such as MS, trafficking of leukocytes across the BBB requires the binding of the adhesion molecule α4β1-integrin (VLA-4) found on lymphocytes and monocytes with its ligand VCAM-1 on the endothelial surface. The blockade of VLA-4 to VCAM-1 binding prevents trafficking of leukocytes into the brain and spinal cord.

Natalizumab, the humanized anti-α4-integrin antibody, has been shown to be safe and well tolerated in a phase I, randomized, placebo-controlled, five-level dose escalation safety and tolerability study. Twenty-eight MS patients received single intravenous doses of natalizumab *(111)*. The drug was found to have a long half-life with sustained plasma levels and good receptor saturation at 28 d. Detectable serum level of the drug was present 8 wk after a single 3 mg/kg injection *(111)*. Two subsequent studies have also shown that the drug is safe and well tolerated in stable relapsing–remitting patients *(112,115)*, and another study demonstrated its effect on acute relapse in relapsing–remitting and secondary progressive patients *(114)*.

A study of MRI lesion activity after two successive monthly intravenous doses of natalizumab was carried out in 72 patients who had active relapsing–remitting and secondary progressive MS. Serial MRI studies were performed and patients were examined monthly for 24 wk. The treated group exhibited significantly fewer new active lesions (1.8) than the placebo group (3) during the first 12 wk, a time when the drug was present in the serum. This benefit seen in the MRI studies was lost in the subsequent 12 wk of the study. A rebound increase in clinical exacerbations was suspected after the benefit from drug infusions had ended *(112)*; however, a 1-yr-long follow-up of our patients from the pharmacokinetic study did not reveal any evidence of a clinical rebound effect following drug administration *(113)*. On the contrary, our patients appeared to have fewer relapses than they had prior to participating in the study.

We hypothesized that natalizumab administration within 36 to 72 h of onset of an MS relapse should accelerate clinical recovery. We expected if continued entry of activated T cells and macrophages into the nervous system were prevented, active plaques would regress and new plaque formation would stop. Concordantly, we predicted cessation of new gadolinium-enhancing brain lesions in brain MRI studies and an acceleration of clinical recovery.

However, the study failed to meet its primary objective. A multicenter, randomized, placebo-controlled, double-blind study of a single intravenous dose of natalizumab administered within 72 h of an exacerbation failed to show an enhanced rate of recovery from exacerbations. As measured by serial Expanded Disability Status Scale and Scripps neurological rating scores, no difference in clinical recovery between natalizumab vs. placebo treatment groups was found *(114)*. Using a visual analog scale, active drug recipients vs placebo did report a "significant" improvement in their sense of well-being. Most importantly, the MRI studies showed a marked inhibition of new T1-weighted gadolinium-enhancing lesion formation during a 14-wk period following treatment *(114)*.

Miller et al. reported a salutary outcome of a multicenter, double-blind, randomized, natalizumab trial of 213 patients with relapsing–remitting or relapsing secondary progressive MS *(115)*. One-third of the study group received 3 mg/kg intravenous natalizumab, one-third 6 mg/kg, and one-third placebo every 28 d for 6 mo. The study's primary end-point was the number of new lesions in monthly gadolinium-enhanced brain MRI. A marked 91% reduction in the mean number of new lesions was seen over 6 mo of treatment in the natalizumab recipients compared with those who received placebo. A subsequent analysis of black-hole formation has shown that active treatment significantly reduced the occurrence of black holes *(116)*. Other secondary outcomes included the number of clinical relapses and self-reporting of well-being using the same visual analog scale as our study employed. Importantly, although the study was not powered to predict such a reduction, the patients in the natalizumab groups experienced a significant 50% lower relapse rate. As seen in the prior relapse treatment study, the study participants reported an improved sense of well-being compared to those who received placebo. Relying on study-defined exacerbations, this reduction was even greater. Remarkably, no significant incidence of adverse experiences was seen in the treatment groups as compared with placebo. There was some indication of a greater risk of urinary tract infections, headache, and fatigue.

Two large phase III studies of natalizumab in MS are presently nearing completion. No new safety concerns have arisen in MS patients. Outcomes for relapse rates at the 52-wk time point of the study have led to early submission for FDA approval. Natalizumab (Tysabri®, previously named Antegren®) was approved in May 2004 for relapse reduction in multiple sclerosis. Approval was based on the first-year results of two large ongoing clinical trials. In both trials, neurological evaluations were performed every 12 wk at the time of suspected relapse. MRI studies were performed annually. The AFFIRM trial (942 patients), where active Tysabri treatment (627 patients) was compared with placebo (315 patents), revealed a 66% reduction of relapses for patients treated with a fixed dose (300 mg) every 4 wk vs placebo. The SENTINEL trial was comprised of Avonex® treatment failures (1171 patients) where Avonex (582 patients) was compared to Avonex plus Tysabri (589 patients). A 54% reduction in relapses with combined drug treatment vs Avonex® was documented. One explanation for the difference in outcomes may be that patients in the second trial were older, had a longer duration of illness, and had more disability. These are all factors associated with a less favorable prognosis. The impressive results achieved in the first year of the study were associated with a favorable safety profile. However, hypersensitivity reactions occurred in 1.4% of the Tysabri-treated patients, but severe reactions such as anaphylaxis occurred in less than 1%. Symptoms associated with these reactions included urticaria, dizziness, fever, rash, rigors, pruritus, nausea, flushing, hypotension, dyspnea, and chest pain. The impact of Tysabri on prevention of sustained disability, the primary outcome from the year 2 data sets is eagerly anticipated.

2.5.2. Lovastatin Clinical Trial

The first clinical trial employing a statin in MS treatment has just been published. The rationale of the study was that statins suppress LFA-1 expression and have had salutary results in EAE. Commercially available lovastatin was administered to 30 study participants in an 80-mg oral daily dosage for 6 mo in a single-armed study. The primary outcome measure was the number of gadolinium-enhancing lesions at 4, 5, and 6 mo of treatment vs pretreatment. MRI studies were enumerated by blinded readers to obtain preliminary efficacy results. Significantly fewer lesions and smaller lesion volumes were found with treatment. There was no change in Th1- and Th2-type cytokines during the course of treatment. Two subjects had increases in liver enzymes, one had an increase in creatine kinase, and two subjects did not complete the study. Based on the outcome of this clinical study, further drug trials can be anticipated.

2.5.3. Other Clinical Trials

A current complete listing of treatment and other clinical trials can be obtained from the National Multiple Sclerosis website. Two clinical phase II trials are now underway for anti-IL12 MAb. No results of clinical studies have been published. Also being studied are T-cell vaccines, which aim to remove immunocompetent cells from patients by immunizing them with antigen analogous to V-β chains of T-cell receptors that are capable recognizing encephalitogenic fragments of MBP. Currently, no real conclusions can be drawn from these complex studies, but a preliminary report was somewhat encouraging.

3. TREATMENT OF MULTIPLE SCLEROSIS

Treatment issues in MS are complex but generally fall into four categories: symptomatic treatment, treatment of acute exacerbations, reducing the risk (prevention) of future exacerbations and disability, and rehabilitation. Patients and the general public focus on recent drug developments for risk reduction (the third category), but important the advances in this area have been modest. In recent years, there have been advances in each of these four areas.

In the past, treatment of MS was limited essentially to empirical management of symptoms, (i.e., symptomatic treatment). At best, most treatments were untested and were of questionable value. Interested readers are referred to Augustus D'Este's diary, which describes treatments. Treatments were generic, ineffective, and sometimes dangerous (e.g., cathartics, enemas, blood-letting). Misguided individuals and quacks continue to offer ineffective empirical treatments. The author believes that removal of amalgam from teeth falls into this area.

3.1. Symptomatic Treatment

Symptomatic treatment covers many areas, but this chapter reviews only a few specific issues. Fatigue, spasticity, and bladder symptoms are among the most important areas. Also important is the management of the paroxysmal disorders: paroxysmal dystonia, paroxysmal akinesia, paroxysmal dysarthria, trigeminal neuralgia, facial myokymia, and hemi-facial spasm. Treatment can be dramatically effective.

Fatigue is a prominent complaint for most patients. In reality, patients complain about fatigability rather than fatigue, although patients who have severe exacerbations may awaken occasionally with overwhelming fatigue. The first drug for fatigue to be evaluated in double blind trials (and shown to be effective) was amantadine HCl (Symmetryl®, Endo) *(117)*. A dose of 100 mg twice daily is an effective antiviral, virtually preventing all influenza type A infections and 90% of type B infections and a lower but important risk reduction for other paramyxovirus infections. The sustained reduction of fatigue observed in the majority of patients taking amantadine HCl presumably is caused by its weak dopamine agonist properties, rather than its antiviral effect.

In addition, a variety of adrenergic drugs have been used to treat fatigue, but quickly developing tolerance and habituation are problems *(118)*. Modafinil (Provigil®, Cephalon), a new more selective member of this family of drugs appears safe and tolerated in small (200 mg) daily doses *(119)*. Unfortunately, in our experience, tolerance also seems to develop quickly with this drug. A matter of concern is that in vitro adrenergic drugs appear to promote cellular immune mechanisms, calling into question their use in fatigue management. Because fatigue and depression commonly coexist, many patients take fluoxetine (Prozac®, E.Y. Lily). Interestingly, fluoxetine has immunomodulatory properties, with resultant increases in the Th2 lymphokines, IL-4, and transforming growth factor-β *(120)*. Fatigue lessens in patients who stabilize clinically, spontaneously, or in conjunction with immunomodulatory therapy.

Spasticity continues to be a major problem for MS patients (2). Diazepam (Valium®, Novartis) was the first drug proven to reduce spasticity in MS, and it continues to be a very helpful drug. The use of single 5-mg oral dose at bedtime is a convenient and cost-effective treatment in a large proportion of patients with mild to moderate spasticity. Occasionally, a small additional dose can be given in the morning, but the long half-life of the drug usually makes that unnecessary or undesirable.

Baclofen (Lioresal®, Novartis) is an important and useful drug that is frequently associated with less sedation than diazepam, even at high doses; however, the oral form of the drug, which is a racemic mixture, does not seem to have a predictable dose response in many patients. In contrast, patients with severe refractory spasticity predictably respond to intrathecal baclofen *(121)*. This partially reflects the addition of l-baclofen to the racemic form of baclofen for intrathecal use. Use of the intrathecal drug requires the implantation of a pump to deliver the drug *(121)*.

Tizanidine (Zanaflex®, Elan), an α-2-adrenergic agonist, is a more recently approved drug that has good dose–response characteristics *(122)*, although tizanidine has a short half-life and 40% of patients experience prominent fatigue and dry mouth as side effects. In some patients, use of tizanidine avoids the necessity of pump implantation and therefore is a welcome alternative. Hopefully, an oral formulation of l-baclofen will advance to phase III studies and become a clinical option.

Bladder dysfunction in the majority of patients is largely owing to hyperreflexia of the detrusor muscle, although dyssynergia accompanies this in 90% of cases. Urinary frequency is usually managed with low doses of anticholinergics and oral baclofen, but treatment is often unsatisfactory. Often, a single dosage of an anticholinergic drug before retiring at night and for occasional social situations is more satisfactory than taking multiple doses. Incomplete emptying usually is best handled by intermittent catheterization.

The management of infections is very important. Avoidance of antibiotics for unproven infections and obtaining bacterial sensitivities for each infection is crucial for avoiding pseudomonas infections. Often, recurrent infections are successfully prevented by chronic use of 2 to 4 g ascorbic acid daily with 2 g hipuric acid daily to acidify the urine, together with six to eight glasses of water.

Once paroxysmal disorders are identified, their management is relatively simple in most patients *(2)*. Paroxysmal dystonia, paroxysmal akinesia, trigeminal neuralgia, facial myokymia and hemi-facial spasm are often successfully managed with modest doses of anticonvulsant drugs, although the response in patients with paroxysmal dysarthria tends to be less predictable. For patients requiring treatment, 100 mg of carbamazepine orally three times daily controls about 70% of these disorders, and 400 mg daily increases the response rate to 80 to 85%. Although higher doses are helpful sometimes, use of a second anticonvulsant is often more effective. Some patients require two or more drugs to control these symptoms, but often carbamazepine can be withdrawn if the second drug is effective. The use of corticotropin (adrenocorticotropic hormone [ACTH]) intravenously or intramuscularly, but not steroids, is sometimes necessary to control paroxysmal disorders *(123)*.

3.2. Treatment of Acute Exacerbations

In the past, management of MS exacerbations consisted principally of continuous enforced rest *(2)*. At the onset of an exacerbation, rest relieves (or prevents) fatigue. Thankfully, the injudicious use of extended periods of rest has given way to the enthusiastic use of physical rehabilitation.

This author's career has spanned the era of validation and FDA approval of corticotrophin *(122)* and the subsequent introduction and use of high-dose intravenous steroids for the management of MS exacerbations. Dr. Leo Alexander of Harvard Medical School initially used corticotrophin because steroids, which he hypothesized should be helpful, were not available. The effectiveness of corticotrophin was established by multiple controlled trials, the first for any MS treatment *(123)*. The pivotal multicenter, double-blind, placebo-controlled trial was published in *Neurology* in 1970 and became the basis of the FDA approval in 1978 *(123)*. No other drug has been validated as an effective treatment for exacerbations of MS.

Thirty years ago, neurologists at the Montreal Neurological Institute, including the author, first prospectively employed high-dose intravenous steroids in patients diagnosed with MS. The use of high-dose parenteral steroids was limited to patients who had vision loss in one or both eyes caused by optic neuritis or who were acutely paraplegic from acute myelitis. On the basis of the analogy with trauma and tumor management, it was hypothesized that that acute severe edematous swelling of the optic nerve or spinal cord resulted in complicating ischemia caused by the limited expansion capacity. Although patients often improved rapidly, frequent complications of high-dose therapy were encountered. Gastrointestinal complications are now rare, but psychiatric disturbances, infectious complications, osteoporosis, and aseptic necrosis of the hip and other bones are side effects that are not rare.

Despite weak evidence of benefit from the single-blind (intravenous) optic neuritis treatment trial, which indicated short-term benefit *(123,124)*, no well-organized appropriately sized, double-blind trials have been carried out. The double-blind oral steroid portion of the optic neuritis trial clearly showed that oral steroids were deleterious to patients with optic neuritis (most of whom would develop clinically definite MS). Patients receiving oral steroids subsequently experienced a doubled relapse rate compared with oral placebo recipients.

We interpret these results as evidence that oral steroids alone should not be used in the management of MS. It is important to note that corticotrophin has a well-established neuroprotective effect on neurons *(125–127)*, although methylprednisolone has recently been shown to induce programmed cell death (apoptosis) of neurons *(128)*. We continue to favor corticotrophin because of its effectiveness and neuroprotective effect.

A trial of natalizumab for the management of acute exacerbations failed to influence the outcome of such clinical exacerbations *(114)*, although it reduced the risk of new MRI brain lesions during the subsequent 12 wk following a single infusion. Despite its failure to induce a more rapid recovery from exacerbations, natalizumab improved the sense of well-being in the drug recipients. This benefit also was observed in a subsequent study. Favorable outcomes from additional studies will be discussed below.

3.3. Reduction of Multiple Sclerosis Exacerbations and Disability

For more than 15 yr, there has been intensive study of the potential value of several drugs in reducing the risk of exacerbations in MS. As a corollary to this outcome, there has been increasing emphasis on potential impact of these drugs on reducing the risk of disability caused by this disease.

IFN-β1b was the first drug approved (1993) for reducing the frequency of MS exacerbations (33% reduction) *(129,130)*. The drug also had a remarkable effect, significantly reducing the burden of disease as measured by brain MRI T2-lesion volumes *(130)*. Unfortunately, use of IFN-β1b is consistently associated with flu-like symptoms and local inflammatory reaction at the injection site.

IFN-β1a is produced using mammalian cell lines and the authentic human genetic sequence, unlike IFN-β1b, which has two genetic alterations and is made using coliform bacteria. INF-β1a is rapidly absorbed from the injection site, and local reactions as well as neutralizing antibody formation are less frequent occurrences than with IFN-β1b. Avonex® (IFN-β1a) was approved in 1996 as a result of a study using 30 μg intramuscularly once weekly *(131)*. Risk of sustained disability, the primary outcome measure, was reduced to 21.9% for drug recipients, compared with 39.7% for placebo recipients. Relapse risk was also reduced (0.61 vs 0.90) for those who completed the 104 wk of the trial. However, data analysis employing intent-to-treat analysis showed a reduction in the risk of relapses with active drug treatment of 0.61 vs 0.82 for placebo. The latter results reflect the fact that 40% of the patients did not complete the study because study drug was not available. Subsequently, the benefits on disability prevention were shown to be sustained *(132)*.

In 2002, a large three-arm pivotal trial (Prevention of Relapses and Disability by Interferon β-1a [REBIF®] Subcutaneously in MS [PRISMS]) was reported, showing results resembling those reported for IFN-β1b *(133)*. After additional studies were performed, a head-to-head trial of Rebif® vs Avonex® was initiated *(134)*. The 16-mo trial benefit favored Rebif® at each time point in the study, although the survival curve of Avonex® appeared to approach that of Rebif® as the study progressed. The PRISMS trial extension did show more benefit for patients at the higher dose who initially had received placebo and who were switched to either 22 or 44 μg three times weekly *(135)*.

Glatiramer acetate (Copaxone®) was approved in 1997 as a result of a double-blind, placebo-controlled trial *(136)*. Compared to those taking placebo, subjects who took glatiramer had a 30% reduction in the risk of relapse, similar to the IFN-β studies. The original investigators have shown during a follow-up of a subset of patients that glatiramer has robust long-term benefits in stabilized subjects. Recently, this information has become part of the package insert.

There is a marked reduction of gadolinium-lesion enhancement following initiation of IFN-β1b *(138)*, IFN-β1a *(131)*, and, more recently, for glatiramer *(139)*. Recently, similar results for natalizumab have been reported *(117)*. Interestingly, the serially studied placebo patients showed that enhancement disappears with steroid administration, returns, and finally disappears about 2 mo after its first appearance *(114)*. Recently, increasing emphasis has been placed on techniques of measuring brain atrophy *(117,140–142)*.

The management of secondary progressive disease is far from satisfactory, but based on prospective studies, mitoxantrone (Novantrone®) *(143,144)* and INF-β1b *(145)* have been approved for this form of MS. The use of INF-β1b varies greatly from one geographic area to another and varies based on the impatience and experience of both physicians and patients. Its use is tempered by the fact that many patients who are seemingly stabilized initially subsequently begin to progress despite continued drug treatment. In retrospect, this is seen in drug trials that have included patients who no longer experienced relapses *(145)*. This observation also matches the findings of the U.S. trial meta-analysis. The use of mitoxantrone resulted in cessation of exacerbations and apparent stabilization in the majority of drug recipients vs controls, although the drug is potentially cardiotoxic *(142,143)*. The published results are difficult to interpret for the nonstatistician, and the specter of cardiotoxicity combined with the risk of myelogenous leukemia has limited the use of this effective drug, despite clear guidelines. It is best used in larger centers where physicians have experience with this drug.

Other nonspecific immunosuppressants have been used in the clinical setting. Some were employed in open-label settings, and limited trials of azathiaprine, methotrexate, and cyclophosphamide have been carried out. These drugs appear to have a desirable effect, but potential infections are real risks, and other problems potentially complicate their use. Hopefully, pivotal trials of one or more of these agents will be organized in the near future. If these immunosuppressants are employed, their use should be limited or guided by neurologists who have experience with them.

3.3.1. Future Directions in Treatment

As this volume goes to press, data from trials employing intravenous natalizumab, an immunomodulatory agent, has been accepted for regulatory approval for the prevention of exacerbations of MS. On the basis of phase III studies, natalizumab, a member of a new class of agents aimed at modulating adhesion molecules, has been shown to be both safe and more effective than currently approved drugs in stabilizing MS. The effect of natalizumab (Tysabri) on disability prevention is unknown. Other drugs administered orally as small molecules have a similar potential benefit for MS and other autoimmune diseases, but their relative safety and effectiveness in MS is unknown.

T-cell vaccines have been a promise for many years. Although some progress has been made *(146,147)*, ongoing trials have not produced important new information. Other immunomodulatory drugs designed as surgical strikes (to use a military parlance) continue to go into clinical trials. Trials of anti-TNF-α, a successful agent in rheumatoid arthritis and Crohn's disease, have shown desirable MRI outcomes in MS but have produced unacceptable toxicities. They also appear to precipitate MS-like illness in some patients who have rheumatoid arthritis. Anti-IL-12 mabs also are under investigation, and no similar problems have been reported so far. In all likelihood, anti-MIF MAb also will be tested. Small molecules with similar or identical properties are already in trials for other diseases. These are exciting times.

3.4. Rehabilitation

Both in the United States and Europe, there is renewed interest in exercise in MS, and rehabilitation strategies are evolving *(148,149)*. Shorter periods of exercise repeated after periods of rest have greatly helped many MS patients greatly. The use of aquatic exercises, in which the patient is cooled during exercise and able to maintain longer periods of sustained effort, also has resulted in more effective rehabilitation.

The use of more modern orthotic devices, which are lighter and reduce fatigue in the MS patient, is a major advance in patient management. Having experienced physicians and therapists fit and monitor these devices is particularly important because it increases their effectiveness. Patients require training and encouragement to adapt to these devices. Similarly, it is insufficient merely to give a patient a prescription for a cane. Early introduction of stretching and judicious use of muscle stretching and antispastic drugs prevents contractures and simplifies management of most patients.

4. CONCLUSIONS

The age of rational therapy for MS has arrived with the successful targeting and blocking of VLA-4, preventing adhesion of circulating $CD4^+$ T cells to their endothelial VCAM-1 counter-receptors. The resulting outcome, the prevention of clinical exacerbations and white matter lesions evidenced by brain MRI, is a scientific success and promises better management for patients. To date, natalizumab therapy has been found quite safe, but greater experience with its use in MS is required, especially in regard to potentially increased infection risks. The level of efficacy and safety demonstrated for natalizumab in earlier studies has been confirmed in the current phase III studies. This agent promises to become the new standard for MS treatment.

Future trials of oral compounds capable of blocking VLA-4 are exciting prospects. Oral drugs must be absorbed, survive circulation through the liver in an active form, and subsequently be transported to sites where they will encounter their unique targets. Thus, they may have difficulty matching the safety documented for natalizumab, an intravascular agent, although the ease of oral administration will result in additional future trials of selected small compounds. Since the specific target for natalizumab is the α-chain of VLA-4, the safety of natalizumab may be greater than small molecules, such as Tanabe (GlaxoSmithkline 683699) and TBC 3486. The results of the ongoing trials of natalizumab and future trials of selected small molecules, such as TBC 3486, are eagerly awaited. It is anticipated that this manipulation of molecular adhesions molecules will constitute a major advance in the management of MS, as well as other T-cell-mediated disorders.

REFERENCES

1. Charcot JM. Histologie de la sclerose en plaques. Gaz Hop (Paris) 1868;41:554–566.
2. Compston A, Ebers G, Lassman H, McDonald I, Mathews B, Wekerle H. McAlpine's Multiple Sclerosis. 3rd ed. London. Churchill Livingstone, 1988.
3. Firth D. The Case of Sir Augustus d'Este. London. Cambridge University Press, 1947.
4. Kurtzke JF. A reassessment of the distribution of MS. Part one. Acta Neurologica Scand 1975;51:110–136.
5. Kurtzke JF. A reassessment of the distribution of MS. Art two. Acta Neurologica Scand 1975;51:137–157.
6. Weinshenker BG, Bass B, Rice GPA, et al. The natural history of MS: a geographically based study. 1. Clinical course and disability. Brain 1989;112:133–146.
7. Noseworthy JH, Luccinetti C, Rodriguez M, Weinschenker BG. Multiple sclerosis. New Engl J Med 2000;343: 938–952.
8. Schumacher GA, Beebe G, Kibler RF, et al. Problems of experimental trials of therapy in MS: report by the panel on the evaluation of experimental trials of therapy in MS. Ann N Y Acad Sci 1965;123:552–568.
9. Poser CM, Paty DW, Scheinberg L, et al. New diagnostic criteria for MS: guidelines for research protocols. Ann Neurol 1983;13:227–231.
10. McDonald WI, Compston A, Edan G, et al. Recommended diagnostic criteria for MS: guidelines from the International Panel on the Diagnosis of Multiple Sclerosis. Ann Neurol 2001;50:121–127.
11. Leibowitz U. Halpern L, Alter M. Clinical studies of MS in Israel. 5. Progressive spinal syndromes and MS. Neurology 1967;17:988–992.

12. Confavreux C, Vukusic S, Moreau T, Adeline P. Relapses and progression of disability in MS. N Engl J Med 2000; 343:1430–1438.

13. Pittock SJ, Mayr WT, McClelland RL, et al. Change in MS–related disability in a population–based cohort: a 10–year follow–up study. Neurology 2004;62:51–59.

14. Berger J, Sheremata WA. Persistent neurological deficit in MS precipitated by hot bath test. J Am Med Assoc 1983;133:1224–1226.

15. Berger JR Sheremata WA. Melmed E. Paroxysmal dystonia as the initial manifestation of MS. Arch. Neurol 1984;41:747–750.

16. Cottrell DA, Kremenchutzky M, Rice GPA, et al. The natural history of MS: a geographically based study. 5. The clinical features and natural history of primary progressive MS. Brain 1999;122:625–689.

17. Sheremata WA, Berger JR, Harrington W Jr, Ayyar R, Stafford JM, Defreitas E. Human lymphotropic (HTLV–I) associated myelopathy: a report of ten cases born in the United States. Arch Neurol 1992;31:34–38.

18. Lowis GW, Sheremata WA, Minagar A. Epidemiologic features of HTLV–II: serological and molecular evidence. Ann Epidemiol 2992;12:46–66.

19. Fink JK. Hereditary spastic paraplegia: the pace quickens. Ann Neurol 1992;51:669–672.

20. Jacobs LD, Beck RW, Simon JH, et al. Intramuscular interferon beta–1a therapy initiated during a first demyelinating event in MS. N Engl J Med 2000:343:898–904.

21. Sadovnick AD, Ebers GC. Epidemiology of MS: a critical overview. Can J Neurol Sci 1993;20:17–19.

22. Confavreux C, Hutchinson M, Hours MM, et al. Rate of pregnancy–related relapse in MS. N Engl J Med 1998;339:285–291.

23. Confavreux C. Infections and the risk of relapse in MS [Editorial]. Brain 2002;125:933–934.

24. Warren S, Greenhill S, Warren KG. Emotional stress and the development of MS: case–control evidence of a relationship. J Chronic Dis 1982;35:821–831.

25. Grant I, Brown GW, Harris T, McDonald WI, Patterson T, Trimble MR. Severely threatening events and marked life difficulties preceding onset or exacerbation of MS. J Neurol Neurosurg Psychiat 1989;52:8–13.

26. Warren S, Warren KG, Cockerill R. Emotional stress and coping in MS and exacerbations. J Psychosom Res 1991;35:37–47.

27. Mohr DC, Goodkin DE, Bacchetti P, Boudewyn AC, Huang L, Marietta P, Cheuk W, Dee B. Psychological stress and he subsequent appearance of new brain MRI lesions in MS. Neurology 2000;55:55–61.

28. Cala LA, Mastaglia FL, Black JL. Computerized tomography of brain and optic nerve in MS: observation in 100 patients including serial studies in 16. J Neurol Sci 1978;36:411–426.

29. Hershey LA, Gado MH, Trotter JL. Computerized tomography in the diagnostic evaluation of MS. Ann Neurol 1979;5:32–39.

30. Barrett L, Drayer B, Shin C. High-resolution computerized tomography in the diagnostic evaluation of MS. Ann Neurol 1985;17:33–38.

31. Bradley WG, Walauch Y, Yadley RA, Wycoff RR. Comparison of CT and MR in 400 patients with suspected disease of the brain and cervical spinal cord. Radiology 1984;152:895–702.

32. Sheldon JJ, Siddharthan R, Tobias J, et al. Magnetic resonance imaging of MS: comparison with clinical, paraclinical, laboratory and CT examination. AJNR 1985:6:683–690.

33. Jacobs L, Kinkel WR, Polachini I, Kinkel RP. Correlations of nuclear magnetic resonance imaging, computerized tomography, and clinical profiles in MS. Neurology 1986;36:27–34.

34. Honig LS, Siddharthan R, Sheremata WA, Sheldon JJ, Sazant A. Multiple sclerosis: correlation of magnetic resonance imaging with cerebrospinal fluid findings. Neurol Neurosurg Psychiat 1988;51:27–280.

35. Honig LS, Sheremata WA. Magnetic resonance imaging of spinal cord lesions in MS. Neurol Neurosurg Psychiat 1989:52:459–466.

36. Brex PA, Ciccarelli O, O'Riordan JI, Sailer M, Thompson AJ, Miller DH. A longitudinal study of abnormalities on MRI and disability from MS. New Engl J Med 2002;348:158–164.

37. Leist TP, Gobbini MI, Frank JA, McFarland HF. Enhancing magnetic resonance imaging lesions and cerebral atrophy in patients with relapsing MS. Arch Neurol 2000;57:57–60.

38. van Walderveen MA, Kamphorst W, Scheltens P, et al. Histopathologic correlate of hypointense lesions on T1-weighted spin-echo magnetic resonance images in MS. Neurology 1998;50:1282–1288.

39. De Stefano N, Narayanan S, Francis GS, et al. Evidence of axonal damage in the early stages of MS and its relevance to disability. Arch Neurol 2001;5:65–70.

40. Sobel RA. The pathology of MS. In: Multiple Sclerosis. Antel J, ed., Neurologic Clinics, Sanders, Philadelphia, 1995;13:1–22.

41. Oppenheimer DR. Demyelinating diseases. In: Greenfield's Neuropathology. 3rd ed. Blackwood W, Corsellis JAN, eds. Edward Arnold, London, 1976:470–499.

42. Lumsden CE. The neuropathology of MS. In: Handbook of Clinical Neurology Vinken PJ, Bruyn GW, eds. Elsevier, New York, 1969:217–309.

43. Adams RD, Kubick CS. The morbid anatomy of the demyelinative disease. Am J Med 1952;12:510–546.

44. Zimmerman HM, Netsky HG. The pathology of MS. Res Publ Res Nerv Ment Dis 1950;28:271–312.
45. Lampert PW. Fine structure of the demyelinating process. In: Hallpike JF, Adams CWM, \Tourtelotte WW, eds. Multiple Sclerosis: Pathology, Diagnosis and Management. Williams and Wilkins, Baltimore, 1983:29–46.
46. Trapp BD, Peterson J, Ransahoff RM, Rudick R, Moerk S, Boe L. Axonal transaction in the lesions of MS. N Engl J Med 1998;338:278–285.
47. Lassmann H, Vass K. Are current immunological concepts of MS reflected by the immunopathology of its lesions? Semin Immunopathol 1995;17:77–87.
48. Lassman H, Raine CS, Antel J, Prineas JW. Immunopathology of MS: report on an international meeting held at the Institute of Neurology of the University of Vienna. J Neuroimmunol 1998;86:213–217.
49. Luccinetti C, Brueck W, Paris J, et al. Heterogeneity of MS lesions: implications for the pathogenesis of demyelination. Ann Neurol 2000;47:707–717.
50. Cannella B, Raine CS. The adhesion molecule and cytokine profile of MS lesions. Ann Neurol 1995;37:424–435.
51. Poser C. The pathogenesis of MS: a commentary. Clin Neurol Neurosurg 2000;102:191–204.
52. Sadovnick AD, Armstrong H, Rice GF, et al. A population based study of MS in twins: an update. Ann Neurol 1993;33:281–285.
53. Sadovnick AD, Baird PA, Ward RH. Multiple sclerosis: update risks for relatives. Am J Genet 1988;29:533–541.
54. Jersild C, Fog T, Hansen GS, Thomsen M, Svejgaard A, Dupont B. Histocompatibility determinants in MS with special reference to clinical course. Lancet 1973;2:1221–1225.
55. Wood DD, Bilbao JM, O'Connor P, Moscarello MA. A highly deiminized form of myelin basic protein in Marburg's disease. Ann Neurol 1996;40:18–24.
56. Schwarz S, Mohr A, Knauth M, Wildemann B, Storch-Hagenlocher B. Acute disseminated encephalomyelitis. A follow-up study of 40 adult patients. Neurology 2001;56:1313–1318.
57. Hartung HP, Grossman RI. ADEM. Distinct disease or part of the MS spectrum? Neurology 2001;56:1257–1260.
58. Murthy JM, Yangala R, Meena AK, Jaganmohan-Reddy J. Acute disseminated encephalomyelitis: clinical and MRI study from South India. J Neurol Sci 1999;165:133–136.
59. Patterson PY. Transfer of allergic encephalomyelitis in rats by means of lymph node cells. J Exp Med 1960;111:119–136.
60. Bornstein MB, Appel SH. Application of tissue culture to the study of experimental allergic encephalomyelitis. 1. Patterns of demyelination. J Neuropath Exp Neurol 1961;20:141–157.
61. Bornstein MB, Raine CS. Multiple sclerosis and experimental allergic encephalomyelitis: Specific demyelination of CNS in culture. Neuropathol Appl Neurobiol 1977;3:359–367.
62. Ben–Nun A, Cohen IR. Genetic control of experimental autoimmune encephalomyelitis at the level of cytotoxic lymphocytes in guinea pigs. Eur J Immunol 1982; 12:709–713.
63. Owens T, Sriram S. The immunology of MS and its animal model experimental allergic encephalomyelitis. Neurology Clinics 1995;13:57–73.
64. Massacesi L, Genain CP, Lee-Parritz D, et al. Active and passively induced experimental autoimmune encephalomyelitis in common marmosets: a new model for MS. Ann Neurol 1995;37:519–530.
65. Uccelli A, Giunti D, Capello E, Roccatagliata L, Mancardi GL. EAE in the common marmoset Callithrix jacchus. Int MS J 2003;10:6–12.
66. Bronstein JM, Lallone RL, Seitz RS, Ellison GW, Myers LW. A humoral response to oligodendrocyte-specific protein in MS. A potential molecular mimic. Neurology 1999;53:154–161.
67. Berger T, Rubner P, Schautzer F, et al. Antimyelin antibodies as a predictor of clinically definite MS after a first demyelinating event. N Engl J Med 2004;349:139–145.
68. Yu T, Ellison GW, Mendoza F, Bronstein JM. T-cell responses to oligodendrocyte-specific protein in MS. J Neurosci Res 2001;66:506–509.
69. Adorini L. Singaglia F. Pathogenesis and immunotherapy of autoimmune disease. Immunol Today 1997;18: 209–211.
70. Yang Y, Tomura M, Ono S, Hamaoka T, Fujiwara H. Requirement for IFN–γ in IL-12 production induced by collaboration between Vα14+NKT cells and antigen–presenting cells. Int Immunol 2000;12:1669–1675.
71. Liu CC, Young LH, Young JD. Lymphocyte-mediated cytolysis and disease. New Engl J Med 2004;335:1651–1659.
72. Minagar A, Alexander JS. Blood-brain barrier disruption in MS. Multiple Sclerosis 2003;9:540–549.
73. Yednock TA, Cannon C, Fritz LC, Sanchez-Madrid F, Steinman L, Karin N. Prevention of experimental autoimmune encephalomyelitis by antibodies against alpha 4 beta 1 integrin. Nature 1992;356:63–66.
74. Carlos TM, Harlan JM. Leukocyte-endothelial adhesion molecules. Blood 1994;84:2068–2101.
75. Frenette PS, Wagner DD. Adhesion molecules—Part 1. N Engl J Med 1996;334:1526–1529.
76. Frenette PS, Wagner DD. Adhesion molecules—Part II: Blood vessels and blood cells. N Engl J Med 1996;335:43–45.
77. von Andrian UH, MacKay CR. T-cell function and migration. Two sides of the same coin. N Engl J Med 2000;343:1020–1034.
78. von Adrian UH, Engelhardt B. α4 integrins as therapeutic targets in autoimmune disease. N Engl J Med 2004;348:68–72.

79. Vestweber D, Blanks JE. Mechanisms that regulate the function of the selectins and their ligands. Physiol Rev 1999;79:181–213.
80. Takada Y, Elices MJ, Crouse C, Hemler ME. The primary structure of the alpha 4 subunit of VLA-4: homology to other integrins and a possible cell-cell adhesion function. EMBO J 1989;8:1361–1368.
81. Hynes RO. Integrins: a family of cell surface receptors. Cell 1987;48:549–554.
82. Hynes RO. Integrins: versatility, modulation, and signaling in cell adhesion. Cell 1992;69:11–25.
83. Piccio L, Rossi B, Scarpini E, et al. Molecular mechanisms involved in lymphocyte recruitment in inflamed brain microvessels: critical roles for P-selectin glycoprotein ligand-1 and heterotrimeric G_i-linked receptors. J Immunol 2002;168:1940–1849.
84. Minagar A, Jy W, Jimenez JJ, et al. Elevated plasma endothelial microparticles in MS. Neurology 2001;56:1319–1324.
85. Qin S, Rottman JB, Myers P, et al. The chemokine receptors CSCR3 and CCR5 mark subsets of T cells associated with certain inflammatory reaction. J Clin Invest 1998:101:746–754.
86. Kent S, Karlik SJ, Cannon C, et al. A monoclonal antibody to α4 integrin suppresses and reverses active experimental allergic encephalomyelitis. J Neuroimmunol 1995;58:1–10.
87. Keszthelyi E, Karlik S, Hyduk S, et al. Evidence for a prolonged role of α3 integrin throughout active experimental allergic encephalomyelitis. Neurology 1996;47:1053–1059.
88. Lin K, Ateeq HS, Hsiung SH, et al. Selective tight binding inhibitors of integrin α4β1 that inhibit allergic airway responses. J Med Chem 1999;42:920–934.
89. Kelly TA, Jeanfavre DD, McNeil DW, et al. Cutting edge: a small molecule antagonist of LFA-1 mediated cell adhesion. J Immunol 1999;163:5173–5177.
90. Cannella B, Gaupp S, Tilton RG, Raine CS. Differential efficacy of a synthetic antagonist of VLA-4 during the course of chronic relapsing experimental autoimmune encephalomyelitis. J Neurosci Res 2003;71:407–416.
91. You TJ, Maxwell DS, Kogan TP, et al. A 3D structure model of integrin alpha 4 beta 1 complex: I. Construction of a homology model of beta 1 and ligand binding analysis. Biophys J 2002;82(Pt 1):447–457.
92. Vanderslice P, Biediger RJ, Woodside DG, Berens KL, Holland GW, Dixon RA. Development of cell adhesion molecule antagonists as therapeutics for asthma and COPD. Pulm Pharmacol Ther 2004;17:1–10.
93. Elices MJ, Osborn L, Takada Y, et al. VCAM-1 on activated endothelium interacts with the leukocyte integrin VLA-4 at a site distinct from the VLA-4/fibronectin binding site. Cell 1990;60:577–584.
94. Dasgupta S, Jana M, Liu X, Pahan K. Myelin basic protein-primed T cells induce nitric oxide synthase in microglial cells. Implications for MS. J Biol Chem 2002;277:39,327–39,333.
95. Dasgupta S, Jana M, Liu X, Pahan K. Role of very-late antigen-4 (VLA-4) in myelin basic protein-primed T cell contact-induced expression of proinflammatory cytokines in microglial cells. J Biol Chem 2003;278: 22,424–22,431.
96. Stanilaus R, Singh AK, Singh I. Lovastatin treatment decreases mononuclear cell infiltration into the CNS of Lewis rats with experimental allergic encephalomyelitis. J Neurosci Res 2001;66:159–162.
97. Pahan K, Sheikh F, Namboodin A, Singh I. Lovastatin and phenylacetate inhibit the induction of nitric oxide synthase and cytokines in rat primary astrocytes, microglial and macrophages. J Clin Invest 1997;100:2671–2679.
98. Vollmer T, Key L, Durkalski V, et al. Oral simvastatin treatment in relapsing-remitting MS. Lancet 2004;363:1607–1608.
99. Denkinger CM, Denkinger M, Kort JJ, Metz C, Forthuber TG. In vivo blockade of macrophage migration inhibitory factor ameliorates acute experimental autoimmune encephalomyelitis by impairing the homing of encephalitogenic T cells to the central nervous system. J Immunol 2003;170:1274–1282.
100. Rocklin RE, Sheremata WA, Feldman RG, Kies MW, David JR. The Guillain-Barre syndrome and MS: in vitro cellular responses. New Engl J Med 1971;284:803–808.
101. Sheremata WA, Cosgrove JBR, Eylar EH. Cellular hypersensitivity to basic myelin (A1) protein and clinical MS. New Engl J Med 1974;291:14–17.
102. Sheremata WA, Cosgrove JBR, Eylar EH. Hypersensitivity to myelin protein preceding attacks of MS. Trans Am Neurol Assoc 1974;99:49–54.
103. Sheremata WA, Wood DD, Moscarello MA, Cosgrove JBR. Sensitization to myelin basic protein in attacks of MS. J Neurol Sci 1978;36:165–170.
104. Sheremata WA., Wood DD, Moscarello MA. Cellular and humoral responses to myelin basic protein in MS: a dichotomy. In: Myelination and Demyelination. Palao J, ed. Plenum, New York, 1978:501–511.
105. Calabresi PA, Pelfrey CM, Tranquill LR, Maloni H, McFarland HF. VLA-4 expression on peripheral blood lymphocytes is downregulated after treatment of MS with interferon beta. Neurology 1997;49:1111–1116.
106. Muraro PA, Leist T, Bielekova B, McFarland HF. VLA-4/CD49d downregulated on primed T lymphocytes during interferon-beta therapy in MS. J Neuroimmunol 2000;111:186–194.
107. Lou J, Gasche Y, Zheng L, et al. Interferon-β inhibits activated leukocyte migration through human brain microvascular endothelial cell monolayer. J Lab Invest 1999;79:1015–1025.
108. Elovaara I, Ukkonen M, Leppakynnas M, et al. Adhesion molecules in MS: relation to subtypes of disease and methylprednisolone therapy. Arch Neurol 2000;47:546–551.

109. Gelati M, Corsini E, de Rossi M, et al. Methylprednisolone acts on peripheral blood mononuclear cells and endothelium in inhibiting migration phenomena in patients with MS. Arch Neurol 2002;59:774–780.

110. Diem R, Hobom M, Maier K, et al. Methylprednisolone increases neuronal apoptosis during autoimmune CNS inflammation by inhibition of an endogenous neuroprotective pathway. J Neurosci 2003;23:6993–7000.

111. Sheremata WA, Vollmer TL, Stone LA, Willmer-Hulme AJ, Koller M. A pharmacokinetic study of intravenous natalizumab in patients with MS. Neurology 1999;52:1072–1074.

112. Tubridy N, Behan PO, Capildo R, et al. The effect of anti-alpha4 integrin antibody on brain lesion activity in MS. The UK Antegren Study Group. Neurology 1999;53:466–472.

113. Minagar A, Sheremata WA, Hume A, Koller M, Vollmer T. Reduction of relapses in MS after Natalizumab (Antegren) treatment. Int MS J (On line) March 15, 2000.

114. O'Connor PW, Goodman A, Willmer-Hulme AJ, et al. Randomized. Multicenter trial of intravenous natalizumab in acute MS relapses: clinical and MRI effects. Neurology 1994;62:2038–2043.

115. Miller DH, Khan OA, Sheremata WA, et al. A controlled trial of natalizumab for relapsing-remitting MS. N Engl J Med 2003;348:15–23.

116. Dalton CM, Miszkiel KA, Barker GJ, et al. The effect of natalizumab on conversion of T1 gadolinium enhancing lesions to T1 hypodense lesions. Neurology 2004;60(Suppl 1):S484.

117. Murray TJ. Amantadine therapy for fatigue in MS. Can J Neurol Sci 1994;21:9–14.

118. Krupp LB, Coyle PK, Doscher C, et al. Fatigue therapy in MS: results of a double-blind, randomized, parallel trial of amantadine, pemoline, and placebo. Neurology 1995;45:1956–1961.

119. Rammohan KW, Rosenberg JH, Lynn DJ, et al. Efficacy and safety of modafinil (Provigil) for the treatment of fatigue in MS: a two centre phase 2 study. J Neurol Neurosurg Psychiatry 2002;72:150–179.

120. Traugott U. Detailed analysis of immunomodulatory properties of fluoxetine (Prozac) in chronic experimental allergic encephalomyelitis in SJL/J mice. Neurology 1998:50:1998. (abstract)

121. Penn RD, Savoy SM, Corcos D, et al. Intrathecal baclofen for severe spinal spasticity. New Engl J Med 1989;320:1517–1521.

122. Nance P, Sheremata WA, Lynch SG, et al. Relationship of the antispasticity effect of tizanidine to plasma concentration in patients with MS. Arch Neurol 1997;54:731–706.

123. Rose AS, Kuzma JW, Kurtzke JF, et al. Cooperative study in the evaluation of therapy in MS: ACTH vs. placebo. Final Report. Neurology 1970;20(Part 2):1–19.

124. Beck BW, Cleary PA, Anderson MM, et al. A randomized controlled trial of corticosteroids in the treatment of acute optic neuritis. N Engl J Med 1992;326:581–588.

125. Botticelli LJ, Wurtman RJ. Septo-hippocampal cholinergic neurons are regulated transynaptically by endorphin and corticotrophin neuropeptides. J Neurosci 1982;2:1316–1321.

126. Spruijt BM, Van Rijzingen I, Masswinkel H. The ACTH (4-9 analog Org2766) modulates the behavioral changes induced by NMDA and the NMDA receptor antagonist AP5. J Neurosci 1994;14:3225–3230.

127. Hol EM, Mandys V, Sodnar P, Gispen WH, Bar PR. Protection by ACTH4-9 analogue against the toxic effects of cisplatin and taxol on sensory neurons and glial cells in vitro. J Neurosci Res 1994;39:178–185.

128. Diem R, Hobom M, Maier K, et al. Methylprednisolone increases neuronal apoptosis during autoimmune CNS inflammation by inhibition of an endogenous neuroprotective pathway. J Neurosci 1993;23:6993–7000.

129. The IFNB Multiple Sclerosis Study Group. Interferon beta-1b is effective in relapsing-remitting MS. 1. Clinical results of a multicenter, randomized, double-blind, placebo-controlled trial. Neurology 1993;43:655–661.

130. Paty DW, Li KDB, the UBC MS/MRI Group and the IFN Multiple Sclerosis Study Group. Interferon beta-1b is effective in relapsing-remitting MS. Neurology 1993;42:662–667.

131. Jacobs LD, Cookfair DL, Rudick RA, et al. Intramuscular interferon beta-1a for disease progression in relapsing MS. Ann Neurol 1996;39:285–294.

132. Rudick RA, Goodkin DE, Jacobs LD, et al. Impact of interferon beta-1a on neurologic disability in relapsing MS. Neurology 1997;49:358–363.

133. PRISMS (Prevention of Relapses and Disability by Interferon β-1a Subcutaneously in MS) Study Group. Randomised double-blind placebo-controlled study of interferon β-1a in relapsing/remitting MS. Lancet 2002;352:1498–1504.

134. Panitch H, Goodin DS, Francis G, et al. Randomized, comparative study of interferon β-1a treatment regimens in MS: The EVIDENCE Trial. Neurology, 2002;59:1496–1506.

135. The PRISMS Study Group and the University of British Columbia MS/MRI Analysis Group PRISMS-4: longer term efficacy of interferon-beta-1a in relapsing MS. Neurology 2001;56:1628–1636.

136. Johnson KP, Brooks BR, Cohen JA, et al. Copolymer 1 reduces relapse rate and improves disability in relapsing-remitting MS: results of a phase III multicenter, double-blind, placebo-controlled trial. Neurology 1995;45:1268–1276.

137. Johnson KP, Brooks BR, Ford CC, et al. Sustained clinical benefits of glatimer acetate (Copaxone) in MS patients observed for 6 years. Mult Scler 2000;6:255–266.

138. Stone LA, Frank JA, Albert PS, et al. Characterization of MRI response to treatment with interferon beta-1b: contrast-enhancing MRI lesion frequency as a primary outcome measure. Neurology 1997;49:862–869.

139. Mancardi GL, Sardanelli F, Parodi RC, et al. Effect of copolymer-1 on serial gadolinium-enhanced MRI in relapsing-remitting MS. Neurology 1998;50:1127–1133.
140. Rudick RA, Fisher E, Lee JC, et al. Us of the brain parenchymal fraction to measure whole brain atrophy in relapsing-remitting MS. Neurology 1999;53:1698–1704.
141. Ge Y, Grossman RI, Udupa JK, et al. Glatiramer acetate (Copaxone) treatment in relapsing-remitting MS. Neurology 2000;54:813–817.
142. Frank JA, Richert N, Bash C, et al. Interferon-β-1b slows progression of atrophy in RRMS. Neurology 2004;62:719–725.
143. Hartung HP, Gonsette R, Koenig N, et al. Mitoxantrone in progressive MS: a placebo controlled, double-blind, randomized, multicentre trial. Lancet 2002;360:2018–2025.
144. Ghalie RG, Edan G, Laurent M, et al. Cardiac adverse effects associated with mitoxantrone (Novantrone) therapy in patients with MS. Neurology 2002;59:909–913.
145. European Study Group on Interferon β-1b in Secondary Progressive MS. Placebo-controlled multicentre randomised trial of interferon β-1b in treatment of secondary progressive MS. Lancet 1998;352:1491–1497.
146. Vandenbark AA, Chou YK, Whitham R, et al. Treatment of MS with T-cell receptor peptides: results of a double-blind pilot trial. Nat Med 1996;2:1109–1115.
147. Goodkin DE, Shulman M, Winkelhake J, et al. A phase I trial of solubilized DR2: MBP84-102 (AG284) in MS. Neurology 2000;54:1414–1420.
148. Aisen ML. Justifying neurorehabilitation [Editorial]. Neurology 1999;52:8.
149. Thompson A. Symptomatic management and rehabilitation in MS. J Neurol Neurosurg Psychiatry 2001;71(Suppl 11): 112–1127.

CME QUESTIONS

1. What is the best definition of multiple sclerosis (MS)?
    A. MS is an immune-mediated disease of unknown etiology that develops in certain genetically suscep-
    tible individuals following exposure to certain environmental antigen(s) and involves only central
    nervous system myelin.
    B. MS affects both peripheral and central myelin and is more common in women than men.
    C. MS is a form of a dysmyelinating disorder
    D. MS is an infectious disease, which affects men more frequently than women.

2. What are the main cell types involved in pathogenesis of MS?
    A. T cells
    B. B cells
    C. T cells, B cells, and macrophages
    D. Eosinophils

3. Major disability in MS patients is usually a result of:
    A. Loss of vision caused by optic neuritis
    B. Transverse myelitis
    C. Brainstem plaques
    D. All of the above

4. Which one of these diseases is in the differential diagnosis of MS?
    A. AIDS
    B. Syphilis
    C. Vitamin B_{12} deficiency
    D. All of the above

5. Urinary incontinence in MS patients:
    A. Is rare
    B. Occurs frequently and is caused by neurogenic bladder from MS
    C. Requires careful urological evaluation
    D. B and C

7

Neuroprotective Effects of Interferon-β in Multiple Sclerosis

Fabrizio Giuliani, Rana Zabad, and V. Wee Yong

1. IMMUNE DYSREGULATION IN MULTIPLE SCLEROSIS

Multiple sclerosis (MS) is considered an immune-mediated, demyelinating, and degenerative disease of the central nervous system (CNS). The immune-mediated pathogenesis is supported by the significant infiltration of leukocytes into the CNS parenchyma and by the finding of a substantial similarity between active MS plaques and lesions in the CNS of animals with experimental autoimmune encephalomyelitis (EAE); EAE is produced by an autoreactive T-cell response. The favorable response of many MS patients to immunomodulatory drugs, including use of β interferons (IFNs) and glatiramer acetate to decrease the number of relapses and reduce magnetic resonance imaging (MRI) disease activity *(1–4)*, also corroborates the hypothesis of immune-mediated injury.

The pathology of MS lesions provides clues to the important role of T cells in the disease. Active MS lesions are characterized by perivascular lymphocyte infiltration that spreads into the parenchyma. A prevailing hypothesis of MS pathogenesis is that T cells are activated in the periphery by unknown antigens *(5,6)* and both myelin and nonmyelin antigens may be involved *(7–9)*. Although auto-antigen specific T cells are present in the immune system of MS patients, they are also found in healthy people, leading to the concept that these cells need to be activated to become mediators of disease. Different mechanisms have been suggested for the activation of autoreactive T cells, such as molecular mimicry, epitope spreading, mistaken self- and bystander activation (Fig. 1).

Molecular mimicry describes conformational similarities between epitopes of myelin proteins and epitopes of foreign antigens (e.g., viral or bacterial origin). For this reason, T cells would recognize self-antigen as non-self. More recently, it has been reported that structural similarities between different proteins of the major histocompatibilty complex (MHC) human leukocyte antigen class II, one recognizing the foreign antigen and the other a self-antigen, can induce an autoimmune response *(10)*. Another proposed mechanism of T-cell activation is epitope spreading; inflammation and tissue destruction would induce antigen presentation of previously hidden epitopes and cause the activation of T cells of different specificities. In this way, the immune response spreads from the first self-antigen to others that induce their own immune responses. Although epitope spreading is documented in EAE, there is still little evidence that this process occurs in MS *(11)*.

In addition to epitope spreading, the same inflammatory environment, because of the high concentration of cytokines, can induce activation of immune cells *per se* by a mechanism called

From: *Current Clinical Neurology: Inflammatory Disorders of the Nervous System: Pathogenesis, Immunology, and Clinical Management*
Edited by: A. Minagar and J. S. Alexander © Humana Press Inc., Totowa, NJ

Periphery   Blood-brain barrier   CNS parenchyn

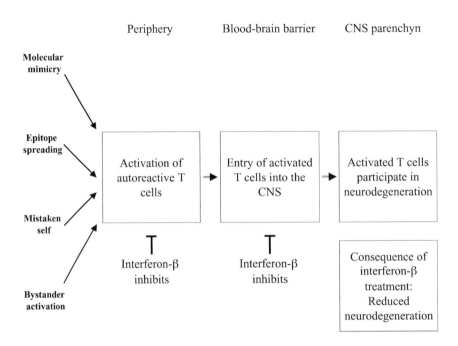

Fig. 1. Proposed mechanisms of neuroprotection by interferon (IFN)-β. By reducing the influx of pathogenic T cells into the central nervous system (CNS), IFN-β would be preventing further insults that these cells can exert in the CNS. The outcome would be neuroprotection, even if this were exerted indirectly be preventing detrimental leukocytes from reaching their sites of action within the CNS parenchyma.

bystander activation. Others have suggested the possibility of a unique MS response called "mistaken self," in which microbial infection of immune cells induces a T-cell response not only against the infective agent but also against a stress protein called B-crystallin, which is expressed in infected immune cells *(12)*; however, this model has not been fully proven in animal studies, and, because of the wide distribution of B-crystallin in human tissues, does not fully explain the organ-specific response in MS.

When activated, T cells cross the blood–brain barrier (BBB) into the CNS parenchyma, where they accumulate and proliferate in response to antigen restimulation *(13–15)*. These activated T cells secrete proinflammatory cytokines that activate resident microglia, infiltrating macrophages and B cells. This inflammatory response is thought to damage axons and myelin through antigen-specific or nonantigen-specific mechanisms.

2. NEURODEGENERATION IN MULTIPLE SCLEROSIS

Although MS is described as a demyelinating disease of the CNS, Charcot *(16)* recognized a neurodegenerative component more than a century ago. Nonetheless, because of the significant and obvious demyelination in MS, the disease was referred to for many years as one with loss of myelin and relative sparing of axons. The pendulum has swung, however, and the concept of significant neurodegeneration in MS has taken hold. Several studies have confirmed axonal loss or injury in MS. For example, immunohistochemical studies of amyloid precursor protein (APP) have demonstrated APP-positive profiles in active MS lesions axons and at the border of chronic active MS lesions. APP is a normal constituent of neurons transported down axons by fast axoplasmic flow; it accumulates in injured neurons to a level detectable by immunohistochemistry and is thus a useful marker of axonal injury. Some of the APP-positive structures in MS lesions resemble the terminal ends of axons and likely represent transected axons *(17)*. Significantly, the number of APP-positive axons correlates with the degree of inflammation *(18)*.

More evidence of neuronal and/or axonal damage in MS arose from clinical outcomes *(19)*. Neurological disability has been correlated with atrophy of the spinal cord, cerebellum, and cerebral cortex *(18,20,21)*. MRI spectroscopy for *N*-acetyl-aspartate (NAA), a marker of axonal integrity, has found reduced levels in brain tissue of MS patients. The decrease of NAA per lesion volume was significantly higher in secondary progressive (SP) MS patients with irreversible neurological disability than in relapsing–remitting (RR) MS patients with little fixed disability *(21)*. More recently, a technique quantifying whole-brain NAA showed that widespread axonal pathology was independent of MRI-enhancement and was present from the earliest clinical stage of the disease *(22)*.

A correlation also exists between the persistence of black holes (described as hypointense lesions on T1-weighted images with low signal intensity compared with the surrounding white matter) and the duration of the inflammatory phase of lesions (measured as length of persistence of the enhancement) *(23)*. Black holes have been interpreted as areas of axonal loss *(24,25)*. Neuronal loss in the thalamus of patients with SPMS *(26)* and RRMS *(27)* has been reported and confirmed by a substantial neocortical volume loss in RR and progressive MS as measured by MRI *(28)*. Neuronal death in cortical MS lesions has also been observed *(29)*.

3. MULTIPLE SCLEROSIS: NEURODEGENERATION INDUCED BY INFLAMMATION?

Because of the correlation between inflammation and signs of axonal injury or loss, it is likely that inflammatory molecules may aggravate and/or cause the degenerative process. If so, it is unknown whether the axonal injury seen in MS lesions results from an immune response against a particular neural antigen, a nonspecific injury related to secretion of soluble factors, or a cell–cell-contact-mediated mechanism. In addition, modification in the CNS microenvironment induced by inflammatory processes, such as axon hyperexcitability following chronic demyelination, may facilitate the neurodegenerative processes *(30)*. Classical proinflammatory cytokines (tumor necrosis factor [TNF]-α and interleukin [IL]-1) can be neurotoxic, whereas anti-inflammatory cytokines (IL-10) may be neuroprotective; however, this is controversial. In one study, TNF-α killed human fetal neurons in culture *(31)*, but in another study, the cytokine had no effect *(32)*. Another study reported that TNF-α killed neurons by preventing the action of a survival factor, insulin-like growth factor-1 *(33)*. IFN-γ, also a proinflammatory cytokine, was shown to induce neurons to express MHC class I on their surface and thus facilitate neuronal recognition and killing by cytotoxic T cells *(34)*.

A number of studies indicate that endogenous IL-1 contributes to experimentally induced neurodegeneration. Administration of recombinant IL-1 receptor antagonist (IL-1ra) into the brain or periphery of rodents markedly inhibits brain damage caused by cerebral ischemia, brain injury, and excitotoxins *(35–37)*. Conversely, injections of IL-1β antibody is neuroprotective *(38)*. We have shown that IL-1β toxicity for oligodendrocytes is mediated by glutamate *(39)*. Glutamate imbalance has been associated with oligodendrocyte and axonal damage in MS lesions *(40)*. Indirect evidence comes from a recent study in which a small number of MS patients were treated with riluzole, an inhibitor of glutamate transmission that is used for treatment of amyotrophic lateral sclerosis, and this reduced the cervical cord atrophy and development of hypointense T1 lesions *(41)*. Although this result is interesting, the number of patients was too small and the study was not randomized.

In addition to cytokines, other molecules elaborated by inflammatory cells can injure axons. This includes free radicals such as nitric oxide, which damages small axons in vitro *(42,43)*, particularly when they are demyelinated. Interestingly, levels of nitric oxide synthase are elevated in MS lesions *(44–46)*.

Matrix metalloproteinases (MMPs), enzymes that can destroy the extracellular matrix (ECM), are associated with the pathogenesis of MS. There is good evidence that T cells and other leukocytes use MMPs to cross the BBB *(47)*. MMP-1 *(48)* and MMP-2 *(49)* are toxic to neurons in vitro, although MMP-2 also has a role in promoting regeneration of denervated nerves in rat peripheral nerve explants *(50)*. These observations confirm the duality of molecules, such as MMPs and cytokines: they can have opposing roles in different environments.

Much attention has recently focused on the possible role of antibodies in MS. Their function in demyelination seems to be important and supported by findings in EAE *(51)*, but there is little data on the role of antibodies in axonal and neuronal injury. Antibodies can cause injury through an antibody-dependent cellular cytotoxicity mechanism or by inducing complement activation. When activated, the complement cascade induces a membrane attack complex (MAC) that breaks the cell membrane. In MS, complement components and activation products have been isolated from cerebrospinal fluid (CSF) *(52)* and brain lesions *(53,54)*. In addition, a good correlation was demonstrated between C9, a component of the MAC, and areas of axonal degeneration *(55)*.

Information on whether and how T cells kill neurons is limited. The first evidence of neuronal susceptibility to T-cell cytotoxicity came from a study using mouse peripheral nervous system neurons in vitro *(56)*; only allogeneic T cells were cytotoxic to neurons. Since then, antigen-specific T cells were found to be toxic to syngeneic mouse neurons but required the neurons to express MHC-I, which was achieved by prior treatment with tetrodotoxin and IFN-γ *(57,58)*.

Neurons in the CNS express minimal or negligible levels of MHC-I *(34,59)*, and given that many infiltrating T cells in MS are probably CNS antigen nonspecific *(60)*, we investigated other means of producing neuronal cytotoxicity. We demonstrated that polyclonally activated T cells have a potent cytotoxic effect on human neurons. This occurred in an allogeneic and syngeneic system in the absence of added antigen, required T-cell activation, and was mediated through contact-dependent non-MHC-I mechanisms. These results show the high and selective vulnerability of human neurons to T cells, and suggest that when enough activated T cells accumulate in the CNS, neuronal cytotoxicity can result *(32)*.

After the initial involvement of an inflammatory insult, neurodegenerative processes of MS can progress for other reasons such as synaptic disconnection and lack of trophic support; possibly, these mechanisms are prevalent in SP and primary progressive (PP)MS. This hypothesis can also explain the absence of any improvement of these forms of MS to the currently available immunomodulatory treatments.

4. INTERFERON-β: A BRIEF REVIEW OF MECHANISMS OF ACTION

IFNs are a family of cytokines that were first described by Isaacs and Lindenmann in 1957 as naturally occurring proteins that interfere with viral replication *(61)*. Subsequently two types of IFNs were identified: type I and type II IFNs. Type I IFN include IFN-α, -β, -ω and -τ, and some IFNs (IFN-α, and -β) are currently used in many therapeutic protocols. On the contrary, IFN-γ, considered a proinflammatory cytokine, is the only type II IFN. Type I and II IFNs engage different receptors expressed on their target cells.

IFN-β has been in clinical use as an immunomodulatory drug for the treatment of MS for more than 10 yr. There are three commercial forms of IFN-β: Betaseron® (IFN-β1b; Berlex Laboratories), Avonex® (Biogen IDEC), and Rebif® (Serono) (both IFN-β1a). All three preparations are referred to in this chapter interchangeably as IFN-β unless otherwise indicated. In MS, the mechanism of the immunomodulatory effect of IFN-β likely occurs at several levels. In the periphery, IFNβ can affect antigen presentation and the cytokine milieu. The activity on antigen presentation is exerted through a mechanism of downregulation of surface molecules involved in this process. IFN-β is effective in preventing the IFN-γ-induced upregulation of MHC-II on antigen-presenting cells *(62)*.

IFN-β can also downregulate the expression of costimulatory molecules and inhibit the activation and proliferation of T cells (Fig. 1). In this regard, IFN-β treatment decreases the expression of CD54 (intercellular adhesion molecule [ICAM-1]) and CD80 (B7.1) on CD14-positive peripheral blood mononuclear cells of MS patients *(63)*. In addition, IFN-β inhibits the expression of FLIP, an antiapoptotic protein, leading to an increased incidence of death of T cells *(64)*. Corresponding with these mechanisms, the frequency of myelin basic protein-reactive T cells in MS patients was found to be reduced following treatment with IFN-β, compared to pretreatment levels *(65)*.

Perhaps predominantly through its effect on antigen presentation, an outcome of IFN-β treatment is its alterations of cytokine levels. Several studies have described an elevation of IL-10 in the mononuclear cells, serum, and CSF of IFN-β-treated MS patients. In addition, the majority of studies have shown that IFN-β decreases IFN-γ, IL-12 and TNF-α (T helper [Th1]1 cytokines) *(62)*, although others found no difference or an increase *(66,67)*. A decrease in both Th1 and Th2 cytokine-producing T cells has also been reported following IFN-β treatment, suggesting a general suppression of T cells. Although the majority of data indicate a diminution of Th1 responses, a clear effect on Th2 cytokines is equivocal.

A major effect of IFN-β therapy seems to involve the BBB. During the migration of leukocytes across the BBB, different adhesion molecules are expressed at the interface between T cells and endothelial cells. An increased expression of some of these adhesion molecules, such as VLA-4, leukocyte function antigen (LFA)-1, vascular cell adhesion molecule (VCAM)-1, and ICAM-1, has been described in MS. Many adhesion molecules are present in two forms: membrane bound and soluble. The soluble form can interact with receptors on the T-cell membrane and prevent the interaction with endothelial cells. The conversion of cell-associated VCAM-1 to its soluble form is facilitated by IFN-β *(68)*. In addition, IFN-β increases soluble ICAM-1 levels in the serum of MS patients *(69)*. Furthermore, IFN-β decreases the expression of several chemokines *(70,71)*, reducing the chemokine gradient that facilitates leukocyte access to the CNS.

When leukocytes traverse the endothelial barrier, they encounter the ECM proteins of the basement membrane. To pass through the basement membrane, digestion of the ECM proteins appears necessary; here, leukocytes employ the action of proteolytic enzymes, such as MMPs. IFN-β reduces the production of MMP-9 by activated T cells *(72,73)*. This decrease impairs the ability of T cells to cross the BBB. Furthermore, MMP-9 serum levels are decreased in RRMS patients treated with IFN-β. *(69)* On the other hand, in PPMS patients treated with IFN-β, serum levels of MMP-9 were not different from those of the placebo-treated group *(74)*. The lack of difference can be related to the reduced inflammatory activity in progressive patients compared to RR ones, and this seems to be confirmed by another observation showing reduced MMP-9 and MMP-7 transcript levels in mononuclear cells of patients with RRMS but not SPMS *(75)*. Overall, IFN-β decreases the number of inflammatory cells infiltrating the CNS parenchyma (Fig. 1) and this appears to be a major mechanism for its clinical effect.

5. IS IFN-β NEUROPROTECTIVE IN MS? ASSESSING CLINICAL OUTCOMES

As the neurodegenerative aspects of MS are strongly correlated with clinical disability, neuroprotection is a primary goal of treatment. A neuroprotective treatment can be defined as one that slows or stops disease progression by protecting, rescuing, or restoring the degenerated neurons and/or axons. In clinical trials, the available treatments for MS have shown some efficacy in reducing the relapse rate and number of gadolinium-enhancing lesions; however evidence for whether these treatments have any neuroprotective effect is weaker.

The progression of disability in MS may be a reflection of the neurodegenerative aspect of MS. IFN-β has a robust effect on inflammation (gadolinium enhancement) on brain MRI *(1)* and a less robust one on the frequency of clinical relapses *(2)*. To assess the effect of these drugs on progression of disability is a challenge, as trials have not been long enough to make such conclusions. Furthermore, MS is a chronic disease, and it takes about 15 yr from onset for a patient with RRMS to reach an Expanded Disability Status Scale (EDSS) of 6 (use of a cane) *(76)*.

The first randomized controlled trial (RCT) of IFN-β used recombinant IFN-β1b at two different doses (1.6 MIU and 8 MIU) subcutaneously every other day and enrolled 372 patients with an EDSS of up to 5.5 inclusive. Patients were followed for 5 yr. Changes in the neurological rating and EDSS were used as secondary outcomes. This trial did not show a change in the neurological rating at 3 yr. The EDSS slightly increased, with a trend for statistical significance only at 3 yr ($p = 0.043$) *(2)*.

IFN-β1a (Avonex) once weekly by intramuscular route was tested in another phase III trial involving 301 patients with a mild to moderate EDSS (1–3.5) who were followed for 2 yr. Because the drop-off rate was lower than expected, the trial was terminated earlier than 2 yr, after 172 patients had completed 2 yr of treatment. The primary outcome in this study, contrary to other trials, was time to onset of sustained worsening of disability instead of relapse rate. There was a 37% reduction in the probability of progression by one EDSS point at 2 yr, analyzing all patients in the study ($p = 0.02$) *(77)*; however, for the patients who completed 2 yr of treatment, the difference in the proportion of patients with progression of disability was 21.1% for the IFN-β1a group, compared with 33.3% in the placebo group ($p = 0.07$) *(78)*.

The third RCT is known as Prevention of Relapses and Disability by Interferon β Subcutaneously in Multiple Sclerosis (PRISMS); this compared 22 and 44 μg IFN-β1a (Rebif) three times a week vs placebo *(79)*. The study (PRISMS-2) enrolled 560 patients with an EDSS of 0 to 5.5 inclusive and followed them for 2 yr. Progression in disability again was a secondary outcome and defined as at least a one-point EDSS increase that was sustained at least for 3 mo. Time to progression was significantly longer in both treatment groups compared to the placebo arm ($p < 0.05$). The Integrated Disability Status Scale (IDSS), defined as the area under the time/EDSS plot, was not increased at 2 yr (median IDSS at 0) in both treated groups and increased by 0.4 in the placebo group. Patients in the placebo group were then rolled over to 22 or 44 μg Rebif and followed for another 2 yr (PRISMS-4). Again, time to progression of disability was significantly longer in the high-dose vs the crossover group (42.1 vs 24.2 mo), and no statistically significant difference was found between the low-dose vs the crossover groups or between the low- vs high-dose groups. IDSS at 4 yr was significantly lower in the high-dose vs the crossover group ($p = 0.034$), and no difference was observed for the low-dose vs the crossover group or low- vs high-dose group. In PRISMS-2, 61.7, 70.3, and 73.2% of patients in the placebo, low-, and high-dose groups, respectively were progression-free, and these were not statistically significant. In PRISMS-4 *(80)*, the percentages of progression-free patients in the aforementioned three groups were 46, 51, and 56%, respectively, and these were also not statistically significant from one another, except for a trend found when comparing the placebo to the high-dose group ($p = 0.07$).

IFN-β was also studied in SPMS. This group might better reveal a neuroprotective effect of IFN-β, as disability in SPMS might be more clearly correlated with axonal loss. In the European SPMS trial, 718 patients were randomized to receive 8 MIU IFN-β1b or placebo. In this trial, 70% of the randomized patients had relapses in addition to progression. The time to confirmed neurological deterioration was statistically significant in the treated group ($p = 0.0008$). About 50% and 39% of the patients progressed in the placebo and treatment group, respectively, representing a 22% decrease in the proportion of treated patients who progressed compared to placebo subjects *(81)*.

Although the above trial did show some therapeutic effect of IFN-β in SPMS, unfortunately, a North American trial failed to replicate these findings. In the North Amercian trial, 939 patients were randomized to receive every other day either placebo, 8 MIU IFN-β1b, or an IFN-β1b dose adjusted to body surface area. This trial was ended early because of the lack of efficacy in reducing disease progression *(82)*.

The above two studies in SPMS were followed by a third one, the Secondary Progressive Efficacy Clinical Trial of Recombinant Interferon-β-1a in MS trial, which randomized patients in North American and Europe to 22 or 44 μg IFN-β1a or placebo. Again, this trial did not show a difference in time to sustained progression in disability. Interestingly, women (62% of the whole population) in the high-dose ($p = 0.006$) and low-dose groups ($p = 0.038$) and men in the placebo group showed a statistically significant delay in progression compared to controls *(19)*.

As noted, the above studies described progression of disability using the EDSS, which relies heavily on ambulation, especially in the higher numerical range; the scale overlooks hand functions and does not include cognitive performance. Therefore, any beneficial effect of immunomodulatory drugs could be an underestimation of their real values. For instance, the last phase III trial in SPMS, the International Multiple Sclerosis Secondary Progressive Avonex Clinical Trial (IMPACT) study, used Avonex at the standard approved dose for 2 yr. The primary objective of IMPACT again was time to disease progression but used the Multiple Sclerosis Functional Composite score (MSFC) based on timing of a patient's ability to walk 25 ft and the nine-hole peg test, which evaluates arm and hand function and ability to perform calculations. The results of the IMPACT study showed a significantly positive effect on the overall MSFC score but not on ambulation *(83)*.

Clinical trials increasingly are relying on MRI of the brain and, very recently, of the spinal cord as a biomarker of the disease. MRI measures used for assessment of neurodegeneration include brain atrophy measurements and T1-hypointense lesions or black T1 *(black holes)*. T2-hyperintense lesions are very sensitive but lack specificity as they reflect edema, demyelination, axonal loss, or gliosis and are therefore not useful as markers for neurodegeneration.

In a longitudinal study of brain atrophy using Avonex, 237 patients had a baseline scan, 124 had a follow-up at yr 1, and 85 at yr 2. This study showed a weak positive correlation between EDSS and third ventricle width ($r = 0.26$, $p = 0.0001$), EDSS and lateral ventricle width ($r = 0.18$, $p = 0.0007$), and EDSS and corpus callosum atrophy ($r = -0.15$, $p = 0.016$) *(84)*. Patients were then randomized to IFN-β1a once weekly vs placebo and followed for at least 2 yr. Brain atrophy was measured using brain parenchymal fraction (BPF), defined as the ratio of brain parenchyma tissue volume over total volume contained within the brain. At 1 yr, the rate of brain atrophy was similar between the two groups but this was significantly different at yr 2 ($p < 0.01$), with less atrophy in the treatment group. In the whole group, BPF decreased as the number of relapses increased. This decrease was statistically significant even in patients with no or a single relapse. Therefore, brain atrophy occurs even without relapses. This could be caused by subclinical inflammation but could also be caused by neurodegenerative aspect of MS, in which axonal loss continues independent of inflammation. This dichotomy could be caused by Wallerian degeneration or lack of trophic support *(85)*. Alternately, the discordance between axonal loss and inflammation could represent a temporal separation, in which axons continue to degenerate slowly some years after the causative inflammatory insult. If so, this could account for the observation that agents, such as CAMPATH-1 *(86,87)* and Linomide *(88)*, reduced gadolinium enhancements but did not affect clinical outcomes.

More recently, an open-label, baseline-vs-treatment crossover study of 30 RRMS patients showed that IFN-β1b slows the progression of brain atrophy during the second and third year of treatment, although 43% of patients had an increase in EDSS of at least 1 point and 70% of at least 0.5 points, consistent with the rate of disease progression observed in other studies. In the same cohort of patients, the presence or absence of neutralizing antibodies had no significant effect on brain atrophy *(89)*.

T1-hypointense lesions or black T1 are markers of destructive pathology, principally of axonal loss. Black holes, however, are not synonymous with destruction in general, as new lesions could present as such, although these new black holes are less hypointense than the persistent lesions, might be reversible, and do enhance with gadolinium. Henceforth, we refer to black T1 as the lesions associated with irreversible damage.

The same group that studied the effect of IFN-β1a on brain atrophy also evaluated the effect of this drug on black holes. Black holes increased by 8% ($p < 0.05$) and 34% ($p < 0.05$) in the treated and placebo group, respectively. The presence of enhancing lesions appeared to be the most important factor determining the future development of T1-hypointense lesions ($r = 0.45$, $p < 0.001$). These enhancing lesions also predicted third ventricle atrophy *(90)*.

T1-hypointense lesions were also studied in a subgroup of SPMS patients *(85)* treated with IFN-β1b in the European trial. Forty-one patients were randomized to placebo and 44 to treatment, and patients were followed-up every 6 mo for 36 mo. At baseline, T1-hypointense lesion volume was 5.1 cc and 4.9 cc in placebo and treatment group and showed a linear increase in volume by 2.4 cc and 0.76 cc, respectively. This increase from baseline was statistically significant for both arms ($p = 0.0002$ and $p = 0.006$, respectively). The average increase of black-hole volume per year was 14% in the placebo group and 7.7% in the treatment group, and this difference was statistically significant ($p = 0.0003$) *(91)*.

As shown above, the correlation between cerebral atrophy and EDSS, although statistically significant, remains weak. It is thought that locomotor disability is more correlated with spinal cord atrophy than with cerebral atrophy *(92,93)*. The assessment of spinal cord atrophy continues to be challenging, as image resolution remains problematic; however, a recent study computed the upper cervical cord area (UCCA) in a series of 38 patients with RRMS (20) and SPMS (18) randomized to IFN-β1a (22 vs 44 µg) matched to nontreated patients. The UCCA decreased by 5.7% and 4.5% at 48 mo in the placebo and IFN-treated group, respectively ($p = 0.35$) *(94)*.

We still have no standardized way to measure the impact of neurodegenerative processes in MS. Characteristics measured by MRI, such as brain atrophy, have not been correlated with disability in MS, and measures of axonal loss, such as the magnetization transfer ratio (MTR) and spectroscopy, have not been used in large-scale clinical trials. The effects of IFN-β on MTR measures in RRMS remain controversial. A recent study of SPMS has shown no effect of IFN-β1b on MTR measures. No data are available for other treatments. In addition, small studies have shown conflicting results regarding the effect of IFN-β on *N*-acetyl-aspartate peak. In one study, 10 patients with RRMS who followed by MRI/MRS for 1 yr pretreatment and 1 yr posttreatment with IFN-β 1b were compared to 6 untreated patients. An increase of *N*-acetyl-aspartate levels in brains of patients with RRMS following IFN-β treatment was noted ($p = 0.03$) *(95,96)*. Another study failed to show an increase in *N*-acetyl aspartate peak following treatment with IFN-β1a, however, the study lasted only 6 mo *(97)*. A third study involving 11 patients taking IFN-β (1 Avonex, 1 Betaseron, and 9 Rebif) for 12 mo showed a decrease in the number of T2 lesions and, contrary to expectations, a decrease in *N*-acetyl-aspartate peak. This study suggested that reduction of new inflammatory activity with IFN-β does not invariably halt progression of axonal injury, although it appeared that an inverse relationship existed between the rate of progression of axonal injury and relapse rate for the preceding 2 yr *(96)*.

In conclusion, what can we learn from these studies? First, IFN-β seems to have a minimal effect on EDSS, as it is mainly used for short-term purposes in clinical trials. Second, if IFN-β has an effect on EDSS, it may reduce disability secondary to inflammation. Third, although their effect on EDSS is less obvious, the IFN-β preparations have a statistically significant effect on brain atrophy and T1-lesion volume, underlining again the weak correlation between EDSS and measures of atrophy. This weak correlation could potentially be improved using measurement of spinal cord atrophy. Fourth, brain atrophy increased as the number of relapses increased and patients with SPMS and superimposed relapses do better on IFN-β than do patients with SPMS without relapses. In these patients without relapses, neurodegeneration might be occurring independently (or as a delayed consequence) of inflammation, and immunomodulators may not provide neuroprotection at this irreversible stage.

6. PROPOSED MECHANISMS OF NEUROPROTECTION BY IFN-β

The clinical studies above suggest a neuroprotective effect for IFN-β in MS, even if it is not robust. What might be the mechanism of neuroprotection? We think it is likely that the neuroprotective mechanism is linked to the neurodegeneration that inflammatory molecules and T cells can effect, as discussed earlier. Thus, by reducing the influx of pathogenic T cells into the CNS, IFN-β would in essence be preventing further CNS insults from these cells. The outcome would be neuroprotection, even if it were exerted indirectly by preventing detrimental leuckocytes from reaching their sites of action within the CNS parenchyma (Fig. 1).

Is there a potential for IFN-β to exert direct neuroprotective effects within the CNS? This seems unlikely, as IFN-β is not thought to cross into the CNS. Although, if it does and the BBB in MS patients is not intact, IFN-β possibly may act within the CNS. In this regard, we have described that IFN-β treatment of astrocytes in culture resulted in the significant upregulation of an important survival factor, nerve growth factor *(98)*; however, it remains to be demonstrated that this occurs in vivo within the CNS.

7. PERSPECTIVES

To design new neuroprotective treatments or confirm the neuroprotection conferred by existing therapeutics, we need to understand the mechanisms responsible for axonal and neuronal loss and find measurable clinical outcomes more related to the neurodegenerative aspects of MS. Furthermore, we need to modify trial designs, which do not adequately reveal the potential beneficial effect of existing immunomodulatory drugs. There is a prospect for drug-related neuroprotection in MS, and medications (e.g., glatiramer acetate) may have this efficacy *(99)*. By decreasing pathogenic inflammation, it appears that some degree of neuroprotection is also afforded by IFN-β, and it is up to the research community to demonstrate this convincingly and to design appropriate strategies to enhance this capacity.

REFERENCES

1. Paty DW, Li DK. Interferon beta-1b is effective in relapsing-remitting multiple sclerosis. II. MRI analysis results of a multicenter, randomized, double-blind, placebo-controlled trial. UBC MS/MRI Study Group and the IFNB Multiple Sclerosis Study Group. Neurology 1993;43:662–667.
2. Interferon beta-1b is effective in relapsing-remitting multiple sclerosis. I. Clinical results of a multicenter, randomized, double-blind, placebo-controlled trial. The IFNB Multiple Sclerosis Study Group. Neurology 1993;43: 655–661.
3. Johnson KP, Brooks BR, Cohen JA, et al. Copolymer 1 reduces relapse rate and improves disability in relapsing-remitting multiple sclerosis: results of a phase III multicenter, double-blind placebo–controlled trial. The Copolymer 1 Multiple Sclerosis Study Group. Neurology 1995;45:1268–1276.
4. Comi G, Filippi M, Wolinsky JS. European/Canadian multicenter, double-blind, randomized, placebo-controlled study of the effects of glatiramer acetate on magnetic resonance imaging-measured disease activity and burden in patients with relapsing multiple sclerosis. European/Canadian Glatiramer Acetate Study Group. Ann Neurol 2001;49:290–297.
5. Lucchinetti C, Bruck W, Rodriguez M, Lassmann G. Distinct patterns of multiple sclerosis pathology indicates heterogeneity on pathogenesis. Brain Pathol 1996;6:800–806.
6. Martin R, Sturzebecher CS, McFarland HF. Immunotherapy of multiple sclerosis: where are we? Where should we go? Nat Immunol 2001;2:785–788.
7. Wekerle H, Kojima K, Lannes-Vieira J, Lassmann H, Linington C. Animal models. Ann Neurol 1994;36(suppl.):S47–53.
8. Hafler DA, Weiner HL. Antigen-specific immunosuppression: oral tolerance for treatment of autoimmune disease. Chem Immunol 1995;60:126–149.
9. Steinman L. Multiple sclerosis: a coordinated immunological attack against myelin in the central nervous system. Cell 1996;85:299–302.
10. Wekerle H, Hohlfeld R. Molecular mimicry in multiple sclerosis. N Engl J Med 2003;349:185–186.
11. Vanderlugt CL, Miller SD. Epitope spreading in immune-mediated diseases: implications for immunotherapy. Nat Rev Immunol 2002;2:85–95.
12. van Noort JM, Bajramovic JJ, Plomp AC, van Stipdonk MJ. Mistaken self, a novel model that links microbial infections with myelin-directed autoimmunity in multiple sclerosis. J Neuroimmunol 2000;105:46–57.
13. Hickey WF, Hsu BL, Kimura H. T-lymphocyte entry into the central nervous system. J Neurosci Res 1991; 28:254–260.
14. Flugel A, Willem M, Berkowicz T, Wekerle H. Gene transfer into CD4+ T lymphocytes: green fluorescent protein-engineered, encephalitogenic T cells illuminate brain autoimmune responses. Nat Med 1999;5:843–847.
15. Qing Z, Sewell D, Sandor M, Fabry Z. Antigen-specific T-cell trafficking into the central nervous system. J Neuroimmunol 2000;105:169–178.
16. Charcot M. Histologie de la sclerose en plaques. Gaz Hosp 1868;141:554–558.

17. Trapp BD, Peterson J, Ransohoff RM, Rudick R, Mork S, Bo L. Axonal transection in the lesions of multiple sclerosis. N Engl J Med 1998;338:278–285.

18. Ferguson B, Matyszak MK, Esiri MM, Perry VH. Axonal damage in acute multiple sclerosis lesions. Brain 1997; 120(Pt 3):393–399.

19. Randomized controlled trial of interferon-beta-1a in secondary progressive MS: Clinical results. Neurology 2001;56:1496–1504.

20. Kuhlmann T, Lingfeld G, Bitsch A, Schuchardt J, Bruck W. Acute axonal damage in multiple sclerosis is most extensive in early disease stages and decreases over time. Brain 2002;125(Pt 10):2202–2212.

21. Tourbah A, Stievenart JL, Gout O, et al. Localized proton magnetic resonance spectroscopy in relapsing remitting versus secondary progressive multiple sclerosis. Neurology 1999;53:1091–1097.

22. Filippi M, Bozzali M, Rovaris M, et al. Evidence for widespread axonal damage at the earliest clinical stage of multiple sclerosis. Brain 2003;126(Pt 2):433–437.

23. Bagnato F, Jeffries N, Richert ND, et al. Evolution of T1 black holes in patients with multiple sclerosis imaged monthly for 4 years. Brain 2003;126:1782–1789.

24. Bruck W, Bitsch A, Kolenda H, Bruck Y, Stiefel M, Lassmann H. Inflammatory central nervous system demyelination: correlation of magnetic resonance imaging findings with lesion pathology. Ann Neurol 1997;42:783–793.

25. Bitsch A, Kuhlmann T, Stadelmann C, Lassmann H, Lucchinetti C, Bruck W. A longitudinal MRI study of histopathologically defined hypointense multiple sclerosis lesions. Ann Neurol 2001;49:793–796.

26. Cifelli A, Arridge M, Jezzard P, Esiri MM, Palace J, Matthews PM. Thalamic neurodegeneration in multiple sclerosis. Ann Neurol 2002;52:650–653.

27. Wylezinska M, Cifelli A, Jezzard P, Palace J, Alecci M, Matthews PM. Thalamic neurodegeneration in relapsing–remitting multiple sclerosis. Neurology 2003;60:1949–1954.

28. De Stefano N, Matthews PM, Filippi M, et al. Evidence of early cortical atrophy in MS: relevance to white matter changes and disability. Neurology 2003;60:1157–1162.

29. Peterson JW, Bo L, Mork S, Chang A, Trapp BD. Transected neurites, apoptotic neurons, and reduced inflammation in cortical multiple sclerosis lesions. Ann Neurol 2001;50:389–400.

30. Smith KJ, Kapoor R, Hall SM, Davies M. Electrically active axons degenerate when exposed to nitric oxide. Ann Neurol 2001;49:470–476.

31. Downen M, Amaral TD, Hua LL, Zhao ML, Lee SC. Neuronal death in cytokine-activated primary human brain cell culture: role of tumor necrosis factor-alpha. Glia 1999;28:114–127.

32. Giuliani F, Goodyer C, Antel JP, Yong VW. Vulnerability of human neurons to T cell-mediated cytotoxicity. J Immunol 2003;171:368–379.

33. Venters HD, Tang Q, Liu Q, VanHoy RW, Dantzer R, Kelley KW. A new mechanism of neurodegeneration: a proinflammatory cytokine inhibits receptor signaling by a survival peptide. Proc Natl Acad Sci USA 1999; 96:9879–9884.

34. Neumann H, Cavalie A, Jenne DE, Wekerle H. Induction of MHC class I genes in neurons. Science 1995; 269:2582–2590.

35. Relton JK, Rothwell NJ. Interleukin-1 receptor antagonist inhibits ischaemic and excitotoxic neuronal damage in the rat. Brain Res Bull 1992;29:243–246.

36. Relton JK, Martin D, Thompson RC, Russell DA. Peripheral administration of interleukin–1 receptor antagonist inhibits brain damage after focal cerebral ischemia in the rat. Exp Neurol 1996;138:206–213.

37. Toulmond S, Parnet P, Linthorst AC. When cytokines get on your nerves: cytokine networks and CNS pathologies. Trends Neurosci 1996;19:409–410.

38. Yamasaki Y, Matsuura N, Shozuhara H, Onodera H, Itoyama Y, Kogure K. Interleukin–1 as a pathogenetic mediator of ischemic brain damage in rats. Stroke 1995;26:676–680, discussion 681.

39. Takahashi JL, Giuliani F, Power C, Imai Y, Yong VW. Interleukin-1beta promotes oligodendrocyte death through glutamate excitotoxicity. Ann Neurol 2003;53:588–595.

40. Werner P, Pitt D, Raine CS. Multiple sclerosis: altered glutamate homeostasis in lesions correlates with oligodendrocyte and axonal damage. Ann Neurol 2001;50:169–180.

41. Kalkers NF, Barkhof F, Bergers E, van Schijndel R, Polman CH. The effect of the neuroprotective agent riluzole on MRI parameters in primary progressive multiple sclerosis: a pilot study. Mult Scler 2002;8:532–533.

42. Smith KJ, Hall SM. Factors directly affecting impulse transmission in inflammatory demyelinating disease: recent advances in our understanding. Curr Opin Neurol 2001;14:289–298.

43. Garthwaite G, Goodwin DA, Batchelor AM, Leeming K, Garthwaite J. Nitric oxide toxicity in CNS white matter: an in vitro study using rat optic nerve. Neuroscience 2002;109:145–155.

44. Bo L, Dawson TM, Wesselingh S, et al. Induction of nitric oxide synthase in demyelinating regions of multiple sclerosis brains. Ann Neurol 1994;36:778–786.

45. Bagasra O, Michaels FH, Zheng YM, et al. Activation of the inducible form of nitric oxide synthase in the brains of patients with multiple sclerosis. Proc Natl Acad Sci USA 1995;92:12,041–12,045.

46. Bitsch A, Schuchardt J, Bunkowski S, Kuhlmann T, Bruck W. Acute axonal injury in multiple sclerosis. Correlation with demyelination and inflammation. Brain 2000;123(Pt 6):1174–1183.

47. Yong VW, Power C, Forsyth P, Edwards DR. Metalloproteinases in biology and pathology of the nervous system. Nat Rev Neurosci 2001;2:502–511.

48. Vos CM, Sjulson L, Nath A, et al. Cytotoxicity by matrix metalloprotease-1 in organotypic spinal cord and dissociated neuronal cultures. Exp Neurol 2000;163:324–330.

49. Johnston JB, Zhang K, Silva C, Shalinsky DR, Conant K, Ni W, et al. HIV-1 Tat neurotoxicity is prevented by matrix metalloproteinase inhibitors. Ann Neurol 2001;49:230–241.

50. Krekoski CA, Neubauer D, Graham JB, Muir D. Metalloproteinase-dependent predegeneration in vitro enhances axonal regeneration within acellular peripheral nerve grafts. J Neurosci 2002;22:10,408–10,415.

51. Linington C, Bradl M, Lassmann H, Brunner C, Vass K. Augmentation of demyelination in rat acute allergic encephalomyelitis by circulating mouse monoclonal antibodies directed against a myelin/oligodendrocyte glycoprotein. Am J Pathol 1988;130:443–454.

52. Mollnes TE, Vandvik B, Lea T, Vartdal F. Intrathecal complement activation in neurological diseases evaluated by analysis of the terminal complement complex. J Neurol Sci 1987;78:17–28.

53. Storch MK, Piddlesden S, Haltia M, Iivanainen M, Morgan P, Lassmann H. Multiple sclerosis: in situ evidence for antibody- and complement-mediated demyelination. Ann Neurol 1998;43:465–471.

54. Lucchinetti C, Bruck W, Parisi J, Scheithauer B, Rodriguez M, Lassmann H. Heterogeneity of multiple sclerosis lesions: implications for the pathogenesis of demyelination. Ann Neurol 2000;47:707–717.

55. Mead RJ, Singhrao SK, Neal JW, Lassmann H, Morgan BP. The membrane attack complex of complement causes severe demyelination associated with acute axonal injury. J Immunol 2002;168:458–465.

56. Manning PT, Johnson EMJ. MHC-specific cytotoxic T lymphocyte killing of dissociated sympathetic neuronal cultures. Am J Pathol 1987;128:395–409.

57. Rall GF, Mucke L, Oldstone MB. Consequences of cytotoxic T lymphocyte interaction with major histocompatibility complex class-1 expressing neurons in vivo. J Exp Med 1995;94:1201–1212.

58. Medana I, Martinic MA, Wekerle H, Neumann H. Transection of major histocompatibility complex class I-induced neurites by cytotoxic T lymphocytes. Am J Pathol 2001;159:809–815.

59. Redwine JM, Buchmeier MJ, Evans CF. In vivo expression of major histocompatibility complex molecules on oligodendrocytes and neurons during viral infection. Am J Pathol 2001;159:1219–1224.

60. Wucherpfennig KW, Newcombe J, Li H, Keddy C, Cuzner ML, Hafler DA. T cell receptor V alpha-V beta repertoire and cytokine gene expression in active multiple sclerosis lesions. J Exp Med 1992;175:993–1002.

61. Isaacs A, Lindenmann J. Virus interference. I. The interferon. Proc R Soc Lond B Biol Sci 1957;147:258–267.

62. Yong VW, Chabot S, Stuve O, Williams G. Interferon beta in the treatment of multiple sclerosis: mechanisms of action. Neurology 1998;51:682–689.

63. Shapiro S, Galboiz Y, Lahat N, Kinarty A, Miller A. The 'immunological-synapse' at its APC side in relapsing and secondary-progressive multiple sclerosis: modulation by interferon-beta. J Neuroimmunol 2003;144:116–124.

64. Sharief MK, Semra YK, Seidi OA, Zoukos Y. Interferon-beta therapy downregulates the anti-apoptosis protein FLIP in T cells from patients with multiple sclerosis. J Neuroimmunol 2001;120:199–207.

65. Zang YC, Yang D, Hong J, Tejada-Simon MV, Rivera VM, Zhang JZ. Immunoregulation and blocking antibodies induced by interferon beta treatment in MS. Neurology 2000;55:397–404.

66. Dayal AS, Jensen MA, Lledo A, Arnason BG. Interferon-gamma-secreting cells in multiple sclerosis patients treated with interferon beta-1b. Neurology 1995;45:2173–2177.

67. Wandinger KP, Sturzebecher CS, Bielekova B, et al. Complex immunomodulatory effects of interferon-beta in multiple sclerosis include the upregulation of T helper 1-associated marker genes. Ann Neurol 2001;50:349–357.

68. Calabresi PA, Pelfrey CM, Tranquill LR, Maloni H, McFarland HF. VLA-4 expression on peripheral blood lymphocytes is downregulated after treatment of multiple sclerosis with interferon beta. Neurology 1997;49:1111–1116.

69. Trojano M, Avolio C, Liuzzi GM, et al. Changes of serum sICAM-1 and MMP-9 induced by rIFNbeta-1b treatment in relapsing-remitting MS. Neurology 1999;53:1402–1408.

70. Iarlori C, Reale M, Lugaresi A, et al. RANTES production and expression is reduced in relapsing-remitting multiple sclerosis patients treated with interferon-beta-1b. J Neuroimmunol 2000;107:100–107.

71. Zang YC, Halder JB, Samanta AK, Hong J, Rivera VM, Zhang JZ. Regulation of chemokine receptor CCR5 and production of RANTES and MIP-1alpha by interferon-beta. J Neuroimmunol 2001;112:174–180.

72. Stuve O, Dooley NP, Uhm JH, et al. Interferon beta-1b decreases the migration of T lymphocytes in vitro: effects on matrix metalloproteinase-9. Ann Neurol 1996;40:853–863.

73. Leppert D, Waubant E, Burk MR, Oksenberg JR, Hauser SL. Interferon beta-1b inhibits gelatinase secretion and in vitro migration of human T cells: a possible mechanism for treatment efficacy in multiple sclerosis. Ann Neurol 1996;40:846–852.

74. Dubois B, Leary SM, Nelissen I, Opdenakker G, Giovannoni G, Thompson AJ. Serum gelatinase B/MMP-9 in primary progressive multiple sclerosis patients treated with interferon-beta-1a. J Neurol 2003;250:1037–1043.

75. Galboiz Y, Shapiro S, Lahat N, Rawashdeh H, Miller A. Matrix metalloproteinases and their tissue inhibitors as markers of disease subtype and response to interferon-beta therapy in relapsing and secondary-progressive multiple sclerosis patients. Ann Neurol 2001;50:443–451.

76. Weinshenker BG, Bass B, Rice GP, et al. The natural history of multiple sclerosis: a geographically based study. I. Clinical course and disability. Brain 1989;112(Pt 1):133–146.

77. Rudick RA, Goodkin DE, Jacobs LD, et al. Impact of interferon beta-1a on neurologic disability in relapsing multiple sclerosis. The Multiple Sclerosis Collaborative Research Group (MSCRG). Neurology 1997;49:358–363.

78. Rice G, Ebers G. Interferons in the treatment of multiple sclerosis: do they prevent the progression of the disease? Arch Neurol 1998;55:1578–1580.

79. Randomised double-blind placebo-controlled study of interferon beta-1a in relapsing/remitting multiple sclerosis. PRISMS (Prevention of Relapses and Disability by Interferon beta-1a Subcutaneously in Multiple Sclerosis) Study Group. Lancet 1998;352:1498–1504.

80. PRISMS-4: long-term efficacy of interferon-beta-1a in relapsing MS. Neurology 2001;56:1628–1636.

81. Placebo-controlled multicentre randomised trial of interferon beta-1b in treatment of secondary progressive multiple sclerosis. European Study Group on interferon beta-1b in secondary progressive MS. Lancet 1998;352:1491–1497.

82. Goodkin DE and the North American Study Group on Interferon Beta-1b in Secondary Progressive MS. Interferon beta-1b in secondary progressive MS: clinical and MRI results of a three-year randomized controlled trial. Neurology 2000;54(suppl.):2352.

83. Cohen JA, Cutter GR, Fischer JS, et al. Benefit of interferon beta-1a on MSFC progression in secondary progressive MS. Neurology 2002;59:679–687.

84. Simon JH, Jacobs LD, Campion MK, et al. A longitudinal study of brain atrophy in relapsing multiple sclerosis. The Multiple Sclerosis Collaborative Research Group (MSCRG). Neurology 1999;53:139–148.

85. Rudick RA, Fisher E, Lee JC, Duda JT, Simon J. Brain atrophy in relapsing multiple sclerosis: relationship to relapses, EDSS, and treatment with interferon beta-1a. Mult Scler 2000;6:365–372.

86. Coles AJ, Wing MG, Molyneux P, et al. Monoclonal antibody treatment exposes three mechanisms underlying the clinical course of multiple sclerosis. Ann Neurol 1999;46:296–304.

87. Paolillo A, Coles AJ, Molyneux PD, et al. Quantitative MRI in patients with secondary progressive MS treated with monoclonal antibody Campath 1H. Neurology 1999;53:751–757.

88. Wolinsky JS, Narayana PA, Noseworthy JH, et al. Linomide in relapsing and secondary progressive MS: part II: MRI results. MRI Analysis Center of the University of Texas-Houston, Health Science Center, and the North American Linomide Investigators. Neurology 2000;54:1734–1741.

89. Frank JA, Richert N, Bash C, et al. Interferon-beta-1b slows progression of atrophy in RRMS: Three-year follow-up in NAb- and NAb+ patients. Neurology 2004;62:719–725.

90. Simon JH, Lull J, Jacobs LD, et al. A longitudinal study of T1 hypointense lesions in relapsing MS: MSCRG trial of interferon beta-1a. Multiple Sclerosis Collaborative Research Group. Neurology 2000;55:185–192.

91. Barkhof F, van Waesberghe JH, Filippi M, et al. T(1) hypointense lesions in secondary progressive multiple sclerosis: effect of interferon beta-1b treatment. Brain 2001;124(Pt 7):1396–1402.

92. Losseff NA, Webb SL, O'Riordan JI, et al. Spinal cord atrophy and disability in multiple sclerosis. A new reproducible and sensitive MRI method with potential to monitor disease progression. Brain 1996;119(Pt 3):701–708.

93. Edwards SG, Gong QY, Liu C, et al. Infratentorial atrophy on magnetic resonance imaging and disability in multiple sclerosis. Brain 1999;122(Pt 2):291–301.

94. Lin X, Tench CR, Turner B, Blumhardt LD, Constantinescu CS. Spinal cord atrophy and disability in multiple sclerosis over four years: application of a reproducible automated technique in monitoring disease progression in a cohort of the interferon beta-1a (Rebif) treatment trial. J Neurol Neurosurg Psychiatry 2003;74:1090–1094.

95. Narayanan S, De Stefano N, Francis GS, et al. Axonal metabolic recovery in multiple sclerosis patients treated with interferon beta-1b. J Neurol 2001;248:979–986.

96. Parry A, Corkill R, Blamire AM, et al. Beta-Interferon treatment does not always slow the progression of axonal injury in multiple sclerosis. J Neurol 2003;250:171–178.

97. Sarchielli P, Presciutti O, Tarducci R, et al. 1H-MRS in patients with multiple sclerosis undergoing treatment with interferon beta-1a: results of a preliminary study. J Neurol Neurosurg Psychiatry 1998;64:204–212.

98. Boutros T, Croze E, Yong VW. Interferon-beta is a potent promoter of nerve growth factor production by astrocytes. J Neurochem 1997;69:939–946.

99. Yong VW. Prospects for neuroprotection in multiple sclerosis. Front Biosci 2004;9:864–872.

CME QUESTIONS

1. All of the following can be direct targets of interferon (IFN)-β except:
   A. T-cell activation
   B. Blood–brain barrier
   C. Major histocompatibilty complex class II expression
   D. Microglia activation
   E. Matrix metalloproteinases production

2. Which of the following is *not* a marker of neuronal injury?
   A. Amyloid precursor protein
   B. Interferon γ
   C. Black holes
   D. *N*-acetyl-aspartate decrease

3. All of the following have been shown to induce neuronal injury *except*:
   A. Tumor necrosis factor-α
   B. activated T cells
   C. Matrix metalloproteinase-1
   D. Complement C9
   E. *N*-acetyl-aspartate

   For questions 4 and 5, choose the correct answer:
   A. If A, B, and C are correct
   B. If A and C are correct
   C. If B and D are correct
   D. If D is correct
   E. If all are correct

4. The reason(s) why IFN-β is not robust on disability/neurodegeneration is:
   A. The lack of sensitivity of the Expanded Disability Status Scale (EDSS)
   B. The lack of methods to assess spinal cord atrophy
   C. IFN-β's lack of a direct neuroprotective effect in the brain
   D. IFN-β might be used too late in the disease degenerative process

5. IFN-β's effect on disability in multiple sclerosis (MS):
   A. Has been shown in all randomized controlled trials
   B. Is strong on the EDSS
   C. Seems to be more obvious in secondary progressive MS
   D. Cannot be assessed reliably because of the relatively short duration of clinical trials

8

Acute Disseminated Encephalomyelitis

Sean J. Pittock and Dean M. Wingerchuk

1. INTRODUCTION

Acute disseminated encephalomyelitis (ADEM) is a rare monophasic inflammatory demyelinating disorder of the central nervous system (CNS) that occurs more often in children or young adults than in older people and has been recognized for more than 200 yr *(1)*. The lack of a universally accepted definition of ADEM is a major impediment to understanding and describing its clinical-pathological boundaries *(2,3)*.

ADEM causes the rapid development of focal or multifocal neurological symptoms and signs in conjunction with an acute meningoencephalitic syndrome. It is often antedated, especially in children, by a febrile prodromal illness, such as infection (postinfectious encephalomyelitis), immunization (postvaccinal encephalomyelitis), exanthema, or even a bee sting *(2,4–8)*. Although ADEM is considered an idiopathic inflammatory demyelinating syndrome, its features may overlap with those of multiple sclerosis (MS), acute transverse myelitis, neuromyelitis optica (NMO), and various focal demyelinating syndromes (e.g., Balo's concentric sclerosis, Marburg variant of MS). Some large retrospective series have used loose criteria for defining ADEM, such as acute neurological symptoms in association with undefined brain magnetic resonance imaging (MRI) white-matter abnormalities compatible with ADEM *(4–6)* or no MRI at all *(9,10)*. Most often, the level of diagnostic uncertainty is highest in adult patients with an initial, acute, multifocal CNS demyelinating syndrome; the overlap of epidemiological, clinical, and imaging features of MS and ADEM may make it difficult to distinguish these disorders.

Interferon (IFN)-β preparations may delay a second attack (and, therefore, confirm a diagnosis of MS) following a clinically isolated demyelinating syndrome accompanied by cranial MRI lesions suggestive of MS *(11–13)*. Patients who present with their first-ever demyelinating event, especially one that involves multifocal symptomatic CNS lesions, may appear to have ADEM and, perhaps, a greater chance of monophasic (nonrecurrent) disease. In these cases, careful clinical and MRI surveillance for development of dissemination in time is mandatory to provide accurate prognostic information and for treatment purposes.

2. EPIDEMIOLOGY

Cases of ADEM have been reported throughout the world. Males and females are affected with equal frequency, whereas in MS, two-thirds of affected people are female. ADEM is commonly antedated by an infectious illness (46–77%) or immunization (0–12%). Table 1 summarizes these reported associations *(14–51)*. In the United States, ADEM was estimated to account

From: *Current Clinical Neurology: Inflammatory Disorders of the Nervous System:*
Pathogenesis, Immunology, and Clinical Management
Edited by: A. Minagar and J. S. Alexander © Humana Press Inc., Totowa, NJ

Table 1
Infections and Immunizations Associated With Acute Disseminated Encephalomyelitis

Viral infections	Reference
Measles, mumps, rubella	*14–16*
Varicella	*17*
Influenza A or B	—
Rocky Mountain Spotted Fever	—
Hepatitis A or B or C	*18*
Herpes Simplex	*19,20*
Human Herpes virus 6	*17*
Ebstein-Barr virus	*21*
Cytomegalovirus	*21*
Vaccinia	—
HIV, HTLV-1	*22–24*
Parainfluenza	*25*
Dengue fever	*26*
Bacterial infections	
Mycoplasma pneumonia	*27–29*
Chlamydia pneumoniae	*30*
Legionella	*31*
Campylobacter	*32*
Pasteurella multocida	*33*
Streptococcus	*34*
Pontiac Fever	*35*
Immunizations	
Rabies	*36–41*
Diptheria-tetanus-polio	*42*
Measles, mumps, rubella	*14,15,43–45*
Vaccinia	*46,47*
Japanese B encephalitis	*48*
Hog vaccine	*49*
Hepatitis B	*50*
Meningococcal A and C	*51*

HIV, human immunodeficiency virus; HTLV-1, human T-cell lymphoma/leukemia virus.

for 30% of encephalitis cases prior to the introduction of vaccines for measles, varicella, and rubella *(52)*. ADEM occurred in about 1 in 1000 measles virus infections, with an associated mortality of 25% and major neurologic sequelae in 25 to 40% *(10,53)*. Other common viral infections, such as varicella zoster (1 in 10,000) and rubella (1 in 20,000), are associated with a relatively low incidence of ADEM.

In developed countries, the advent of immunizations has reduced the incidence of infectious ADEM. Currently, ADEM most commonly is associated with measles, mumps, and rubella vaccinations. The incidence of 1 to 2 per 1 million for live measles vaccine immunizations is much lower than for ADEM associated with measles itself. The generalized use of vaccines in the developed world has resulted in a decrease in the incidence of postinfectious ADEM. In developing countries with incomplete immunizations, these infections remain poorly controlled *(7)*. ADEM after smallpox vaccination occurs in 2.2 to 3.5 cases per 1 million children *(54)*.

Changes in vaccine characteristics can affect ADEM incidence. Neurological complications occurred with a frequency of up to 1 in 400 after use of rabies vaccine produced from virus grown in rabbit brain and about 1 in 1000 with the Semple type; these complications are now rare, as non-neural-tissue-based vaccines are used.

3. IMMUNOPATHOLOGY

The most important pathological feature of ADEM (also known as *perivenous encephalomyelitis* and *acute perivascular myelinoclasis*) is perivenous inflammation with infiltration of predominantly macrophages (reactive microglia) and associated demyelination occurring in the cerebral hemispheres, brainstem, cerebellum, and spinal cord *(55)*. A cell-mediated autoimmune response to myelin proteins triggered by infection or immunization may be a possible etiological factor.

In patients who die of fulminant ADEM, the brain is swollen and congested and may show signs of herniation. The freshly sliced brain reveals little apart from swelling and occasional petechial hemorrhages, in contrast to acute MS, in which lesions are visible macroscopically (Table 2). The pathological hallmark of ADEM is the sleeve-like distribution of demyelination in the hypercellular perivenous zones. Lymphocytes, and to a lesser extent neutrophils, may be seen outside the Virchow-Robin spaces. Other changes include vessel wall invasion by inflammatory cells, perivascular edema, petechial hemorrhage, and endothelial swelling.

ADEM lesions are of similar histological age and are most evident in the small blood vessels of the white matter, although they may involve the deeper layers of the cerebral cortex, thalamus, hypothalamus, and basal ganglia and also blood vessels in the walls of the lateral and third ventricle. Lesions are often multiple and may be concentrated in a particular area, such as a lobe (especially the occipital lobe), brainstem, or spinal cord *(2,7,55)*. Axons are relatively preserved and tend to be tortuous and swollen. Reactive astrocytes are relatively uncommon. Narrow zones of subpial demyelination in spinal cord and brainstem may be present. There is no convincing evidence of inflammatory cells in spinal roots, ganglia, or peripheral nerves. Cases of acute hemorrhagic leukoencephalitis (AHL), a form of ADEM, reveal a greater degree of polymorphonuclear cell infiltrates than in typical ADEM and include perivenous hemorrhages. The neuropathology of relapsing ADEM has also been described; these rare cases show scattered sleeve-like perivenous demyelinating lesions with little or no similarities to MS pathology. The limited extent and pattern of demyelination helps distinguish ADEM from MS pathologically. Pathological features that can help distinguish ADEM, MS, AHL, and NMO are shown in Table 2.

In contrast to ADEM pathological characteristics, standardized pathological examination of MS biopsy and autopsy specimen materials demonstrate four different immunopathological patterns of disease *(56)*. Patterns I and II are similar and are characterized by oligodendrocyte survival and remyelination, suggesting that myelin is the target of injury. T cells and macrophages are present within lesions, and pattern II has complement activation and immunoglobulin (Ig) deposition at sites of myelin breakdown. Patterns III and IV also involve T cells and macrophages but, in contrast to patterns I and II, are characterized by oligodendrocyte loss with limited remyelination. Oligodendrocytes appear to be the target of injury. Pattern III has preferential loss of myelin-associated glycoprotein (MAG) localized in the interglial loop, a finding interpreted as oligodendrocyte dystrophy with associated apoptosis. These patterns are heterogenous among patients but homogenous within multiple active lesions for individual patients *(56)*. Similar detailed immunopathological studies will determine the common and differentiating characteristics of ADEM and typical forms of MS.

Identifiable demyelinating disorders that may be confused with ADEM include NMO, Balo's concentric sclerosis, and the Marburg variant of MS. NMO usually can be readily differentiated from ADEM by features summarized in Table 2. Balo's concentric sclerosis consists of large demyelinating plaques that show alternating rings of myelin preservation and loss, giving the lesions the macroscopic and microscopic appearance of onion bulbs. The Marburg variant of MS is characterized by lesions that are more destructive than typical MS or ADEM, with massive macrophage infiltration, acute axonal injury, and necrosis.

Though ADEM usually occurs as a consequence of an antecedent infection (usually viral), in contrast to viral encephalitis, virus proteins or genome could not be recovered from cerebrospinal fluid (CSF) or brain biopsies, suggesting that ADEM is a postinfectious, autoimmune disorder *(15,16,57)*. Autoimmunity may be triggered by several mechanisms, including molecular mimicry,

Table 2
Comparison of Acute Disseminated Encephalomyelitis, Acute Multiple Sclerosis, Acute Hemorrhagic Leukoencephalitis and Neuromyelitis Optica

	Acute disseminated encephalomyelitis	Multiple sclerosis	Acute hemorrhagic leukoencephalitis	Neuromyelitis optica
Antecedent virus/immunization	+	–	+	–
Macroscopically: Number and location of lesions	Lesions inconspicuous or multiple small perivenous lesions throughout white and grey matter of brain, spinal cord and optic nerves.	Variable lesions (several mm to several cm in diameter) throughout white and grey matter of brain, spinal cord and optic nerves.	Lesions in centrum ovale, internal capsule and cingulate gyrus extending to corpus callosum, spreading to involve grey and white matter in brainstem and cerebellar peduncles. Rarely involves spinal cord.	Lesions restricted to optic nerves, spinal cord grey and white matter (extending over multiple spinal segments).
Perivascular Infiltrates	Prominent, perivenular	Scant, variable	Variable	Variable
• Macrophages	+	+	++	++
• Lymphocytes	++	++	++	++
• Polymorphs	±	±	++ (also frequently in the leptomeninges)	++
• Eosinophils	–	– (rare)	–	++
Perivascular immunoglobulin-G and complement	+	–	++	++
Perivacular hemorrhage	–	–	++	–
Perivascular demyelination	++	±	+	++
Age of lesions	Uniform	Different ages	Uniform	Different ages
Astrocytic reaction	Less prominent than in MS	Large, numerous Creutzfeld cells	Less prominent than in MS	Less prominent than in MS
Acute axonal injury	++	+	++	+++
Necrosis of blood vessel walls ± fibrinous exudates	±	–	++	±

MS, multiple sclerosis.

bystander activation, epitope spreading, and mistaken self *(58,59)*. The Thieler's murine encephalomyelitis model of experimental autoimmune encephalomyelitis (EAE) mimics the neuropathological lesions of ADEM and, to a lesser extent, of MS. The initial injury caused by the infecting agent is followed by a secondary autoimmune response. Rodriguez et al. have shown that in this virus model, CD4 and CD8 cells each show reactivity to myelin autoantigens after viral infection, and mice with severe combined immunodeficiency do not develop demyelination *(60–64)*.

The neuropathology of another animal model of EAE induced by exposure to myelin antigens (e.g., myelin basic protein [MBP], proteolipid protein, myelin oligodendrocyte glycoprotein) in complete Freund's adjuvant results in a diffuse white-matter encephalomyelitis that is also used as a model of MS, although it has greater similarity to ADEM *(14,53,65–68)*. MBP-reactive T cells have previously been reported in patients with ADEM by single-cell cloning of T cells with phytohemagglutinin *(69)*. Similarly, patients with postmeasles encephalomyelitis have increased immune responses to MBP *(14)*. In EAE, tissue destruction is associated with the predominance of myelin reactive T helper 1 (Th1)-type T cells *(70,71)*. In the recovery phase of EAE, Th2-type T cells are observed and may have a protective role *(72)*. Patients in the recovery phase of ADEM have a significantly higher frequency of MBP-reactive T cells than patients with viral encephalitis and normal subjects *(67)*. In addition, there was no significant IFN-γ secretion (marker of Th1-cell response), but the MBP-reactive T cells were characterized as interleukin (IL)-4-secreting Th2 cells, further supporting the similarity between ADEM and EAE. Others have suggested a role for B cells and GM1 and GD1a antibodies *(73)*.

There are few studies of cytokines in ADEM *(74)*. Intense expression of tumor necrosis factor (TNF)-α and IL-1β, along with absence of IL-6 *(75)*, has been reported. In vitro and human pathological studies have shown that TNF-α and IL-1β are toxic to myelin and oligodendrocytes and can induce expression of human lymphocyte antigen II and adhesion molecules, further promoting microglial activation and demyelination. The detection of these cytokines supports the concept that T-cell-mediated autoimmune responses have a role in ADEM and may suggest novel therapeutic approaches, such as neuroimmunomodulation with anticytokine treatments.

AHL is a hyperacute, severe, and often fatal form of ADEM, although successful recovery has been described *(76–79)*. Cranial MRI demonstrates that, compared with ADEM, AHL lesions tend to be larger and associated with more edema and mass effect. The infiltrates in AHL are predominantly neutrophilic, with pericapillary ball-and-ring hemorrhages surrounding necrotic venules; sometimes fibrinous exudates within the vessel or extending into adjacent tissue may be seen (Table 2).

It should be noted that some patients have lesions with histologic features of both ADEM and MS. The presence of these transitional forms suggests a spectrum of inflammatory demyelinating diseases that share a common pathogenic relationship.

4. CLINICAL FEATURES

The clinical presentation of ADEM is determined by the location and severity of the inflammatory process. The clinical characteristics of predominantly pediatric patients from five recent large ADEM series are shown in Table 3 *(4–6,80,81)*. Impairment of consciousness, with occasional progression to coma, is the most common presentation, followed by fever and headache. Other clinical features include rapid onset of multifocal neurologic disturbances, such as optic neuritis (sometimes bilateral), visual field deficits, aphasia, cranial neuropathy, motor and sensory dysfunction, ataxia, involuntary movements, seizures, psychiatric disturbance, and signs of an acute meningoencephalopathy with meningismus, a reduced level of consciousness. Maximal deficits usually occur within the first week, and recovery, although sometimes rapid, may take weeks to months. Neuropsychiatric features have also been described *(82,83)*.

Table 3
Clinical Characteristics of Patients From Acute Disseminated Encephalomyelitis Series[a]

	Dale et al. (4)	Hynson et al. (6)	Murthy et al. (80)	Tenembaum et al. (5)	Schwarz et al. (81)
Study sample	Pediatric	Pediatric	Pediatric	Pediatric	Pediatric
Country of origin	United Kingdom	Australia	United States	Argentina	Germany
Patients, n	35	31	18	84	26
Age range (yr)	3–15	2–16	2.5–22	0.4–16	19–61
Female sex, n (%)	16 (46)	18 (58)	7 (39)	30 (36)	17 (65)
Antecedent infection, n (%)	22 (63)	24 (77)	13 (72)	52 (62)	12 (46)
Antecedent vaccination	2 (6)	2 (6)	0	10 (12)	0
Time (mean) from prodrome to onset in days	13	Not stated	10	12	Not stated
Seasonal occurrence	Winter	Not stated	Winter/spring	Not stated	Not stated
Meningoencephalitic features, %					
Fever	43	52	39	Not stated	15
Headache	58	45	23	32	Not stated
Meningism	31	26	6	43	15
Alteration in or loss of consciousness	69	74	45	69	19
Focal neurological features, %					
Optic neuritis (ON)	23 (all bilateral)	13	Unclear	23	Not stated
Cranial neuropathy	51	45	23 (includes ON)	44	Not stated
Pyramidal/focal motor signs	71	23	39	85	77
Sensory deficit	17	3	28	Unclear	65
Aphasia/language deficit	0	26	6	21	8
Seizure	17	13	17	35	4
Ataxia	49	65	39	50	38
Movement disorder	3	Not stated	Not stated	12	Not stated
Spinal cord syndrome	23	Not stated	Unclear	24	15

[a]Modified from Wingerchuk DM. Post infectious encephalomyelitis. Curr Neurol Neurosci Rep 2003;3:256–264. Reprinted with permission.

A novel clinical phenotype has been reported in 10 children with poststreptococcal ADEM characterized by basal ganglia involvement, dystonic movement disorders (50%), behavioral disturbance (70%), and the presence of defining autoreactive antibodies against the basal ganglia *(34)*. This form of ADEM occurred within 18 d of acute pharyngitis/tonsillitis and was distinct from rheumatic fever and Sydenham's chorea. In addition, 80% of the patients had basal ganglia lesions on MRI.

ADEM has also been described in the posttransplantation population *(84,85)*. It remains unclear as to whether these cases represent postinfectious encephalomyelitis in an immunocompromised host or are related to use of drugs, such as methotrexate or cyclosporine, that are known to cause white-matter disease.

The classification of these syndromes is further complicated by other unusual ADEM-like cases, such as that described in eight South African patients with features of NMO, ADEM, and MS *(86)*. These findings suggest that certain phenotypes may be associated with specific infectious agents, as well as genetic and environmental factors.

The clinical manifestations of adult ADEM are generally similar to those seen in children, though certain differences do exist *(81,87)*. In the largest contemporary series of adult ADEM, there was a greater proportion of women (65%) to men, compared with the pediatric series *(81)*. Antecedent infection was less likely (46% vs 62–77% in children), and alteration in consciousness and meningism were also less common (Table 3).

Although generally considered to be a monophasic disorder, ADEM cases with a polyphasic course (recurrent attacks) have been described *(10,88–93)*. In the first few weeks after clinical onset, it is important to differentiate a definite new relapse from reactivation of the same lesions with tapering or withdrawal of therapy (e.g., corticosteroids). Beyond this timeframe, clinical and/or MRI evidence of new disease activity is more suggestive of MS than of ADEM.

One series of 84 patients with a mean follow-up of 7 yr reported that 10% had a single relapse (all polysymptomatic and considered biphasic ADEM) within a mean of 3 yr after the first attack *(5)*. To qualify as a definite relapse, the new clinical episode required at least an interval of 1 mo from the initial symptom, in addition to different symptoms and radiologic evidence of new lesions at a different site. The authors argued that the lack of dissemination in time, the absence of further clinical relapses, and new lesions on MRI scans repeated during the mean follow-up of 8.2 yr, in addition to the lack of oligoclonal bands in CSF on presentation and during relapse, allowed differentiation of relapsing ADEM from MS.

Another study of 21 patients given a diagnosis of ADEM based on clinical signs, disease course, and imaging and laboratory data found that 8 of 21 patients had between two and four relapses; these recurrences took place in the same brain region in 60% of patients. Some of the relapses were recurrent events of large tumor-like lesions that were steroid responsive *(94)*. Two were finally diagnosed as MS, and one developed both a central and peripheral nervous system disorder resulting from a systemic autoimmune process. In the other five patients, biopsy supported the diagnosis of ADEM. The difficulties in distinguishing this form of ADEM from MS are further discussed later.

5. CEREBROSPINAL FLUID

Results of CSF examination in five large ADEM series are shown in Table 4. Lymphocytic pleocytosis (up to 1000 leukocytes/mm^3) and elevated protein levels are common in the acute phase. Oligoclonal bands are identified in a minority of children (<30%) but are found in most adults (58%) after prolonged follow-up. The prevalence of oligoclonal bands is 80% in patients with an initial diagnosis of ADEM but who subsequently develop a clinical course consistent with MS. Other markers such as IgG and myelin basic protein are sometimes detectable but are not specific. One preliminary report suggests that CSF β-1 globulin may be a useful early marker in differentiating MS from ADEM *(95)*. Overall, a prominent CSF pleocytosis, especially if polymorphonuclear cells are present, favors a diagnosis other than typical MS (especially ADEM or NMO), but the immunoglobulin markers and oligoclonal banding results overlap too much to provide much diagnostic assistance.

Table 4
Diagnostic Imaging and Laboratory Characteristics of Patients From Recent Large ADEM Case Series

	Dale et al. (4)	Hynson et al. (6)	Murthy et al. (80)	Tenembaum et al. (5)	Schwarz et al. (81)
Number with MRI[b], n (%)	32 (91)	31 (100)	15 (83)	79 (94)	26 (100)
Lesion site on MRI					
White matter	91	90	93	Not stated	100
Periventricular	44	29	60	Not stated	54
Corpus callosum	Not stated	29	7 (splenium)	Not stated	23
Subcortical/deep	91	80	93	Not stated	38
Cortical gray matter	12	Not stated	80	Not stated	8
Brainstem	56	42	47	Not stated	57
Cerebellum	31	Not stated	13	Not stated	31
Thalamus	41	32	27	13 (bilateral, symmetrical)	15 (± basal ganglia)
Basal ganglia	28	39	20	Not stated	15 (± thalamus)
Spinal cord	Not stated	67	71	Not stated	Not stated
Gadolinium enhancement, n (%)	Not stated	8 (29)	7 (47)	10 (37)	20 (95)
Follow-up brain MRI, n (%)	19 (59)	8 (26)	14 (93)	Not stated	20 (77)
Mean MRI follow-up, yr (range)	1.5 (0.2–9)	0.2–2 (range only)	0.04–1.5 (range only)	Not stated	Not stated
Original brain lesion change, %					
Complete resolution	37	Unclear	7	Not stated	30
Partial resolution	53	6	57	Not stated	55
No change	10	Unclear	21	Not stated	0
New lesions	0	3 (all relapsed)	14	0	15 (no clinical relapses)
Cerebrospinal fluid, %					
Pleocytosis	64	62	39	28 (combined with protein)	81
Elevated protein	60	48	55	28 (combined with pleocytosis)	Not stated
Oligoclonal bands	29	3	13	4	58

[a]Modified from ref. 2. Reprinted with permission. MRI, magnetic resonance imaging.

154

6. DIAGNOSTIC IMAGING

Brain MRI is highly sensitive in detecting demyelinating white-matter lesions in ADEM; however, many disorders can have a similar appearance, including progressive multifocal leukoencephalopathy, MS, leukodystrophies, leukoencephalitis, neurosarcoidosis, vasculitis, and lymphoma. Up to a 2-wk delay may occur between the onset of clinical signs and appearance of MRI lesions *(96–102)*. Typical findings include multifocal lesions, usually bilateral, that vary in size and number in the subcortical white matter, brain stem, middle cerebellar peduncle, and periventricular white matter *(103,104)*. Gray-matter involvement, particularly in the basal ganglia, is not unusual and deep gray structures may also be affected (61% in the study by Hynson et al.) *(6)*. The spinal cord is frequently involved *(105)*. Distribution of MRI lesions in five recent large case series is shown in Table 4.

Cranial MRI is sensitive for lesion detection in both ADEM and MS but does not reliably distinguish them. More than half of patients with ADEM have periventricular lesions and up to one-third have corpus callosum involvement, findings considered highly suggestive of MS. Although uniform lesion enhancement may occur in ADEM, about half of patients present with no enhancing lesions. When present, thalamic or basal ganglia lesions favor ADEM over MS, particularly in cases in which there is no involvement of the corpus callosum. In poststreptococcal ADEM with associated antibasal ganglia antibodies, 80% of patients had basal ganglia lesions, which was greater than the serial nonstreptococcal ADEM controls (18%) *(34)*.

The utility of other radiological techniques in the diagnosis of ADEM is unknown. Abnormal cortical metabolism on two fluoro-2-deoxyglucose positron emission tomography and magnetic resonance spectroscopic imaging findings have been described in the affected brain in ADEM *(106,107)*. The variability in timing, distribution, number, size, and appearance of lesions warrants emphasis and suggests that diagnostic criteria based on specific findings will not be possible.

7. TREATMENT

There have been no controlled therapeutic trials in ADEM. Once a putative diagnosis of ADEM is made, the first-line therapeutic approach is use of high-dose intravenous corticosteroids *(44,96,108–110)*, although patients with ADEM can recover rapidly and spontaneously, clouding the benefit attributed to steroids in uncontrolled studies *(6,14)*. Treatment consists of high-dose intravenous methylprednisolone (10–30 mg/kg/d for children weighing less than 30 kg and 1000 mg/d for those weighing more than 30 kg) for 3 to 10 d, followed by an oral prednisone taper for 4 to 8 wk. Intravenous dexamethasone (1 mg/kg/d) can be substituted for a similar duration, followed by the same oral prednisone taper.

In patients who do not respond to parenteral corticosteroids, there are alternative treatments. Patients with disabling, corticosteroid treatment-resistant attacks of CNS demyelination caused by MS, NMO, and severe isolated demyelinating events, such as acute transverse myelitis or Marburg MS variant, benefit from plasma exchange, as demonstrated in a small randomized, controlled, crossover trial of true vs sham plasma exchange *(111,112)*. The response rate in patients treated with true plasma exchange was 42%, compared with 6% in the sham group. Benefit of plasma exchange had been previously reported in uncontrolled observations *(113–115)*. Plasma exchange should be implemented in patients with steroid-resistant ADEM and seven treatments should be administered on alternate days for 14 d. Intravenous γ-globulin may also be beneficial *(116–122)*. Less frequent anecdotal successes have been reported with use of cyclophosphamide *(81)* and hypothermia *(123)*.

8. ADEM VS MS

The advent of immunomodulatory drugs in the treatment of relapsing–remitting MS (RRMS) and secondary progressive MS highlights the importance of careful diagnosis of CNS white-matter disease *(11,124–129)*. The National Multiple Sclerosis Society (United States) recommends initiation of disease-modifying therapy with an INF-β or glatiramer acetate "as soon as possible following a definite diagnosis of multiple sclerosis and determination of a relapsing course" *(130)*. The US Food and Drug Administration recently approved the use of INF-β1a (Avonex®, Biogen Inc.) for patients who experience a first-ever clinically isolated episode and have MRI features consistent with MS. Therefore, the clinician is faced not only with difficult prognostic and counseling questions at disease onset but also must help the patient and family understand the possible risk of MS and the advantages and disadvantages of initiating long-term immunotherapy under a cloud of uncertainty.

It is not known what proportion of cases most clinicians diagnose at onset as ADEM, rather than a typical clinically isolated syndrome, yet later term MS. As discussed previously, some clinical and imaging features favor, but are not diagnostic of ADEM at disease onset.

Some investigators have reported longitudinal data describing patients originally diagnosed with ADEM. Diagnostic criteria in these studies were not standardized and were rather indistinct. In a follow-up study of 40 adult patients diagnosed with ADEM, 14 of 40 (35%) had developed clinically definite MS during a mean period of 38 mo *(81)*. Patients with a final long-term diagnosis of ADEM were younger, had more acute onset of symptoms, frequently had a preceding infection, and presented more often with clinical and radiological signs of infratentorial lesions. Despite these differences, no clinical, laboratory, or radiological feature clearly helped differentiate the two disorders. Nearly 50% of patients that did not convert to MS during the follow-up period had MRI findings compatible with MS. Some developed new lesions without clinical relapse, calling into question the diagnosis of ADEM. Thus, decisions regarding diagnosis based on the initial MRI may be incorrect. The McDonald criteria *(131)* for MS diagnosis recommend that initial judgment be suspended but state that MS can be confirmed if new clinical or MRI abnormalities occur more than three months after the sentinel event. It is not clear how relapsing forms of ADEM fit into this scheme in the absence of readily available pathological data.

The underlying immunopathology of ADEM and MS appear to be different, and pathological data may represent a gold standard for validation of clinical criteria. A clear and consistent ADEM definition that allows confident between-study comparisons is lacking. Information from developing countries would be informative because of the large number of infectious and postinfectious cases of ADEM, especially in children, that generally have not been reported to convert to MS *(7)*. Clinicians should be cautious in diagnosing relapsing ADEM, since it remains unclear whether it represents a distinct separate entity from RRMS *(132,133)*.

Although ADEM is typically multifocal throughout the CNS and often involves impaired consciousness, a few cases are characterized predominantly by spinal cord pathology, which can sometimes result in difficulty distinguishing ADEM from other causes of myelitis (e.g., NMO or lupus myelitis). Humoral mechanisms were recently implicated in NMO and a recent NMO-specific auto-antibody marker has been identified *(134,135)*. It is plausible that immunological or genetic biological markers will eventually allow more diagnostic precision within the CNS demyelinating disease spectrum.

9. OUTCOME

The reported outcome of ADEM is highly variable. Mortality reported in recent studies is low. The mortality from ADEM associated with measles was previously as high as 20%, much greater than that of rubella or varicella *(4,136,137)*. The reason for the apparent reduction in mortality is unclear but may have been caused by changes in the type of prodromal illness, treatment with steroids, increased use of antibiotics, change in supportive care, and diagnosis of milder cases with the advent of MRI.

In one series of 31 children with ADEM, 81% of patients recovered completely and the remainder had only mild neurological sequelae; none of the children died *(4)*. A separate study of 35 children with ADEM (mean age = 6 yr), all survived and 57% had no long-term impairment. Neurological deficits included motor dysfunction (17%), cognitive impairment (11%), epilepsy (9%) with resolution in two- thirds on extended follow-up, visual loss (11%), and behavioral problems (11%). Comparing patients with monophasic ADEM with those who subsequently develop MS revealed that the MS patients had a greater frequency of moderate-to-severe deficits *(81)*. Similar findings were reported in a large Argentinian follow-up series of 84 patients *(5)*. Eighty-nine percent of patients (*n* = 75) had either complete recovery, with normal neurological examination findings in most or abnormal signs without disability (Expanded Disability Status Scale of 0 to 2.5). They corresponded to 96% of patients with small lesions on MRI, 80% of those showing large lesions on MRI, 80% of those with bithalamic involvement, and one of the two patients with hemorrhagic disease.

In a recent review of 360 children with ADEM from nine studies between 1987 and 2002, no patients died and 75% had excellent recovery, usually within months *(138)*. Permanent neurological sequelae were more common in severely ill patients (those with coma or hemiplegia) and included mental retardation, weakness, spasticity, seizures, and ataxia. Relapses occurred in 14% of patients, some of whom may have had MS.

10. CONCLUSION

The syndrome of ADEM is generally accepted, but there is no agreement on formal diagnostic criteria. No studies have attempted to validate clinical diagnostic criteria against a pathological gold standard. Acute, fulminant, multifocal CNS presentations associated with meningeal symptoms and signs, especially following a well-defined infectious or inflammatory stimulus, are usually diagnosed as ADEM, if they are accompanied by enhancing white-matter lesions on cranial MRI and an inflammatory CSF profile. Clearly, cases that are ultimately diagnosed as MS, NMO, or other disorders may be mistaken for ADEM at disease onset. Although biopsy might reveal the typical but not necessarily pathognomonic perivenular lesions that seem to characterize ADEM, clinicians must use all available diagnostic information, in addition to observation over time to determine the best clinical diagnosis within the uncertain nosological structure of CNS demyelinating diseases.

REFERENCES

1. Lucas J. An account of uncommon symptoms succeeding the measles; with some additional remarks on the infection of measles and smallpox. London Med J 1790;11:325.
2. Wingerchuk DM. Postinfectious encephalomyelitis. Curr Neurol Neurosci Rep 2003;3:256–264.
3. Hollinger P, Sturzenegger M, Mathis J, Schroth G, Hess CW. Acute disseminated encephalomyelitis in adults: a reappraisal of clinical, CSF, EEG, and MRI findings. J Neurology 2002;249:320–329.
4. Dale RC, de Sousa C, Chong WK, Cox TCS, Harding B, Neville BGR. Acute disseminated encephalomyelitis, multiphasic disseminated encephalomyelitis and multiple sclerosis in children. Brain 2000;123:2407–2422.
5. Tenembaum S, Chamoles N, Fejerman N. Acute disseminated encephalomyelitis. A long-term follow-up study of 84 pediatric patients. Neurology 2002;59:1224–1231.
6. Hynson JL, Kornberg AJ, Coleman LT, et al. Clinical and neuroradiologic features of acute disseminated encephalomyelitis in children. Neurology 2001;56:1308–1312.
7. Garg RK. Acute disseminated encephalomyelitis. Postgrad Med J 2003;79:11–17.
8. Boz C, Velioglu S, Ozmenoglu M. Acute disseminated encephalomyelitis after bee sting. Neurol Sci 2003;23:313–315.
9. Rust RS, Dodson W, Prensky A, et al. Classification and outcome of acute disseminated encephalomyelitis. *In*: Program and Abstracts of the 26th Annual Meeting of the Child Neurology Society, Phoenix. Ann Neurol 1997;42:49.
10. Miller HG, Evans MJL. Prognosis in acute disseminated encephalomyelitis; with a note on neuromyelitis optica. Q J Med 1953;22:347–349.
11. Jacobs LD, Beck RW, Simon JH, et al. Intramuscular interferon beta-1a therapy initiated during a first demyelinating event in multiple sclerosis. CHAMPS Study Group. N Engl J Med 2000;343:898–904.
12. CHAMPS Study Group. Interferon beta-1a for optic neuritis patients at high risk for multiple sclerosis. Am J Ophthalmol 2001;132:463–471.
13. Comi G, Filippi M, Barkhof F, et al. Effect of early interferon treatment on conversion to definite multiple sclerosis: a randomised study. Lancet 2001;357:1576–1582.
14. Johnson RT, Griffin DE, Hirsch RL, et al. Measles encephalomyelitis: clinical and immunologic studies. N Engl J Med 1984;310:137–141.
15. Johnson RT. Pathogenesis of acute viral encephalitis and post infectious encephalomyelitis. J Infect Dis 1987;155:359–364.

16. Johnson RT. Postinfectious demyelinating diseases. *In*: Johnson RT. Viral infections of the nervous system. 2nd ed. Philadelphia, Lippincott–Raven, 1998;181–210.

17. An SF, Groves M, Martinian L, Kuo LT, Scaravilli F. Detection of infectious agents in brain of patients with acute hemorrhagic leukoencephalitis. J Neurovirol 2002;8:439–446.

18. Sacconi S, Salviati L, Merelli E. Acute disseminated encephalomyelitis associated with hepatitis C virus infection. Arch Neurol 2001;58:1679–1681.

19. Kaji M, Kusuhara T, Ayabe M, Hino H, Shoji H, Nagao T. Survey of herpes simplex virus infections of the central nervous system, including acute disseminated encephalomyelitis, in the Kyushu and Okinawa regions of Japan. Multiple Sclerosis 1996;2:83–87.

20. Ito T, Watanabe A, Akabane J. Acute disseminated encephalomyelitis developed after acute herpetic gingivostomatitis. Tohoku J Exp Med 2000;192:151–155.

21. Revel-Vilk S, Hurvitz H, Klar A, Virozov Y, Korn-Lubetzki I. Recurrent acute disseminated encephalomyelitis associated with acute cytomegalovirus and Epstein-Barr virus infection. J Child Neurol 2000;15:421–424.

22. Bhigjee AI, Patel VB, Bhagwan B, et al. HIV and acute disseminated encephalomyelitis. S Afr Med J 1999;89: 283–284.

23. Narisco P, Galgani S, Del Grosso B, et al. Acute disseminated encephalomyelitis as manifestation of primary HIV infection. Neurology 2001;57:1493–1496.

24. Tachi N, Watanabe T, Wakai S, et al. Acute disseminated encephalomyelitis following HTLV–1 associated myelopathy. J Neurol Sci 1992;110:234–235.

25. Au WY, Lie AK, Cheung RT, et al. Acute disseminated encephalomyelitis after para-influenza infection post bone marrow transplantation. Leukemia & Lymphoma 2002;43:455–457.

26. Yamamoto Y, Takasaki T, Yamada K, et al. Acute disseminated encephalomyelitis following dengue fever. J Infection Chemotherapy 2002;8:175–177.

27. Yamashita S, Ueno K, Hashimoto Y, Teramoto H, Uchino M. A case of acute disseminated encephalomyelitis accompanying Mycoplasma pneumoniae infection (Japanese). Brain Nerve 1999;51:799–803.

28. Riedel K, Kempf VA, Bechtold A, Klimmer M. Acute disseminated encephalomyelitis (ADEM) due to Mycoplasma pneumoniae infection in an adolescent. Infection 2001;29:240–242.

29. Yamamoto K, Takayanagi M, Yoshihara Y, et al. Acute disseminated encephalomyelitis associated with Mycoplasma pneumoniae infection. Acta Paediatrica Japonica 1996;38:46–51.

30. Heick A, Skriver E. Chlamydia pneumoniae-associated ADEM. Eur J Neurol 2000;7:435–438.

31. Sommer JB, Erbguth FJ, Neundorfer B. Acute disseminated encephalomyelitis following Legionella pneumophila infection. Eur Neurol 2000;44:182–184.

32. Nasralla CA, Pay N, Goodpasture HC, Lin JJ, Svoboda WB. Postinfectious encephalopathy in a child following Campylobacter jejuni enteritis. Am J Neuroradiology 1993;14:444–448.

33. Proulx NL, Freedman MS, Chan JW, Toye B, Code CC. Acute disseminated encephalomyelitis associated with Pasteurella multocida meningitis. Can J Neurol Sci 2003;30:155–158.

34. Dale RC, Church AJ, Cardoso F, et al. Poststreptococcal acute disseminated encephalomyelitis with basal ganglia involvement and auto-reactive antibasal ganglia antibodies. Ann Neurol 2001;50:588–595.

35. Spieker S, Petersen D, Rolfs A, et al. Acute disseminated encephalomyelitis following Pontiac fever. Eur Neurol 1998;40:169–172.

36. Held JR, Adros HL. Neurological disease in man following administration of suckling mouse brain antirabies vaccine. Bull World Health Organ 1972;46:321–327.

37. Label LS, Batts DH. Transverse myelitis caused by duck embryo rabies vaccine. Arch Neurol 1982;39:426–430.

38. Swamy HS, Shankar SK, Chandra PS, et al. Neurological complications due to beta–propiolactone (BPL) inactivated antirabies vaccination. J Neurol Sci 1984;63:111–128.

39. Hemchudha T, Griffin DE, Giffels JJ, et al. Myelin basic protein as an encephalitogen in encephalomyelitis and polyneuritis following rabies vaccination. N Engl J Med 1987;316:369–374.

40. Murthy JMK. MRI in acute disseminated encephalomyelitis following Semple antirabies vaccine. Neuroradiology 1998;40:420–423.

41. Chakrawarty A. Neurologic illness following post-exposure prophylaxis with purified chick embryo cell antirabies vaccine. J Assoc Physicians India 2001;44:927–928.

42. Gout O. Vaccinations and multiple sclerosis. Neurol Sci 2001;22:151–154.

43. Fenichel GM. Neurological complications of immunization. Ann Neurol 1982;12:119–128.

44. Karelitz S, Eisenberg M. Measles encephalitis: evaluation of treatment with adrenocorticotropin and corticosteroids. Pediatrics 1961;27:811–818.

45. Nalin DR. Mumps, measles, and rubella vaccination and encephalitis. BMJ 1989;299:1219.

46. Centers for Disease Control and Prevention. Vaccinia (smallpox) vaccine: recommendations of the Advisory Committee on Immunization Practices 2001. MMWR Morb Mortal Wkly Rep 2001;50:1–24.

47. Gurvich EB, Vilesova IS. Vaccinia virus in postvaccinal encephalitis. Acta Virologic 1983;27:154–159.

48. Ohtaki E, Matsuishi T, Hirano Y, Maekawa K. Acute disseminated encephalomyelitis after treatment with Japanese B encephalitis vaccine (Nakayama-Yoken and Beijing strains). J Neurol Neurosurg Psychiatry 1995;59:316–317.

49. Dodick DW, Silber MH, Noseworthy JH, et al. Acute disseminated encephalomyelitis after accidental injection of a hog vaccine: successful treatment with plasmapheresis. Mayo Clin Proc 1998;73:1193–1195.

50. Ascherio A, Zhang SM, Hernan MA, et al. Hepatitis B vaccination and the risk of multiple sclerosis. N Engl J Med 2001;344:327–332.

51. Py MO, Andre C. Acute disseminated encephalomyelitis and meningococcal A and C vaccine: case report. Arquivos de Neuro-Psiquiatria 1997;55:632–635.

52. Scott TFM. Post infectious and vaccinal encephalitis. Med Clin North Am 1967;51:701–716.

53. Litvak AM, Sands IJ, Gibel H. Encephalitis complicating measles: report of 56 cases with follow-up studies in 32. Am J Dis Child 1943;65:265–295.

54. Lane JM, Ruben FL, Neff JM, Millar JD. Complications of smallpox vaccination, 1968. N Engl J Med 1969;281:1201–1208.

55. Prineas JW, McDonald, WI, Franklin, RJM. Demyelinating diseases. *In*: Greenfield's Neuropathology. 7th ed. Graham DI, Lantos PL, eds. London, Arnold, 2002:471–535.

56. Lucchinetti C, Bruck W, Parisi J, Scheithauer B, Rodriguez M, Lassmann H. Heterogeneity of multiple sclerosis lesions: implications for the pathogenesis of demyelination. Ann Neurol 2000;47:707–717.

57. Cherry JD, Shields WD. Encephalitis and meningoencephalitis. *In*: Feigin RD, Cherry JD, eds. Textbook of Pediatric Infectious Diseases. Philadelphia, W.B. Saunders, 1992:445–454.

58. Stocks M. Genetics of childhood disorders:XXIX. Autoimmune disorders, part 2: molecular mimicry. J Am Acad Child Adolescent Psychiatry 2001;40:977–980.

59. Miller SD, Vanderlugt CL, Begolka WS, et al. Persistent infection with Theiler's virus leads to autoimmunity via epitope spreading. Nat Med 1997;3:1133–1136.

60. Murray PD, Pavelko KD, Leibowitz J, Lin X, Rodriguez M. CD4$^+$ and CD8$^+$ T cells make discrete contributions to demyelination and neurologic disease in a viral model of multiple sclerosis. J Virol 1998;72:7320–7329.

61. Lin X, Pease LR, Murray PD, Rodriguez M. Theiler's virus induced infection of genetically susceptible mice induces central nervous system-infiltrating CTLs with no apparent viral or major myelin antigenic specificity. J Immunol 1998;160:5661–5668.

62. Rodriguez M, Dunkel AJ, Thiemann RL, Leibowitz J, Zijlstra M, Jaenisch R. Abrogation of resistance to Theiler's virus-induced demyelination in H-2b mice deficient in beta 2-microglobulin. J Immunol 1993;151:266–276.

63. Rivera-Quinones C, McGavern D, Schmelzer JD, Hunter SE, Low PA, Rodriguez M. Absence of neurologic deficits following extensive demyelination in a class I-deficient murine model of multiple sclerosis. Nat Med 1998;4:187–193.

64. Njenga MK, Murray PD, McGavern D, Lin X, Drescher KM, Rodriguez M. Absence of spontaneous central nervous system remyelination in class II-deficient mice infected with Theiler's virus. J Neuropathol Exp Neurol 1999;58:78–91.

65. Gold R, Hartung HP, Toyka KV. Animal models for autoimmune demyelinating disorders of the nervous system. Mol Med Today 2000;62:88–91.

66. Ben-Nun A, Wekerle H, Cohen IR. The rapid isolation of clonable antigen specific T lymphocyte lines capable of mediating autoimmune encephalomyelitis. Eur J Immunol 1981;11:195–199.

67. Pohl-Koppe A, Burchett SK, Thiele EA, Hafler DA. Myelin basic protein reactive Th2 T cells are found in acute disseminated encephalomyelitis. J Neuroimmunol 1998;19–27.

68. Kuchroo VK, Sobel RA, Yamamura T, et al. Induction of experimental allergic encephalomyelitis by myelin proteolipid-protein-specific T cell clones and synthetic peptides. Pathobiology 1991;59:305–312.

69. Hafler DA, Benjamin DS, Burks J, Weiner HL. Myelin basic protein and proteolipid protein reactivity of brain and cerebrospinal fluid derived T cell clones in multiple sclerosis and post infectious encephalomyelitis. J Immunol 1987;139:69–72.

70. Miller A, Al-Sabbagh A, Santos LMB, Prabhu-Das M, Weiner HL. Epitopes of myelin basic protein that trigger TGF-β release after oral tolerization are distinct from encephalitogenic epitopes and mediate epitope-driven bystander suppression. J Immunol 1993;151:7307–7315.

71. Wucherpfennig KW, Weiner HL, Hafler DA. T cell recognition of myelin basic protein. Immunol Today 1991;12:277–282.

72. Kuchroo VK, Prabhu-Das M, Brown JA, et al. B7-1 and B7-2 costimulatory molecules activate differentially the Th1/Th2 developmental pathways: application to autoimmune disease therapy. Cell 1995;80:707–718.

73. Laouini D, Kennou MF, Khoufi S, Dellagi K. Antibodies to human myelin proteins and gangliosides in patients with acute neuroparalytic accidents induced by brain-derived rabies vaccine. J Neuroimmunol 1998;91:63–72.

74. Ichiyama T, Shoji H, Kato M, et al. Cerebrospinal fluid levels of cytokines and soluble tumour necrosis factor receptor in acute disseminated encephalomyelitis. Eur J Pediatr 2002;161:133–137.

75. Kadhim H, De Prez C, Gazagnes MD, Sebire G. In situ cytokine immune responses in acute disseminated encephalomyelitis: insights into pathophysiologic mechanisms. Human Pathology 2003;34:293–297.

76. Hurst EW. Acute hemorrhagic leukoencephalitis: a previously undefined entity. Med J Aust 1941;1:1–6.

77. Klein C, Wijdicks EFM, Earnest IVF. Full recovery after acute hemorrhagic leukoencephalitis (Hurst's disease). J Neurol 2000;247:977–979.

78. Rosman NP, Gottlieb SM, Bernstein CA. Acute hemorrhagic leukoencephalitis: recovery and reversal of magnetic resonance imaging findings in a child. J Child Neurol 1997;12:448–454.

79. Seales D, Greer M. Acute hemorrhagic leukoencephalitis: a successful recovery. Arch Neurol 1991;48:1086–1088.

80. Murthy SN, Faden HS, Cohen ME, Bakshi R. Acute disseminated encephalomyelitis in children. Pediatrics 2002;110:e21.

81. Schwarz S, Mohr A, Knauth M, Wildemann B, Storch-Hagenlocher B. Acute disseminated encephalomyelitis: a follow-up study of 40 patients. Neurology 2001;56:1313–1318.

82. Patel SP, Friedman RS. Neuropsychiatric features of acute disseminated encephalomyelitis: a review. J Neuropsychiatr Clin Neurosci 1997;9:534–540.

83. Nasr JT, Andriola MR, Coyle PK. ADEM: literature review and case report of acute psychosis presentation. Pediatr Neurol 2000;22:8–18.

84. Horowitz MB, Comey C, Hirsch W, Marion D, Griffith B, Martinez J. Acute disseminated encephalomyelitis (ADEM) or ADEM-like inflammatory changes in a heart-lung transplant recipient: a case report. Neuroradiology 1995;37:434–437.

85. Re A, Giachetti R. Acute disseminated encephalomyelitis (ADEM) after autologous peripheral blood stem cell transplant for non-Hodgkin's lymphoma. Bone Marrow Transplantation 1999;24:1351–1354.

86. Modi G, Mochan A, Modi M, Saffer D. Demyelinating disorder of the central nervous system occurring in black South Africans. J Neurol Neurosurg Psychiatry 2001;70:500–505.

87. Wang PN, Fuh JL, Liu HC, Wang SJ. Acute disseminated encephalomyelitis in middle-aged or elderly patients. Eur Neurol 1996;36:219–223.

88. Walker RW, Gawler J. Serial cerebral CT abnormalities in relapsing acute disseminating encephalomyelitis. J Neurol Neurosurg Psychiatry 1989;52:1100–1102.

89. Shoji H, Kusuhara T, Honda Y, et al. Relapsing acute disseminated encephalomyelitis associated with chronic Epstein-Barr virus infection: MRI findings. Neuroradiology 1992;34:340–342.

90. Mancini J, Chabrol B, Moulene E, Pinsard N. Relapsing acute encephalopathy: a complication of diphtheria-tetanus-poliomyelitis immunization in a young boy. Eur J Pediatr 1996;155:136–138.

91. Durston JHJ, Milnes JN. Relapsing encephalomyelitis. Brain 1970;93:715–730.

92. Tsai ML, Hung KL. Multiphasic disseminated encephalomyelitis mimicking multiple sclerosis. Brain Dev 1996;18:412–414.

93. Apak RA, Anlar B, Saatci I. A case of relapsing acute disseminated encephalomyelitis with high dose corticosteroid treatment. Brain Dev 1999;21:279–282.

94. Cohen O, Steiner-Birmanns B, Biran I, Abramsky O, Honigman S, Steiner I. Recurrence of acute disseminated encephalomyelitis at the previously affected brain site. Arch Neurol 2001;58:797–801.

95. Chopra B, Abraham R, Abraham A. CSF beta-1 globulin—a potential marker in differentiating multiple sclerosis and acute disseminated encephalomyelitis: a preliminary study. Neurology India 2000;50:41–44.

96. Caldemeyer KS, Smith RR, Harris TM, Edwards MK. MRI in acute disseminated encephalomyelitis. Neuroradiology 1994;36:216–220.

97. Murray BJ, Apetauerova D, Scammell TE. Severe acute disseminated encephalomyelitis with normal MRI at presentation. Neurology 2000;55:1237–1238.

98. Honkaniemi J, Dastidar P, Kähärä V, Haapasalo H. Delayed MR imaging changes in acute disseminated encephalomyelitis. Am J Neuroradiol 2001;22:1117–1124.

99. Epperson LW, Whitaker JN, Kapila A. Cranial MRI in acute disseminated encephalomyelitis. Neurology 1988;38:332–333.

100. O'Riordan JI, Gomez-Anson B, Moseley IF, Miller DH. Long term MRI follow-up of patients with post infectious encephalomyelitis: evidence for a monophasic disease. J Neurol Sci 1999;167:132–136.

101. Kimura S, Nezu A, Ohtsuki N, Kobayashi T, Osaka H, Uehara S. Serial magnetic resonance imaging in children with postinfectious encephalitis. Brain Dev 1996;18:461–465.

102. Kesselring J, Miller DH, Robb SA, et al. Acute disseminated encephalomyelitis. MRI findings and the distinction from multiple sclerosis. Brain 1990;113:291–302.

103. Murthy JM, Yangala R, Meena AK, Jaganmohan-Reddy J. Acute disseminated encephalomyelitis: clinical and MRI study from South India. J Neurol Sci 1999;165:133–138.

104. Singh S, Alexander M, Korah IP. Acute disseminated encephalomyelitis: MR imaging features. AJR Am J Roentgenol 1999;173:1101–1107.

105. Baum PA, Barkovich AJ, Koch TK, Berg BO. Deep gray matter involvement in children with acute disseminated encephalomyelitis. Am J Neuroradiol 1994;15:1275–1283.

106. Tan TXL, Spigos DG, Mueller CF. Abnormal cortical metabolism in acute disseminated encephalomyelitis. Clin Nucl Med 1998;23:629–630.

107. Bizzi A, Ulug AM, Crawford TO, et al. Quantitative proton MR spectroscopic imaging in acute disseminated encephalomyelitis. Am J Neuroradiol 2001;22:1125–1130.

108. Pasternak JF, De Vivo DC, Prensky AL. Steroid-responsive encephalomyelitis in childhood. Neurology 1980;30:481–486.

109. Straub J, Chofflon M, Delavelle J. Early high-dose intravenous methylprednisolone in acute disseminated encephalomyelitis: a successful recovery. Neurology 1997;49:1145–1147.

110. Hindley DT, Newton RW, Clarke MA, et al. Steroid-responsive relapsing encephalopathy presenting in young children. Neuropediatrics 1993;24:182.

111. Weinshenker BG, O'Brien PC, Petterson TM, et al. A randomized trial of plasma exchange in acute central nervous system inflammatory demyelinating disease. Ann Neurol 1999;46:878–886.

112. Keegan M, Pineda AA, McClelland RL, Darby CH, Rodriguez M, Weinshenker BG. Plasma exchange for severe attacks of CNS demyelination: predictors of response. Neurology. 2002;58:143–146.

113. Kanter DS, Horensky D, Sperling RA, Kaplan JD, Malachowski ME, Churchill WH Jr. Plasmapheresis in fulminant acute disseminated encephalomyelitis. Neurology 1995;45:824–827.

114. Rodriguez M, Karnes WE, Bartleson JD, Pineda AA. Plasmapheresis in acute episodes of fulminant CNS inflammatory demyelination. Neurology 1993;43:1100–1104.

115. Miyazawa R, Hikima A, Takano Y, et al. Plasmapheresis in fulminant acute disseminated encephalomyelitis. Brain Dev 2001;23:424–426.

116. Kleiman M, Brunquell P. Acute disseminated encephalomyelitis: response to intravenous immunoglobulin? J Child Neurol 1995;10:481–483.

117. Pittock SJ, Keir G, Alexander M, Brennan P, Hardiman O. Rapid clinical and CSF response to intravenous gamma globulin in acute disseminated encephalomyelitis. Eur J Neurol 2001;8:725.

118. Finsterer J, Grass R, Stollberger C, Mamoli B. Immunoglobulins in acute, parainfectious, disseminated encephalomyelitis. Clin Neuropharmacol 1998;21:258–261.

119. Hahn JS, Siegler DJ, Enzmann D. Intravenous gammaglobulin therapy in recurrent acute disseminated encephalomyelitis. Neurology 1996;46:1173–1174.

120. Sahlas DJ, Miller SP, Guerin M, Veilleux M, Francis G. Treatment of acute disseminated encephalomyelitis with intravenous immunoglobulin. Neurology 2000;54:1370–1372.

121. Pradhan S, Gupta RP, Shashank S, Pandey N. Intravenous immunoglobulin therapy in acute disseminated encephalomyelitis. J Neurol Sci 1999;165:56–61.

122. Marchioni E, Marinou-Aktipi K, Uggetti C, et al. Effectiveness of intravenous immunoglobulin treatment in adult patients with steroid-resistant monophasic or recurrent acute disseminated encephalomyelitis. J Neurol 2002;249:100–104.

123. Takata T, Hirakawa M, Sakurai M, Kanazawa I. Fulminant form of acute disseminated encephalomyelitis: successful treatment with hypothermia. J Neurol Sci 1999;165:94–97.

124. European Study Group on Interferon (beta)-1b in Secondary Progressive MS. Placebo-controlled multicentre randomized trial of interferon (beta)-1b in treatment of secondary progressive multiple sclerosis. Lancet 1998;352:1491–1497.

125. Johnson KP, Brooks BR, Cohen JA, et al. Copolymer 1 reduces relapse rate and improves disability in relapsing-remitting multiple sclerosis: results of a phase III multicenter, double-blind, placebo-controlled trial. Neurology 1995;45:1268–1276.

126. Jacobs LD, Cookfair DL, Rudick RA, et al. Intramuscular interferon beta-1a for disease progression in relapsing multiple sclerosis. Ann Neurol 1996;39:285–294.

127. The IFNB Multiple Sclerosis Study Group. Interferon beta-1b is effective in relapsing-remitting multiple sclerosis. I. Clinical results of a multicenter, randomized, double blind, placebo-controlled trial. Neurology 1993;43:655–666.

128. PRISMS (Prevention of Relapses and Disability by Interferon (beta)-1a Subcutaneously in Multiple Sclerosis) Study Group. Randomized double-blind placebo-controlled study of interferon (beta)-1a in relapsing/remitting multiple sclerosis. Lancet 1998;352:1498–1504.

129. Noseworthy JH, Lucchinetti C, Rodriguez M, Weinshenker BG. Multiple sclerosis. N Engl J Med 2000;343:938–952.

130. van den Noort S, Eidelman B, Rammohan K, et al. National Multiple Sclerosis Society (NMSS): Disease management consensus statement. New York, NY: National MS Society; 1998.

131. Mc Donald WI, Compston DAS, Edan G, et al. Recommended diagnostic criteria in multiple sclerosis: guidelines from the International Panel on the Diagnosis of Multiple Sclerosis. Ann Neurol 2001;50:121–127.

132. Stuve O, Zamvil SS. Pathogenesis, diagnosis, and treatment of acute disseminated encephalomyelitis. Curr Opin Neurol 1999;12:395–401

133. Hartung HP, Grossman RI. ADEM: distinct disease or part of the MS spectrum? Neurology 2001;56:1257–1260.

134. Lucchinetti CF, Mandler RN, McGavern D, et al. A role for humoral mechanisms in the pathogenesis of Devic's neuromyelitis optica. Brain 2002;125:1450–1461.

135. Lennon VA, Lucchinetti CF, Weinshenker BG. Identification of a marker autoantibody of neuromyelitis optica. Neurology 2003;60:A519–A520.

136. Boe J, Solberg CO, Saeter T. Corticosteroid treatment for acute meningoencephalitis: a retrospective study of 346 cases. BMJ 1965;1:1094–1095.

137. Sriram S, Steinman L. Post infectious and postvaccinial encephalomyelitis. Neurol Clin 1984;2:341–353.

138. Davis LE. Booss J. Acute disseminated encephalomyelitis in children: a changing picture. Pediatr Infect Dis J 2003;22:829–831.

CME QUESTIONS

1. Which of the following statements is *false*?
   A. Brain MRI is highly sensitive in detecting the demyelinating white-matter lesions of acute disseminated encephalomyelitis (ADEM)
   B. Gray matter involvement is rare in ADEM
   C. Many patients with ADEM have periventricular lesions and corpus callosum involvement
   D. Basal ganglia lesions occur in about 80% of patients with poststreptococcal ADEM associated with antibasal ganglia antibodies

2. The incidence of ADEM after measles vaccination is approx:
   A. 1 in 1000
   B. 1 in 100,000
   C. 1 in 1 million
   D. 1 in 10 million

3. The pathological hallmark of ADEM is:
   A. Perivenous inflammation with infiltration of eosinophils with immunoglobulin-G and complement deposition
   B. Perivascular neutrophil infiltration and presence of numerous reactive lymphocytes
   C. Perivenous demyelination with infiltration by predominantly macrophages and an inconspicuous astrocytic reaction
   D. Concentric, lamellated pattern of myelin loss, alternating with zones of myelin preservation.

4. Which of the following statements regarding ADEM is true?
   A. The clinical, radiological, and laboratory findings in ADEM make it easy to distinguish it from MS
   B. In a small randomized controlled crossover trial, plasma exchange has been shown to be beneficial in patients with steroid-resistant disabling attacks of CNS demyelination
   C. Randomized controlled trials of intravenous immunoglobulin support its use as a second-line treatment in steroid-resistant ADEM
   D. There are well-defined criteria for the diagnosis of ADEM

9

Ingested Type I Interferon in Experimental Autoimmune Encephalomyelitis

Staley A. Brod

1. OVERVIEW OF MULTIPLE SCLEROSIS

Multiple sclerosis (MS) is a chronic demyelinating disease of the central nervous system (CNS), which has been postulated to be a T-cell-mediated autoimmune disease *(1,2)*. Although the etiology of MS is unknown, most investigators believe that the immune system is intimately involved in the progression of the disease *(3)*. MS is clinically associated with periods of disability (relapse) alternating with periods of recovery *(4)* but often leading to progressive neurological disability *(2,5)*. The lesions in the CNS are similar to the lesions produced by T-lymphocyte delayed-type hypersensitivity (DTH) reactions.

Studies of the cellular immune system in tissue compartments have suggested a sequestration of antigen-specific T-cell populations in the cerebrospinal fluid (CSF) *(6)*. A major hypothesis concerning the CNS inflammation is that T lymphocytes are reacting to an (un)identified self-antigens intrinsic to myelin (e.g., myelin basic protein [MBP], proteolipid protein [PLP] and these T lymphocytes damage myelin directly or by activating macrophages and other agents of inflammation, although microglia may have an important role in MS pathogenesis *(7)*. Progression or recurrence of immune damage appears to result from a failure of normal regulatory mechanisms that suppress the immune process in MS *(8)*. There is a CD3 pathway defect *(9)*, and secretion of interferon (IFN)-γ was significantly decreased and transforming growth factor (TGF)-β was significantly increased in stable relapsing–remitting MS (RRMS) patients compared to controls *(10)*.

2. TYPE I INTERFERONS

In 1957, Isaacs and Lindenmann described a factor (IFN) produced by virus-infected cells that had rapid antiviral activity *(11)*. Type I IFN is composed primarily of two highly homologous proteins that have similar biological properties, IFN-α (leukocyte IFN) and IFN-β (fibroblast IFN) *(12–14)*. IFN-α and IFN-β have relatively similar actions and interact with the same cell receptor *(15)*. The natural IFN-α family contains 165 to 166 amino acids with about an 80% sequence homology to each other *(16)*. IFN activates cellular-oligoadenylate synthetase (2, 5 OAS) *(17)*, β_2-microglobulin *(18)*, or other proteins (IRF-1, PI/eIF-2a protein kinase, Mx, MHC) *(19)*, thus providing markers indicating IFN–IFN receptor interaction. IFN-α can also decrease T-cell function and T-cell-dependent antibody production in humans when it is given parenterally *(20)*.

From: *Current Clinical Neurology: Inflammatory Disorders of the Nervous System: Pathogenesis, Immunology, and Clinical Management*
Edited by: A. Minagar and J. S. Alexander © Humana Press Inc., Totowa, NJ

2.1. Interferons in Disease: Present Parenteral and Oral Therapeutic Use

In view of the immunoregulatory and antiviral properties of the type I IFN, its response and production has been assessed in autoimmune diseases. Inactive rheumatoid arthritis (RA) is marked by augmented inducibility to IFN-α stimulus, whereas active RA is associated with low inducibility of peripheral blood mononuclear lymphocytes (PMNC) to IFN stimulus and no evidence of IFN production in vivo *(21)*. Active RA patients exhibited a significantly reduced IFN-α/β production compared to normal donors *(22)*. Other autoimmune diseases, such as psoriasis and atopic dermatitis, showed decreased type I IFN production *(22–24)*. PMNC in patients with MS show a similar ineffective production of type I IFN in response to viral or mitogenic stimulus *(25,26)* that parallels the severity of the disease *(27)*. Defects in natural killer (NK) cell activity and renormalization after IFN-α treatment have also been observed in Sjogren's syndrome *(28)*, type 1 diabetes mellitus *(29)*, RA *(21,30)*, and MS *(27,31,32)*, which has correlated with disease severity by some, but not all, investigators *(33)*. Human IFN-β (hIFN-β) reportedly augments suppressor cell function in vitro and in vivo in progressive MS *(34,35)*.

The reported abnormalities of production or response to type I IFN in autoimmune diseases have prompted several small pilot studies of parenteral type I IFN as therapeutic agents in MS. *(36–38)* Although the results have not been conclusive, the studies showed a clear trend toward fewer relapses during IFN treatment *(39)* and a decreased capacity to synthesize native IFN *(40)*, but they were without a clear marker for either MS activity or therapeutic effect *(41)*. Other studies used subcutaneous or intrathecal type I IFN but did not show significant clinical improvement *(40,42–44)*, reduced relapses *(45)*, stabilization of disease progression *(46,47)*, therapeutic efficacy *(48)*, or a relationship of IFN treatment to MS disease activity *(49)*; however, there was an increase in mean circulating NK cells *(50)*. Studies of parenterally administered human recombinant type I IFN (hrIFN) in RRMS demonstrated decreases in relapses *(51)*, brain inflammation *(52)*, and spontaneous in vitro IFN-γ production *(53)*, as well as reductions in progression, relapse rate, and active lesions on MRI *(54)*.

Oral administration of type I IFN may avoid the inconvenience and side effects of intrathecal and systemic administration and may have a unique and more effective mode of action than the other methods. Natural hIFN-α has been orally administered at low doses in the treatment of viral disease in animals. The first report suggesting that orally administered IFN could exert a protective effect showed that 500 U/mL IFN protected suckling mice from orally administered lethal virus challenge *(55)*. Orally administered natural hIFN-α can prevent experimental development of feline leukemia *(56)* and bovine *Theileria parva* infection *(57)*. Stanton found that low doses of hrIFN-α A/D (which is highly active in mouse cells *[58]*) or mouse IFN-α/β [mIFN-α/β] given orally in drinking water protected mice from encephalitis and death from intraperitoneal injection of Semliki Forest virus *(59)*. Importantly, this response was biphasic; higher levels of IFN were not protective nor were high or low intraperitoneal doses. Recent studies indicate that systemic IFN effects can be achieved with comparatively very low doses (approx 100–1000 units) of natural hIFN-α *(56,60–62)*. Therefore, systemic effects may be obtained through oral administration, and the therapeutic effect may not require transit of intact IFN across the bowel. Proteins that might not survive transit through the alimentary canal may still exhibit immunomodulatory activity via the gut-associated lymphoid tissue (GALT) in the oropharynx and beyond via paracrine activity *(63–66)*.

Several early studies of the pharmacokinetics of IFN delivered by various routes reported that orally administered IFN failed to appear in the bloodstream *(67–69)*. There are no reports of orally administration of IFN peptides or the presence of IFN breakdown products in the lumen of the gut or in the bloodstream, although IFN-α amino acids 9–18 and 26–40 in vitro inhibit antigen receptor-stimulated proliferation or viral activity in human cells *(70,71)*; however, several investigations have shown that small but measurable amounts of IFN can be absorbed from the oral pharynx or large intestine in rats *(70,72)*.

More recent studies demonstrate that oral administration of IFN-α in mice *(73)*, dogs *(74)*, green monkeys *(75)*, or humans *(76)* does not result in detectable levels of IFN-α in the blood, in contrast to parenteral administration nor can its effect be blocked by circulating anti-IFN antibodies in mice *(73)*. The inability to detect orallyadministered IFN in blood may be caused by its modest spillover in a rapidly turning over lymphatic pool *(72)*. The absence of increases in biological markers (β_2-microglobulin, neopterin or 2, 5 OAS) after orally administration *(76)* and their presence with subcutaneous or intravenous IFN-β *(77)* suggests that orally adminsitered IFN acts through a different mechanism. The neutropenic effect of orally administered IFN can be transferred by injection of blood cells but not serum from IFN-fed animals to recipient animals *(73)*. Activated monocytes and lymphocytes, by virtue of their circulatory ability, potentially can transfer their biological activities throughout the body in the absence of circulating cytokines after contacting IFN or IFN-induced cells in GALT *(72,78)*. Therefore, the evaluation of type I IFN therapy administered orally compared to parenterally in experimental autoimmune encephalomyelitis (EAE) may be relevant to the therapy of early autoimmune disease, including RRMS and other chronic non-neurological autoimmune diseases.

3. INGESTED INTERFERON IN ACUTE EXPERIMENTAL AUTOIMMUNE ENCEPHALOMYELITIS

Acute EAE is a T-cell mediated inflammatory autoimmune process of the CNS that resembles the human disease MS *(79)*. It provides a model for assessing the ability of ingested immunoactive substances to influence the course of an autoimmune disease; however, despite the parenteral IFN-β trials in MS, limited information exists about the effect of type I IFN on EAE. Previous investigators have demonstrated that parenteral TGF-β can decrease clinical disease and inflammation in brain and spinal cord in EAE *(80)* and that rat IFN-β decreases the severity of symptoms in rat EAE *(81)*. CD4[+] T cells from the spleens of rats that have recovered from EAE inhibit the in vitro production of IFN-γ by effector cells cultured with MBP, and this inhibition can be abrogated by anti-TGF-β_2 antibodies *(82)*. Parenteral (intravenous) natural rat IFN (10^5 U) can partially suppress acute EAE in male Lewis rats *(83)* and inhibits passive hyperacute, localized EAE *(84)* when administered on the same day as inoculation with immunogen. Investigation of cytokine evolution in the CNS during the natural course of EAE suggests that interleukin (IL)-2, IL-6, and IFN-γ mRNA are elevated in acute disease, but during stabilization of symptoms, these cytokines decrease with increasing IL-10 mRNA levels *(85)*.

Because IFN-β proved useful in MS, an understanding of the mechanism of action of parenterally administered type I IFN on cytokine profiles would be important and might determine whether an immune response can be inhibited by orally administered cytokines. Studies cited above *(56,60–62,86)* indicate that systemic IFN effects can indeed be achieved with natural hIFN-α administered orally. We therefore examined whether the oral administration of type I IFN would inhibit the clinical expression of attacks, decrease pathological sequellae, and inhibit inflammatory cytokine IFN-γ secretion in a model of acute autoimmune disease, EAE.

3.1. Ingested Natural Rat Interferon α /β Can Modify Clinical Disease, Inhibit Proliferation, and Decrease Inflammation

For 7 d preceding immunization with MBP (d –7) and for 21 d thereafter (d +14 postimmunization), three groups of Lewis rats were fed daily either mock IFN or 1000 or 5000 U rat type I IFN-α/β in 0.1 mL phosphate-buffered saline (PBS) *(87)*. All animals were scored for clinical disease until d 16 after immunization (Fig. 1). Results from blinded examination of daily group clinical scores demonstrated significant differences in clinical outcome in rats fed mock IFN vs those fed 5000 U IFN-α/β on d 14–16 and in the animals fed 1000 U at d 14 only. Rats treated with 5000 U rat natural

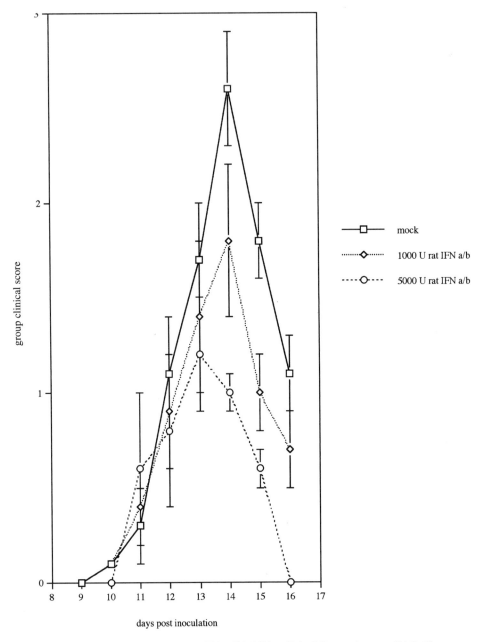

Fig. 1. Oral administration of 5000 U rat IFN-α/β inhibits clinical disease in acute EAE. Three groups of six 8–10-wk-old Lewis rats were immunized with equal parts MBP and CFA and subsequently had attacks beginning by d 9 and were followed until d 16. Seven days preceding immunization (d −7) and for 21 d thereafter (d +14), each group of animals were fed either mock IFN, 1000, or 5000 U rat-type I IFN-α/β (Cytimmune Rat IFN α + β, 4.0×10^5 IRU/mL, Lee Biomolecular Research, Inc., San Diego, CA) daily in 0.1 mL PBS. All animals were scored for clinical disease until d 16 after immunization. Results are shown from blinded examination of daily group clinical scores. Results are expressed as average clinical score for each group on each d of disease postinoculation ± SEM. Combined data from at least two experiments are shown ($p < 0.001$ between mock IFN- and 5000 U IFN-α/β-fed animals on d 14 and between mock IFN- and 5000 U IFN-α/β-fed animals on d 14, 15, and 16 by nonpaired *t* test).

Table 1
**Inhibition of Disease in Rat Acute EAE by Oral Rat and Human rIFN-α Correlates
With Decreased Inflammation in the Spinal Cord**[a]

	Mock	1000 U IFN[b] PO	5000 U IFN PO	5000 U IFN SC
Rat IFN	50 ± 2 [$n = 3$]	ND	26 ± 2 [$n = 3$]	—
hrIFNα PO	52 ± 6 [$n = 7$]	62 ± 8 [$n = 7$]	32 ± 6^c [$n = 7$]	—
hrIFN-α PO/SC	60 ± 4 [$n = 5$]	—	40 ± 10^d [$n = 5$]	82 ± 12 [$n = 5$]

[a]Following sacrifice, spinal cords were removed and immersion fixed in 10% neutral buffered formalin for a minimum of 2 wk. After fixation, cords were sectioned in entirety in the horizontal plane at approx 3 mm intervals and processed to paraffin. Paraffin blocks were sectioned at 6–8 μ, and step sections were stained with hematoxylin, eosin, and Luxol-fast blue/PAS/hematoxylin and examined by light microscopy. Cord sections were evaluated independently for foci of inflammation by a blinded observer, who did not have knowledge of the treatment status of the animals prior to sacrifice. Spinal cord tissue was sampled in an identical fashion for each animal and numbers of inflammatory foci per section (>20 inflammatory cells) in the parenchyma were counted. Results are expressed as number of inflammatory foci per cord ± SEM. Values represent combined data of two separate experiments.

[b]IFN = interferon; PO = orally administered; SC = subcutaneous; ND = not detected; hrIFN-α = human recombinant interferon-α; SEM = standard error of mean.

[c]$p < 0.05$ compared to control.

[d]$p < 0.01$ compared to control.

IFN-α/β had peak disease that was less severe than in the mock group, and the 5000 U IFN-α/β-treated group recovered more quickly and returned to baseline sooner than the mock-treated group. Rats treated with 1000 U rat natural IFN-α/β had peak disease that was less severe than in the mock group, but neither recovered nor returned to baseline as quickly as the 5000 U-fed group. The overall mean cumulative clinical score (area under the curve) of the animals treated with 5000 U rat natural IFN-α was significantly less than in mock IFN-fed controls (0.8 ± 0.2, 5000 U-fed vs 1.2 ± 0.2, mock IFN-fed; $p < 0.02$). Animals were also examined histologically 16 d following immunization. There were less inflammatory foci in the animals treated with IFN-α/β as compared to the control mock IFN group, although this did not attain statistical significance because of the small number of spinal cords examined per group (Table 1; 5000 IFN orally vs mock IFN; $p < 0.06$).

Sixteen days after immunization, draining popliteal lymph node (PLN) Con A proliferation was inhibited from $16,209 \pm 1234$ cycles per minute (cpm) from mock-fed animals to 8120 ± 765 cpm in 5000 U IFN-α/β-fed animals ($p < 0.05$). Draining PLN cells from mock- and 5000 U-treated animals were stimulated with ionomycin plus phorbol myristate acetate (PMA), and demonstrated decreasing proliferation from animals treated with mock IFN ($20,505$ cpm ± 505) to animals treated with 5000 U IFN (6111 cpm ± 636; $p < 0.05$). No consistent differences in MBP or mycobacterium tuberculosis (MT) proliferation between fed and mock-fed animals was demonstrated in draining PLN (data not shown). There was also no inhibition in spleen or nondraining mesenteric lymph nodes to Con A or ionomycin/PMA in IFN-treated animals (data not shown).

These data suggest that species-specific type I IFN can inhibit the severity of acute clinical disease when given at adequate dosages. Inhibition of proliferation from ingested IFN-α/β could be caused by a direct action of IFN that enters the bloodstream through the gut or indirectly. We examined whether in vitro type I IFN treatment of draining PLN and spleen cells from immunized mock-treated animals would demonstrate effects similar to in vivo treatment. There was no clear effect on Con A proliferation in draining PLN or spleen cells exposed to IFN in vitro (Fig. 2), because in contrast to in vivo IFN oral administration, neither draining PLN nor spleen in vitro Con A proliferation was decreased. This implies a unique effect of type I IFN delivered via the GALT.

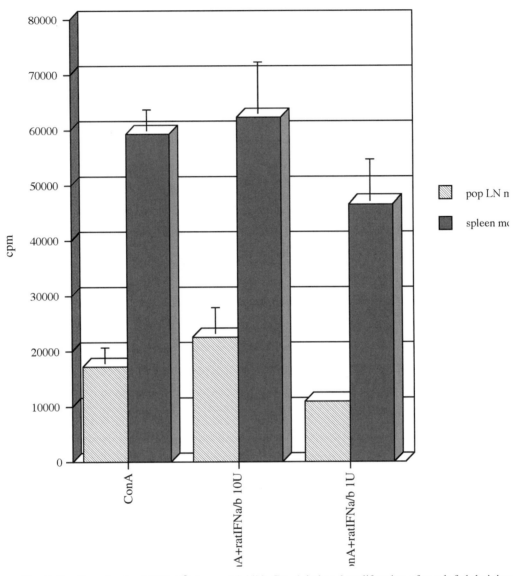

Fig. 2. In vitro rat natural IFN-α/β does not inhibit Con A induced proliferation of mock-fed draining popliteal LN (pop LN) or spleen in acute EAE. Following clinical attack, rats were sacrificed, and spleen and draining lymph node cells were pooled and cultured in vitro with Con A ± 1 or 10 U rat natural IFN-α/β. Cultures were run in triplicate and the results expressed as ΔCPM ± SEM. Cell preparation and proliferation is as described in ref. *87.*

3.2. Modification of Acute Rat Experimental Autoimmune Encephalomyelitis by Ingested hrIFN-α

Because type I hIFN can show cross-species activity in mice *(88)*, guinea pigs *(89)*, gnotobiotic calves *(90)*, horses, pigs *(91)*, and cats *(92,93)*, we also used hrIFN-α, a uniform material that would eliminate the possibility that disease was modified by non-IFN rat immunoactive proteins induced during manufacturing by induction of rat fibroblast cultures with Newcastle disease virus. Recombinant human IFN-αIIb (human recombinant Schering IFN-α used in these experiments) was used because of the high degree of homology between human and murine type I IFN gene products *(94)*, type I IFN can induce viral resistance in cultured heterologous cells thus demonstrating trans-species activity *(95,96)*, and hIFN has been successfully used in cats *(56)* and pigs *(62)*. In addition, hrIFN-α may also provide more immunosuppression per unit of activity than natural preparations. Because both 1000 and 5000 U natural rat IFN-α/β administered orally for 7 d preceding immunization (d –7) and for 21 d thereafter (d +14) demonstrated some effectiveness in inhibiting acute disease, each group of animals was fed either 1000 U mock PBS or 5000 U hrIFN-α daily. Three groups of seven 8- to 10-wk-old Lewis rats were immunized and subsequently had an attack beginning by d 10 and extending through d 16. All animals were scored for clinical disease until d 16 after immunization. Results from blinded examination of daily group clinical scores demonstrated significant differences in clinical outcome in the mock-fed vs 5000 U hrIFN-α-fed animals at d 12 to 15 but not in the animals fed 1000 U (Fig. 3A). Animals fed 5000 U hrIFN-α showed delayed attack onset, decreased severity at peak, and earlier resolution of the attack. The overall mean cumulative clinical score of the animals treated with either PBS control-fed (1.8 ± 0.2) or 1000 U-fed animals (2.1 ± 0.3) was significantly greater than 5000 U hrIFN-α (0.5 ± 0.2; $p < 0.001$). There was a trend for decreased Con A proliferation in draining PLN from 56,209 ± 5386 cpm in mock PBS-fed animals to 37,438 ± 8862 cpm in 5000 U IFN-α/β-fed animals ($p < 0.06$). This suggests that ingested hrIFN-α can inhibit clinical attacks of EAE in the Lewis rat when administered before inoculation. Following sacrifice 16 d postimmunization, animals were also examined histologically. There were significantly more inflammatory foci in the mock PBS group or 1000 U hrIFN-α-fed group compared to the 5000 U hrIFN-α-fed group (*see* Table 1, hrIFN-α administered orally).

3.3. Ingested Inequivalent Doses of Parenterally Administered hrIFN-α Modifies Clinical Disease

The above data suggests that ingested hrIFN-α can modify clinical disease and decrease inflammation in the spinal cord. Experiments were performed to examine equivalent amounts of ingested vs parenterally administered hrIFN-α. Three groups of 10 Lewis rats were immunized and either not treated, fed 5000 U hrIFN-α, or injected with 5000 U hrIFN-α subcutaneously for 7 d preceding immunization (d –7) and for 21 d thereafter (d +14). All animals were scored for clinical disease until d 18 after immunization. Results from blinded examination of daily group clinical scores demonstrated significant differences in clinical outcome in the mock-fed vs 5000 U hrIFN-α-fed animals at d 12 to 15 and 17 but not in the animals injected subcutaneously with 5000 U hrIFN-α (Fig. 3B). Rats treated with oral 5000 U hrIFN-α had a less severe disease at peak of the disease, and more rapid recovery compared to the untreated group. Indeed, the untreated and the subcutaneously treated groups had similar clinical curve scores, suggesting that subcutaneous hrIFN-α had little or no effect on clinical disease. Overall mean cumulative clinical scores demonstrated significant differences in clinical outcome in the untreated (1.5 ± 0.2), and subcutaneously treated (1.8 ± 0.4) vs fed animals (0.6 ± 0.2; $p < 0.005$, fed vs untreated/-subcutaneously treated). There was no significant difference between untreated and subcutaneously treated animals. There was no significant difference in draining PLN Con A proliferation between untreated and 5000 U subcutaneously-treated animals (untreated: 30,854 ± 2142 cpm vs 5000 U subcutaneous: 38,242 ± 4476 cpm). Eighteen days following immunization, animals were sacrificed and examined histologically. There were significantly more inflammatory foci in the 5000 U subcutaneously treated group and untreated group compared to the 5000 U-fed (*see* Table 1, hrIFN-α orally adminstered/subcutaneous).

Experiments using PBS-fed and PBS subcutaneously injected controls demonstrated similar findings. In this case four groups of six Lewis rats were either fed PBS, injected subcutaneously with PBS, fed 5000 U hrIFN-α, or injected with 5000 U hrIFN-α for 7 d preceding immunization (d –7) and for 21 d thereafter (d +14). All animals were immunized on d 0. Animals were scored for clinical disease until d 18 after immunization and sacrificed. Mean cumulative clinical scores

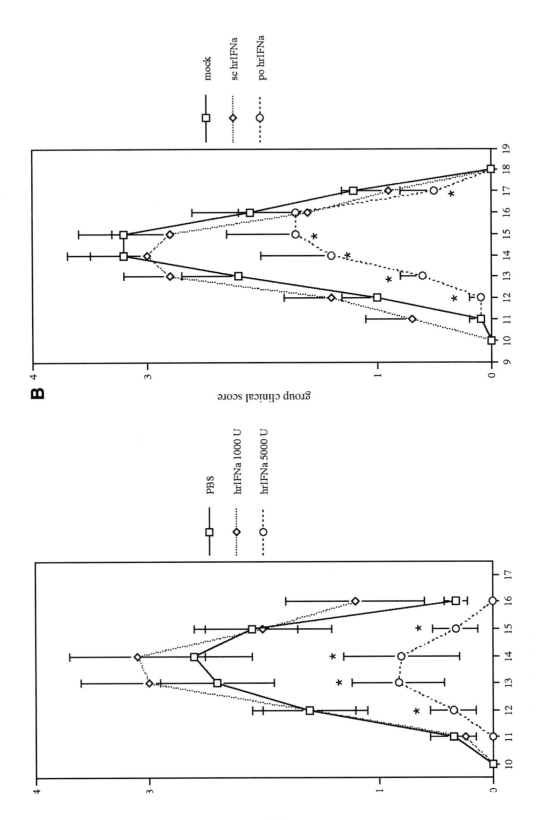

were significantly less in hrIFN-α-fed animals (1.0 ± 0.2) compared to PBS-fed (2.5 ± 0.4) ($p < 0.005$) animals. There was no significant difference between mock subcutaneously fed animals (1.7 ± 0.4) and 5000 U subcutaneous hrIFN-α-fed animals (2.1 ± 0.4), even though subcutaneously treated animals did have higher mean cumulative clinical scores. This suggests that subcutaneous hrIFN-α cannot modify the onset of acute clinical disease when given at clinically preventive ingested dosages.

3.4. Ingested IFN-α Inhibits the Mitogen-Induced Production of IFN-γ in Draining Popliteal Lymph Nodes

The intensity of disease in EAE has been associated with IFN-γ secretion after Con A stimulation *(97)*. We assessed IFN-γ secretion at 9 d postimmunization, at d 16 before disease onset and when there was significant clinical difference between mock IFN- and 5000 U hrIFN-α-fed animals, and at d 18 postimmunization, after clinical attack had subsided. Spleen and draining PLN cells from mock-fed, 5000 U hrIFN-α-fed, or 5000 U subcutaneous hrIFN-α-treated rats were stimulated with Con A (2.5 µg/mL) for 2 d. At d 9 preceding clinical disease, but during the generation of antigen-specific T cells in draining popliteal lymph nodes, draining PLN cells from mock IFN-treated animals demonstrated detectable IFN-γ production when there was no IFN-γ production from 5000 U hrIFN-α-fed animals (Table 2). At d 16, when clinical differences persisted in animals, and at d 18 postimmunization, after clinical attack had subsided, draining PLN cells from mock PBS-treated animals continued to demonstrate significantly greater IFN-γ production compared to 5000 U-fed animals (Table 2). There was no difference between mock- and 5000 U-treated spleen cells (data not shown). There were no differences in draining PLN IFN-γ secretion between animals subcutaneous mock-treated vs injected subcutaneously treated with 5000 U hrIFN-α. The results show that ingested, not subcutaneous hrIFN-α, decreased IFN-γ, a mediator of inflammation, in draining popliteal lymph nodes.

Ingested type I IFNs, as opposed to identical subcutaneous doses, can be used to modify biological response to MBP in acute EAE in Lewis rats when it is administered before sensitization and clinical attack. Ingested type I IFN modifies clinical attacks, decreases the number of inflammatory foci in spinal cord, decreases nonspecific proliferation by Con A and ionomycin/PMA, and decreases the production of IFN-γ in draining popliteal lymph nodes. This suggests that IFN-α is more active by the oral route compared to the parenteral route and has definable immunological effects and confirms that specific cytokines are capable of inhibiting clinical disease when given via the gastrointestinal tract. Both hrIFN-α and species-specific rat natural IFN worked in our experiments. Natural IFN is a mixture of 14 separate subspecies, including the IFN-αII subtype, which may be only a small component of the natural type *(98)*. Human IFN shows cross-species activity when used at larger doses (5000 U), compared to rat species-specific type I IFN, which showed some activity at 1000 U administered orally. The IFN αII subtype may provide a

---

Fig. 3. Oral administration of 5000 U hrIFN-α in rat acute EAE, not SC administration, decreases the severity and speeds the recovery of clinical attacks. A. Three groups of seven Lewis rats were inoculated with MBP and CFA on d 0 and orally administered PBS, 1000 U or 5000 U hrIFN-α (Schering hrIFN-αIIb, 3×10^6 IU/ml, Schering Pharmaceuticals, Kenilworth, NJ) daily starting 7 d preceding immunization (d −7) and for 14 d thereafter (d +14). Values represent mean clinical scores for each group of seven animals ± SEM. Combined data from at least two experiments are shown ($p < 0.05$ between mock PBS/1000 U IFN-α-fed vs 5000 U IFN-α-fed animals on d 12–15 by nonpaired *t* test). B. Oral administration of 5000 U hrIFN-α, not SC administration, decreases the severity of clinical attacks. Three groups of 10 Lewis rats were inoculated with MBP and CFA on d 0 and untreated, fed 5000 U, or injected SC with 5000 U hrIFN-α daily starting 7 d preceding immunization (d −7) and for 21 d thereafter (d +14). Values represent mean daily clinical scores for each group of 10 animals + SEM. Combined data from at least two experiments are shown ($p < 0.005$ between mock PBS/5000 U SC IFN-α- vs 5000 U IFN-α fed animals on d 12–14; $p < 0.05$ on d 15 and 17 by nonpaired *t* test).

Table 2
Orally Administered Human Recombinant Inteferon-α Inhibits the Mitogen-Induced Production of Interferon-γ in Draining Popliteal Lymph Nodes[a]

Day postimmunization	Mock PO[b] PBS	5000 U PO IFN	Mock SC PBS	5000 U SC IFN
9	50 ± 14	ND	—	—
16	1140 ± 6	68 ± 22^c	—	—
18	460 ± 60	96 ± 32^c	540 ± 80	421 ± 38^d

[a]Draining popliteal lymph node cells from mock and 5000 U IFN-treated immunized rats were cultured with Con A (2.5 µg/mL) at 1×10^6 cells/mL in 75 cm² tissue culture flasks for 48 h in a humidified 5% CO_2/95% air incubator at 37°C. Supernatants were collected at 48 h after Con A activation and frozen at −70°C after centrifugation. IFN-γ was measured using a solid phase ELISA assay. Anti-IFN-γ (PharMingen, San Diego, CA) was incubated on 96 polyvinyl plastic well microtiter plates with 0.01 M carbonate buffer (pH 9.6) overnight at 4°C. The plate was blocked with 3% BSA in phosphate-buffered saline for 3 h. 100 µL of supernatants was added at various dilutions that were titered to the linear portion of the absorbance/concentration curve in triplicate and incubated for 1 h at room temperature. After the plate was washed five times with phosphate buffered saline Tween (0.05%; Sigma), 100 µl peroxidase conjugated IFN-γ monoclonal antibody (with a different epitopic determinant than the first antibody used to coat the polyvinyl plate) at a 1:1000 concentration was added for 60 min. Subsequently, the peroxidase substrate O-phenylenediamine dihydrochloride was added, and the absorbance measured at 450 nm. Standard curves with various amounts of the IFN-γ were generated. Results are expressed as IFN-γ ng/mL ± SEM. Values represent combined data of two separate experiments.
[b]PO = orally administered; PBS = phosphate-buffered saline; IFN = interferon; SC = subcutaneous; ND = not detected; ELISA = enzyme-linked immunosorbent assay; BSA = bovine serum albumin; SEM = standard error of mean.
[c]$p < 0.05$ compared to mock PO PBS control.
[d]$p < 0.05$ compared to mock SC PBS.

relatively greater amount of inhibitory activity/total units of antiproliferative activity of the most important component for immunosuppression in the rat.

Antiproliferative effects of ingested IFN α/β were greater in draining popliteal lymph nodes than in nondraining mesenteric lymph nodes *(99)*. Oral administration of IFN-α, as opposed to subcutaneous administration, inhibited the production of IFN-γ in draining popliteal lymph nodes. Draining popliteal lymph nodes are the natural draining areas for subcutaneously administered antigens and are presumably the reservoir of high frequencies of sensitized MBP-specific T cells. Ingested cytokines may preferentially affect proliferation and cytokine production at sites of immune activation, compared to equivalent systemic doses. Inhibition of IFN-γ secretion in an activated regional immune compartment by IFN-α may cause a decreased inflammatory effect of MBP-specific cells in the CNS.

4. INGESTED IFN IN CHRONIC EXPERIMENTAL AUTOIMMUNE ENCEPHALOMYELITIS

One major difficulty in treating autoimmune disease in humans is that the immune system has already been sensitized to autoantigen at the time of clinical presentation. An animal model that mimics clinical disease and previous immunological sensitization is useful in the evaluation of potential therapies for human disease. Chronic EAE (CR-EAE) is such a disease because it involves a chronic inflammatory CNS autoimmune process that more closely resembles MS *(100–102)*. After immunization, animals cycle repeatedly through manifest clinical attacks; thus, CR-EAE provides an excellent model to test the modulation of clinical, immunological, and histological sequelae in orally or parenterally administered IFN.

4.1. Effects of Murine Type I IFNs on Clinical Disease

Initial experiments suggested that 1 to 10 U of ingested type I hIFN had an immunological effect on CR-EAE but was not adequate to suppress clinical relapses (data not shown); thus,

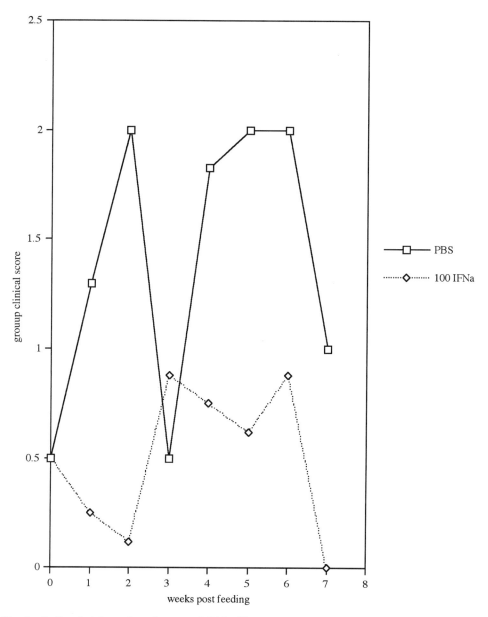

Fig. 4. Orally administered murine natural IFN-α/β suppresses clinical relapse in murine CR-EAE. Two groups of six animals were inoculated and, following the first attack, were fed either mock IFN or 100 U murine natural IFN-α/β (Cytimmune Mouse IFN-α + β, 4.0×10^5 IRU/mL, Lee Biomolecular Research, Inc., San Diego, CA), or mock mIFN-α/β (Cytimmune <2 IRU/ml, Lee Biomolecular Research, Inc., San Diego, CA. [generated identically to IFN-α/β except cultures are mock induced]) three times per week for 7 wk. One of two representative experiments are shown. SEM is <10% and is not shown.

experiments were performed in which two groups of six immunized SJL/J mice (using the method of Brown and McFarlin *[103]*, modified by Miller *[104]*) were fed mock IFN or 100 U natural mIFN-α/β three times per week beginning on d 30, following recovery from the first clinical attack. Group clinical scores after the initial attack were not significantly different among the different groups. Clinical relapses began approx 40 d after inoculation. Clinical scores demonstrated significant differences in outcome in the mock IFN-fed vs 100 U natural mIFN-α/β-fed animals ($p < 0.03$; *see* Fig. 4). Two major relapses occurred in the mock IFN-fed group during the 7-wk course with a resultant increased neurological deficit. The oral natural mIFN-α/β group underwent a delayed single attack without residual neurological deficit. Ingested natural mIFN-α/β blunted the severity and decreased the group score during clinical relapse (oral administration of IFN-γ has no effect on EAE [unpublished results, Brod SA]).

Con A activation of draining inguinal lymph node cells was inhibited in mice fed 100 U natural mIFN-α/β compared to those fed mock IFN (38,095 cpm ± 3160 vs 88,222 cpm ± 1910; $p < 0.05$). Lymph node cells from mock IFN-fed mice tested with MBP generated a robust proliferative response, but that response was profoundly inhibited in natural mIFN-α/β-fed animals (14,052 cpm ± 842 vs 448 cpm ± 50; $p < 0.05$).

To determine whether another sensitized antigen was inhibited, we examined antigen-specific proliferation of draining inguinal lymph nodes to a second sensitized antigen, *Mycobacterium tuberculosus hominis* (MT), a component of mouse spinal cord homogenate (MSCH) inoculum. Lymph node cells from mock IFN-fed animals generated a robust proliferative response to MT but that response was profoundly decreased in 100 U natural mIFN-α/β-fed animals (52,401 cpm ± 857 vs 5214 cpm ± 808; $p < 0.05$).

Animals were also examined histologically 65 d following immunization and after clinical relapse. There were significantly fewer inflammatory foci in the IFN-fed group (0.5 ± 0.1) compared to the mock IFN group (1.8 ± 1.1; $p < 0.05$). The data above suggests that orally administered natural type I mIFN can suppress clinical relapse disease, decrease inflammation, and inhibit proliferation to mitogen, MBP, and MT.

4.2. Suppression of Relapse by Ingested IFN-α/β Correlates With Decreased IFN-g Secretion

The intensity of disease in EAE has been associated with IFN-γ secretion after Con A stimulation of spleen cells *(97)*; therefore, pooled spleen cells were stimulated from mice that were mock-fed ($n = 5$) or 100 U-fed ($n = 5$) mIFN-α/β with Con A (2.5 µg/mL) at 1×10^6 cells/mL for 2 d, and supernatants were assayed by solid-phase enzyme-linked immunosorbent assay (ELISA; IL-2, IL-10, IFN-γ). Oral mIFN-α/β consistently decreased IFN-γ, a mediator of inflammation (Table 3; $p < 0.001$). There was also a decrease in IL-2, a T-cell growth factor, and increased IL-10 production, although these changes did not attain statistical significance (data not shown).

As in the rat system, available natural type I mIFN is manufactured by viral induction in murine fibroblasts and could contain non-IFN immunoactive proteins responsible for disease modification. Others have found that hIFN-α1 and IFN-α2 have 1 to 50% of antiviral activity in L929 mouse cells, compared to human WISH or HEp2 cell lines *(58,97,105,106)*. Thus, suppression of actively induced relapses and prevention of adoptive transfer with pure human preparations would eliminate the possibility that non-IFN murine proteins modify disease but might require higher doses relative to mIFN to show effects. Accordingly, we examined whether the oral administration of hrIFN-α and lower doses of murine species-specific IFN-α would prevent clinical relapses of EAE.

4.3. Ingested hrIFN-α Suppresses Clinical Experimental Autoimmune Encephalomyelitis and Inhibit Proliferative Responses to MBP

Three groups of six SJL/J 6- to 8-wk-old female mice that were immunized with MSCH subsequently had an attack beginning by d 16 and ending by d 30. Each group of animals had comparable scores after the initial clinical attack had subsided. On d 30 following immunization, groups were either mock-fed PBS, 100 U hrIFN-α, or 1000 U hrIFN-α three times per week during the following 5 wk *(107)*. Mean weekly clinical relapse scores demonstrated significant differences in outcome in the mock PBS-fed vs 100 U and 1000 U hrIFN-α-fed animals (Fig. 5). The mock PBS-fed group incurred increasing disease severity during the course of 5 wk, as shown by increasing neurological deficit *(108)* over time. The 1000 U-fed hrIFN-α animals underwent a

Table 3
Orally Administered Murine Interferon-α/β Inhibits Mitogen-Induced Production of Interferon-γ in Spleen Cells[a]

	Mock IFN[b]	100 U IFN
Exp 1	2500 ± 300	1100 ± 200[c]
Exp 2	2180 ± 100	247 ±143[c]

[a]Spleen cells from mock and 100 U murine IFN-α/β treated mice were cultured with Con A (2.5 µg/mL) for 2 d and interleukins (IL-2, IL-10, and IFN-γ) were measured as described in table 2. Results are expressed as IFN-γ ng/mL ± SEM. Values represent combined data of two separate experiments.
[b]IFN = interferon; SEM = standard error of mean.
[c]$p < 0.001$ compared to mock IFN control.

mild single attack with decreasing neurological deficit. Overall, ingested hrIFN-α decreased the groups' scores during relapse. Thus, ingested hrIFN-α is active by the oral route and suppresses clinical relapses.

Following clinical relapse, mice were sacrificed, and spleen and draining inguinal lymph node cells were pooled into hrIFN-α-fed ($n = 6$) and mock PBS-fed ($n = 6$) groups, respectively, and cultured in vitro to determine antigen-specific T-cell proliferation. There was a significant decrease in proliferation in draining inguinal lymph node cells to GP-MBP in mice fed 1000 U hrIFN-α compared with mock PBS-fed controls ($p < 0.05$), and in spleen cells in mice fed 100 U hrIFN-α to GP-MBP and MT compared to mock PBS fed animals (*see* Table 4, exp. 1).

4.4. Lower Doses of Ingested Murine Species-Specific IFN-α Suppress Clinical Disease and Decrease Inflammation and Cytokine Secretion

We have previously shown that 100 U of ingested mIFN-α/β *(104)* and 100 U of hrIFN-α can suppress clinical relapse attacks *(109–111)*. A dose-response-ranging experiment for ingested type I IFN treatment is critical for designing clinical trials in patients with MS. Therefore, we examined whether one-tenth of the dose (10 U) of orally administered mIFN-α would suppress relapse attacks. Animals were immunized, and after 30 d at the completion of the initial attack, fed mock mIFN or 10 or 100 U mIFN-α. The mock IFN-fed group incurred relapse during the course of 5 wk. Clinical scores demonstrated significant differences in outcome in the mock mIFN-fed vs 10 and 100 U mIFN-α-fed animals (Fig. 6). Histological examination showed decreased inflammation in animals with decreased clinical scores (mock IFN: 2.2 ± 0.1; 10 U mIFN-α: 0.9 ± 0.4; $p < 0.01$; 100 U mIFN-α: 0.8 ± 0.6; $p < 0.05$). Orally administered mIFN-α is effective at an order of magnitude less than the effective hrIFN dose, consistent with data for cross species antiviral activity *(109–111)*. Phenotyping at the time of sacrifice demonstrated no significant differences in CD3-, CD4-, or CD8-cell surface expression in pooled lymph node or pooled spleen cells from mock IFN-fed animals compared to mIFN-α-fed animals in two separate experiments (data not shown). Con A activation of draining PLN cells was inhibited in mIFN-α-fed animals compared to mock IFN-fed animals (*see* Table 4, exp 3). There was a significant decrease in proliferation in spleen cells to PLP 139–151 in mice fed 10 U mIFN-α compared to mock IFN-fed mice (*see* Table 4, exp 3). Con A-stimulated spleen cells from mIFN-α-fed animals demonstrated decreased secretion of IFN-γ and IL-2 (*see* Table 5, exp. 3) compared to mock IFN-fed animals.

5. INGESTED IFN IN ADOPTIVE OR PASSIVE TRANSFER OF EXPERIMENTAL AUTOIMMUNE ENCEPHALOMYELITIS

EAE can be adoptively or passively transferred by using in vitro antigen-activated lymph node or spleen cells from actively immunized mice *(112)* that have been immunized with

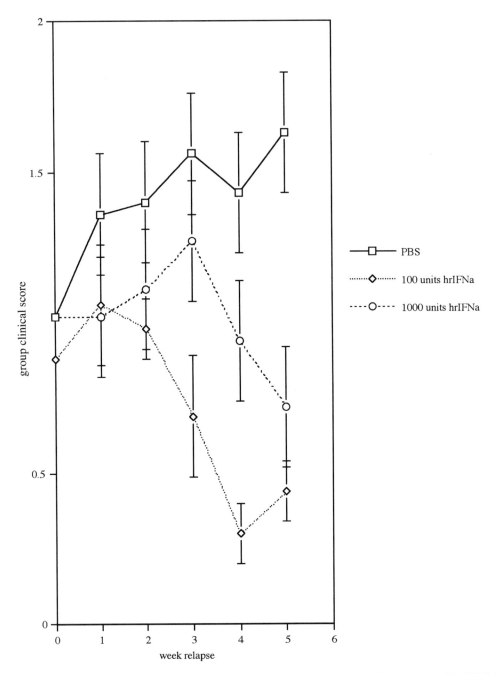

Fig. 5. Oral administration of hrIFN-α in murine CR-EAE suppresses relapses. Three groups of six SJL/J 6- to 8-wk-old female mice were immunized with MSCH in CFA. On d 40 postimmunization, one group was fed PBS, another group 100 U hrIFN-α, and a third group was fed 1000 U hrIFN-α three times per week over the following 5 wk. All animals were scored by a blinded observer for clinical disease until d 75 after immunization. Values represent combined data of two separate experiments of mean weekly group clinical scores ± SEM (mock PBS-fed vs 100 U hrIFN α-fed for wk 2–5 [$p < 0.001$] vs 1000 U hrIFN-α fed animals for wk 4–5 [$p < 0.01$ by nonpaired *t* test]).

Table 4
Oral Interferon-α Inhibits Proliferation to GP-Myelin Basic Protein,
Proteolipid Protein 139–151, MT and Con A[a]

Exp 1	GP-MBP[b] LN	GP-MBP Spleen	MT Spleen
Mock PBS	6105 ± 705	11,357 ± 948	14,086 ± 1385
100 U hrIFN	3330 ± 595	5841 ± 1846[c]	8396 ± 948[c]
1000 U hrIFN	1182 ± 121[c]	ND	ND
Exp 2	Con A Spleen	PLP 139–151 LN	
Mock PBS	40,822 ± 1803	46,187 ± 2836	
100 U hrIFN	2,406 ± 436[c]	25,966 ± 929[c]	
Exp 3	Con A LN	PLP 139–151 Spleen	
Mock mIFN	94,770 ± 2783	5360 ± 262	
10 U mIFN	31,943 ± 7840[c]	2,166 ± 93[c]	
Exp 4	Con A LN: IFN-γ		
Mock mIFN	126,625 ± 10,743		
10 U mIFN	85,900 ± 7,153[c]		

[a]Following clinical acute (exp 2 and 4) or relapse (exp 1 and 3) attack, mice were sacrificed, spleen and draining inguinal LN were pooled and cultured in vitro to determine mitogen- or antigen-specific T-cell proliferative responses. All antigen stimulation was carried out by incubating whole spleen/popliteal draining LN populations at 2×10^5 cells/well with antigen at 10 µg/mL (GP-MBP, PLP 139–151 [PLP 139–151 HSLGKWLGHPDKF (119)], or MT) in standard media for 4 d and cultured as described in methods. Cultures were run in triplicate and results are expressed as cycles per minute minus background with cells alone ± SEM.

[b]GP-MBP = GP-myelin basic protein; PLP = proteolipid protein; MT = mycobacterium tuberculosis; PBS = phosphate-buffered saline; hrIFN = human recombinant interferon; ND = not done.

[c]$p < 0.05$ compared to mock control. Values represent combined data from two separate experiments.

spinal cord *(113)*. Transfer of disease can also be performed by activation with Con A and pokeweed mitogens *(114)*. CR-EAE in SJL/J mice can be adoptively transferred following the IV injection of an MBP peptide 89–100-specific T-cell line *(115)* or in vitro PLP-stimulated lymph node cells from SJL/J mice immunized with human myelin PLP *(116)*. The immunodominant epitopes of PLP in the SJL/J mouse are PLP peptide 139–151 and 178–191 *(117–119)*. Treatment of mice with splenocytes coupled with mouse spinal cord homogenate or PLP after immunization with MSCH suppressed the onset and severity of clinical and histologic signs of relapsing EAE *(120,121)*. This suggests that PLP is a major encephalitogen in MSCH-induced CR-EAE in the SJL/J mouse.

5.1. Activated Donor Cells From Animals Orally Administered hrIFN-α Are Less Effective in Transferring Clinical Disease Than Cells From Mock PBS-Fed Mice

Adoptive transfer experiments were performed to determine if activated spleen cells from hrIFN-α fed animals could transfer disease *(109–111)*. Con A-activated T cells from mock PBS-fed or 100 U hrIFN-α-fed immunized SJL/J mice, followed for 5 wk after initiation of feeding during relapse, were transferred adoptively IP to recipient mice that were then followed for evidence of disease. Mice that received Con A-activated mock PBS T cells had a significant clinical attack starting at d 5, whereas recipients of Con A-activated hrIFN-α T cells had a much less severe clinical attack (Fig. 7). In contrast, Con A-activated spleen cells from animals treated with hrIFN-α in vitro, as opposed to in vivo, feeding did not prevent adoptive disease transfer (data not shown). Con A induced spleen-cell proliferation from mock PBS-fed recipients was significantly greater compared to hrIFN-α-fed recipients (*see* Table 4, exp. 2). Pooled spleen cells from immunized recipients of either mock-fed or 100 U-fed hrIFN-α donor cells were stimulated with PLP 139–151 (10 µg/mL) for 2 d, and supernatants were assayed by ELISA. The results combined from two separate

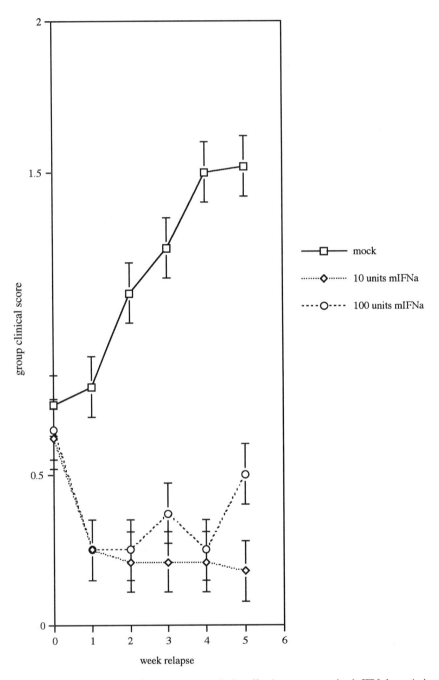

Fig. 6. Oral mIFN-α suppresses relapses at one-tenth the effective cross-species hrIFN dose. Animals (*n* = 8/group) were immunized, followed as described in Fig. 4, and treated with mock mIFN, 10, or 100 U mIFN-α. Animals were scored by a blinded observer for clinical disease for 5 wk after feeding. Values represent combined data of two separate experiments of mean weekly group clinical scores ± SEM (mock IFN-fed vs 10 U mIFN-α-fed animals for wk 1–5 [*p* < 0.001] vs 100 U mIFN-α for wk 1–5 [*p* < 0.001 by nonpaired *t* test]).

experiments (*see* Table 5, exp. 2) show that cells from oral hrIFN-α-treated donors secrete less IFN-γ, a mediator of inflammation.

Because PLP is the major encephalitogen in the SJL/J mouse *(117–121)*, adoptive transfer experiments were performed to determine if PLP 139–151-activated spleen cells from IFN-α-fed

Table 5
Oral Interferon-α Inhibits Interferon-γ and Interleukin-2 Secretion[a]

Exp 2	PLP[b] 139–151: Interferon-γ	
Mock PBS	30 ± 2	
100 U hrIFN	12 ± 2^{c}	
Exp 3	Con A spleen: IFN-γ	Con A: IL-2
Mock mIFN	42 ± 1	112 ± 3
10 U mIFN	14 ± 1^{c}	61 ± 3^{c}
Exp 4	Con A LN: IFN-γ	
Mock mIFN	26 ± 1	
10 U mIFN	6 ± 1^{c}	

[a]Following clinical acute (exp 2 and 4) or relapse (exp 3) attack, mice were sacrificed, and spleen cells were pooled and cultured in vitro for cytokine production. Antigen stimulation was carried out as described in Table 4 and interleukin assayed as described in Table 3.
[b]PLP = proteolipid protein; INF-γ = interferon-γ; PBS = ; hrIFN = human recombinant interferon; IL-2 = interleukin-2; mIFN = murine interferon; LN = lymph node.
[c]$p < 0.05$ compared to mock control. Values represent combined data of two separate experiments.

animals could transfer disease. CR-EAE was induced in SJL/J mice with MSCH and CFA. Following recovery, animals were fed mock or hrIFN-α three times per week for 6 wk. 10×10^{6} 3 d PLP 139–151-activated T cells from mock-fed or 10 U hrIFN-α-fed immunized SJL/J mice were adoptively transferred IP to nonfed recipient SJL/J mice and followed for evidence of disease (Fig. 8). The recipient mice that received PLP 139–151-activated T cells from a mock-fed donor had a significant clinical attack starting at d 4–5, whereas recipients of PLP 139–151-activated T cells from hrIFN-α-fed donors had a much less severe clinical attack (Con A: 3.0 ± 0.3 mock IFN vs 0.5 ± 0.2 100 U IFN; $p < 0.01$; PLP 139–151: 1.7 ± 0.2 mock IFN vs 0.7 ± 0.1 100 U IFN; $p < 0.01$). Pooled spleen cells stimulated with PLP 139–151 (10 µg/mL) from recipients of IFN-α-fed donor cells secreted less IFN-γ compared to mock-fed mice (donor mock IFN: 30 ng/mL ± 2 donor; 100 U IFN: 10 ng/mL ± 2, $p < 0.05$). There were no changes in IL-2 or IL-4 secretion between mock PBS- and hrIFN-α-fed animals (data not shown). Activated cells from IFN-α-fed animals do not transfer disease as well as cells from mock-fed animals and secrete less IFN-γ in recipients than cells from mock-fed animals.

5.2. Activated Donor Cells From Animals Orally Administered mIFN-α Are Less Effective in Transferring Clinical Disease Than Are Cells From mIFN-Fed Mice

Adoptive transfer experiments were performed to determine if activated spleen cells from 10 U mIFN-α-fed animals could prevent transfer of disease. Con A-activated mock mIFN-fed or 10 U mIFN-α-fed T cells from immunized SJL/J mice, followed for 5 wk after initiation of feeding during relapse, were transferred adoptively intraperitoneally to recipient mice and followed for evidence of disease. Mice that received activated mock IFN T cells had significantly more severe clinical attacks starting at d 13 compared to mIFN-α recipients (Fig. 9). Con A-stimulated proliferation of draining lymph nodes was significantly less from mIFN-α recipients than from mock IFN recipients (*see* Table 4, exp 4). Con A-induced IFN-γ secretion by lymph node cells was inhibited in mIFN-α compared to mock IFN-recipient animals (*see* Table 5, exp. 4), although there was no significant difference in the number of lesions between mock recipients and mIFN-α recipients (mock IFN: 1.8 ± 0.6 [$n = 6$]; 10 U mIFN-α: 1.5 ± 0.5, [$n = 6$]).

5.3. T Cells/T-Cell Subsets From Actively Immunized mIFN-α-Fed Donors Could Transfer Protection to EAE in Actively Immunized Recipients

It is unclear from these experiments whether splenocytes from IFN-fed donors were unable to transfer disease because they were suppressor-like populations. The induction of disease by active

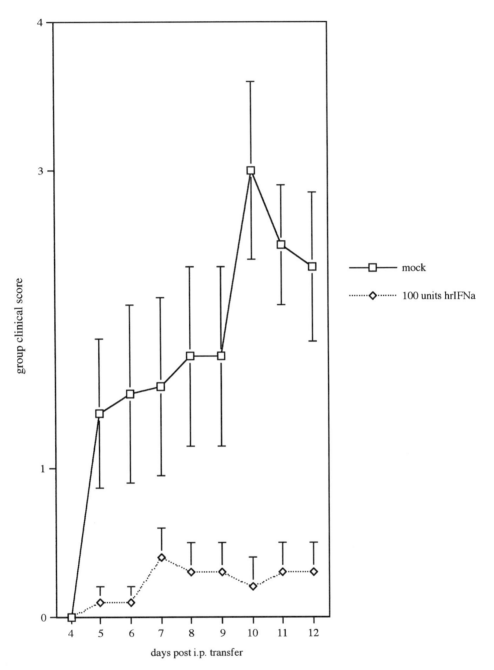

Fig. 7. hrIFN-α-fed animals do not adoptively transfer disease. 10×10^6 3 d-Con A-activated T cells from mock PBS-fed or 100 U hrIFN-α-fed immunized donor SJL/J mice, which had undergone relapse attacks 5 wk earlier, were transferred adoptively IP to naive SJL/J mice ($n = 6$, mock donor; $n = 6$, 100 U hrIFN-α donor) and followed for evidence of disease. Values represent combined data of two separate experiments of mean group daily blinded clinical scores ± SEM (mock PBS-fed donors vs hrIFN-α-fed donors for d 5–12; $p < 0.01$ by nonpaired t test).

immunization can be prevented by the intraperitoneal administration of activated CD8+ T lymphocytes from orally tolerized animals *(122)*. Passive immunization against EAE provides a method to investigate the mechanism of adoptively transferred protection induced by donor cells

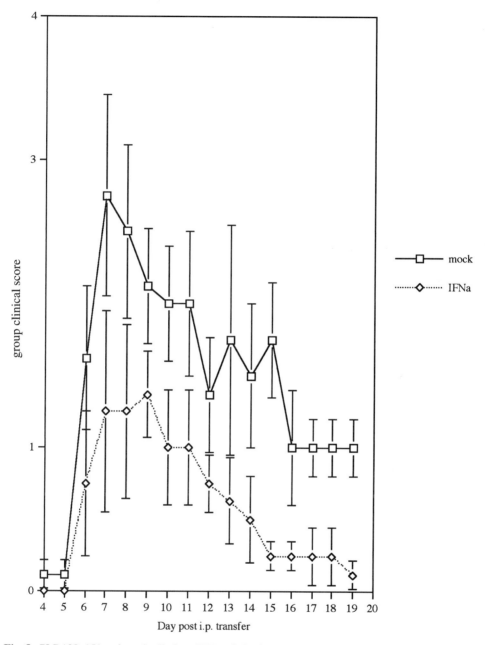

Fig. 8. PLP 139–151 activated cells from IFN-α-fed animals do not transfer disease passively. 10×10^6 3 d PLP 139–151-activated T cells from mock-fed or 100 U hrIFN-α-fed immunized SJL/J mice, which had undergone relapse attacks, were adoptively transferred IP to previously nonfed immunized SJL/J mice (recipient $n = 3$, mock donor; recipient $n = 3$, 100 U IFN donor) and followed for evidence of disease. Values represent mean group daily blinded clinical scores ± SEM ($p < 0.05$ by nonpaired t test at d 7–8, 10–11, 14–19).

through the ingestion of type I IFN to immunized recipient mice. Therefore, we performed experiments with active immunization in recipients and concurrent adoptive transfer of T cells or CD8[+] T-cell subsets from mock-fed or mIFN-α-fed immunized donors to the actively immunized mice. If immunized donor T or CD8[+] T cells from IFN-α donors modulate active induced EAE, the donor cells must be acting as immunomodulatory cells induced by the oral IFN.

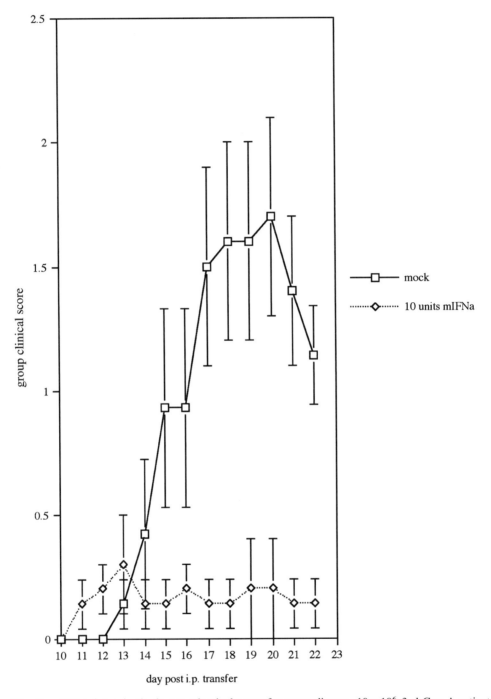

Fig. 9. mIFN-α-fed animals do not adoptively transfer acute disease. 10×10^6 3 d-Con A-activated T cells from mock IFN- or 10 U mIFN-α-fed immunized SJL/J mice that had undergone relapse attacks 35 d earlier were transferred adoptively IP to naive SJL/J mice ($n = 6$, mock IFN donor; $n = 6$, 10 U mIFN-α donor) and followed for evidence of disease. Values represent combined data of two separate experiments of mean group daily blinded clinical scores $\pm$ SEM (mock IFN recipients vs mIFN-α-treated recipients d 15–22; $p < 0.01$ by nonpaired t test).

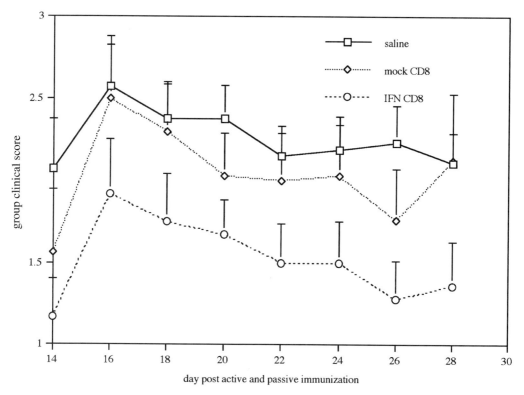

Fig. 10. Concurrent adoptive transfer of activated CD8+ T cells from mIFN-α fed donors inhibits clinical attack in actively immunized recipient mice. Two groups of donor SJL/J 6- to 8-wk-old female mice were actively immunized with MSCH and MT in IFA. After 4 wk and after acute attack, one group was fed mock IFN and the other group fed mIFN-α for at least 4 wk. The spleens were harvested, and purified CD8+ T-cell populations were obtained and activated with PLP 139–151 for 48 h, and 5 × 10^6 injected IP (adoptive transfer) into recipient animals (d 0) that received concurrently MSCH with MT in IFA (d 0 and d 7 active immunization; *n* = 15/group). Clinical scores were determined in a blinded fashion. Results are expressed as the combined results from four separate experiments ± SEM. Individual clinical scores for mice in each treatment group from d 14 through 28 are shown in the figure.

Chronic EAE was induced in 7- to 10-wk-old female SJL/J or SWR mice as described above. On d 30 postimmunization and after the initial clinical attack had subsided, donor mice ingested 10 U of natural mIFN-α or mock mIFN-α *(110)* three times per week (Monday, Wednesday, Friday) for at least 4 wk. Donor SJL/J mice were sacrificed at least 8 wk after immunization and at least 4 wk after initiation of mock IFN or mIFN-α feeding for the CR-EAE experiments. T cells, CD4+ and CD8+ T cells were purified and pulsed with irradiated PLP 139–151 (100 μg/mL) antigen-presenting cells (ratio 1:1). CD4+ and CD8+ T cells were adjusted to 5–16 × 10^6 cells/0.5 mL Dulbecco's phosphate-buffered saline (DPBS) immediately prior to intraperitoneal injection into simultaneously (d 0) actively immunized recipient mice.

Concurrent adoptive transfer of activated CD8+ T cells from mIFN-α-fed donors, sensitized to neuroautoantigen after undergoing initial clinical attack, inhibited acute clinical attack in actively immunized recipient SJL/J mice. Donor CD8+ T-cell subsets from mock-fed (mock CD8) and from mIFN-α-fed mice (IFN CD8) T cells or saline control were injected intraperitoneally, and simultaneously all recipient mice were also actively immunized with MSCH and MT in incomplete Freund's adjuvant (IFA) (Fig. 10). The immunized mice (*n* = 15 in each group) were monitored by blinded examination for the next 28 d. The saline intraperitoneally injected recipients demonstrated severe clinical disease starting on d 14, peaking on d 16, and subsequently plateauing during the next 12 d. Mice adoptively transferred with $CD8^+$ T cells from mock-fed donors showed no improvement in actively induced disease throughout the course of clinical examinations compared to the intraperitoneal saline control. There was a significant modulation of active disease by adoptively transferred $CD8^+$ T cells from IFN-α-fed donors compared to intraperitoneal saline control ($p < 0.0005$ by analysis of variance [ANOVA]) and compared to mock-fed $CD8^+$ donor T cells ($p < 0.0006$ by ANOVA). Mice adoptively transferred with $CD4^+$ T cells from IFN-fed donors showed no improvement in actively induced disease throughout the course of clinical examinations compared to intraperitoneal saline control or mock-fed $CD4^+$ donor T cells (data not shown). Actively immunized animals receiving adoptively transferred $CD8^+$ T cells from IFN-α-fed donors demonstrated decreased peak disease and disease score throughout the period of observation compared to all other sample groups.

5.4. T Cells/T-Cell Subsets From Naive mIFN-α-Fed Donors Could Transfer Protection to EAE in Actively Immunized Recipients

Acute EAE protocols using MBP usually demonstrate a more robust effect of protective donor T-cell populations. To examine the mechanism of protection optimally by donor $CD8^+$ T cells and to determine if ingested IFN-α activates natural immunomodulatory cell populations, we used the acute EAE model and naïve-fed donor animals as sources of T and $CD8^+$ T cells, asking whether donor activated spleen T cells from naive nonimmunized IFN-α-fed mice suppress actively induced EAE in recipients. Donor mice were 6- to 8-wk-old female SWR mice treated with 10 U ingested mIFN-α for 7 consecutive days. Two groups of seven recipient mice were actively immunized with 200 µg bovine MBP and 400 ng pertussis toxin intravenously and either mock injected intraperitoneally with 16×10^6 Con A-activated splenic T cells from naive nonimmunized SWR mock-fed donors (active/mock T) or with Con A-activated splenic T cells from naive nonimmunized SWR donors fed 10 U mIFN-α for 7 d (active/IFN fed T). Results from blinded examination demonstrated significant differences in clinical outcome in the active/mock T vs active/IFN-fed T-cell transferred group (d 11–21; $p < 0.01$ by nonpaired t test; Fig. 11). Con A-activated spleen T cells from naive mIFN-α-fed donors inhibited actively induced disease in actively immunized recipients. The mechanism of the suppressor-like function is unclear.

In an attempt to isolate which subpopulation of T cells might be responsible for the effect found above, and because $CD8^+$ T cells adoptively transfer protection in other EAE paradigms of orally administered immunomodulators, experiments were performed to examine immunomodulation of acute EAE after passively transferring activated $CD8^+$ T cells. The donors were SWR mice treated with 10 U orally mIFN-α for 7 consecutive days. Two groups of five recipient mice were actively immunized as described above and either injected with Con A-activated splenic $CD8^+$ T cells from mice fed mock IFN for 7 d (active/mock $CD8^+$) or injected with Con A-activated splenic $CD8^+$ T cells from mice fed 10 U mIFN-α for 7 d (active/IFN fed $CD8^+$). Results from blinded examinations performed every day demonstrated significant differences in clinical outcome in the active/mock $CD8^+$ vs active/IFN-fed $CD8^+$ group (d 10–19; $p < 0.01$ by nonpaired t test) (Fig. 12). Donor-activated spleen $CD8^+$ T cells from naive nonimmunized IFN-α fed animals can suppress actively induced EAE in recipients.

5.5. Which Cytokines Are Responsible for the T-Cell Protection?

The proinflammatory cytokines IFN-γ and TNF-α have been shown to participate in the induction and pathogenesis of EAE *(123)*. EAE demonstrates high mRNA expression for proinflammatory cytokines IFN-γ and TNF-α in PMNC and in the CNS with classical signs of inflammation *(124)*.

Recipient spleen cells were isolated at the end of the clinical attack from the mock-fed donor T-cell injected or IFN-fed donor T-cell adoptive transfer group. The respective recipient splenocytes were stimulated with either MBP (Fig. 13) or Con A (Fig. 14), and supernatants were

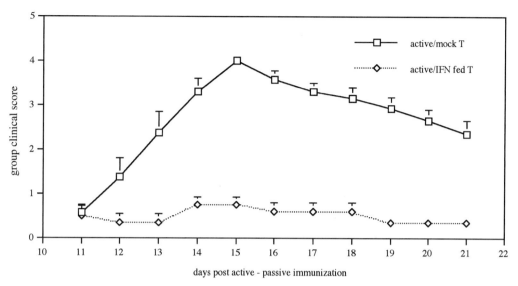

Fig. 11. T-Con A-activated spleen T cells from naive mIFN-α-fed donors inhibited actively induced disease in recipients. The donors were 6- to 8-wk-old female SWR mice treated with 10 U oral mIFN-α for 7 consecutive d. Two groups of seven recipient mice were actively immunized with 200 μg bovine MBP (d 0) and 400 ng PT IV (d 0 and d 2) and either injected IP (d 0) with 16×10^7 Con A-activated splenic T cells from naive nonimmunized mice fed mock IFN (active/mock T) or injected IP with 16×10^7 Con A-activated splenic T cells from naive nonimmunized mice fed 10 U mIFN-α for 7 d (active/IFN-fed T). Results from blinded examination performed every day demonstrated significant differences in clinical outcome in the active vs IFN-fed T-cell transferred group (d 11–21 [$p < 0.01$ by nonpaired t test]).

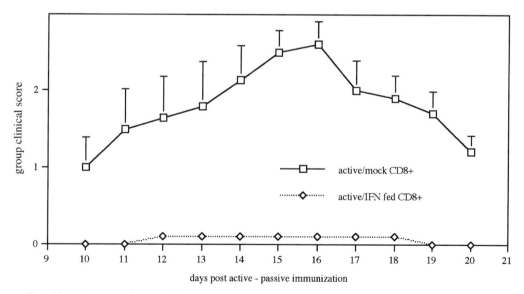

Fig. 12. The respective recipient splenocytes were stimulated with either MBP at 20 μg/mL (Fig. 12) or Con A (2.5 mg/mL; Fig. 13) at 2×10^6 cells/mL for 2 d, and supernatants were assayed by solid phase ELISA for IL-1β, IL-2, IL-4, IL-6, IL-10, TGF-β, TNF-α, and IFN-γ. Results of the individual assays were grouped for purposes of analysis (pg/mL ± SEM). Recipients of T cells from IFN-α-fed donors (active/IFN-fed T—white columns) demonstrated decreased IL-1 and TNF-α proinflammatory secretion after Con A or MBP activation compared to recipients of T cells from mock-fed donors (active/mock T—black columns [$p < 0.05$ by t test]). TGF-β secretion also decreased after Con A and MBP activation.

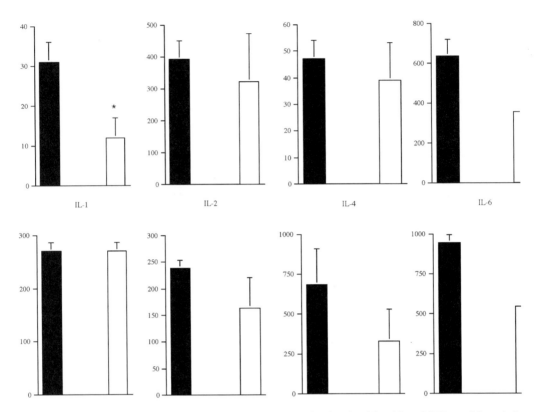

Fig. 13. The respective recipient splenocytes were stimulated with either MBP at 20 μg/mL (Fig. 12) or Con A (2.5 mg/mL; Fig. 13) at 2×10^6 cells/mL for 2 d, and supernatants were assayed by solid phase ELISA for IL-1β, IL-2, IL-4, IL-6, IL-10, TGF-β, TNF-α, and IFN-γ. Results of the individual assays were grouped for purposes of analysis (pg/mL ± SEM). Recipients of T cells from IFN-α-fed donors (active/IFN-fed T—white columns) demonstrated decreased IL-1 and TNF-α proinflammatory secretion after Con A or MBP activation compared to recipients of T cells from mock-fed donors (active/mock T—black columns [$p < 0.05$ by t test]). TGF-β secretion also decreased after Con A and MBP activation.

assayed by solid-phase ELISA for IL-1β, IL-2, IL-4, IL-6, IL-10, TGF-β, TNF-α, and IFN-γ. Recipients of T cells from IFN-α-fed donors demonstrated decreased IL-1 and TGF-β secretion after both Con A and MBP activation, decreased TNF-α secretion after Con A activation, and decreased IL-6 secretion after MBP activation compared to recipients of T cells from mock-fed donors. There were no significant changes in IL-2, IL-4, IL-10, or IFN-γ secretion, although in all cases, mice receiving cells from IFN-fed donors demonstrated less cytokine secretion compared to the mock-fed T cell control.

The respective splenocytes from recipients of mock CD8+-fed or IFN-fed CD8+ T cells were stimulated with either MBP (Fig. 15) or Con A (Fig. 16), and supernatants were assayed for cytokines as above. Recipients of T cells from IFN-α-fed donors demonstrated decreased IFN-γ and TNF-α proinflammatory secretion after both Con A or MBP activation, compared to recipients of CD8+ T cells from mock-fed donors. TGF-β secretion also decreased after Con A activation. IL-4 secretion was increased in recipients of T cells from IFN-α-fed donors after Con A, but not after MBP, activation. There were no significant changes in IL-2, IL-6, and IL-10 secretion in the recipient splenocytes, although there was a trend for decreased IL-1 secretion.

T cells and CD8+ T cells from mock-fed and IFN-fed naive donors were analyzed for Con A-induced IL-1, IL-2, IL-4, IL-6, IL-10, TNF-α, TGF-β, and IFN-γ secretion to determine if the functional state of the adoptively transferred cell populations could explain the alteration of proinflammatory

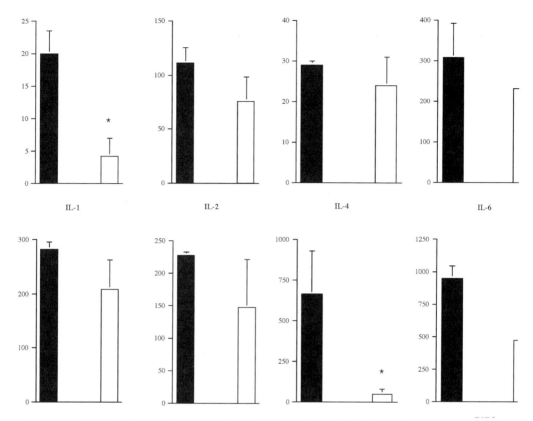

Fig. 14. Donor-activated spleen CD8[+] T cells from mIFN-α-fed animals inhibited actively induced disease in recipients. The donors were 6- to 8-wk-old female SWR mice treated with 10 U oral mIFN-α for 7 consecutive days. Two groups of five recipient mice were actively immunized with 200 μg bovine MBP (d 0) and 400 ng PT IV (d 0 and d 2) and either injected IP with 5×10^6 Con A-activated splenic CD8[+] T cells from mice fed mock IFN-α for 7 d (active/mock CD8[+]), or injected IP with 5×10^6 Con A-activated splenic CD8[+] T cells from mice fed 10 U mIFN-α for 7 d (active/IFN-fed CD8[+]). Results from blinded examinations performed every day demonstrated significant differences in clinical outcome in the active/mock CD8[+] vs active/IFN-fed CD8[+] group (d 10–20; $p < 0.01$ by nonpaired t test).

cytokine expression in protected recipients. Although there was a trend for decreased proinflammatory IL-2 and IL-6 secretion, there was also a trend for decreased counter-regulatory anti-inflammatory IL-10 and TGF-β secretion in the IFN-fed donor T and CD8[+] T-cell splenocytes. There was no effect on IL-1, IL-4, TNF-α,and IFN-γ secretion in T and CD8[+] T cell populations in the IFN-fed donors (data not shown).

Our experiments demonstrate that adoptive transfer of antigen- or mitogen-activated T cells or T-cell subsets from IFN-fed donors can modulate clinical disease expression in actively immunized recipient mice. The clinical modulatory effect is seen in both activated T cells and CD8[+] T-cell populations from IFN-α-fed donors, demonstrating that CD8[+] T cells are most likely the immunomodulatory cell. Most Con A- and MBP-stimulated splenocyte cytokine production is decreased in recipients of T cells and CD8[+] T cells from IFN-fed donors compared to recipients of mock-fed T cells or mock-fed CD8[+] T cells. There is decreased Con A and MBP induced IFN-γ secretion after CD8[+] T-cell transfer but not after T-cell transfer. The inhibition of cytokine secretion extends to a potential counter-regulatory anti-inflammatory TGF-β, which is responsible for recovery from EAE in other models. Con A- and MBP-activated splenocytes from both IFN-fed CD8[+] T-cell recipients and MBP-activated splenocytes from IFN-fed T-cell recipients demon-

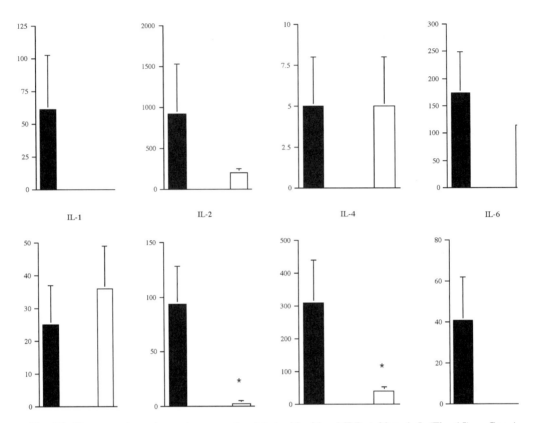

Fig. 15. The respective splenocytes were stimulated with either MBP at 20 μg/mL (Fig. 15) or Con A (2.5 μg/mL) (Fig. 16) as described in Figs. 12 and 13. Recipients of T cells from IFN-α-fed donors (active/IFN fed-T—white columns) demonstrated decreased IFN-γ and TNF-α proinflammatory secretion after Con A or MBP activation compared to recipients of T cells from mock IFN-fed donors (active/mock CD8+—black columns; $p < 0.05$ by t test). TGF-β secretion also decreased after Con A activation.

strated decreased TNF-α secretion. This result suggests, regardless of the underlying immunomodulatory mechanism of T-cell populations from IFN-fed donors, that the inhibition of proinflammatory cytokine secretion in recipients is paramount. Decrease TNF-α and IFN-γ secretion correlates best with the disease protection from IFN-fed T and CD8+ T cells.

5.6. Which Cytokines Are Responsible for Protection in the Target Organ?

We have previously demonstrated that activated donor cells from mice ingesting IFN-α did not passively transfer clinical disease, although there was no significant difference in the number of lesions in the CNS between mice receiving cells from mock- or IFN-fed donors (109). This suggests that the ingested IFN does not decrease the ability of disease to migrate to the CNS but may well decrease the local levels of proinflammatory cytokines produced at the target organ. Because antigen-specific activation occurs peripherally in actively immunized recipient mice with subsequent trafficking into the CNS, the data from experiments mentioned above suggests that the immunomodulatory cells from IFN-fed donors inhibit MBP-reactive cells that are already primed. The protective cells may well work in the target organ locally to suppress inflammation and encephalitogenicity. A remaining question is whether protective cells decrease proinflammatory cytokines or produce anti-inflammatory cytokines. We examined alterations in the CNS with cytokine-competitive polymerase chain reaction (PCR) techniques in severe combined immunod-

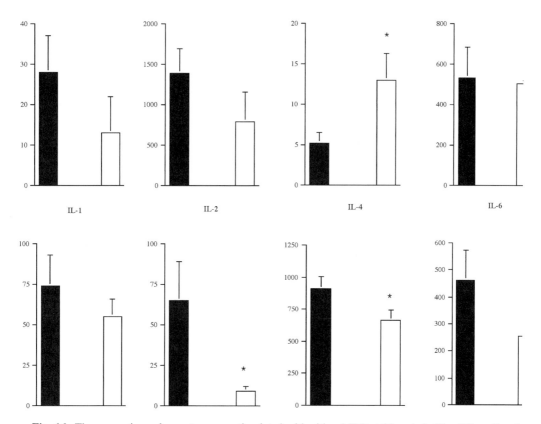

Fig. 16. The respective splenocytes were stimulated with either MBP at 20 μg/mL (Fig. 15) or Con A (2.5 μg/mL) (Fig. 16) as described in Figs. 12 and 13. Recipients of T cells from IFN-α-fed donors (active/IFN fed-T—white columns) demonstrated decreased IFN-γ and TNF-α proinflammatory secretion after Con A or MBP activation compared to recipients of T cells from mock IFN-fed donors (active/mock CD8+—black columns; $p < 0.05$ by t test). TGF-β secretion also decreased after Con A activation.

eficiency (SCID) EAE-susceptible mice after adoptive transfer of encephalitogenic and protective T-cell populations.

Twenty C57BL/6 6- to 8-wk-old females were actively immunized with 200 μg myelin oligo-dendrocyte glycoprotein (MOG) peptide 35–55 (MEVGWYRSPFSRVVHLYRNGK) and 800 μg MT on d 0 and 7, followed with pertussis toxin 200 ng intraperitoneally on d 0 and 2, and watched for evidence of disease *(125)*. Nonimmunized donor B6 mice ingested 100 IU of natural mIFN-α ($n = 20$) or mock mIFN-α ($n = 20$) daily for at least 14 d before spleen cells were harvested. On d 23 postinoculation, splenocytes from the MOG-immunized donor mice were restimulated in vitro with 30 μg/mL MOG peptide 35–55. A second set of splenocytes from the saline (mock; $n = 20$) or IFN-α-fed ($n = 20$) nonimmunized donor mice were activated in vitro with 2.5 μg/mL Con A 100 ×10⁶ MOG-restimulated cells were passively transferred intraperitoneally into 8- to 10-wk-old female B6 SCID recipients ($n = 6$). At the same time (d 0), three recipients received 70 × 10⁶ Con A-activated splenocytes from saline-fed donors (control group), and three recipients received 70 × 10⁶ Con A-activated splenocytes from IFN-α-fed donors (active treatment group). Thereafter, the reconstituted SCID recipients were followed for clinical disease as described above.

The recipients of MOG peptide *and* Con A-activated saline-fed splenocytes (control group) all showed clinical signs of disease starting by d 6 and progressing over the next 2 wk to peak scores of 2, 2.5, and 3.0. The recipients of MOG peptide *and* Con A-activated IFN-α-fed splenocytes (active treatment group) showed mild nonpersistent clinical signs of EAE (Fig. 17).

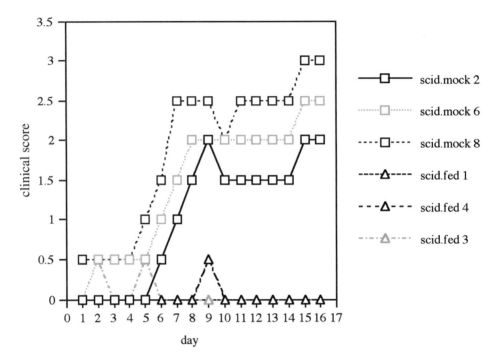

Fig. 17. Nonimmunized donor B6 mice ingested 100 IU of natural mIFN-α or mock mIFN-α as previously described *(109)*. Daily feeding of 20 B6 mice with 100 IU mIFN-α (active-treatment donors) or saline (mock donors) was started and continued for at least 14 d before spleen cells were harvested. On d 23 postinoculation, splenocytes from the MOG-immunized donor mice were restimulated in vitro with 30 µg/mL MOG peptide 35–55. A second set of splenocytes from the saline- ($n = 20$) or IFN-α-fed ($n = 20$) nonimmunized donor mice were activated in vitro with 2.5 µg/mL Con A. 100×10^6 MOG-restimulated cells were passively transferred IP into 8- to 10-wk-old female B6 SCID recipients ($n = 6$). At the same time (d 0), three recipients received 70×10^6 Con A-activated splenocytes from saline-fed donors (control group) and three recipients received 70×10^6 Con A-activated splenocytes from IFN-α-fed donors (active-treatment group). Thereafter, the reconstituted SCID recipients were followed for clinical disease.

Cytokine production by stimulated lymphocytes in vitro may not reflect in vivo activity. Ex vivo analysis avoids the problems of in vitro restimulation with antigen or mitogen. As such, cytokine production from CNS tissue samples measurable by ELISA may not accurately reflect the activity of the cells in vivo. In addition, extraction of relatively small numbers of lymphocytes from CNS tissue is potentially difficult and may result in loss of significant number of cells. Quantitative PCR (Q-PCR) for cytokine mRNA from cells directly from the target CNS tissue can circumvent this difficulty. The Q-PCR system has numerous advantages, including ease of operation, speed, and the capability of handling large numbers of samples. Therefore, we determined whether we could measure β-actin, IL-2, and IFN-γ mRNA from control (mock donor) and active treatment (IFN-fed donor) groups in a Q-PCR system. Mice were followed up to the point at which it was clear that they had achieved the peak of their disease. The relative numbers of transcripts for murine β-actin, IL-2, and IFN-γ were measured. The mean measured cytokine-of-interest transcript levels were normalized to the β-actin control (normalized mean = cytokine of interest [COI] mean/β-actin × 100) and expressed as the percentage of β-actin molecules.

At d 23 postpassive immunization, whole spinal cords were processed for total RNA, DNase-treated, and amplified for IFN-γ signal. Even at this late stage in the evolution of the clinical course of disease, there were clear differences in the levels of proinflammatory IL-2 (Table 6b) and IFN-γ (Table 6a) transcript (Th1-like cytokines) in the CNS in the SCID recipients of IFN-α-fed

Table 6 a/b
SCID Recipients Adoptively Immunized With IFN-α-Fed Donor Cells Generate Less Target Organ IL-2 and IFN-γ

		Peak score	IFNγ	SD	β-Actin	SD	Normalized
Mock recipient	SCID #2	2	290	136	218889	30636	0.13
Mock recipient	SCID #6	2.5	535	145	138431	32804	0.39
Mock recipient	SCID #8	3	1078	359	304282	111948	0.35
IFN-fed recipient	SCID #1	0.5	<20	—	59180	6560	—
IFN-fed recipient	SCID #3	0.5	<20	—	83015	5721	—
IFN-fed recipient	SCID #4	0.5	<20	—	186833	28679	—
		Peak score	IL-2	SD	β-Actin	SD	Normalized
Mock recipient	SCID #2	2	<20	136	218889	30636	—
Mock recipient	SCID #6	2.5	651	208	138431	32804	0.47
Mock recipient	SCID #8	3	590	208	304282	111948	0.19
IFN-fed recipient	SCID #1	0.5	<20	—	59180	6560	
IFN-fed recipient	SCID #3	0.5	<20	—	83015	5721	—
IFN-fed recipient	SCID #4	0.5	<20	—	186833	28679	—

IFN-γ = interferon-γ; SD = ; IL-2 = interleukin-2.

cells compared to the SCID recipients of saline-fed cells. There were detectable levels of IL-2 (two of three) and IFN-γ (three of three) transcripts in the mock recipients respectively but no detectable (below the threshold of detection = 20 transcripts) IL-2 and IFN-γ transcripts in the IFN-fed donor recipients. These differences were seen as late as d 23 postimmunization, when clinical disease had peaked for more than 7 d (SCID mock no. 6 and 8) or was resolving (SCID mock no. 2—loss of detectable IL-2 signal in least diseased control recipient). The mock-fed recipients had more severe clinical disease than the IFN-fed recipients had. These differences in IL-2 and IFN-γ transcripts correlated with the clinical outcome.

This is consistent with our previous experiments in acute rat EAE, in which proinflammatory cytokine decreased after peak disease *(87)*. At d 9 preceding clinical disease, draining PLN cells from mock IFN-treated rats showed detectable IFN-γ production (50 ng/mL). At d 16 with peak clinical disease, PLN cells from mock-treated rats demonstrated greater IFN-γ production (1140 ng/mL). At d 18 postimmunization, after clinical attack had subsided, PLN from mock treated rats showed less IFN-γ (460 ng/mL). Sampling may miss cytokines if delayed long after peak EAE. These data suggest that Q-PCR can: (a) detect IL-2 and IFN-γ transcript in whole spinal cord; (b) differentiate control- from active-treatment recipients, according to their clinical outcomes; (c) and detect difference between groups as late as 7 d after peak disease. We suspect that recipients of mock-fed cells will produce more IL-2 and IFN-γ and that recipients of IFN-α-fed cells may produce counter-regulatory cytokines at some point in their clinical EAE course if assayed early during the onset of peak disease. In conclusion, the use of whole spinal cord homogenates can provide useful data on important proinflammatory cytokines critical for EAE pathogenesis.

6. DISCUSSION

These data document that ingested mIFN and hrIFN can suppress relapses and prevent adoptive transfer of EAE. The inhibition of an established and ongoing immune response by ingested immunoactive proteins is an important therapeutic issue. Animals administered 100 to 1000 U hrIFN-α exhibited less severe relapses than mock-fed animals, although 1000 U was marginally

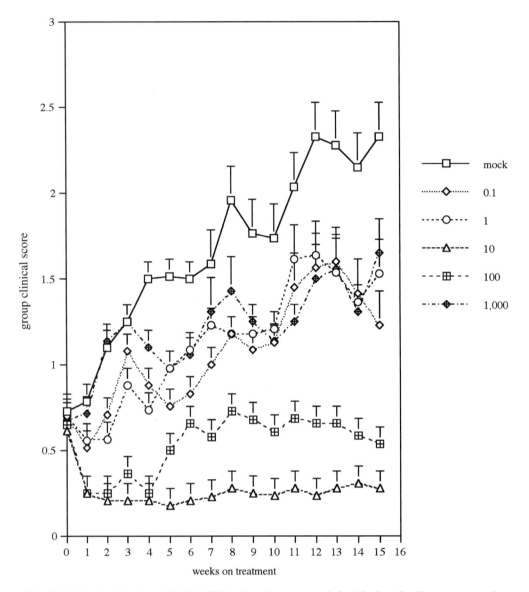

Fig. 18. Oral administration of 10 U mIFN-α three times per week for 15 wk optimally suppresses relapse attacks in murine CR-EAE. Six groups of eight SJL/J 6- to 8-wk-old female mice were immunized as described in earlier. Values represent mean weekly group clinical scores ± SEM (mock mIFN vs. 10 U PO mIFN-α, wk 1–15; $p < 0.001$ by ANOVA and Wilcoxon signed rank test; mock mIFN vs 0.1, 1 and 1000 U PO mIFN-α, wk 4–6, 9–10, 12–15; $p < 0.01$ by t test; animals fed 0.1, 1, and 1000 U were significantly worse compared to 10 U PO [10 U PO mIFN-α vs 0.1, 1, 1000 U PO mIFN-α, wk 1–15; $p < 0.01$ by ANOVA and Wilcoxon signed rank test]).

less effective compared to 100 U. Animals fed species-specific mIFN at only 10 to 100 U had suppressed clinical relapse attack. Thus, species-specific mIFN-α decreased the overall neurological deficits from baseline values at one order of magnitude less than hrIFN-α. This is consistent with experiments suggesting a therapeutic dose-response window with the optimal dose being 10 to 100 U species-specific oral mIFN-α, and 0.1, 1 and 1000 U being significantly less effective in suppressing clinical relapse disease in murine CR-EAE (data not shown) (Fig. 18) *(111)*.

Proinflammatory cytokines are thought to be critical in the pathogenesis of EAE. The proin-flammatory cytokine TNF-α has been demonstrated in various autoimmune diseases and is thought to participate in the induction and pathogenesis of EAE. TNF-α is cytotoxic for oligoden-drocytes in vitro and has been implicated in the pathology of EAE. TNF mRNA expression in brain tissue sections appeared early and peaked at the height of clinical signs in acute EAE *(123)*. EAE demonstrates high mRNA expression for proinflammatory cytokine TNF-α in PMNC *(124)*. The TNF inhibitor, dimeric polyethylene glycol-linked form of the type I soluble receptor of TNF, inhibited clinical signs in active EAE, suggesting that TNF is a pivotal mediator of inflammation resulting from immunization *(126)*. TNF-α is made by both CNS-resident microglia and infiltrating macrophages in EAE, and this production is tightly controlled by cytokines secreted by infiltrating T cells *(127)*. Anti-TNF antibodies can inhibit passively transferred EAE by preventing the upreg-ulation of VCAM-1 *(128)*, interfering with the effector phase of the disease *(129)*. Therefore, TNF-α is critical in EAE, and the inhibition of recipient TNF-α secretion by IFN-fed donor T cells and CD8$^+$ T cells is important for protection in our model.

IFN-γ is also an important pro-inflammatory cytokine in the development of EAE. Secretion of the inflammatory cytokine IFN-γ is characteristic of encephalitogenic T helper 1 (Th1) cells in animals and humans *(130–138)*. In acute EAE, Con A-stimulated spleen cell IFN-γ production in vitro increases during peak incidence of disease on d 13–14 *(97)*. Cytokine mRNA analysis of the CNS in EAE suggests that IFN-γ is elevated in acute disease *(85)*. Although anti-IFN-γ antibody results in more severe EAE *(139–141)*, suggesting that systemic IFN-γ activates suppression *(142)*, our experi-ments have all demonstrated that inhibition of IFN-γ correlates with EAE remission *(87,109–111)*.

There were decreased levels of TGF-β levels in protected mice in our experiments. In most instances, TGF-β reduces the clinical severity and inhibits adoptive transfer of EAE *(82,143–145)*; however, as noted above, the neutralization of TGF-β activity does not exacerbate disease *(146)* and TGF-β can be absent peripherally in EAE *(124)*. In our model ,the absence of TGF-β apparently does not preclude protection.

The transduction of ingested IFN-α signal and its therapeutic effect does not require transit of intact IFN-α across the bowel. Oral administration of IFN-α in mice does not result in serum IFN-α *(147)*. We have demonstrated increased relative type I IFN-induced Mx mRNA levels, a type I IFN-specific-induced message, using RT-PCR in splenocytes and human PMNC after IFN-α ingestion. Murine T cells and CD8$^+$ T cells also demonstrated upregulation of Mx mRNA after IFN-α ingestion of 10 and 100 U but not after 0, 1000, or 5000 U, suggesting a dose response effect *(148)*.

The immunomodulatory mechanism of ingested IFN-α may result not only in the reduction of proinflammatory cytokines but also in the generation of suppressor factors by T cells. Modulatory effects of Con A-activated lymphocytes on the mitogen responses of normal responder cells can be abrogated by addition of antihuman leukocyte IFN serum in vitro *(149)*, which may prevent the production of inhibitory factors induced by IFN-α (e.g., soluble immune response suppressor [SIRS]) *(150)* and macrophage-derived suppressor factor (MØ-SF; e.g., TGF-β) by CD8$^+$ T cells *(151,152)*. Peripheral T cells are required for IFN production after such mitogen stimulation *(153)*. Other cytokines may be important because both IFN-α and IFN-β stimulate the production of a multitude of new cellular proteins *(154,155)*. Type I IFN may induce suppressor factors inhibiting responses to immunogenic antigens, such as MBP and PLP. IFN-α may be an immunomodulatory molecule pro-duced by activated CD8$^+$ T and other immune cells that induce suppressor factors, such as IL-4, IL-10 or SIRS, which in turn induce hyporesponsiveness to immunized antigens, such as MBP and MT.

The GALT has multiple types of constituent immune cells. It consists of lymphoid nodules termed *Peyer's patches* (PP), villi-containing epithelial cells, intraepithelial lymphocytes (IEL), and lympho-cytes scattered throughout the lamina propria (LP) *(156)*. PP contain T and B lymphocytes, macrophages, dendritic cells, and a germinal center with B lymphocytes. T lymphocytes in PP are predominantly composed of the CD4$^+$ Th1 and Th2 phenotypes, whereas parafollicular cells are both

CD4$^+$ and CD8$^+$ (157,158). Regulatory cells can be generated in PP (159–161). T cells in lymphoid organs draining from nonmucosal sites, such as inguinal lymph nodes, secrete IL-2 as the primary T-cell growth factor after activation, whereas T cells from mucosal sites, such as PP, produce IL-4 (162). The lymphoid microenvironment can determine the pattern of T-cell responses in different immune organs (163). An integrin receptor molecule termed *lymphocyte high endothelial venule* (HEV) *adhesion molecule* (LPAM-1) can mediate organ-specific adhesion of lymphocytes to specialized HEVs found in PP (164). TGF-β and IL-4 regulate the adhesiveness of PP HEV for lymphocytes on HEVs possibly through LPAM-1 expression (165). IELs are distinct from other lymphocyte populations because monoclonal antibodies raised against human IEL, termed *human mucosal lymphocytes* (HML-1, β7-integrin family), react with virtually all IELs and 40% of LP lymphocytes but less than 2% of PBL, suggesting they are specific GALT addressins. IELs include 75% CD8$^+$ in humans and 40–65% CD8$^+$ T cells in mice. Some IEL CD8$^+$ T cells use the γδ T-cell receptor and express the CD8 α chain without the β chain (166). The CD8$^+$ IELs that express the αβ TCR are of thymic origin and arrive from nearby PP (167). LP lymphocytes have CD4$^+$/CD8$^+$ ratios resembling PP and PBL (156). In oral tolerance, antigen-specific regulatory cells migrate to lymphoid organs and suppress immune responses by inhibiting the generation of effector cells (168). Therefore, there are diverse cell populations in the GALT that may potentially become immunoregulatory via ingested IFN and suppress peripheral immune Th1-like T-helper-cell function.

Previous studies in the EAE model suggested that orally administered MBP suppressed the afferent limb of the immune response (169,170). This suppression may be mediated by CD8$^+$ T cells (122) and provides an organ-specific immune hyporesponsiveness. Cells responsible for prevention of sensitization after intragastric administration of sheep red blood cells have been tracked from PP (2 d) to mesenteric lymph nodes (4 d) and subsequently to the spleen (7 d) (160). These data suggest active and antigen-specific suppression as the mechanism of orally induced tolerance. More recent studies suggest that mucosal derived MBP-specific CD4$^+$ Th2-like T-cell clones producing TGF-β suppressed EAE (171). These data suggest that migrating pools of different cell populations originating in the GALT transfer acquired immunoregulation in the systemic efferent immune system. Moreover, the tolerizing antigen does not need to cause the autoimmune disease; MBP-specific suppressor cells would home to the CNS in MS even if MBP were not the MS antigen.

For ingested low-dose IFN to be effective, there should be a fantastic amplification system. IFN-induced activities could be either transferred between adjacent epithelial cells and from these to lymphocytes or could be directly transferred from lymphocytes to other cells and other lymphoid sites (172). Subsequent antiviral and immunomodulatory activities could be achieved by either cell to cell communication (78), or be transported and generalized by lymphocytes that home via lymph to lymphoid and nonlymphoid organs (173) without having any accompanying side effects caused by circulating IFN (64). At their destination, activated cells can release cytokines in a paracrine fashion (72,174,175) and in turn stimulate either neighboring or circulating cells. This suggests that biological response modifiers (BRM), such as ingested type I IFN, are drugs that act outside the realm of classical pharmocological parameters (66) and suppress autoimmune disease by activating a unique natural immune system originating in the mucosa that involves cellular communication and amplification.

Mice receiving T cells adoptively from mIFN-α-fed animals do exhibit inflammation (*vide supra*). Others have shown that adoptively transferred MOG peptide-specific T cells can demonstrate inflammation in the CNS without inducing a neurological deficit (176). We might speculate that ingested IFN-α generates immunoregulatory CD8$^+$ T cells via the gut immune system that can traffic to the recipient's peripheral lymphoid system or CNS. These cells would not cause clinical disease but instead might suppress inflammation by either generating suppressor factors locally in the CNS compartment or by decreasing responsiveness to immunizing antigens by inhibiting IFN-γ secretion.

These data document that ingested murine, rat species-specific, and human recombinant type I IFN can inhibit disease, inflammation, and decrease proliferation of activated and antigen-specific cells in EAE in mice and rats when administered after or before sensitization. Type I IFN is active by the oral route and has significant immunological effects at very low dosages. Specific cytokines, in particular type I IFN lacking a protective matrix to prevent protein digestion and directly delivered to the distal esophagus, stomach, and proximal small intestine (determined experimentally by injecting Evans blue during routine feeding and subsequent sacrifice), are capable of producing immunomodulation, but not tolerance, to previously sensitized antigens. Ingested IFN-α therapy in EAE appears to be more effective than equivalent doses of parenteral IFN-α. In vitro IFN did not inhibit Con A proliferation in contrast to the strong inhibition seen after in vivo orally administration. Thus, route of administration is critical in the determination the specific immunological mechanism for IFN. Ingested IFN-α may activate immunomodulatory cell populations in the GALT and thereby function by a different mechanism, in contrast to subcutaneous administration, which did not directly act on similar cell subsets.

Passive immunization provides a method to investigate the mechanism of ingested type I IFN on different cell populations in adoptively transferred disease, eliminating the role of potential suppressor antigen-presenting cells in actively immunized animals. Adoptive transfer of mitogen-activated splenic T cells from IFN-fed mice to recipients suppresses EAE induced by active immunization. Ingested IFN-α acts through an active mechanism of suppression induced by oral IFN-α on effector encephalitogenic T cells. If so, ingestion of selected cytokines may provide a more effective delivery system compared to the parenteral route to produce organ-blind immunomodulation to sensitized antigen, regardless of haplotypic background, for the treatment of human autoimmune diseases. Ingested BRM, such as type I IFN, potentially provides a continuous means of generating immunomodulation of autoreactive T-cell populations. BRM delivered by the oral route may also provide a means of treating autoimmune diseases, such as MS, and other chronic non-neurological autoimmune diseases, such as RA *(177)* and type I diabetes mellitus *(148,178)*, by the possible generation of immunoregulatory cells via the esophageal/gut immune system. The oral route is a convenient drug delivery system that may allow the use of lower doses of cytokines, minimize side effects, and provide enhanced efficacy via potent immunoregulatory circuits.

ACKNOWLEDGMENT

Supported by a grant from the Clayton Foundation.

REFERENCES

1. Hafler DA, Brod SA, Weiner HL. Immunoregulation in multiple sclerosis. Res Immunol 1989;140:233.
2. Wolinsky J. Multiple sclerosis. *In:* Appel S. Current Neurology, Vol. 13. New York, Mosby-Year Book, 1993:167.
3. Hafler DA, Brod SA, Weiner HL. Experimental approaches to specific immunotherapy in multiple sclerosis. *In:* Rudick R, Goodkin D. Treatment of Multiple Sclerosis: Trial Design, Results, and Future Perspectives. London, Springer-Verlag, London, 1992;301.
4. Agner T, Damm P, Binder C. Remission in IDDM: prospective study of basal C-peptide and insulin dose in 268 consecutive patients. Diabetes Care 1987;10:164.
5. McFarlin D, McFarland H. Multiple Sclerosis. N Eng J Med 1987;307:1183.
6. Waksman B, Reynolds WE. Multiple sclerosis as a disease of immune regulation. Proc Soc Exp Biol Med 1987;175:282.
7. Sriram S, Rodriguez M. Indictment of the microglia as the villain in multiple sclerosis. Neurology 1997;48:464.
8. Antel JP, Freedman MS, Brodsovsky S, Francis GS, Duquette P. Activated suppressor cell function in severely disabled patients with multiple sclerosis. Ann Neurol 1989;25:204.
9. Brod SA, Scott M. Defective CD3 mediated proliferation and LPS responsiveness in multiple sclerosis. Autoimmunity 1994;17:143.
10. Brod SA, Khan M, Bright J, et al. Decreased CD3-mediated interferon-gamma production in relapsing-remitting multiple sclerosis. Ann Neurol 1995;37:546.
11. Isaacs A, Lindenmann J. Virus interference. I. The interferon. Proc R Soc Lond [Biol] 1957;147:258.
12. Johnson HM, Baron S. Evaluation of the effects of interferon and interferon inducers on the immune response. Pharmac Ther 1977;1:349.
13. Tyrrell DA. Research on interferon: a review. J R Soc Med 1981;74:145.
14. Stanton, GJ, Weigent DA, Fleischmann DA, Jr, Dianzani F, Baron S. Interferon review. Invest Radiol 1987;22:259.
15. Aguet M, Mogensen KE. Interferon receptors. *In:* Gresser I. Interferons, Vol. 5. New York, Academic Press, 1983;1.

16. Rashidbaigi A, Pestka S. Interferons: protein structure. *In:* Baron S, Dianzani F, Stanton GJ. Fleischmann WR. Interferon System. Austin, Texas, UT Press, 1987;149.

17. Baglioni, C. 2',5'-oligo(A) pathway of interferon action. *In:* Baron S, Dianzani F, Stanton GJ, Fleischmann WR. Interferon System. Austin, Texas, UT Press, 1987;365.

18. Dolei A, Ameglio F. Effects of IFN on phenotypic expression by cells. *In:* Baron S, Dianzani F, Stanton GJ, Fleischmann WR. Interferon System. Austin, Texas, UT Press, 1987:271.

19. Pestka S, Langer J, Zoon KC, Samuel CE. Interferons and their actions. Ann Rev Biochem 1987;56:727.

20. Balkwill FR. The regulatory role of interferons in the human immune response. *In:* Taylor-Papadimitriou J. Interferons: Their Impact in Biology of Medicine. Oxford, Oxford Medical Publications, 1985;61.

21. Hertzog, PJ, Emery P, Cheetham BF, MacKay IR, Linnane AW. Interferons in rheumatoid arthritis: alterations of production and response related to disease activity. Clin Immunol Immunopathol 1988;48:192.

22. Seitz M, Napierski I, Augustin R, Hunstein W, Kirchner H. Reduced production of interferon alpha and interferon gamma in leucocyte cultures from patients with active rheumatoid arthritis. Scand J Rheumatol 1987.16:257.

23. Kapp A, Gillitzer R, Kirchner H, Schopf E. Production of interferon and proliferative response in whole blood cultures derived from patients with atopic dermatitis. Arch Dermat Res 1987;279(suppl S):S55.

24. Kapp A, Gillitzer R, Kirchner H, Schopf E. Decreased production of interferon in whole blood cultures derived from patients with psoriasis. J Invest Dermat 1988;90:511.

25. Hertzog PJ, Wright A, Harris G, Linnane AW, Mackay IR. Intermittent interferonemia and interferon responses in multiple sclerosis. Clin Immunol Immunopath 1991;58:18.

26. Neighbour PA, Bloom BR. Absense of virus-induced lymphocyte suppression and interferon production in multiple sclerosis. Proc Natl Acad Sci USA 1979;76:476.

27. Maruo, Y. Interferon production and natural killer activity of peripheral blood lymphocytes obtained from patients with multiple sclerosis. Hokkaido J Med Sci 1988;63:521.

28. Struyf NJ, Snoeck HW, Bridts CH, Clerck LSD, Stevens WJ. Natural killer cell activity in Sjogren's syndrome and systemic lupus erythematosis: stimulation with interferons and interleukin-2 and correlation with immune complexes. Ann Rheum Dis 1990;49:690.

29. Negishi KG, Gupta KG, Chandy N, et al. Interferon responsiveness of natural killer cells in type I diabetes mellitus. Diabetes Res 1988;7:49.

30. Theon, J, Waalen L, Forre O. Natural killer (NK) cells at inflammatory sites of patients with rheumatoid arthritis and IgM rheumatoid factor positive polyarticular juvenile rheumatoid arthritis. Clin Rheumatol 1987;6:215.

31. Kastrukoff LF, Mogan NG, Aziz TM, Zecchini D, Berkowitz J, Paty DW. Natural killer (NK) cells in chronic progressive multiple sclerosis patients treated with lymphoblastoid interferon. J Neuroimmunol 1988;20:15.

32. Vranes Z, Paljakovic Z, Marucic M. Natural killer cell number and activity in multiple sclerosis. J Neurol Sci 1989;94:115.

33. Rice G, Casali P, Merigan T, Oldstone M. Natural killer cell activity in patients with multiple sclerosis given alpha interferon. Ann Neurol 1983;14:333.

34. Noronha A, Toscas A, Arnason BG, Jensen MA. Interferon beta augments in vivo suppressor function in multiple sclerosis. Neurology 1994;44(suppl 2):212.

35. Noronha A, Toscas A, Jensen MA. Interferon beta augments suppressor cell function in multiple sclerosis. Neurology 1990;27:207.

36. Ververken D, Carton H, Billiau A. Intrathecal administration of interferon in MS patients? *In*: Karcher D, Lowenthal A, Strosberg AD. Humoral Immunity in Neurological Disease. New York, Plenum, 1979;625.

37. Montezuma-de-Carvalho MJ. A treatment for the chronic disabilities of stable multiple sclerosis. Acta Medicotechnica 1983;31:155.

38. Fog T. Interferon treatment of multiple sclerosis patients: a pilot study. *In*: Boese A. Search for a Cause of Multiple Sclerosis and Other Chronic Diseases of the CNS. A. Boese, Weinheim, Verlag Chemie, 1980;491.

39. Knobler RL, Panitch HS, Braheny SL, et al. Controlled clinical trial of systemic alpha interferon in multiple sclerosis. Neurology 1983;34:1273.

40. Kamin-Lewis RM, Panitch HS, Johnson KP. Leucocytes from MS patients respond to alpha and gamma interferons. J Neuroimmunol 1985;9:221.

41. Panitch HS, Francis GS, Hooper CJ, Merigan TC, Johnson KP. Serial immunological studies in multiple sclerosis patients treated systemically with human interferon alpha. Ann Neurol 1985;18:434.

42. Panitch HS. Systemic alpha-interferon in multiple sclerosis. Long-term patient follow-up. Arch Neurol 1987;44:61.

43. Knobler RL. Systemic interferon in multiple sclerosis: the pros. Neurology 1988;38:58.

44. Kastrukoff LF, Oger JJ, Hashimoto SA, et al. Systemic lymphoblastoid interferon therapy in chronic progressive multiple sclerosis. I. Clinical and MRI evaluation. Neurology 1990;40:479.

45. Jacobs L, O'Malley J, Freeman A, Murawski J, Ekes R. Intrathecal interferon in multiple sclerosis. Arch Neurol 1982;39:609.

46. Jacobs L, O'Malley JA, Freeman A, Ekes R, Reese PA. Intrathecal interferon in the treatment of multiple sclerosis. Patient follow-up. Arch Neurol 1985;42:841.

47. Jacobs L, Herndon R, Salazar RM, et al. Intrathecally administered natural human fibroblast interferon reduces exacerbations of multiple sclerosis. results of a multicenter, double blinded study. Arch Neurol 1987;44:589.
48. Camenga DL, Johnson KP, Alter M, et al. Systemic recombinant alpha-2 interferon therapy in relapsing multiple sclerosis. Arch Neurol 1986;43:1239.
49. Hirsch RL, Johnson KP. Placebo induced enhancement of natural killer cell activity in a double blind trial of recombinant alpha-2 interferon in multiple sclerosis. *In*: Spector NH. Neuroimmunomodulation: Vol. Proceedings of the first International Workshop of Neuroimmunomodulation. Bethesda, Maryland, IWGN, 1986;219.
50. Hirsch RL. Defective autologous mixed lymphocyte reactivity in multiple sclerosis. Clin Exp Immunol 1986;64:107.
51. Group TIMSS. Interferon beta-1b is effective in relapsing-remitting multiple sclerosis. I. Clinical results of a multicenter, randomized, double-blind, placebo-controlled trial. Neurology 1993;43:655.
52. Paty DW, Li DK. Interferon beta-1b is effective in relapsing-remitting multiple sclerosis. II. MRI analysis results of a multicenter, randomized, double-blind, placebo-controlled trial. UBC MS/MRI Study Group and the IFNB Multiple Sclerosis Study Group. Neurology 1993;43:662.
53. Durelli L, Bongioanni MR, Cavallo R, et al. Chronic systemic high-dose recombinant interferon alfa-2a reduces exacerbation rate, MRI signs of disease activity, and lymphocyte interferon gamma production in relapsing-remitting multiple sclerosis. Neurology 1994;44:406.
54. Jacobs L, Cookfair D, Rudick R, et al. Intramuscular interferon beta-1a for disease progression in relapsing multiple sclerosis. The Multiple Sclerosis Collaborative Research Group (MSCRG). Ann Neurol 1994;39:285.
55. Schafer TW, Lieberman M, Cohen M, Came PE. Interferon administered orally: protection of neonatal mice from lethal virus challenge. Science 1972;176:1326.
56. Cummins JM, Tompkins MB, Olsen RG, Tompkins WA, Lewis MG. Oral use of human alpha interferon in cats. J Biol Response Mod 1988;7:513.
57. Young AS, Maritim AC, Kariuki DP, et al. Low-dose oral administration of human interferon alpha can control the development of Theileria parva infection in cattle. Parasitology 1990;101(Pt 2):201.
58. Streuli M, Hall A, Boll W, Stewart WE, Nagat S, Weissman C. Target cell specificity of two species of human interferon-α produced from *Escherichia coli* and of hybrid molecules derived from them. Proc Natl Acad Sci USA 1981;78:2848.
59. Stanton G. Hughes T, Heard H, Georgiades J, Whorton E. Modulation of a natural virus defense system by low concentration of interferons at mucosal surfaces. J Interferon Res 1990;10:(S99).
60. Young A, Cummins J. The history of interferon and its use in animal therapy. East African Med J 1990;67:SS31.
61. Koech DK, Obel AO, Minowada J, Hutchinson VA, Cummins JM. Low dose oral alpha-interferon therapy for patients seropositive for human immunodeficiency virus type-1 (HIV-1). Mol Biother 1990;2:91.
62. Lecce JG, Cummins JM, Richards AB. Treatment of rotavirus infection in neonate and weanling pigs using natural human interferon alpha. J Mol Biotherapy 1990;2:211.
63. Bocci V. Is interferon effective after oral administration? J Biol Reg Homeostasis Agents 1990;4:81.
64. Bocci V. Immunomodulators as local hormones: new insights regarding their clinical utilization. J Biol Res Mod 1985;4:340.
65. Bocci V. Catabolism of therapeutic proteins and peptides with implications for drug delivery. Adv Drug Del Rev 1990;4:149.
66. Bocci V. Absorption of cytokines via the oropharyngeal associated lymphoid tissues—Does an unorthodox route improve the therapeutic index of interferon. Clin Pharmacokinet 1991;21:411.
67. Cantell K, Pyhala L. Circulating interferon in rabbits after administration of human interferon by different routes. J Gen Virol 1973;20:97.
68. Hanley D, Wirowowska-Stewart M, Stewart W II. Pharmacology of interferons. I. Pharmacologic distinctions between human leucocyte and fibroblast interferons. Int J Immunopharmacol 1979;1:219.
69. Stewart WE, Wirowowska-Stewart M. Characterization of human interferon types and subtypes. *In:* Khan A, Hill NO, Dorn GL. Interferon: Properties and Clinical Uses. Dallas, Texas, L. Fikes Press, 1980;111.
70. Paulesu L, Corradeschi F, Nicoletti C, Bocci V. Oral administration of human recombinant interferon-α_2 in rats. Int J Pharmaceutics 1988;46:199.
71. Ruegg CL, Strand M. Identification of a decapeptide region of human interferon α with antiproliferative activity and homology to an immunosuppressive sequence of the retroviral transmembrane protein P15E. J Interferon Res 1990;10:621.
72. Bocci V. Roles of interferon produced in physiological conditions. A speculative review. Immunology 1988;64:1.
73. Fleischmann WR Jr, Koren S, Fleischmann CM. Orally administered interferons exert their white blood cell suppressive effects via a novel mechanism. Proc Soc Exp Biol Med 1992;201:200.
74. Gibson DM, Cotler S, Spiegel HE, Colburn WA. Pharmacokinetics of recombinant leukocyte A interferon following various routes and modes of administration to the dog. J Interferon Res 1985;5:403.
75. Wills RJ, Spiegel HE, Soike KF. Pharmacokinetics of recombinant alpha A interferon following I.V. infusion and bolus, I.M., and P.O. administrations to African green monkeys. J Interferon Res 1984;4:399.
76. Witt, PJ, Goldstein D, Storer BE, et al. Absense of biological effects of orally administered interferon-β_{ser}. J Interferon Res 1992;12:411.

77. Goldstein D, Sielaff KM, Storer BE, et al. Human biologic response modification by interferon in the absence of measurable serum concentrations: a comparative trial of subcutaneous and intravenous interferon-β serine. J Natl Cancer Inst 1989;81:1061.

78. Blalock JE, Baron S, Johnson HM, Stanton GJ. Transmission of interferon-induced activities by cell to cell communication. Texas Rep Biol Med 1982;41:344.

79. Alvord EC, Shaw CM, Huby S, Kies MK. Encephalitogen-induced inhibition of experimental allergic encephalomyelitis: prevention, suppression, and therapy. Ann N Y Acad Sci 1965;122:333.

80. Adams J, Stein R. Ann Rep Med Chem 1996;31:279.

81. Hertz F, Deghenghi R. Effect of rat and beta interferons on hyperacute experimental allergic encephalomyelitis in rats. Agents Actions 1985;16:397.

82. Karpus WJ, Swanborg RH. CD4+ suppressor cells inhibit the function of effector cells of experimental autoimmune encephalomyelitis through a mechanism involving transforming growth factor-β. J Immunol 1991;146:1163.

83. Abreu SL. Suppression of experimental allergic encephalomyelitis by interferon. Immunol Commun 1982;11:1.

84. Abreu SL, Thampoe L, Kaplan P. Interferon in experimental autoimmune encephalomyelitis: intraventricular administration. J Interferon Res 1986;6:627.

85. Kennedy MK, Torrance DS, Picha KS, Mohler KM. Analysis of cytokine mRNA expression in the central nervous system of mice with experimental autoimmune encephalomyelitis reveal that IL-10 mRNA expression correlates with disease. J Immunol 1992;149:2496.

86. Hutchinson V, Angenend J, Mok W, Cummins J, Richards A. Chronic recurrent aphthous stomatitis: oral treatment with low-dose interferon alpha. Molecular Biotherapy 1990;2:160.

87. Brod SA, Scott M, Burns DK, Phillips JT. Modification of acute experimental autoimmune encephalomyelitis in the Lewis rat by oral administration of type 1 interferons. J Interferon Cytokine Res 1995;15:115.

88. Tabata Y, Uno K, Yamaoka T, Ikada Y, Muramatsu S. Effects of recombinant alpha interferon gelatin conjugate on in vivo murine tumor growth. Cancer Res 1991;51:5532.

89. Shibita M, Blatteis M. Human recombinant tumor necrosis factor and interferon affect the activity of neurons in the organum vasculosum lamina terminalis. Brain Res 1991;562:323.

90. Dennis MJ, Thomas LH, Scott EJ. Effects of recombinant human alpha A interferon in gnotobiotic calves challenged with respiratory syncytial virus. Res Veterinary Sci 1991;50:222.

91. Horisberger MA, Gunst MC. Interferon induced proteins: identification of Mx proteins in various mammalian species. Virology 1991;180:185.

92. Weiss RC, Cummins JM, Richards AB. Low-dose orally administered alpha interferon treatment for feline leukemia virus infection. J Am Vet Med Assoc 1991;199:1477.

93. Weiss RC, Oostrom-Ram T. Effects of recombinant human interferon alpha in vitro and in vivo on mitogen induced lymphocyte blastogenesis in cats. J Clin Immunol Immunopathol 1990;24:147.

94. Kawade Y. The interferon system in the mouse. In: Baron S, Dianzani F, Stanton GJ, Fleischmann WR. The Interferon System. Austin, Texas, UT Press, 1987;169.

95. Blalock J, Baron S. The transfer of interferon-induced viral resistance between animal cells. Texas Rep Biol Med 1977;35:307.

96. Blalock JE, Baron S. Interferon induced transfer of viral resistance between animal cells. Nature 1977;269:422.

97. McDonald AH, Swanborg RH. Antigen-specific inhibition of immune interferon production by suppressor cells of autoimmune encephalomyelitis. J Immunol 1988;140:1132.

98. Brod SA. Ingested type I interferon: a potential treatment for autoimmunity. J Interferon Cytokine Res 2002;22:1153.

99. Randomised double-blind placebo-controlled study of interferon beta-1a in relapsing/remitting multiple sclerosis. PRISMS (Prevention of Relapses and Disability by Interferon beta-1a Subcutaneously in Multiple Sclerosis) Study Group [see comments]. Lancet 1998;352:1498.

100. Wisnewski HM, Keith AB. Chronic relapsing experimental allergic encephalomyelitis: an experimental model of multiple sclerosis. Ann Neurol 1977;1:144.

101. Raine CS, Snyder DH, Stone SH, Bronstein MB. Suppression of acute and chronic experimental allergic encephalomyelitis in Strain 13 guinea pigs. A clinical and pathological study. J Neurol Sci 1977;31:355.

102. Feuer C, Prentice DE, Cammisuli S. Chronic relapsing experimental allergic encephalomyelitis in the lewis rat. J Neuroimmunol 1985;10:159.

103. Brown AM, McFarlin DE. Relapsing experimental allergic encephalomyelitis in the SJL/J mouse. Lab Invest 1981;45:278.

104. Miller SD, Clatch RJ, Pevear DC, Trotter JL, Lipton HL. Class II restricted T cell response in Theiler's murine encephalomyelitis virus induced demyelinating disease. J Immunol 1987;138:3776.

105. Weber H, Valenzuela D, Lujger G, Gubler M, Weissman C. Single amino acid changes that render human IFN-α_2 biologically active on mouse cells. EMBO J 1987;6:591.

106. McInnes M, Chambers PJ, Cheetham BF, Beilharz MJ, Tymms MJ. Structure function studies of interferons-α: amino acid substitutions at the conserved residue tyrosine 123 in human interferons-α. J Interferon Res 1989;9:305.

107. Diabetes Prevention Trial—Type 1 Diabetes Study Group. Effects of insulin in relatives of patients with type 1 diabetes mellitus. N Engl J Med 2002;46:1685.

108. Neutralizing antibodies during treatment of multiple sclerosis with interferon beta-1b: experience during the first three years. The IFNB Multiple Sclerosis Study Group and the University of British Columbia MS/MRI Analysis Group. Neurology 1996;47:889.

109. Brod SA, Khan M, Kerman RH, Pappolla M. Oral administration of human or murine interferon alpha suppresses relapses and modifies adoptive transfer in experimental autoimmune encephalomyelitis. J Neuroimmunol 1995;58:61.

110. Brod SA, Burns DK. Suppression of relapsing experimental autoimmune encephalomyelitis in the SJL/J mouse by oral administration of type I interferons. Neurology 1994;44:1144.

111. Brod SA, Khan M. Oral administration of IFN-alpha is superior to subcutaneous administration of IFN-alpha in the suppression of chronic relapsing experimental autoimmune encephalomyelitis. J Autoimmunol 1996;9:11.

112. Lublin F. Adoptive transfer of murine relapsing experimental autoimmune encephalomyelitis. Ann Neurol 1985;17:188.

113. Whitham RH, Bourdette DN, Hashim GA, et al. Lymphocytes from SJL/J mice immunized with spinal cord respond selectively to a peptide of proteolipid protein and transfer demyelinating relapsing experimental autoimmune encephalomyelitis. *J Immunol* 1991;146:101.

114. Peters BA, Hinrichs DJ. Passive transfer of experimental allergic encephalomyelitis in the Lewis rat with activated spleen cells: differential activation with mitogens. Cell Immunol 1982;69:175.

115. Fallis RJ, Raine CE, McFarlin DE. Chronic relapsing experimental allergic encephalomyelitis in SJL/J mice following the adoptive transfer of an epitope-specific T cell line. J Neuroimmunol 1989;22:93.

116. van der Veen RC, Trotter JL, Clark HB, Kapp JA. The adoptive transfer of chronic experimental allergic encephalomyelitis with lymph nodes sensitized to myelin proteolipid protein. J Neuroimmunol 1989;21:183.

117. Tuohy VK, Lu Z, Sobel RA, Laursen RA, Lees MB. Identification of an encephalitogenic determinant of myelin proteolipid protein for SJL/J mice. J Immunol 1989;142:1523.

118. Sobel RA, Tuohy VK, Lu Z, Laursen RA, Lees MB. Acute experimental allergic encephalomyelitis in the SJL/J mouse induced by a synthetic peptide of myelin proteolipid protein. J Neuropath Exp Neurol 1990;49:468.

119. Greer JM, Kuchroo VJ, Sobel RA, Lees MB. Identification and characterization of a second encephalitogenic determinant of myelin proteolipid protein (residues 178-191) for SJL/J mice. J Immunol 1992;149:783.

120. Kennedy MK, Tan LJ, Canto MCD, Miller SD. Regulation of the effector stages of experimental autoimmune encephalomyelitis via neuroantigen-specific tolerance induction. J Immunol 1990;145:117.

121. Kennedy MK, Tan LJ, Canto MCD, et al. Inhibition of murine autoimmune encephalomyelitis by immune tolerance to proteolipid protein and its encephalitogenic peptides. J Immunol 1990;144:909.

122. Lider O, Santos LMB, Lee CSY, Higgins PJ, Weiner HL. Suppression of experimental autoimmune encephalomyelitis by oral administration of myelin basic protein. II. Suppression of disease and in vitro immune responses is mediated by antigen-specific CD8[+] T lymphocytes. J Immunol 1989;142:748.

123. Diab A, Zhu J, Xiao B, Mustafa M, Link H. High IL-6 and low IL-10 in the central nervous system are associated with protracted relapsing EAE in DA rats. J Neuropathol Exp Neurol 1997;56:641.

124. Issazadeh S, Lorentzen J, Mustafa M, Hojeberg B, Mussener A, Olsson T. Cytokines in relapsing experimental autoimmune encephalomyelitis in DA rats: persistent mRNA expression of proinflammatory cytokines and absent expression of interleukin-10 and transforming growth factor-beta. J Neuroimmunol 1996;69:103.

125. Tompkins SM, Padilla K, Dal Canto MC, Ting JP, Van Kaer L, Miller SD. De novo central nervous system processing of myelin antigen is required for the initiation of experimental autoimmune encephalomyelitis. J Immunol 2002;168:4173.

126. Martin D, Near S, Bendele A, Russell D. Inhibition of tumor necrosis factor is protective against neurologic dysfunction after active immunization of Lewis rats with myelin basic protein. Exp Neurol 1995;131:221.

127. Renno T, Krakowski M, Piccirillo C, Lin L, Owens T. TNF-alpha expression by resident microglia and infiltrating leukocytes in the central nervous system of mice with experimental allergic encephalomyelitis. Regulation by Th1 cytokines. J Immunol 1995;154:944.

128. Barten DM, Ruddle NH. Vascular cell adhesion molecule-1 modulation by tumor necrosis factor in experimental allergic encephalomyelitis. J Neuroimmunol 1994;51:123.

129. Selmaj K, Raine CS, Cross AH. Anti-tumor necrosis factor therapy abrogates autoimmune demyelination. Ann Neurol 1991;30:694.

130. Mosmann TR, Cherwinski H, Bond MW, Giedlin MA, Coffman RL. Two types of murine helper T cell. I. Definition according to profiles of lymphokine activities and secreted proteins. J Immunol 1986;136:2348.

131. Kim J, Woods A, Becker-Dunn E, Bottomly K. Distinct functional phenotypes of cloned Ia-restricted helper T cells. J Exp Med 1985;162:188.

132. Cher DJ, Mosmann TR. Two types of murine helper T cells. II. Delayed-type hypersensitivity is mediated by Th1 clones. J Immunol 1987;138:3688.

133. Boom WH, Liano D, Abbas AK. Heterogeneity of helper/inducer T lymphocytes. II. Effects of interleukin-4 and interleukin-2 producing T cells clones on resting B cells. J Exp Med 1988;167:1350.

134. Street N, Schumacher JH, Fong TAT, et al. Heterogeneity of mouse helper T cells: evidence from bulk cultures and limiting dilution cloning for precursors of Th1 and Th2 cells. J Immunol 1990;144:1629.

135. Merrill JE, Kono DH, Clayton J, Ando DG, Hinton DR, Hofman FM. Inflammatory leukocytes and cytokines in the peptide-induced disease of experimental allergic encephalomyelitis in SJL and B10.PL mice. Proc Natl Acad Sci USA 1992;89:574. [published erratum appears in Proc Natl Acad Sci USA 1992;89:10,562]

136. Brod SA, Benjamin D, Hafler DA. Restricted T cell expression of IL-2/IFN-gamma mRNA in human inflammatory disease. J Immunol 1991;147:810.

137. Haanen J, Malefijt R, Res P, et al. Selection of a human T helper type-1 T cell subset by Mycobacteria. J Immunol 1991;174:583.

138. Yssel H, Shanafelt MC, Soderberg C, Schneider PV, Anzola J, Peltz G. Borrelia burgdorferai activates a T helper type-1 like T cell subset in Lyme arthritis. J Exp Med 1991;174:593.

139. Voorthuis JA, Uitdehaag BM, De Groot CJ, Goede PH, van der Meide PH, Dijkstra CD. Suppression of experimental allergic encephalomyelitis by intraventricular administration of interferon-gamma in Lewis rats. Clin Exp Immunol 1990;81:183.

140. Heremans H, Dillen C, Groenen M, Martens E, Billiau A. Chronic relapsing experimental autoimmune encephalomyelitis (CREAE) in mice: enhancement by monoclonal antibodies against interferon-gamma. Eur J Immunol 1996;26:2393.

141. Duong TT, St. Louis J, Gilbert JJ, Finkelman FD, Strejan GH. Effect of anti-interferon-gamma and anti-interleukin-2 monoclonal antibody treatment on the development of actively and passively induced experimental allergic encephalomyelitis in the SJL/J mouse. J Neuroimmunol 1992;36:105.

142. Lublin FD, Knobler RL, Kalman B, et al. Monoclonal anti-gamma interferon antibodies enhance experimental allergic encephalomyelitis. Autoimmunity 1993;16:267.

143. Stevens D, Gould K, Swanborg R. Transforming growth factor-beta 1 inhibits tumor necrosis factor-alpha/lymphotoxin production and adoptive transfer of disease by effector cells of autoimmune encephalomyelitis. J Neuroimmunol 1994;51:77.

144. Racke M, Sriram S, Carlino J, Cannella B, Raine C, McFarlin D. Long-term treatment of chronic relapsing experimental allergic encephalomyelitis by transforming growth factor-beta 2. J Neuroimmunol 1993;46:175.

145. Johns L, Sriram S. Experimental allergic encephalomyelitis: neutralizing antibody to TGF beta 1 enhances the clinical severity of the disease. J Neuroimmunol 1993;47:1.

146. Crisi G, Santambrogio L, Hochwald G, Smith S, Carlino J, Thorbecke G. Staphylococcal enterotoxin B and tumor-necrosis factor-alpha-induced relapses of experimental allergic encephalomyelitis: protection by transforming growth factor-beta and interleukin-10. Eur J Immunol 1995;25:3035.

147. Baron S, Coppenhaver DH, Dianzani F, et al. Introduction to the interferon system. *In*: Baron S, Coppenhaver DH, Dianzani F, et al. Interferon: Principles and Medical Applications. Galveston, Texas, UT-Galveston, 1992;1.

148. Brod S, Darcan S, Malone M, Pappolla M, Nelson L. Ingested IFN-α suppresses IDDM in the NOD mouse. Diabetologia 1998;41:1227.

149. Kadish AS, Tansey FA, Yu GSM, Doyle AT, Bloom BR. Interferon as a mediator of human lymphocyte suppression. J Exp Med 1980;151:637.

150. Devens BH, Semenuk G, Webb DR. Antipeptide antibody specific for the N-terminal of soluble immune response suppressor neutralizes concanavalin A and IFN-induced suppressor cell activity in an in vitro cytotoxic T lymphocyte response. J Immunol 1988;141:3148.

151. Aune TM, Pierce CW. Activation of a suppressor T-cell pathway by interferon. Proc Natl Acad Sci USA 1982;79:3808.

152. Schnaper HW, Pierce CW, Aune TM. Identification and initial characterization of concanavalin A- and interferon-induced human suppressor factors: evidence for a human equivalent of murine soluble immune response suppressor (SIRS). J Immunol 1984;132:2429.

153. Stobo J, Green I, Jackson L, Baron S. Identification of a subpopulation of mouse lymphoid cells required for interferon production after stimulation with mitogens. J Immunol 1974;112:1589.

154. Weil J, Epstein C, Epstein LB, Sedmek JJ, Sabran JL, Grossberg SE. A unique set of polypeptides is induced by gamma interferon in addition to those induced in common with alpha and beta interferon. Nature 1983;301:437.

155. de Veer MJ, Holko M, Frevel M, et al. Functional classification of interferon-stimulated genes identified using microarrays. J Leukoc Biol 2001;69:912.

156. Brandtzaeg P. Overview of the mucosal immune system. Curr Topics Microbiol Immunol 1989;146:13.

157. Ermak TH, Owen RL. Differential distribution of lymphocytes and accessory cells in Peyer's patch. Anat Rev 1986;215:144.

158. Witmer MD, Steinman RM. The anatomy of peripheral lymphoid organs with emphasis on accessory cells: light-microscopic immunocytochemical studies of mouse spleen, lymph node, and Peyer's patch. Am J Anat 1984;170:465.

159. Santos LM, al-Sabbagh A, Londono A, Weiner HL. Oral tolerance to myelin basic protein induces regulatory TGF-beta-secreting T cells in Peyer's patches of SJL mice. Cell Immunol 1994;157:439.

160. Mattingly JA. Immunologic suppression after oral administration of antigen. III. Activation of suppressor-inducer cells in the Peyer's patches. Cell Immunol 1984;86:46.

161. MacDonald TT. Immunosuppression caused by antigen feeding II. Suppressor T cells mask Peyer's patch B cell priming to orally administered antigen. Eur J Immunol 1983;13:138.

162. Xu-Amano J, Aicher WK, Tagichi T, Kiyono H, McGhee JR. Selective induction of Th2 cells in murine Peyer's patches by oral immunization. Int Immunol 1992;4:433.

163. Daynes RA, Araneo BA, Dowell TA, Huang K, Dudley D. Regulation of murine lymphokine production in vivo. III. The lymphoid tissue microenvironment exerts regulatory influences over T helper cell function. J Exp Med 1990;171:979.

164. Hu MCT, Crowe DT, Weissman IL, Holzmann B. Cloning and expression of mouse integrin β_p [β_7]: A functional role in Peyer's patch-specific lymphocyte homing. Proc Natl Acad Sci USA 1990;89:8254.

165. Chin YH, Cai JP, Hieselaar T. Lymphocyte migration into mucosal lymphoid tissues: mechanism and modulation. Immunol Res 1991;10:271.

166. Lefrancois, L. Intraepithelial lynmphocytes of the intestinal mucosa: curiouser and curiouser. Semin Immunol 1991;3:99.

167. Sydora BC, Mixter PF, Holcombe HR, et al. Intestinal intraepithelial lymphocytes are activated and cytolytic but do not proliferate as well as other T cells in response to mitogenic stimulation. J Immunol 1993;150:2179.

168. Weiner HL, Mackin GA, Matsui M, et al. Oral tolerance: immunologic mechanisms and treatment of animal and human organ-specific autoimmune diseases by oral adminstration of autoantigens. Ann Rev Immunol 1994;12:809.

169. Higgins P, Weiner HL. Suppression of experimental autoimmune encephalomyelitis by oral administration of myelin basic protein and its fragments. J Immunol 1988;140:440.

170. Fuller KA, Pearl D, Whitacre CC. Oral tolerance in experimental autoimmune encephalomyelitis: serum and salivary antibody responses. J Neuroimmunol 1988;28:15.

171. Chen Y, Kuchroo VJ, Inobe JI, Hafler DA, Weiner HL. Regulatory T cell clones induced by oral tolerance: suppression of autoimmune encephalomyelitis. Science 1994;265:1237.

172. Georgiades JA, Kruzel ML, Seman G. Transfer of antiviral resistance by spleen and blood cells of mice receiving low doses of IFN alpha or gamma. J Interferon Res 1989;9:S213.

173. Butcher EC. The regulation of lymphocyte traffic. Curr Topics Microbiol Immunol 1986;128:85.

174. Boccoli G, Masciulli R, Ruggeri EM, et al. Adoptive immunotherapy of human cancer: the cytokine cascade and monocyte activation following high-dose interleukin 2 bolus treatment. Cancer Res 1990;50:5795.

175. Dinarello C, Cannon JG, Wolff SM, et al. Tumor necrosis factor [cachetin] is an endogenous pyrogen and induces production of interleukin-1. J Exp Med 1986;163:1433.

176. Linington C, Berger T, Perry S, et al. T cells specific for myelin oligodendrocyte glycoprotein mediate an unusual autoimmune inflammatory response in the central nervous system. Eur J Immunol 1993;23:1364.

177. Brod SA, Friedman AW, Appleyard J, Warner NB, Henninger EM. Ingested IFN-α has biological effects in rheumatoid arthritis. Int J Immunother 2001;16:53.

178. Brod SA, Orlander P, Lavis P, et al. Ingested IFN-α prolongs the "honeymoon" period in newly diagnosed type I diabetes mellitus. J Interferon Cyt Res 2001;21:1021.

CME QUESTIONS

1. In which aspect does ingested type I IFN inhibit experimental autoimmune encephalomyelitis?
   A. By blocking inflammatory T helper 1 (Th1)-like cytokines
   B. By upregulating counterregulatory cytokines
   C. By decreasing migration of adoptively transferred lymphocytes.
   D. By causing apoptosis of encephalitogenic cells.

2. Which of the following statements is *false*?
   A. Ingested interferon is absorbed into the body from the gut
   B. Interferons are defined by their antiviral activity
   C. Both interferon-α and interferon-β have activity in multiple sclerosis
   D. Experimental autoimmune encephalomyelitis resembles a type IV immune response

3. The immunopathogenesis of type 1 diabetes is *not* similar to the following diseases?
   A. Rheumatoid arthritis
   B. systemic lupus erythematosus
   C. Multiple sclerosis
   D. Sjogren's syndrome

4. Ingested interferon may have an effect in multiple sclerosis by reducing magnetic resonance imaging new enhancing lesions if:
   A. More interferon is administered at more frequent intervals
   B. Antibody formation could be inhibited
   C. Less interferon is given compared to the previously tested doses
   D. Induction of MxA mRNA or protein can be demonstrated

Neuromyelitis Optica

Dean M. Wingerchuk

1. BACKGROUND AND NOSOLOGICAL OVERVIEW

Idiopathic inflammatory demyelinating central nervous system (CNS) diseases include the various clinical types of multiple sclerosis (MS), acute transverse myelitis (TM), optic neuritis (ON), recurrent forms of TM and ON, the Marburg variant of MS, Balo's concentric sclerosis, and neuromyelitis optica (NMO; Devic's syndrome or Devic's disease) *(1)*. The association of spinal cord disease and visual impairment was first recognized in 1870 by Allbutt *(2)*. In 1894, Devic reported a case of bilateral ON and myelitis occurring in rapid succession, leading to the eponymous designation of *Devic neuromyelitis optica (3)*. Stansbury's extensive 1949 review influenced the clinical concept of NMO; thereafter, the term was typically applied to patients with a monophasic disorder consisting of acute or subacute, usually bilateral, ON occurring in close temporal association with severe myelitis *(4–7)*.

The definition of NMO has been frequently revisited *(8–10)*. Contemporary case series have expanded the spectrum of idiopathic NMO to encompass otherwise typical cases allowing any of the following features:

1. unilateral ON
2. a more protracted initial course with no restrictions on the timeframe during which the initial defining events of ON and myelitis occur
3. a relapsing course *(10)*.

The long-term natural history of relapsing NMO, as diagnosed with broader criteria, is similar between patients with unilateral vs bilateral ON and between those with rapid onset vs those with more protracted disease development *(10)*. It is not clear whether idiopathic syndromes of recurrent ON *(11)* or myelitis (in both Caucasians and non-Caucasians *[12–14]*) are pathophysiologically related, but some cases of apparently isolated TM eventually convert to NMO *(15)*.

The nosology of NMO is complicated by the fact that people with systemic autoimmune diseases, such as Sjögren's syndrome or systemic lupus erythematosus, may develop NMO *(16–18)*. Furthermore, many people with MS present with ON or myelitis, and some may have clinically restricted opticospinal disease for several years. The clinical course, imaging, and laboratory results help differentiate NMO from typical forms of MS, although current diagnostic criteria remain arbitrary and have not been rigorously validated against a gold standard. Furthermore, they require the occurrence of two or more clinical events. Diagnosis immediately following a first-ever attack is desirable because the treatment approach in idiopathic NMO differs from that of MS and could plausibly require modification in the setting of a systemic autoimmune disease

From: *Current Clinical Neurology: Inflammatory Disorders of the Nervous System:*
Pathogenesis, Immunology, and Clinical Management
Edited by: A. Minagar and J. S. Alexander © Humana Press Inc., Totowa, NJ

(16,19). The discovery of an objective biological marker that allows discrimination of idiopathic NMO from MS and other entities at the time of initial presentation with ON or myelitis would signal tremendous progress in the treatment and research of each disorder.

2. CLINICAL FEATURES AND DIAGNOSIS

The core feature of NMO is clinically restricted opticospinal disease. Patients typically present with acute, severe unilateral or bilateral ON or a severe attack of acute myelitis. Attacks of myelitis are often fulminant episodes of *complete transverse myelitis* and are associated with pain and substantial residual neurological impairment. The observation that attacks tend to be more severe in NMO than in typical MS is integrated into a current NMO diagnostic scheme (Table 1). The presence of bilateral ON or a severe, permanent deficit as a residual effect of an attack (visual acuity worse than 20/200 or severe limb weakness) favor NMO over MS. Some NMO patients, especially those with established relapsing disease, may experience milder attacks. Progressive disease, manifested by gradual loss of visual function or a chronic progressive myelopathy, is a rare NMO manifestation. Most cases characterized by gradually worsening myelopathy, even in the setting of a negative cranial MRI, are primary progressive MS rather than NMO.

NMO may follow a monophasic course (unilateral or bilateral ON in close temporal association with myelitis, followed by apparently permanent clinical remission), but at least 80% of patients have relapsing disease characterized by recurrent attacks of ON, myelitis, or both *(10,20)*. Therefore, the phasic characteristics of NMO are similar to those of MS, often leading to a diagnosis of severe atypical MS and treatment with standard MS disease-modifying therapies by clinicians unaware of the distinct NMO phenotype.

Although very severe attacks of ON or myelitis suggest NMO, there is substantial overlap in clinical severity between NMO and MS; therefore, the diagnosis is best supported by the presence of imaging and laboratory features that are characteristic of NMO and not of typical MS. Although a recently discovered serum auto-antibody, NMO-immunoglobulin (NMO-IgG), seems a promising diagnostic tool, the most useful indicators are neuroimaging and cerebrospinal fluid (CSF) findings, and a number of investigators have combined these into arbitrary but clinically useful diagnostic criteria (Table 1).

Magnetic resonance imaging (MRI) studies of the head and spinal cord are the most powerful tools for distinguishing NMO from MS. During acute ON attacks, brain MRI studies may demonstrate optic nerve enhancement with gadolinium, but this is not specific to NMO. Cranial MRI is very useful for NMO diagnosis because it reveals either normal brain parenchyma or only a few nonspecific subcortical white matter abnormalities that do not fulfill radiological criteria for MS *(10)*. This result pattern is especially helpful in cases in which a patient has experienced multiple ON or myelitis attacks. During years of follow-up, serial imaging studies may reveal an increasing number of cerebral white matter lesions, but very few appear to meet MRI criteria for MS.

The most specific diagnostic result for NMO is a contiguous, longitudinally extensive lesion that spans three or more vertebral segments on spinal cord MRI (Fig. 1) *(10)*. Such lesions are virtually never seen in typical MS, in which plaques are visible as small dorsal lesions less than one vertebral segment in craniocaudal length *(21,22)*. During acute NMO attacks, these lengthy cord lesions usually exhibit gadolinium enhancement. On follow-up, the affected area may develop a syrinx with or without focal atrophy.

Although spinal cord and brain MRI findings are the most useful diagnostic aids, several other less common laboratory features are also helpful. Only 20 to 40% of NMO patients have oligoclonal bands present in CSF, compared with 80 to 90% of those with MS (even when MS case samples are derived by different methods) *(8–10,23,24)*. During acute myelitis exacerbations in NMO, the CSF may reveal a brisk pleocytosis (more than 50 leukocytes/mm^3), a rare finding in typical MS *(10)*. The cell differential is also very useful; whereas in MS all CSF leukocytes are mononuclear, a minority of NMO cases is associated with a predominance of polymorphonuclear cells.

Table 1
Proposed Diagnostic Criteria for Neuromyelitis Optica

Diagnosis requires all absolute criteria *and* one major supportive criterion *or* two minor supportive criteria.

Absolute criteria:
1. ON
2. Acute myelitis
3. No clinical disease outside of the optic nerves and spinal cord

Major supportive criteria:
1. Negative brain MRI at disease onset (normal or not meeting radiological diagnostic criteria for MS)
2. Spinal cord MRI with T2-signal abnormality extending over ≥3 vertebral segments
3. CSF pleocytosis (>50 WBC/mm^3) OR >5 neutrophils/mm^3

Minor supportive criteria:
1. Bilateral ON
2. Severe ON with fixed visual acuity worse than 20/200 in at least one eye
3. Severe, fixed, attack-related weakness (MRC grade 2 or less) in one or more limbs

ON, optic neuritis; MRI, magnetic resonance imaging; MS, multiple sclerosis; CSF, cerebrospinal fluid; WBC, white blood cell; MRC Medical Research Council. (From ref. *10*.)

Prospective validation studies of current diagnostic criteria are needed. Nevertheless, some preliminary studies suggest that these criteria consistently distinguish cases of NMO from typical forms of MS, especially when MRI criteria are applied *(25–27)*. This is consistent with observations colleagues and I have made about the discriminative ability of the spinal cord MRI features.

Identification of a biological or pathological marker associated with NMO but not with MS would greatly enhance clinical practice and research. A recent important advance in this direction was the discovery of NMO-IgG, which may have excellent specificity and good sensitivity for distinguishing NMO from typical MS *(28)*. NMO-IgG seropositive rates were 54.2% for NMO ($n = 48$) and 0% for MS ($n = 20$). This indirect immunofluoresence assay reveals a distinct staining pattern that appears to selectively bind a target associated with CNS capillaries, pia, and subpia *(29)*. If validated, NMO-IgG represents the first specific biological marker for NMO within the spectrum of CNS demyelinating syndromes.

Once NMO is diagnosed, the next important feature to consider is the disease course. Because patients with relapsing disease require ongoing interventions aimed at attack prevention, and those with monophasic disease do not, methods are needed to differentiate these groups as early as possible. Imaging findings and CSF abnormalities are not independently predictive, but some clinical features are useful. Patients who experience a course similar to the *historical* NMO definition (acute ON and myelitis occurring simultaneously or within a few days) are much more likely have a monophasic course. In the largest modern case series *(20)*, the median interval between the first clinical event and achievement of NMO diagnosis was much shorter in the monophasic group compared with the relapsing group (5 d [range 0–151 d] vs 166 d [range 2–730 d]). The relative risk of relapsing disease is increased by 2.16 for every month increase in the first interattack interval, making this the strongest clinical predictor of disease course. Other significant independent variables include female sex (relative risk [RR] = 10.0; female vs male) and less severe motor impairment with the initial myelitis event (RR = 0.48 for every point decrease on a motor weakness scale). These prognostic variables may be useful when considering implementation of chronic, aggressive immunotherapy early in the disease course and in planning therapeutic clinical trials.

Although not independently predictive, initial ON and myelitis attack severity are greater in those patients destined to have a monophasic course. Complete paraplegia at the nadir of the first

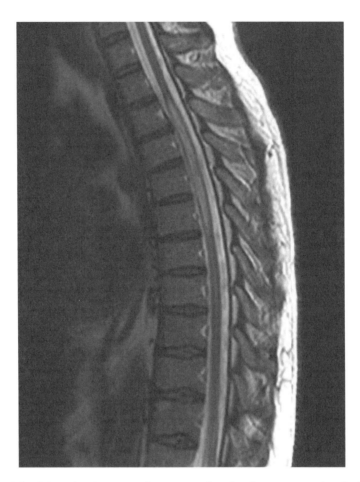

Fig. 1. T2-weighted thoracic spine magnetic resonance imaging demonstrates a longitudinally extensive cord lesion characteristic of neuromyelitis optica.

myelitis attack (70% monophasic patients vs 31% relapsing patients) and complete loss of light perception (>50% monophasic vs about 28% relapsing patients) (10,20). Despite this, long-term neurological impairment and disability is measurably less in monophasic NMO because patients with relapsing disease continue to accrue visual, motor, sensory, and sphincter impairment in a stepwise fashion. Long-term follow-up of patients with monophasic NMO revealed that although 22% had permanent serious visual loss (<20/200 visual acuity) in at least one eye, more than 50% experienced visual improvement to at least 20/30. Most serious disability was caused by the residual effects of myelitis; permanent monoplegia or paraplegia occurred in 31%. Five-year survival of this group was approx 90%; deaths were usually unrelated to NMO.

Outcomes in relapsing NMO are decidedly worse than for monophasic disease. Relapsing NMO follows an unpredictable course consisting of clusters of attacks months or years apart. Relapsing NMO is usually evident relatively early; after meeting NMO criteria, 55% relapse within 1 yr, 78% by 3 yr, and 90% within 5 yr (10). Relapse timing and frequency is as unpredictable in NMO as it is in MS. Many patients experience clusters of several attacks over a few months, whereas others enjoy remissions lasting more than a decade. The median number of relapses was five (range 1 to 18) in the Mayo Clinic series (median follow-up 16.9 yr). Disability mounts accordingly, and only 5 yr from NMO onset, more than 50% have monocular blindness or cannot ambulate without assistance. This attack-related disability starkly contrasts the usual course of relapsing–remitting MS (RRMS), in which significant gait impairment does not usually occur until the 10- to 15-yr mark, when a secondary progressive course is well established. Progressive disease is a rare finding in NMO.

Longitudinal data revealed the disturbing fact that the relapsing NMO survival rate may be curtailed by as much as one-third because of respiratory failure resulting from attacks of severe, ascending cervical myelitis *(10,20)*. Predictors of mortality in relapsing NMO include a history of systemic autoimmune disease (RR = 4.15), greater exacerbation frequency during the first 2 yr of disease (RR = 1.21 per attack), and better motor recovery following the first myelitis attack. With the expansion of the NMO spectrum and improvements in medical supportive care, these estimates will undoubtedly be lowered, but the findings emphasize the importance of early and aggressive therapies to prevent attacks in relapsing NMO.

3. EPIDEMIOLOGY AND DISEASE ASSOCIATIONS

The clinical combination of ON and myelitis can occur as an idiopathic syndrome (Devic's syndrome) or in association with systemic autoimmune disorders, infectious diseases (pulmonary tuberculosis and a myriad of viral illnesses), or immunizations. The list of associations is extensive and suggests that the opticospinal axis may be selectively vulnerable to immunological injury under certain circumstances. There are comprehensive reviews of diseases, infections, and immunizations associated with NMO *(5,6)*. This chapter focuses on idiopathic NMO, especially epidemiological and genetic factors, with recognition that there may be overlap among the idiopathic and parainfectious/postimmunization types.

3.1. Epidemiology

The prevalence of NMO in the general population and compared with typical forms of MS is not known. The disorder is almost certainly under-recognized and usually misdiagnosed as MS; therefore, medical record reviews will underestimate any attempts at prevalence figures. Women comprise at least two-thirds of patients with NMO and perhaps more than 80% of relapsing cases. The median onset age in North American cases is late in the fourth decade, about 10 yr later than for typical MS. Although most North American NMO patients are Caucasian, there is a distinct over-representation of people with Asian and African ancestry compared with typical MS *(10)*.

Racial and genetic factors may assume a large role in susceptibility to the NMO phenotype. For instance, reports of demyelinating disease from Asia, African, and Caribbean nations and in African-American and indigenous (Native) American populations consistently reveal a tendency to an opticospinal phenotype that meets diagnostic criteria for NMO *(30–34)*. The best documented example comes from Japan, where cases of *opticospinal* or *Asian* MS have been distinguished from *Western* MS for decades *(35,36)*. The term *Devic's disease* was reserved for cases similar to the historical definition referred to earlier, whereas relapsing cases were diagnosed as MS. In the Japanese population, CNS demyelinating disease is associated with lower overall prevalence, a more common opticospinal pattern, more frequent and severe involvement of the visual system, lower familial co-occurrence, and low incidence of a progressive course. Kira summarized the Japanese literature and descriptions of opticospinal MS for comparison with more recent series of relapsing NMO and found that the racial predilections, age of onset, gender, clinical imaging, CSF, and pathological descriptions were very similar *(36)*. The sole qualitative difference is that NMO, unlike Japanese opticospinal MS, is frequently associated with the presence of a systemic autoimmune disease or positive autoimmune serological studies. Furthermore, the characteristics of a *pure* Japanese opticospinal MS subgroup (clinical opticospinal disease, normal cranial MRI excluding optic nerves, and more than 5 yr of follow-up) are virtually identical to cases of relapsing NMO *(37)*. These findings suggest that opticospinal MS and relapsing NMO are the same disorder or at least have similar pathogenic mechanisms.

4. GENETICS

Although familial cases have been reported in North America, NMO is largely a sporadic disease *(38–40)*. Familial Japanese NMO cases have been reported *(41)*, but a national survey of MS in Japan demonstrated that the frequency of multiplex families in opticospinal MS was less than 1% *(42)*.

There are few genetic data derived from North American patients with NMO. Studies of mitochondrial DNA, performed because of a speculative link between NMO and genetically based visual loss (Leber's hereditary optic neuropathy), were negative *(43,44)*.

Most immunogenetic information about the NMO phenotype comes from studies of Japanese opticospinal MS. In people of European descent and Japanese with *conventional* or *Western* MS, disease susceptibility is associated with the human lymphocyte antigen (HLA)-DRB1*1501 haplotype *(45–50)*. Several studies have shown that Japanese opticospinal MS, however, is strongly associated with the HLA-DPB1*0501 allele *(46–49)*, the most common DPB1 allele in Asia but an infrequent one in Caucasians. The same allele has been associated less strongly with conventional MS in Japanese *(48)*. A recent study in Caucasians found no difference in prevalence of DRB1*1501 between opticospinal and typical forms of MS *(51)*. Clearly, future immunogenetic studies of Caucasian and non-Caucasians patients with the relapsing NMO phenotype are needed to further study this association and other potential genetic factors that may explain clinical heterogeneity.

5. IMMUNOLOGY

There are few immunological studies of serum and CSF from NMO patients. Immunopathological abnormalities from tissue samples are discussed in Section 6.

The detection of a putative serum auto-antibody marker of NMO is of great interest *(28,29)*. The indirect immunofluoresence staining pattern of NMO-IgG is associated with capillaries in the cerebellar cortex and midbrain. Its target antigen is not known, but efforts at identifying it and determining whether it has a primary role in NMO pathophysiology or simply reflects a secondary immune response to optic nerve and spinal cord injury may provide important insights into whether NMO is a distinct disease.

Until such target antigens, pathogenic antibodies, and animal models of NMO are developed and refined, we will continue to make inferences about NMO immunological mechanisms from disease associations and basic serum and CSF analyses. As previously outlined, the NMO syndrome may occur in the context of infectious and systemic inflammatory illnesses. North American series increasingly reveal the coexistence of one or more pre-existing autoimmune diseases or positive serological studies in most patients with relapsing NMO. For example, autoimmune thyroid dysfunction or sicca or Sjögren's syndrome may precede the development of NMO. Frequently, comprehensive serological testing reveals the presence of one or more autoantibodies, such as antinuclear antibodies, antidouble-stranded DNA, extractable nuclear antigen (ENA), anticardiolipin antibodies, and antiparietal cell antibodies. These associations have not been commonly noted in Japanese patients, but prospective systematic analyses have not been reported. This evidence supports the contention that NMO may be a B-cell-mediated disorder, in contrast to MS, which is postulated to be driven by T-cell processes.

Immunological studies from peripheral blood in Japanese opticospinal MS patients demonstrate further differences compared to typical MS. Analysis of production of interferon (IFN)-γ and interleukin (IL)-4 by peripheral CD4-positive T cells demonstrated a shift towards a T helper 1 (Th1) phenotype (increased intracellular ratio of IFN-γ to IL-4) during both the relapse and remission phases of opticospinal MS. In contrast, this Th1 shift occurred only in the relapse phase in conventional MS *(52,53)*. Increased IFN-γ from CD8-positive T cells and upregulation of chemokine receptors (a Th1-type response) have been detected in both the relapse and remission phases in opticospinal MS *(53,54)*. Again, conventional MS differed in that chemokine upregulation occurred only in the relapse stage. Such Th1-shifts were associated with decreased serum IgE concentrations that were interpreted as possibly contributing to relapse generation in opticospinal MS *(36,52)*. These results require replication in Japanese and non-Japanese populations, and it is not clear how to put them in context with the pathological findings of Th2-predominance.

Immunological CSF studies in NMO are also somewhat limited. Many studies have replicated the finding that oligoclonal banding is less prevalent in NMO (about 35%) and Japanese opticospinal MS (35–45%) than in conventional MS in people of European descent (85–90%) *(36)*. This association is consistent and revealed even when consecutive MS patients in Japan were compared based on whether they had CSF oligoclonal banding; of those who were negative, 50% had opticospinal MS, and 78% had no or few MRI lesions *(55)*. The reason for oligoclonal banding absence in most NMO and Japanese opticospinal MS patients is not clear. Nakashima et al. recently found that both NMO and MS patients have higher CSF IgG concentrations than controls and the IgG1 percentage and IgG1 index were elevated only in the MS cases *(56)*. Because oligoclonal bands typically are restricted to IgG, the authors speculated that lack of IgG1 response may explain the absence of oligoclonal banding in NMO. Furthermore, because IgG1 is associated with Th1 autoimmunity, this finding is congruent with immunological and immunopathological findings that suggest that Th2 mechanisms are of primary importance in NMO. Other investigators found that higher CSF IL-10 levels were associated with the presence of oligoclonal banding and that these levels were much lower in NMO than in MS *(57)*.

Mandler et al. compared levels of matrix metalloproteinases (MMP) in NMO and MS *(58)*. These markers of inflammation, such as MMP-9, are elevated in CSF during the acute phase of MS but are reduced in NMO. Furthermore, tissue inhibitor of metalloproteinases (TIMP-1) was reduced in CSF from RRMS patients but not in NMO CSF. These differences in inflammatory markers suggest that the basic inflammatory reaction differs in MS and NMO.

Immunological or biochemical CSF markers that correlate with clinical outcome would be clinically useful. The degree of pleocytosis, protein level, and presence or absence of CSF oligoclonal bands are not independent predictors of disease course or outcome. The level of 14-3-3 protein was associated with disability and other CSF abnormalities suggestive of severe CNS tissue injury in Japanese opticospinal and myelitis patients *(59)*, a finding compatible with previous reports in transverse myelitis and MS *(60,61)*. Further study of such markers is an area of active study in all CNS demyelinating syndromes.

6. PATHOLOGY

6.1. *General Pathology*

Human pathological studies of NMO are rather limited. Optic nerve specimens reveal nonspecific but rather extensive demyelination and various degrees of remyelination in inactive lesions *(4)*. Brain white matter may be normal or contain scattered areas of small perivascular infiltrates, patchy demyelination, or gliosis.

Acute myelitic lesions usually expand the spinal cord and, depending on attack severity, pathological findings range from modest perivascular inflammatory demyelination to necrotic destruction of both gray and white matter. Destructive inflammatory infiltrates often included a high proportion of polymorphonuclear cells, which were detected in CSF analysis. In many cases, cell infiltrates contain large numbers of eosinophils *(62)*. This pattern of destructive, polymorphonuclear inflammation is distinct from typical MS.

An interesting pathological observation in NMO is the hyalinization of medium-caliber spinal cord arteries *(62–64)*. This vascular feature is not a feature of typical MS and is usually associated with cord necrosis and a macrophage-predominant inflammatory infiltrate. It is not known whether these vascular changes reflect a primary vascular immunological target or are a secondary and nonspecific effect of the severe and destructive spinal cord lesion.

6.2. Immunopathology

Detailed immunopathological study of spinal cord lesions at various stages of activity and maturity has provided strong evidence supportive of humoral disease mechanisms in NMO. Lucchinetti et al. studied early and late active demyelinating lesions, remyelinating lesions, and inactive demyelinated lesions using spinal cord biopsy and autopsy tissue samples from patients with established NMO. They confirmed intense perivascular and meningeal spinal cord infiltration with eosinophils and neutrophils. Lesions with active myelin destruction contained prominent IgG- and C9-neoantigen deposits; these were also present around vessel walls associated with vascular proliferation and fibrosis *(62)*. Overall, the results were strongly suggestive of humorally mediated, Th2-predominant mechanisms.

The immunological target in NMO is not known. Experimental autoimmune encephalomyelitis (EAE), a putative animal model of MS, can express a variety of clinical and pathological phenotypes by manipulating factors, such as the genetic strain of the animal and characteristics of the antigen exposure (antigen type, timing, and route of administration). The antigen myelin oligodendrocyte glycoprotein (MOG) can result in EAE phenotypes that encompass the spectrum of clinically recognizable human CNS demyelinating syndromes, such as prototypic MS, optic neuritis, and the acute Marburg variant *(65,66)*. In addition, MOG can produce inflammatory lesions highly restricted to the optic nerve and spinal cord. The genetic and/or environmental factors that dictate the phenotypic expression are largely unknown. The role of MOG as a putative target antigen in human NMO warrants further investigation.

The discovery of the NMO-IgG serum autoantibody marker described earlier may provide an avenue for directed immunopathological investigation. Further studies to elucidate the target autoantigen and its distribution will help clarify whether this specific autoantibody represents a primary effector of the disease or an epiphenomenon.

The reasons for restriction of the NMO phenotype to the optic nerves and spinal cord are not understood. It is possible that antibody-mediated injury may occur more readily in sites with a less effective blood–brain barrier; various EAE models with a predominance of optic nerve and spinal cord lesions indirectly support this idea.

7. THERAPY

7.1. Acute Exacerbations

Many patients with NMO are diagnosed during or shortly after a severe episode of myelitis, and acute therapeutic options may be the foremost consideration, especially if the scenario includes quadriplegia, respiratory failure, or clinical deterioration, despite treatment. Anecdotal evidence supports the first-line use of parenteral corticosteroids; there are no controlled trials of therapy for NMO attacks. Intravenous (iv) 1000 mg methylprednisolone daily for 5 consecutive days is a typical regimen; in the current era of methylprednisolone shortage, 200 mg/d iv dexamethasone may be substituted. Following the parenteral dose, it is reasonable to begin oral prednisone, approximately 1 mg/kg/d, to initiate chronic immunosuppression for long-term attack prophylaxis (*see* Section 7.2.).

Second-line treatment options are necessary because clinical worsening of myelitis often occurs despite methylprednisolone therapy. The only existing evidence from controlled trials supports intervention with plasmapheresis in this circumstance (seven exchanges, each of about 55 mL/kg, administered every other day). In a randomized, double-blind, crossover trial of patients with various forms of severe, idiopathic inflammatory demyelinating disease (including NMO) and corticosteroid-refractory attacks, meaningful clinical improvement occurred in significantly more plasmapheresis patients (42%) than sham exchange patients (6%) *(67)*. A retrospective review of plasmapheresis experience in NMO found that 6 of 10 patients with severe, treatment-refractory attacks experienced moderate or marked clinical improvement within days after the onset of therapy

(68). Early treatment initiation, male gender, and preserved muscle-stretch reflexes were independent predictors of a favorable response. These findings suggest that one should have a low threshold for intervening with plasmapheresis when patients with severe attacks worsen depsite corticosteroid therapy or do not begin to show objective clinical improvement shortly after completion of the steroid course. This is particularly important in cases of ascending cervical myelitis, which puts patients are at risk of neurogenic respiratory failure.

Other immune-based interventions, such as intravenous immune globulin, have been used with anecdotal success but currently represent third-line therapy.

Patients with severe myelitis attacks may require lengthy hospitalization or rehabilitation unit stays. They acquire the usual risks of new-onset immobility, and clinicians must be vigilant in prevention of and surveillance for thromboembolic events, nosocomial or aspiration pneumonia, and urinary tract infections.

7.2. *Immunotherapy for Attack Prevention*

MS and NMO require different long-term therapeutic approaches *(6,16).* The treatments of choice for attack prevention in MS are the IFN-β and glatiramer acetate *(69).* Despite some exceptions (e.g., a report that IFN-β1b seemed to benefit Japanese opticospinal MS *[70]* and a case report of clinical stability associated with glatiramer acetate treatment *[71]*), most clinicians who treat and follow a substantial number of patients with NMO believe that these immunotherapies are ineffective or minimally effective in this disorder.

There have been no randomized and properly controlled therapeutic trials aimed at attack suppression in NMO. In the only published prospective case series, seven newly diagnosed patients began combination therapy with azathioprine (2 mg/kg/d) and oral prednisone (1 mg/kg/d) *(72).* Two months into this protocol, the dosage of prednisone was reduced by 10 mg every 3 wk to 20 mg/d, then reduced more slowly to a target maintenance dose of 10 mg/d. Most patients took maintenance doses of 75–100 mg azathioprine and 10 mg prednisone daily. No patient experienced a clinical attack during the 18-mo observation period and neurological impairment scores improved slightly. A reasonable regimen starts azathioprine 50 mg/d and prednisone 60–80 mg/d (depending on the proximity to a recent exacerbation). The daily azathioprine dosage is increased by 50 mg every week to a target dose of 2.5 to 3 mg/kg/d. If clinical stability persists for more than 8 wk, the prednisone dosage may be slowly tapered on alternate days (e.g., 5 mg every 2 wk) to minimize adverse effects. The prednisone dosage may be reduced again (e.g., 5 mg every 4 wk) with a goal of discontinuation once azathioprine has demonstrated a laboratory effect (mild decrease in leukocyte count and increase in mean corpuscular volume). Unfortunately, some patients are unable to sustain clinical remission with azathioprine monotherapy and remain steroid dependent, either because of perceived neurological worsening or documented new exacerbations during attempts at prednisone dosage reduction.

Various other immunosuppressive drugs have been used but in limited numbers and outside the realm of a structured study. Mycophenolate mofetil is not associated with the idiosyncratic gastrointestinal symptoms that can occur with azathioprine, although its onset of action may be no more rapid. Some clinicians use mitoxantrone, a chemotherapeutic agent approved for use in rapidly worsening secondary progressive or RRMS *(73,74),* perhaps perceiving that NMO is simply severe MS. There are no published data concerning the use of mitoxantrone in NMO. The chimeric monoclonal antibody rituximab targets CD20-positive cells and seems a logical agent to study given its ability to cause B-cell clearance *(75).* Future therapeutic investigations aimed at humoral mechanism modulation would seem profitable based on current understanding of immunopathological mechanisms.

As discussed earlier, relapsing NMO carries a poor prognosis because of early attack-related disability. Therefore, early consideration and confirmation of the diagnosis should be followed immediately by initiation of closely monitoring immunotherapy.

8. CONCLUSION

Data from studies around the world are converging to provide a better understanding of the nosology, natural history, and treatment of NMO. Modern immunopathological techniques have provided additional important insights that, together with the clinical observations, strongly suggest that NMO and opticospinal MS are the same disorder and that they are distinct from typical MS. Relapsing NMO needs to be recognized early in its course to allow early initiation of therapy and to prevent attack-related disability. The recently discovered serum auto-antibody marker, if validated, may facilitate earlier and more precise diagnosis of relapsing NMO and, ultimately, earlier and more effective treatment for patients who have this unusual and disabling disorder.

REFERENCES

1. Weinshenker BG, Miller D. MS: one disease or many? *In:* Siva A, Kesselring J, Thompson A, eds. Frontiers in Multiple Sclerosis. London, Martin Dunitz, 1999:37–46.
2. Allbutt TC. On the ophthalmoscopic signs of spinal disease. Lancet 1870;1:76–78.
3. Devic E. Myélite subaiguë compliquée de néurite optique. Bull Med 1894;8:1033–1034.
4. Stansbury FC. Neuromyelitis optica (Devic's disease). Presentation of five cases with pathological study and review of the literature. Arch Ophthalmol 1949;42:292–335.
5. Cree BA, Goodin DS, Hauser SL. Neuromyelitis optica. Semin Neurol 2002;22:105–122.
6. Wingerchuk DM, Weinshenker BG. Neuromyelitis optica. *In:* McDonald WI, Noseworthy JH, eds. Multiple Sclerosis 2. Woburn, MA, Butterworth-Heinemann, 2003:243–258.
7. de Seze J. Neuromyelitis optica. Arch Neurol 2003;60:1336–1338.
8. Mandler RN, Davis LE, Jeffery DR, Kornfeld M. Devic's neuromyelitis optica: a clinicopathological study of 8 patients. Ann Neurol 1993;34:162–168.
9. O'Riordan JI, Gallagher HL, Thompson AJ, et al. Clinical, CSF, and MRI findings in Devic's neuromyelitis optica. J Neurol Neurosurg Psychiatry 1996;60:382–387.
10. Wingerchuk DM, Hogancamp WF, O'Brien PC, Weinshenker BG. The clinical course of neuromyelitis optica (Devic's syndrome). Neurology 1999;53:1107–1114.
11. Kidd D, Burton B, Plant, GT, Graham EM. Chronic relapsing idiopathic optic neuropathy. Brain 2003;126:276–284.
12. Tippett DS, Fishman PS, Panitch HS. Relapsing transverse myelitis. Neurology 1991;41:703–706.
13. Pandit L, Rao S. Recurrent myelitis. J Neurol Neurosurg Psychiatry 1996;60:336–338.
14. Kim K. Idiopathic recurrent transverse myelitis. Arch Neurol 2003;60:1290–1294.
15. Wingerchuk DM. Delayed evolution of recurrent transverse myelitis into relapsing neuromyelitis optica. Can J Neurol Sci 2002;29(Suppl 1):S87.
16. Weinshenker BG. Neuromyelitis optica: what it is and what it might be. Lancet 2003;361:889–890.
17. Bonnet F, Mercie P, Morlat P, et al. Devic's neuromyelitis optica during pregnancy in a patient with systemic lupus erythematosus. Lupus 1999;8:244–247.
18. Mochizuki A, Hayashi A, Hisahara S, Shoji S. Steroid-responsive Devic's variant in Sjogren's syndrome. Neurology 2000;54:1391–1392.
19. Wingerchuk DM. Neuromyelitis optica: update. Front Biosci 2004;9:834–840.
20. Wingerchuk DM, Weinshenker BG. Neuromyelitis optica: clinical predictors of a relapsing course and survival. Neurology 2003;60:848–853.
21. Thielen KR, Miller GM. Multiple sclerosis of the spinal cord: magnetic resonance appearance. J Comput Assist Tomogr 1996;20:434–438.
22. Filippi M, Rocca MA, Moiola L, et al. MRI and magnetization transfer imaging changes in the brain and cervical cord of patients with Devic's neuromyelitis optica. Neurology 1999;53:1705–1710.
23. Andersson M, Alvarez-Cermeno J, Bernardi G, et al. Cerebrospinal fluid in the diagnosis of multiple sclerosis: a consensus report. J Neurol Neurosurg Psychiatry 1994;57:897–902.
24. Rudick RA, Cookfair DL, Simonian NA, et al. Cerebrospinal fluid abnormalities in a phase III trial of Avonex (IFNbeta-1a) for relapsing multiple sclerosis. The Multiple Sclerosis Collaborative Research Group. J Neuroimmunol 1999;93:8–14.
25. Papais-Alvarenga RM, Miranda-Santos CM, Puccioni-Sohler M, et al. Optic neuromyelitis syndrome in Brazilian patients. J Neurol Neurosurg Psychiatry 2002;73:429–435.
26. de Seze J, Stojkovic T, Ferriby D, et al. Devic's neuromyelitis optica: clinical, laboratory, MRI and outcome profile. J Neurol Sci 2002;197:57–61.
27. de Seze J, Lebrun C, Stojkovic T, Ferriby D, Chatel M, Vermersch P. Is Devic's neuromyelitis optica a separate disease? A comparative study with multiple sclerosis. Multiple Sclerosis 2003;9:521–525.

28. Weinshenker BG, Wingerchuk DM, Lucchinetti CF, Lennon VA. A marker autoantibody discriminates neuromyelitis optica from multiple sclerosis. Neurology 2003;60(Suppl 1):A520.

29. Lennon VA, Lucchinetti CF, Weinshenker BG. Identification of a marker autoantibody of neuromyelitis optica. Neurology 2003;60(Suppl 1):A519–A520.

30. Mirsattari SM, Johnston JB, McKenna R, et al. Aboriginals with multiple sclerosis: HLA types and predominance of neuromyelitis optica. Neurology 2001;56:317–323.

31. Phillips PH, Newman NJ, Lynn MJ. Optic neuritis in African Americans. Arch Neurol 1998;55:186–192.

32. Osuntokun BO. The pattern of neurological illness in tropical Africa: experience at Ibadan, Nigeria. J Neurol Sci 1971;12:417–442.

33. Cabre P, Heinzlef O, Merle H, et al. MS and neuromyelitis optica in Martinique (French West Indies). Neurology 2001;56:507–514.

34. Jain S, Maheshwari MC. Multiple sclerosis: Indian experience in the last thirty years. Neuroepidemiology 1985;4:96–107.

35. Okinaka S, Tsubaki K, Kuroiwa Y, Toyokura Y, Imamura Y, Yoshikawa M. Multiple sclerosis and allied diseases in Japan: clinical characteristics. Neurology 1958;8:756–763.

36. Kira J. Multiple sclerosis in the Japanese population. Lancet Neurology 2003;2:117–127.

37. Misu T, Fujihara K, Nakashima I, et al. Pure optico-spinal form of multiple sclerosis in Japan. Brain 2002;125: 2460–2468.

38. McAlpine D. Familial neuromyelitis optica: its occurrence in identical twins. Brain 1938;61:430–438.

39. Ch'ien LT, Medeiros MO, Belluomini JJ, Lemmi H, Whitaker JN. Neuromyelitis optica (Devic's syndrome) in two sisters. Clinical Electroencephalography 1982;13:36–39.

40. Keegan BM, Weinshenker B. Familial Devic's disease. Can J Neurol Sci 2000;27(Suppl 2), S57–S58.

41. Yamakawa K, Kuroda M, Fujihara K, et al. Familial neuromyelitis optica (Devic's syndrome) with late onset in Japan. Neurology 2000;55:318–320.

42. Kuroiwa Y, Igata A, Itahara K, et al. Nationwide survey of multiple sclerosis in Japan: clinical analysis of 1,084 cases. Neurology 1975;25:845–851.

43. Cock H, Mandler R, Ahmed W, Schapira AH. Neuromyelitis optica (Devic's syndrome): no association with the primary mitochondrial DNA mutations found in Leber hereditary optic neuropathy. J Neurol Neurosurg Psychiatry 1997;62:85–87.

44. Kalman B, Mandler RN. Studies of mitochondrial DNA in Devic's disease revealed no pathogenic mutations, but polymorphisms also found in association with multiple sclerosis. Ann Neurol 2002;51:661–662.

45. Herrera BM, Ebers GC. Progress in deciphering the genetics of multiple sclerosis. Curr Opin Neurol 2003;16:253–258.

46. Ono T, Zambenedetti MR, Yamasaki K, et al. Molecular analysis of HLA class (HLA-A and -B) and HLA class II (HLA-DRB1) genes in Japanese patients with multiple sclerosis (Western type and Asian type). Tiss Antigens 1998;52:539–542.

47. Yamasaki K, Horiuchi I, Minohara M, et al. HLA-DPB1*0501-associated opticospinal multiple sclerosis: clinical, neuroimaging and immunogenetic studies. Brain 1999;122:1689–1696.

48. Fukazawa T, Kikuchi S, Sasaki H, Yabe I, Miyagishi R, Hamada T, Tashiro K. Genomic HLA profiles of MS in Hokkaido, Japan: important role of DPB1*0501 allele. J Neurol 2000;247:175–178.

49. Fukazawa T, Yamasaki K, Ito H, et al. Both the HLA-DPB1 and -DRB1 alleles correlate with risk for multiple sclerosis in Japanese: clinical phenotypes and gender as important factors. Tiss Antigens 2000;55:199–205.

50. Kikuchi S, Fukazawa T, Niino M, et al. HLA-related subpopulations of MS in Japanese with and without oligoclonal IgG bands. Neurology 2003;60:647–651.

51. Hensiek AE, Sawcer SJ, Feakes R, Deans J, Mander A, Akesson E, et al. HLA-DR 15 is associated with female sex and younger age at diagnosis in multiple sclerosis. J Neurol Neurosurg Psychiatry 2002;72:184–187.

52. Horiuchi I, Kawano Y, Yamasaki K, et al. Th1 dominance in HAM/TSP and the optico-spinal form of multiple sclerosis versus Th2 dominance in mite antigen-specific IgE myelitis. J Neurol Sci 2000;172:17–24.

53. Ochi H, Wu X-M, Osoegawa M, et al. Tc1/Tc2 and Th1/Th2 balance in Asian and Western types of multiple sclerosis, HTLV-I-associated myelopathy/tropical spastic paraparesis and hyperIgEaemic myelitis. J Neuroimmunol 2001;119: 297–305.

54. Wu X-M, Osoegawa M, Yamasaki K, et al. Flow cytometric differentiation of Asian and Western types of multiple sclerosis, HTLV-1-associated myelopathy/tropical spastic paraparesis (HAM/TSP) and hyperIgEaemic myelitis by analyses of memory CD4 positive T cell subsets and NK cell subsets. J Neurol Sci 2000;177:24–31.

55. Nakashima I, Fujihara K, Misu T, et al. A comparative study of Japanese multiple sclerosis patients with and without oligocolonal IgG bands. Multiple Sclerosis 2002;8:459–462.

56. Nakashima I, Fujihara K, Fujimori J, Narikawa K, Misu T, Itoyama Y. Absence of IgG1 response in the cerebrospinal fluid of relapsing neuromyelitis optica. Neurology 2004;62:144–146.

57. Nakashima I, Fujihara K, Misu T, Okita N, Takase S, Itoyama Y. Significant correlation between IL-10 levels and IgG indices in the cerebrospinal fluid of patients with multiple sclerosis. J Neuroimmunol 2000;111:64–67.

58. Mandler RN, Dencoff JD, Midani F, Ford CC, Ahmed W, Rosenberg GA. Matrix metalloproteinases in cerebrospinal fluid differ in multiple sclerosis and Devic's neuromyelitis optica. Brain 2001;124:493–498.

59. Satoh J, Yukitake M, Kurohara K, Takashima H, Yasuo K. Detection of the 14-3-3 protein in the cerebrospinal fluid of Japanese multiple sclerosis patients presenting with severe myelitis. J Neurol Sci 2003;212:11–20.

60. Irani DN, Kerr DA. 14-3-3 protein in the cerebrospinal fluid of patients with acute myelitis. Lancet 2000;355:901.

61. Martinez-Yelamos A, Saiz A, Sanchez-Valle R, et al. 14-3-3 protein in the CSF as a prognostic marker in early multiple sclerosis. Neurology 2001;57:722–724.

62. Lucchinetti CF, Mandler RN, McGavern D, et al. A role for humoral mechanisms in the pathogenesis of Devic's neuromyelitis optica. Brain 2002;125:1450–1461.

63. Ortiz de Zarate JC, Tamaroff L, Sica RE, Rodriguez JA. Neuromyelitis optica versus subacute necrotic myelitis. II. Anatomical study of two cases. J Neurol Neurosurg Psychiatry 1968;31:641–645.

64. Lefkowitz D, Angelo JN. Neuromyelitis optica with unusual vascular changes. Arch Neurol 1984;41:1103–1105.

65. Stefferl A, Brehm U, Storch M, et al. Myelin oligodendrocyte glycoprotein induces experimental autoimmune encephalomyelitis in the 'resistant' Brown Norway rat: disease susceptibility is determined by MHC and MHC-linked effects on the B cell response. J Immunol 1999;163:40–49.

66. Storch MK, Stefferl A, Brehm U, et al. Autoimmunity to myelin oligodendrocyte glycoprotein in rats mimics the spectrum of multiple sclerosis pathology. Brain Pathol 1998;8:681–694.

67. Weinshenker BG, O'Brien PC, Petterson TM, et al. A randomized trial of plasma exchange in acute central nervous system inflammatory demyelinating disease. Ann Neurol 1999;46:878–886.

68. Keegan M, Pineda AA, McClelland RL, Darby CH, Rodriguez M, Weinshenker BG. Plasma exchange for severe attacks of demyelination: predictors of response. Neurology 2001;58:143–146.

69. Noseworthy JH, Weinshenker BG, Lucchinetti C, Rodriguez M. Multiple sclerosis. N Engl J Med 2000;343:938–952.

70. Itoyama Y, Saida T, Tashiro K, Sato T, Ohashi Y, The Interferon-beta Multiple Sclerosis Research Group in Japan. Japanese multicenter, randomized, double-blind trial of interferon beta-1b in relapsing-remitting multiple sclerosis: two year results. Ann Neurol 2000;48:487.

71. Bergamaschi R, Uggetti C, Tonietti S, Egitto MG, Cosi V. A case of relapsing neuromyelitis optica treated with glatiramer acetate. J Neurol 2003;250:359–361.

72. Mandler RN, Ahmed W, Dencoff JE. Devic's neuromyelitis optica: a prospective study of seven patients treated with prednisone and azathioprine. Neurology 1998;51:1219–1220.

73. Hartung HP, Gonsette R, Konig N, et al. Mitoxantrone in progressive multiple sclerosis: a placebo-controlled, double-blind, randomized, multicenter trial. Lancet 2002;360:2018–2025.

74. Goodin DS, Arnason BG, Coyle PK, Frohman EM, Paty DW. The use of mitoxantrone (Novantrone) for the treatment of multiple sclerosis: report of the Therapeutic and Technology Assessment Subcommittee of the American Academy of Neurology. Neurology 2003;61:1332–1338.

75. Silverman GJ, Weisman S. Rituximab therapy and autoimmune disorders. Prospects for anti-B cell therapy. Arthritis Rheum 2003;48:1484–1492.

CME QUESTIONS

1. Which cerebrospinal fluid finding is more suggestive of neuromyelitis optica than of typical multiple sclerosis?
   A. A leukocyte count of less than 10 white blood cells/mm^2
   B. Presence of oligoclonal banding
   C. Presence of neutrophils
   D. Increased immunoglobulin-G index

2. The strongest independent clinical predictor of a relapsing disease course in neuromyelitis optica is:
   A. Severity of initial myelitis attack
   B. Increased interval between the first and second attacks
   C. Bilateral optic neuritis at disease onset
   D. Male gender

3. Which of the following pathological features of the spinal cord is *not* characteristic of neuromyelitis optica?
   A. Deposition of complement
   B. Vascular hyalinization
   C. Polymorphonuclear cell infiltrate
   D. Vasculitis

4. A 45-yr-old woman with relapsing neuromyelitis optica experiences an attack of ascending cervical myelitis and develops neurogenic respiratory failure despite intravenous corticosteroids. The most appropriate rescue therapy at this point is:
   A. A second course of intravenous corticosteroids
   B. Plasmapheresis
   C. Intravenous immune globulin
   D. Mitoxantrone

11

Transverse Myelitis

Clinical Manifestations, Pathogenesis, and Management

Chitra Krishnan, Adam I. Kaplin, Deepa M. Deshpande, Carlos A. Pardo, and Douglas A. Kerr

1. INTRODUCTION

First described in 1882, and termed *acute transverse myelitis* (TM) in 1948 *(1)*, TM is a rare syndrome with an incidence of between one and eight new cases per million people per year *(2)*. TM is characterized by focal inflammation within the spinal cord and clinical manifestations are caused by resultant neural dysfunction of motor, sensory, and autonomic pathways within and passing through the inflamed area. There is often a clearly defined rostral border of sensory dysfunction and evidence of acute inflammation demonstrated by a spinal magnetic resonance imaging (MRI) and lumbar puncture. When the maximal level of deficit is reached, approx 50% of patients have lost all movements of their legs, virtually all patients have some degree of bladder dysfunction, and 80 to 94% of patients have numbness, paresthesias, or band-like dysesthesias *(2–7)*. Autonomic symptoms consist variably of increased urinary urgency, bowel or bladder incontinence, difficulty or inability to void, incomplete evacuation or bowel, constipation, and sexual dysfunction *(8)*. Like multiple sclerosis (MS) *(9)*, TM is the clinical manifestation of a variety of disorders with distinct presentations and pathologies *(10)*. Recently, we proposed a diagnostic and classification scheme that has defined TM as either idiopathic or associated with a known inflammatory disease (i.e., MS, systemic lupus erythematosus [SLE], Sjogren's syndrome, or neurosarcoidosis) *(11)*. Most TM patients have monophasic disease, although up to 20% will have recurrent inflammatory episodes within the spinal cord (Johns Hopkins Transverse Myelitis Center [JHTMC] case series, unpublished data) *(12,13)*.

2. DIAGNOSTIC CLASSIFICATION OF TRANSVERSE MYELITIS

TM exists in a series of neuroinflammatory central nervous system (CNS) conditions, characterized by abrupt neurological deficits associated with inflammatory cell infiltrates and demyelination. This can occur as a single episode (e.g., TM, optic neuritis [ON], or acute disseminated encephalomyelitis [ADEM]) or as a multiphasic condition (e.g., recurrent TM, recurrent ON, neuromyelitis optica [NMO], and MS). The pathophysiological cause of recurrence is unknown but of obvious clinical significance. This spectrum of neuroinflammatory CNS conditions also varies based on regional involvement of the CNS, ranging from monofocal involvement (e.g., TM involving the spinal cord, isolated ON involving the optic nerve, and ADEM involving the brain and spinal cord) to multifocal involvement (e.g., NMO involving the optic nerve and spinal cord and MS involving any area in the central neuraxis). Because there is no consensus

From: *Current Clinical Neurology: Inflammatory Disorders of the Nervous System: Pathogenesis, Immunology, and Clinical Management*
Edited by: A. Minagar and J. S. Alexander © Humana Press Inc., Totowa, NJ

Table 1
Diagnostic Criteria for Transverse Myelitis

Inclusion criteria
- Motor, sensory, or autonomic dysfunction attributable to the spinal cord
- Bilateral signs and/or symptoms
- Clearly defined sensory level
- Inflammation defined by CSF pleocytosis *or* elevated IgG index *or* gadolinium enhancement
- Progression to nadir between 4 h and 21 d

Exclusion criteria
- Radiation to spine in the past 10 yr
- Clear arterial distribution clinical deficit consistent with thrombosis of the anterior spinal artery
- Extra-axial compressive etiology by neuroimaging
- Abnormal flow voids on the surface of the spinal cord consistent with AVM
- Serologic or clinical evidence of connective tissue disease, such as sarcoidosis, Behcet's disease, Sjogren's syndrome, SLE, and mixed connective tissue disorder (diagnostic of connective-tissue-associated TM)
- History of clinically apparent optic neuritis (diagnostic of neuromyelitis optica)
- CNS manifestations of syphilis, Lyme disease, HIV, HTLV-1, mycoplasma, or other viral infection such as HSV-1, HSV-2, VZV, EBV, CMV, HHV-6, and enteroviruses (diagnostic of infectious myelitis)
- Brain and spinal cord MRI abnormalities suggestive of MS and presence of oligoclonal bands in CSF (suggestive of TM associated with MS. Apply McDonald criteria to define MS)

CSF, cerebrospinal fluid; IgG, immunoglobulin-G; AVM, arteriovenous malformation; SLE, systemic lupus erythematosus; TM, transverse myelitis; HIV, human immunodeficiency virus; HTLV-1, human T-cell lymphotropic virus-1; HSV, herpes simplex virus; VZV, varicella zoster virus; EBV, Epstein-Barr virus; CMV, cytomegalovirus; HHV, human herpes virus; MRI, magnetic resonance imaging; MS, multiple sclerosis.

explanation, the cause for this regional specificity is a subject of considerable research interest. We speculate that this regional specification could result from differences inherent in CNS tissue at different sites (e.g., varying threshold for injury or distinct localization of signal transduction machinery or antigens) or from differential access to distinct regions of the CNS by exogenous pathogenic mechanisms.

Acute transverse myelopathy (which includes noninflammatory causes) and TM have often been used interchangeably throughout the published literature. Most recently, we proposed diagnostic criteria for distinguishing TM from noninflammatory myelopathies and for distinguishing idiopathic TM from TM associated with multifocal CNS and multisystemic inflammatory disorders. These criteria are summarized in Table 1. A diagnosis of TM requires confirmation of inflammation within the spinal cord by MRI and lumbar puncture. Markers of inflammation include gadolinium-enhanced spinal MRI, cerebrospinal fluid (CSF) pleocytosis and/or elevated immunoglobulin-G (IgG) index *(11)*. If none of the inflammatory criteria are met at symptom onset, MRI and lumbar puncture evaluation should be repeated between 2 and 7 d following symptom onset. IgG synthesis rate is a less specific indicator of CNS inflammation than is CSF IgG index *(14,15)* and should not be used in diagnosis. Vascular myelopathies can be differentiated from TM by a progression of symptoms to maximal severity in less than 4 h and the lack of inflammation as defined above; however, these criteria do not completely distinguish vascular myelopathies from TM, because myelopathies associated with venous infarcts or vascular malformations may progress more slowly and may meet the other criteria for TM.

Differentiating idiopathic TM from TM attributed to an underlying disease is also important. Many systemic inflammatory disorders (e.g., sarcoidosis, SLE, Behçet's disease, Sjögren's syndrome) may involve the nervous system, and TM may be one of the possible presentations. Therefore, all patients presenting with TM should be investigated for the presence of systemic inflammatory disease. Important historical information should be obtained from the patient regarding the presence of rashes, night sweats, oral or genital ulcers, sicca symptoms, shortness of breath, pleuritic pain, and hematuria. Examination should attempt to detect the presence of uveitis or retinitis, decreased lacrimation or salivation, skin rash (malar, livedo reticularis, erythema nodosum), oral or genital ulcers, adenopathy, pleuritic or pericardial friction rub, and organomegaly. Laboratory studies should include a complete blood count with differential and smear, antinuclear antibodies (ANA), SS-A, SS-B, erythrocyte sedimentation rate , and complement. Additional laboratory testing may be required if signs of systemic vasculitis are detected.

From this evaluation, it may be possible to distinguish idiopathic TM from disease-associated TM (i.e., TM associated with multifocal CNS disease or systemic inflammatory disease). This distinction is important because patients at high risk of developing MS may be evaluated more closely or may be offered immunomodulatory treatment *(16)*. Similarly, patients with disease-associated TM may need to be closely followed for recurrent systemic and neurological complications and should be offered immunosuppressive treatment to decrease the risk of recurrence.

3. CLINICAL MANIFESTATIONS OF TM

3.1. Epidemiology

TM affects individuals of all ages with bimodal peaks between the ages of 10 and 19 yr and 30 and 39 yr *(2–5)*. There are approx 1400 new cases diagnosed in the United States each year, and approx 34,000 people have chronic morbidity from TM at any given time. About 28% of reported TM cases are in children (JHTMC case series). There is no gender or familial predisposition to TM.

A preceding illness including nonspecific symptoms, such as fever, nausea, and muscle pain, has been reported in about 40% of pediatric cases within 3 wk of the onset of the disorder *(17,18,JHTMC)*. Thirty percent of pediatric TM cases referred to an academic center had a history of an immunization with 1 mo of the onset of symptoms (JHTMC case series). Although a history of an immunization preceding the onset of TM is commonly reported, there is insufficient information about the relationship between immunization and TM.

3.2. Clinical Symptoms

TM is characterized clinically by acute or subacute signs of neurological dysfunction in motor, sensory, and autonomic nerves and nerve tracts of the spinal cord. Weakness is described as a rapidly progressive paraparesis starting with the legs and occasionally progresses to involve the arms. Flaccidity may be noted initially with gradually appearing pyramidal signs by the second week of the illness. A sensory level can be documented in most cases. In adults, the most common sensory level is the midthoracic region, although children may have a higher frequency of cervical spinal cord involvement and a cervical sensory level (JHTMC case series). Pain may occur in the back, extremities, or abdomen. Paresthesias are a common initial symptom in adults with TM but are unusual for children *(19)*. Autonomic symptoms consist variably of increased urinary urgency, bowel or bladder incontinence, difficulty or inability to void, incomplete evacuation, or bowel constipation *(8)*. Another common result of sensory and autonomic nervous system involvement in TM is sexual dysfunction *(20,21)*. Genital anesthesia from pudendal nerve involvement (S2–S4) results in impaired sensation in men and women. Additional male sexual problems involving parasympathetic (S2–S4) and sympathetic (T10–L2) dysfunction in TM patients include erectile dysfunction, ejaculatory disorders, and difficulty reaching orgasm. Corresponding female sexual problems include reduced lubrication and difficulty reaching orgasm.

In addition to the signs and symptoms of direct spinal cord involvement by the immune system in TM, there also appears to be indirect effects, such as depression and selective cognitive impairment that are reminiscent of that described in MS (unpublished observations) *(22)*. This depression or cognitive impairment does not correlate significantly with the patient's degree of physical disability and can have lethal consequences resulting in suicide in severe cases, if left untreated. In fact, in our case series, depression resulting in suicide was the leading cause of mortality, accounting for 60% of the deaths we have seen in our clinic (unpublished observations).

When the maximal level of deficit is reached, approx 50% of patients have lost all movements of their legs, virtually all patients have some degree of bladder dysfunction, and 80 to 94% of patients have numbness, paresthesias, or band-like dysesthesias *(2–7)*. More than 80% of the patients reach their clinical nadir within 10 d of the onset of symptoms *(18)*. Although the temporal course may vary, neurological function usually progressively worsens during the acute phase, typically d 4–21 *(11)*.

A spinal MRI and lumbar puncture often show evidence of acute inflammation *(2–4,7,10,23,24)*. In our case series of 170 idiopathic TM patients, spinal MRI showed a cervical T2-signal abnormality in 44% and a thoracic T2-signal abnormality in 37% of cases. Five percent of patients had multi-focal lesions, and 6% showed a T1 hypointense lesion. This corresponded to the following clinical sensory levels: 22% cervical, 63% thoracic, 9% lumbar, 6% sacral, and no sensory level in 7%. The rostral-caudal extent of lesions ranged from one vertebral segment in many to spanning the entire spinal cord in two patients. In 74% of patients, the T2 lesion also enhanced with gadolinium. Forty-two percent of patients had a CSF pleocytosis with a mean white blood cell count of 38 ± 13 cells (range 0–950 cells).Fifty percent of patients revealed an elevated protein level (mean protein level 75 ± 14 g/dL).

3.3. TM Differs From Guillain-Barré Syndrome

TM is often misdiagnosed as acute inflammatory demyelinating polyradiculoneuropathy (AIDP) or Guillain-Barré syndrome (GBS) because both conditions may present with rapidly progressive sensory and motor loss principally involving the lower extremities. Table 2 illustrates key differences between these conditions. A pure paraplegia or paraparesis with a corresponding distribution of sensory loss may favor TM, whereas GBS may present with a gradient of motor and sensory loss involving the lower extremities more than the upper extremities. When weakness and sensory loss involves both the upper and lower extremities equally with a distinct spinal cord level, TM involving the cervical region is more likely than GPS. Pathologically brisk deep tendon reflexes are supportive of TM, although patients with fulminant TM that includes significant destruction of spinal cord gray matter may present with hypotonia and have decreased or absent deep tendon reflexes. Urinary urgency or retention is a common early finding in TM and is less common in GBS. In GBS, dysesthetic pain, involvement of the upper extremity and cranial nerve 7, and absent deep tendon reflexes involving the upper extremities are more common findings. An MRI of the spinal cord may show an area of inflammation in TM but not in GBS. Although CSF fluid findings in TM are not consistent and an elevated cell count may be absent, there is usually a moderate lymphocytic pleocytosis and elevated protein level. This contrasts the albumino-cytologic dissociation of the CSF seen in GBS *(18)*.

3.4. Distinction From Noninflammatory Myelopathies

Vascular myelopathy may be fairly easy to recognize in the setting of an anterior spinal artery infarct (sudden onset of symptoms with relative preservation of posterior column function). On the other hand, it may be more difficult to recognize in the setting of a venous infarct or vascular malformation. Venous infarct may be suspected when a clinical history and serologic studies suggest a prothrombotic state (deep venous thrombosis, pulmonary embolus, livedo reticularis,

Table 2
Distinguishing Features of Transverse Myelitis and Guillain-Barré

Characteristics	Transverse myelitis	Guillain-Barré syndrome
Motor	Paraparesis or quadriparesis	Ascending weakness (greater in lower extremities than in upper extremities in the early stages)
Sensory	Usually can identify a spinal cord level	Ascending sensory loss (greater in lower extremities than in upper extremities in the early stages)
Autonomic	Early loss of bowel and bladder function	Dysfunction of the cardiovascular system
Cranial nerve	No involvement	EOM palsies or facial weakness
Electrophysiology	EMG/NCV may be normal or may implicate the spinal cord: prolonged central conduction on SEP latencies or missing SEP in conjunction with normal sensory nerve action potentials	EMG/NCV confined to the PNS: motor and/or sensory nerve conduction velocity reduced, and distal latencies prolonged, conduction block, reduced H reflex usually present
MRI	Usually a focal area of increased T2 signal with or without gadolinium enhancement	Normal
CSF	Usually CSF pleocytosis and/or increased IgG index	Usually elevated protein in the absence of CSF pleocytosis

EOM, extra-ocular muscle; EMG, electromyography; NCV, nerve conduction velocity; SEP, somatosensory evoked potential; PNS, peripheral nervous system; MRI, magnetic resonance imaging; CSF, cerebrospinal fluid; IgG, immunoglobulin-G.

antiphospholipid antibodies, factor V Leiden mutation, antigen-presenting *cell* resistance, or pro-thrombin gene mutation). A vascular malformation (dural arteriovenous [AV] fistula, arteriovenous malformation [AVM], cavernous angioma) may be suspected if imaging suggests the presence of flow voids or bleeding into the spinal cord. A dural AV fistula is most likely to occur in men older than 40 and may present with a *stuttering* or progressive myelopathy. Patients with a dural AV fistula may report a postural dependence of symptoms, and pain is usually a prominent feature. Spinal angiography is the diagnostic study of choice to define the presence of a vascular malformation. Surgical or endovascular treatment may result in stabilization or clinical improvement in a substantial proportion of patients *(25–27)*.

Fibrocartilagenous embolism is a rare (although likely underreported) cause of acute myelopathy *(28–31)*. In most reports, there has been a sudden increase in intrathoracic or intra-abdominal pressure prior to the onset of symptoms, and in several autopsies, fibrocartilagenous material was found to have embolized to the spinal cord. The most likely explanation for these findings is that the nucleus pulposis herniated vertically into the vertebral body sinusoids in response to markedly elevated pressure, followed by further herniation through vascular channels into the spinal cord parenchyma. Fibrocartilagenous embolism should be suspected when a patient has a sudden onset of myelopathy that reaches its maximal severity within hours or if a patient has an antecedent elevation of intra-abdominal or intrathoracic pressure. Imaging may show acute loss of intervertebral disk height and vertebral body end-plate changes adjacent to an area of T2-signal abnormality within the spinal cord. Table 3 lists some of the radiological features that distinguish various acute myelopathies.

Radiation myelopathy may develop at any time up to 15 yr after ionizing radiation. Pathological studies show preferential involvement of myelinated tissue and blood vessels, and it is likely that cellular death of oligodendrocytes and endothelial cells contributes to the clinical disorder *(32)*.

Table 3
Differential Diagnoses Based on Radiologic Features

Differential Diagnosis	Radiologic Features
Cavernous angioma or dural AV fistula	Blood within the spinal cord (bright and dark T1 and T2 signal)
Dural AV fistula or AVM	Flow voids within spinal cord
Venous hypertensive myelopathy	Central T2 signal abnormality
Infection or tumor	Ring-enhancing lesion
Fibrocartilagenous embolism	Acute loss of vertical intervertebral disc height and corresponding T2 signal abnormality
Neuromyelitis optica or disease-associated TM	Fusiform lesion extending over >3 spinal cord segments
MS	T2 bright lesion in white matter occupying <2 spinal cord segments in rostral-caudal extent and less than 50% of the cord diameter
Dynamic spinal cord compression only during flexion or extension	T2 spinal cord lesion adjacent to disk herniation or spondylitic ridge, but lack of spinal cord compression (flexion-extension x-ray to determine the presence of abnormal spinal column mobility; MRI in flexion or extended position instead of in neutral position)

AV, arteriovenous; AVM, arteriovenous malformation; TM, transverse myelitis; MS, multiple sclerosis; MRI, magnetic resonance, imaging.

Patients may present with slowly progressive spasticity, weakness, hyperreflexia, and urinary urgency. There is often a corresponding T2-signal abnormality that is nonenhancing and preferentially affects the more superficial spinal cord white matter. Although anticoagulation (*33,34*) or hyperbaric oxygen (*35–37*) have been proposed as treatment options, neither has been clearly shown to be effective in patients with radiation myelopathy.

3.5. Monophasic vs Recurrent TM

Of TM patients, 75–90% experience monophasic disease and have no evidence of multisystemic or multiphasic disease. Most commonly, symptoms stop progressing after 2–3 wk, and CSF and MRI abnormalities stabilize and begin to resolve. There are several features, however, that predict recurrent disease (Table 4). Patients with multifocal lesions within the spinal cord, demyelinating lesions in the brain, oligoclonal bands in the spinal fluid, mixed connective tissue disorder, or serum auto-antibodies (most notably SS-A) are at a greater risk of recurrence (*38*) compared to patients who do not have these findings. Preliminary studies suggest that patients who have persistently abnormal CSF cytokine profiles (notably interleukin [IL]-6) may also be at increased risk for recurrent TM, although these findings must be validated before they are used clinically (unpublished data). We do not understand the relative contribution of these factors and thus cannot gauge whether chronic immunomodulatory treatment is warranted in high-risk patients.

3.6. Discrimination From Multiple Sclerosis

TM can be the presenting feature of MS. Patients who are ultimately diagnosed with MS are more likely to have asymmetric clinical findings, predominant sensory symptoms with relative sparing of motor systems, MR lesions extending over fewer than two spinal segments, abnormal brain MRI, and oligoclonal bands in the CSF (*23,39–43*). A patient with monofocal CNS demyelination (TM or ON) whose brain MRI shows lesions consistent with demyelination (*44*) has an 83% chance of meeting clinical criteria for MS over the subsequent decade compared with 11% of such patients with normal brain MRI (*45*).

Table 4
Distinguishing Features of Monophasic and Recurrent Transverse Myelitis

Characteristics	Monophasic	Recurrent
MRI		
• Spine	• Single T2 lesion	• Multiple distinct lesions or fusiform lesion extending over ≥3 spinal cord segments
• Brain	• Normal	• T2/FLAIR abnormalities
Blood		
• Serology	• Normal	• Presence of autoantibodies (ANA, dsDNA, phospholipids, c-ANCA)
• SS-A	• Negative	• Positive
CSF		
• Oligoclonal Bands	• Negative	• Positive
Other		
• Systemic disease	• None	• Connective tissue disorder
• Involvement of the optic nerve	• None	• Likely

MRI, magnetic resonance imaging; FLAIR, fluid attenuated inversion recovery; ANA, anti-nuclear antibody; dsDNA, double-stranded DNA; c-ANCA, c-anti-neutrophil cytoplasmic antibody; CSF, cerebrospinal fluid.

4. IMMUNOPATHOGENESIS OF TM

4.1. Pathogenesis of TM

Much of the pathology of acute myelopathies has been described in clinicopathological case reports *(46–48)*. Pathological data from autopsies and biopsies of suspicious spinal cord lesions from patients later found to have TM studied at the JHTMC (unpublished data) revealed inflammatory changes. These pathologic abnormalities invariably included focal infiltration by monocytes and lymphocytes into segments of the spinal cord and perivascular spaces and astroglial and microglial activation (Fig. 1) *(49)*. The magnitude and extension of these inflammatory features vary and are determined by the etiological factors and the temporal profile of the myelopathic changes. The presence of white matter changes, demyelination, and axonal injury is prominent in postinfectious myelitis, although involvement of the central compartment of the cord, gray matter, or neurons is also prominent in some cases, a finding that supports the view that both gray- and white-matter compartments may be equally affected in TM. In some biopsies obtained during the acute phases of myelitis, infiltration of CD4+ and CD8+ lymphocytes, along with an increased presence of monocytes, is quite prominent. In biopsies obtained during subacute phases of myelopathic lesions, prominent monocyte and phagocytic-macrophage infiltration is observed. In some cases, autoimmune disorders, such as SLE, lead to vasculitic lesions that produce focal areas of spinal cord ischemia without prominent inflammation *(50)*. These immunopathological observations further confirm that TM is an immune-mediated disorder that involves cellular reactions and perhaps humoral factors that injure compartments of the spinal cord.

4.2. Immunopathogenesis of TM

The immunopathogenesis of TM varies. Several potential mechanisms have been proposed *(51)* to describe idiopathic TM. TM patients likely have abnormal activation of the immune system resulting in inflammation and injury within the spinal cord. An understanding of the immunopathogenesis of TM must account for abnormal or excessive incitement of immune activation and effector mechanisms by which immune activation leads to CNS injury.

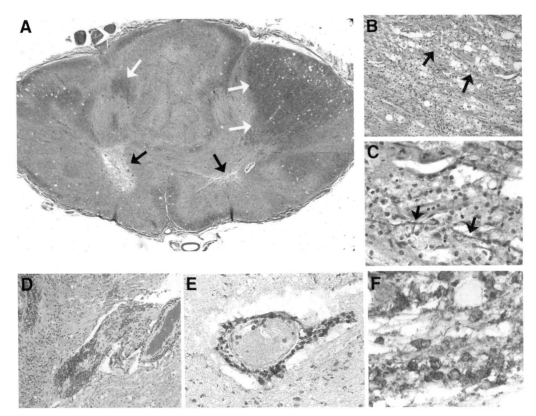

Fig. 1. Histology of TM. (**A**) Myelin staining of cervical spinal cord section from a patient who died during a subacute stage of TM. There are a few myelinated areas left (asterisk) and foci of cystic degeneration in the anterior horns (arrow). The remaining spinal cord shows chronic inflammation and demyelination (Luxol Fast Blue/hematoxyline eosin [LFB/HE] stain). (**B**) An area of demyelination from the same spinal cord as A that shows areas of active myelin and fiber degeneration (LFB/HE stain). (**C**) High magnification view of the few myelinated fibers left in areas of active inflammation (LFB/HE stain). (**D**) Focal area of acute inflammation and perivascular accumulation of inflammatory cells seen in a biopsy obtained from a patient with acute TM (H&E stain). (**E**) Perivascular infiltration by T lymphocytes as demonstrated by immunocytochemistry in an area of active inflammation in a patient with TM (CD3 immunostaining). (**F**) Infiltration by macrophages in an area of myelitis (HLA–Dr immunostaining). (Reproduced with permission, published in Front Biosci, 2004;9:1483–1499.)

4.2.1. Postvaccination TM

Several recent published reports note TM followed vaccination, including influenza *(52)* and booster hepatitis B vaccination *(53)*. Autopsy evaluation of patients with postvaccination TM revealed lymphocytic infiltration of the spinal cord with axonal loss and demyelination. The suggestion from these studies is that a vaccination may induce an autoimmune process resulting in TM; however, it should be noted that extensive data continues to show overwhelmingly that vaccinations are safe and are not associated with an increased incidence of neurological complications *(54–58)*. Therefore, such case reports must be viewed with caution, as it is entirely possible that two events occurred in close proximity by chance alone or for reasons that are only incidentally related to the vaccination procedure.

4.2.2. Parainfectious TM

In 30 to 60% of idiopathic TM cases, there is an antecedent respiratory, gastrointestinal, or systemic illness *(3,4,7,10,17)*. The term *parainfectious* has been used to suggest that the neurological injury may be associated with direct microbial infection and injury as a result of the infection, direct microbial infection with immune-mediated damage against the agent, or remote infection followed by a systemic response that induces neural injury. An expanding list of antecedent infections is now recognized, including herpes viruses and *Listeria monocytogenes,* although in the vast majority of these cases, causality has not been established.

Although in these cases, the infectious agent is required within the CNS, other mechanisms of autoimmunity discussed below, such as molecular mimicry and superantigen-mediated disease, require only peripheral immune activation and may account for other cases of TM.

4.2.3. Molecular Mimicry

Molecular mimicry as a mechanism to explain an inflammatory nervous system disorder has been best described in GBS. First referred to as an *acute postinfectious polyneuritis* by W. Osler in 1892, GBS is preceded 75% of the time by an acute infection *(59–62)*. *Campylobacter jejuni* infection has emerged as the most important antecedent event in GBS, occurring in up to 41% of cases *(63–66)*. Human neural tissue contains several subtypes of ganglioside moieties within its cell walls *(67,68)*. A characteristic component of human gangliosides, sialic acid *(69)* is also found as a surface antigen within the lipopolysaccharide outer coat of *C. jejuni (70)*. Antibodies against *C. jejuni* that crossreact with gangliosides have been found in serum from patients with GBS *(71–73)* and have been shown to bind peripheral nerves, fix complement, and impair neural transmission in experimental conditions that mimic GBS *(67,74–76)*. Susceptibility to the development of GBS also depends on host genetic factors, which are at least partly mediated by human leukocyte antigen alleles *(63,77)*.

Molecular mimicry in TM may be associated with the development of auto-antibodies in response to an antecedent infection. This etiology was postulated to be involved in the case of a patient who contracted TM following infection with *Enterobium vermicularis* (perianal pinworm) and was found to have elevated titers of crossreacting antibodies *(78)*.

4.2.4. Microbial Superantigen-Mediated Inflammation

Another link between an antecedent infection and the development of TM may be the fulminant activation of lymphocytes by microbial superantigens (SAGs). SAGs are microbial peptides that have a unique capacity to stimulate the immune system and may contribute to a variety of autoimmune diseases. The best-studied SAGs are staphylococcal enterotoxins A through I, toxic shock syndrome toxin-1, and *Streptococcus pyogenes* exotoxin, although many viruses also encode SAGs *(79–82)*. SAGs activate T lymphocytes in a unique manner compared to conventional antigens: instead of binding to the highly variable peptide groove of the T-cell receptor (TCR), SAGs interact with the more conserved $V\beta$ region *(83–86)*. Additionally, unlike conventional antigens, SAGs are capable of activating T lymphocytes in the absence of costimulatory molecules. As a result of these differences, a single SAG may activate between 2 and 20% of circulating T lymphocytes compared to 0.001 to 0.01% with conventional antigens *(87–89)*. Stimulation of large numbers of lymphocytes may trigger autoimmune disease by activating autoreactive T-cell clones *(90,91)*.

4.2.5. Humoral Derangements

Either of the above processes may result in abnormal immune function with blurred distinction between self and nonself. The development of abnormal antibodies potentially may then activate other components of the immune system or recruit additional cellular elements to the spinal cord. Recent studies have emphasized distinct autoantibodies in patients with NMO *(92–96)* and recurrent TM *(12,13,97)*. The high prevalence of various autoantibodies seen in such patients suggests polyclonal derangement of the immune system. Additionally, some auto-antibodies may initiate a direct and selective injury of neurons that contain antigens that crossreact with antibodies directed against infectious pathogens.

In addition to auto-antibodies, high levels of normal circulating antibodies may have a causative role in TM. A case of TM was described in a patient with extremely high serum and CSF antibody levels to hepatitis B surface antigen (HbsAg) following booster immunization *(98)*. Such circulating antibodies may form immune complexes that deposit in focal areas of the spinal cord. Such a mechanism has been proposed to describe a patient with recurrent TM and high titers of HbsAg *(99)*. Circulating immune complexes containing HbsAg were detected in the serum and CSF during the acute phase, and the disappearance of these complexes following treatment correlated with functional recovery.

Several Japanese patients with TM were found to have much higher serum IgE levels than MS patients or controls (360 vs 52 vs 85 U/mL) *(100)*. Virtually all of the patients in this study had specific serum IgE to household mites (*Dermatophagoides pteronyssinus* or *Dermatophagoides farinae*), whereas less than one-third of MS and control patients did. One potential mechanism to explain the TM in such patients is the deposition of IgE with subsequent recruitment of cellular elements. Indeed, biopsy specimens of two TM patients with elevated total and specific serum IgE revealed antibody deposition within the spinal cord, perivascular lymphocyte cuffing, and infiltration of eosinophils *(101)*. It was postulated that eosinophils recruited to the spinal cord degranulated and induced the neural injury in these patients.

4.3. Disease-Associated TM

The immunopathogenesis of disease associated TM has been described in the literature. For example, pathological data confirms that many cases of lupus-associated TM are associated with a CNS vasculitis *(102–104)*, whereas others may be associated with thrombotic infarction of the spinal cord *(105,106)*. Neurosarcoid is often associated with noncaseating granulomas within the spinal cord *(107)*, whereas TM associated with MS often has perivascular lymphocytic cuffing and mononuclear cell infiltration and with variable complement and antibody deposition *(108)*. Because these diseases have such varied (albeit poorly understood) immunopathogenic and effector mechanisms, we will not further discuss instances of disease-associated TM; rather, the subsequent discussion focuses on findings potentially related to idiopathic TM.

4.4. Putative Mechanisms of Immune-Mediated Central Nervous System Injury

We recently carried out a series of investigations that describe immune derangements in TM patients (Kaplin et al., unpublished). We found that IL-6 levels in the spinal fluid of TM patients were markedly elevated compared to control patients and to MS patients. Although relatively low levels of IL-6 in patients with MS did not correlate with disability, IL-6 levels in patients with TM strongly correlated with and were highly predictive of disability. IL-6 levels in a TM patient's CSF correlated with nitric oxide (NO) metabolites, which also correlated with disability. Thus, we suggest that marked upregulation of IL-6 as a result of immune system activation correlates with increased NO production and that this elevation is etiologically related to tissue injury leading to clinical disability in TM.

5. MANAGEMENT OF TM

5.1. Intravenous Steroids

Intravenous steroid treatment is often instituted for patients with acute TM. Corticosteroids have multiple mechanisms of action including anti-inflammatory activity, immunosuppressive properties, and antiproliferative actions *(109,110)*. Although there is no randomized double-blind placebo-controlled study that supports this approach, evidence from related disorders and clinical experience supports this treatment *(111–115)*. Additionally, there are several small studies that support intravenous steroid administration in patients with TM *(116–119)*. A study of five children with severe TM who received methylprednisolone (1 g/1.73 m^2/d) for 3 or 5 consecutive days followed by oral prednisone for 14 d reported beneficial effects compared to 10 historic controls *(118)*. In the steroid-treated group, the median time to walking was 23 d vs 97 d, full recovery occurred in 80% vs 10%, and full motor recovery at 1 yr was present in 100% vs 20%. No serious adverse effects from the steroid treatments occurred.

Other investigations have suggested that intravenous steroid administration may not be effective in TM patients *(18,19,120)*. The most significant of these reports *(120)* compared 12 TM patients seen between 1992 and 1994 who did not receive steroids to nine steroid-treated patients seen between 1995 and 1997. Although the authors claimed that there was no statistically significant difference in the outcomes between the groups, it is evident that the TM patients who received steroids were more likely to recover, and fewer had a poor outcome on the Barthel Index (33% vs 67%). Therefore, the available evidence suggests that intravenous steroids are somewhat effective if given in the acute phase of TM; however, these studies did not rigorously define TM and therefore likely included patients with noninflammatory myelopathies.

At our center, we routinely offer intravenous methylprednisolone (1000 mg) or dexamethasone (200 mg) for 3 to 5 d, unless there are compelling reasons to avoid this therapy. The decision to offer continued steroids or add a new treatment is often based on the clinical course and MRI appearance at the end of 5 d of steroids.

5.2. Plasma Exchange

Plasma exchange (PLEX) is often initiated in patients that have moderate to severe TM (i.e., inability to walk, markedly impaired autonomic function, and sensory loss in the lower extremities) and exhibit little clinical improvement within 5–7 d of intravenous steroids. PLEX is believed to work in autoimmune CNS diseases through the removal of specific or nonspecific soluble factors that are likely to mediate, be responsible for, or contribute to inflammatory-mediated target organ damage. PLEX has been shown to be effective in adults with TM and other inflammatory disorders of the CNS *(121–123)*. Predictors of good response to PLEX include early treatment (<20 d from symptom onset), male sex, and a clinically incomplete lesion (i.e., some motor function in the lower extremities, intact or brisk reflexes) *(124)*. It is our experience that PLEX may significantly improve outcomes of patients with severe (although incomplete) TM who have not significantly improved with intravenous steroids.

5.3. Other Immunomodulatory Treatment

No controlled information exists regarding the use of other treatment strategies in patients with acute TM. Some clinicians consider pulse-dose intravenous cyclophosphamide (500–1000 mg/m^2) for patients with TM who continue to progress despite intravenous steroid therapy. Cyclophosphamide, a bifunctional alkylating agent, forms reactive metabolites that crosslink DNA. This results in apoptosis of rapidly dividing immune cells and is believed to underlie the immunosuppressive properties of this medication. At our center, we have found that some patients will respond significantly to intravenous cyclophosphamide; thus, this treatment is worthy of consideration while we await double-blind placebo trials. However, cyclophosphamide should be administered under the auspices of an experienced oncology team, and caregivers should monitor the patient carefully for hemorrhagic cystitis and cytopenias.

CSF filtration is a new therapy, not yet available in the United States, in which spinal fluid is filtered for inflammatory factors (e.g., cells, complement, cytokines, and antibodies) prior reinfusion into the patient. In a randomized trial of CSF filtration vs PLEX for AIDP, CSF filtration was better tolerated than and at least as effective as PLEX *(125)*. Clinical trials for CSF filtration are currently being initiated.

Chronic immunomodulatory therapy should be considered for the small subgroup of patients with recurrent TM. Although the ideal treatment regimen is not known, we consider a 2-yr course of oral immunomodulatory treatment in patients with two or more distinct episodes of TM.

We most commonly treat patients with azathioprine (150–200 mg/d), methotrexate (15–20 mg/wk), or mycophenolate (2–3 g/d), although oral cyclophosphamide (2 g/kg/d) may also be used in patients with systemic inflammatory disease. On any of these medicines, patients must be followed for transaminitis or leukopenias.

5.4. Long-Term Management

It is important to begin occupational and physical therapies early during the course of recovery to prevent the inactivity related problems of skin breakdown and soft tissue contractures that lead to loss of range of motion. The principles of rehabilitation in the early and chronic phases of TM are summarized in Table 5. During the early recovery period, family education is essential to develop a strategic plan for dealing with the challenges to independence following return to the community.

The long-term management of TM requires attention to a number of issues. These are the residual effects of any spinal cord injury including TM. Patients should be educated about the effect of TM on mood regulation and routinely screened for the development of symptoms consistent with clinical depression. Patient warning signs that should prompt a complete evaluation for depression include failure to progress with rehabilitation and self-care, worsening fixed low mood, pervasive decreased interest, and social and professional withdrawal. A preoccupation with death or suicidal thoughts constitutes a true psychiatric emergency and should lead to prompt evaluation and treatment.

There are three main points related to depression. First, patients should be educated that depression in TM is similar to other neurologic symptoms patients endure, since it is mediated by the effects of the immune system on the brain. Depression is remarkably prevalent in TM, occurring in up to 25% of patients at any given time and is largely independent of the patient's degree of physical disability. Depression is not caused by personal weakness or the inability to cope. Second, depression in TM can have devastating consequences; not only can depression worsen physical disability (e.g., fatigue, pain, decreased concentration) but also has lethal consequences. Suicide is the leading cause of death in TM, accounting for 60% of the deaths in the JHTMC since its inception. Third, despite the severity of the clinical presentation of depression in many patients with TM, these patients generally show a very robust response to the combined interventions of aggressive psychopharmacological and psychotherapeutic interventions. Complete symptom remission is the rule rather than the exception with appropriate recognition and treatment of TM depression.

Spasticity is often a difficult problem to manage. The goal is to maintain flexibility with a stretching routine using exercises for active stretching and a bracing program with splints for a prolonged stretch. These splints are commonly used at the ankles, wrists, or elbows. An appropriate strengthening program for the weaker of the spastic muscle acting on a joint and an aerobic conditioning regimen are also recommended. These interventions are supported by adjunctive measures that include antispasticity drugs (e.g., diazepam, baclofen, dantrolene, tiagabine), therapeutic botulinum toxin injections, and serial casting. The therapeutic goal is to improve the patient's ability to perform specific activities of daily living (e.g, feeding, dressing, bathing, hygiene, mobility) through improving the available joint range of motion, teaching effective compensatory strategies, and relieving pain.

Another major area of concern is effective management of bowel function. A high-fiber diet, adequate and timely fluid intake, and medications to regulate bowel evacuations are the basic components to success. Regular evaluations by medical specialists for adjustment of the bowel program are recommended to prevent potentially serious complications.

Bladder function is almost always at least transiently impaired in patients with TM. Immediately after the onset of TM, as in the aftermath of traumatic spinal cord injury, there is frequently a period of transient loss or depression of neural activity below the involved spinal cord lesion. This phenomenon is often referred to as *spinal shock* and lasts about 3 wk, during which there is an interruption of descending excitatory influence with resultant bladder flaccidity. Following this period, bladder dysfunction can be classified into two syndromes involving either upper motor neurons (UMN) or lower motor neurons (LMN). Sympathetic input to the bladder, which promotes

Table 5
Long-Term Management of Transverse Myelitis

Features	Rehabilitation
General	• Provide inpatient rehabilitation initially • Prescribe daily land-based and/or water-based therapy for 8–12 wk • Prescribe daily weight-bearing exercise for 45–90 min, essential in the early phase • Examine for scoliosis • Perform a serial flexion/extension x-ray of back to follow angle • For fatigue, administer amantidine, methylphenidate, modafinil, coenzyme Q10 • To increase bone density, administer vitamin D, calcium, bisphosphonates
Depression	• Treat depression with antidepressants and talk therapy. SSRIs are common first-line agents • Refer to a psychiatrist if diagnosis is in doubt, if initial trials of antidepressant treatment are unsuccessful, or if there is concern about suicide potential
Autonomic dysfunction—bladder	• If postvoid residual is >80 cc, consider clean intermittent catheterization • Perform urodynamics study • Prescribe an anticholinergic drug if the detrusor is hyperactive and an adrenergic blocker if there is sphincter dysfunction • Give cranberry juice or vitamin C for urine acidification • Consider sacral nerve stimulation
Autonomic dysfunction—bowel	• Recommend a high-fiber diet, increased fluid intake • Perform digital disimpaction • Prescribe colace, senokot, dulcolax, docusate PR, bisacodyl in water base, miralax, enemas as needed
Autonomic dysfunction—aexual	• Prescribe phosphodiesterase V inhibitors
Motor dysfunction—weakness	• Administer passive and active ROM • Splint or give orthoses when necessary • Recommend continued land and water therapy • Prescribe ambulation devices • Recommend daily weightbearing for 45–90 min • Perform an orthopedics evaluation if there is joint imbalance
Motor dysfunction—spasticity	• Recommend ROM exercises • Recommend aquatherapy • Prescribe baclofen, tizanidine, diazepam, botulinum toxin, tiagabine • Perform an intrathecal baclofen trial
Sensory dysfunction—pain or dysesthesias	• Recommend ROM exercises • Prescribe gabapentin, carbamazepine, nortriptyline, tramadol • Prescribe topical lidocaine (patch or cream) • Prescribe intrathecal baclofen or opioids

ROM, range of motion.

urine storage, originates at levels T10–L2 of the spinal cord and travels via the hypogastric nerve. Afferent input to the urinary tract is provided by the sacral (S2–S4) spinal cord through the pelvic nerve. Efferent parasympathetic input to the bladder, which mediates detrusor contractions, is carried by the pelvic nerve (S2–S4). UMN bladder dysfunction results from lesions above S1–S2 and is characterized by reflexive emptying with bladder filling if the injury is complete, and urge incontinence if the neurologic involvement is incomplete. In addition, detrusor-sphincter dyssynergia results from impaired communication between the sacral and brain stem micturition centers. In the case of UMN dysfunction, anticholinergic medications, α-blockers, or electric stimulation are used to restore adequate bladder storage and drainage. LMN bladder dysfunction, with either direct involvement of S2–S4 or indirect involvement of the conus medullaris and cauda equina, results in detrusor areflexia and requires clean intermittent self-catheterization.

TM-induced sexual dysfunction involves similar innervation and analogous syndromes as those found in bladder dysfunction. Spinal cord segments S2–S4 relay afferent sensory fibers from the genitalia via the pudendal nerves and supply parasympathetic input via the pelvic nerves. Parasympathetic stimulation initiates and maintains penile erection in men and clitoral and labial engorgement and vaginal lubrication in women. Sympathetic fibers from T10–L2 provide the major stimulus for ejaculation and orgasm but can also mediate erections through less-understood mechanisms. Reflex erections in response to tactile stimulation are parasympathetically mediated through a local sacral (S2–S4) reflex arc and tend to occur in patients with UMN lesions. Psychogenic erections are sympathetically mediated through sympathetic pathways that exit the spinal cord at T10–T12 and allow many patients with LMN lesions of the sacral reflex arc to achieve erections through psychogenic stimulation. Treatment of sexual dysfunction should take into account baseline function before the onset of TM and begins with adequate education and counseling about the known physical and neurologic effects that TM has on sexual functioning. Patients should be encouraged to discuss their concerns with their doctors as well as their partners. Because of the similarities in innervation between sexual and bladder function, patients with UMN-mediated sexual dysfunction should be encouraged to empty their bladders before sexual stimulation to prevent untimely incontinence. The mainstays of treatment for erectile dysfunction in men are inhibitors of cGMP phosphodiesterase, type 5, which will allow the vast majority of men with TM to achieve adequate erections for success in intercourse through a combination of reflex and/or psychogenic mechanisms. Although less effective in women, these same types of medications have been shown capable of enhancing sexual functioning in women.

6. PROGNOSIS OF TM

Some patients with TM may experience recovery in neurological function regardless of whether specific therapy has been instituted. Recovery, if it occurs, should begin within 6 mo, and the vast majority of patients show some restoration of neurologic function within 8 wk *(19)* (JHTMC case series). Recovery may be rapid during 3–6 mo after symptom onset and may continue, albeit at a slower rate, for up to 2 yr *(18)* (JHTMC case series). Longitudinal case series of TM reveal that approximately one-third of patients recover with little to no sequelae, one-third are left with a moderate degree of permanent disability, and one-third have severe disabilities *(4,5,10,17,18)*. Knebusch estimated that a good outcome with normal gait, mild urinary symptoms, and minimal sensory and upper motor neuron signs occurred in 44% of patients. A fair outcome with mild spasticity but independent ambulation, urgency, and/or constipation, and some sensory signs occurred in 33%, and a poor outcome with the inability to walk or severe gait disturbance, absence of sphincter control, and sensory deficit occurred in 23%. The patient cohort we follow at Johns Hopkins is more severe, with only 20% experiencing a good outcome by those definitions and is likely a reflection of referral bias to a tertiary care center. Symptoms associated with poor outcome include back pain as an initial complaint, rapid progression to maximal symptoms within hours of onset, spinal shock, and sensory disturbance up to the cervical level *(19)*.

The presence of 14-3-3 protein, a marker of neuronal injury, in the CSF during the acute phase may also predict a poor outcome *(126)*. Our recent studies suggest that CSF IL-6 levels at acute presentation are proportional to, and highly predictive of, long-term disability (unpublished data). If confirmed by future studies, the finding that IL-6 levels are proportional to disability in untreated subjects could provide a much needed biomarker to help guide the aggressiveness of interventions employed in treating patients presenting with acute TM.

7. SPECULATIONS ON FUTURE THERAPIES

Over the last few years, research has begun to reveal fundamental immune abnormalities in patients with TM and related neuroimmunologic disorders. The generation of autoantibodies and the presence of abnormally elevated cytokine levels in the spinal fluid are likely to be important immunopathogenic events in many patients with TM. Although TM is a heterogeneous syndrome that is associated with distinct pathologies, recent classification strategies have attempted to identify patients with likely similar immunopathogenic events. Although current therapies are largely non-specific, future therapies will be more specifically targeted to those critical immunopathogenic events in TM. For example, evolving strategies will more effectively identify autoantibodies and the antigen to which they respond *(127,128)*, making it possible to develop specific targets to block the effects of these autoantibodies. Additionally, several strategies exist and more are being developed that specifically alter cytokine profiles or the effects of these cytokines within the nervous system. However, a cautionary note exists from recent studies examining tumor necrosis factor (TNF)-α modulation in patients with MS or systemic rheumatologic disease: paradoxical demyelination may be triggered by TNF-α reduction in the blood *(129)*. These findings may suggest that secondary alterations in immune system function may occur in response to blockade of any single pathway and that a *cocktail approach* aimed at halting multiple proinflammatory pathways may be ideal.

Future research will attempt to elucidate individual predispositions and environmental triggers to immune overactivation. A more comprehensive understanding of the mechanisms of tissue insult will lead to the development of rational therapeutics geared to intervention at various steps of the signal transduction pathways leading to injury. For those patients who have already undergone extensive neurologic injury as a result of TM, neurorestorative treatments (perhaps involving stem cells) offer the best hope for meaningful functional recovery.

8. CONCLUSION

TM is a clinical syndrome caused by focal inflammation of the spinal cord. Many cases are postinfectious and are thought to be caused by a transient abnormality in the immune system that results in injury to a focal area of the spinal cord. Recent studies have emphasized the need to classify TM according to whether there is evidence of systemic disease or multifocal CNS disease. The importance of this may be that distinct treatment strategies are offered to patients with distinct forms of TM. Although the causes of TM remain unknown, recent advances have suggested specific cytokine derangements that likely contribute to sustained disability caused by injury of motor, sensory, or autonomic neurons within the spinal cord. Future research will attempt to define triggers for the immune system derangements, effector mechanisms that propagate the abnormal immune response, and cellular injury pathways initiated by the inflammatory response within the spinal cord. Ultimately, this may allow us to identify patients at risk for developing TM, specifically treat the injurious aspects of the immune response, and/or offer neuroprotective treatments that minimize neural injury that occurs in response to the inflammation.

ACKNOWLEDGMENTS

We acknowledge the support and efforts of the Transverse Myelitis Association (TMA) and its president Sanford Siegel. The TMA serves a critical role to the TM community and to researchers striving to understand and treat this disorder. We also acknowledge financial support of Katie Sandler Fund for TM research and the Claddagh Foundation to the Johns Hopkins TM Center.

REFERENCES

1. Suchett-Kaye AI. Acute transverse myelitis complicating pneumonia. Lancet 1948;255:417.
2. Berman M, Feldman S, Alter M, Zilber N, Kahana E. Acute transverse myelitis: incidence and etiologic considerations. Neurology 1981; 31:966–971.

3. Jeffery DR, Mandler RN, Davis LE. Transverse myelitis. Retrospective analysis of 33 cases, with differentiation of cases associated with multiple sclerosis and parainfectious events. Arch Neurol 1993; 50:532–535.

4. Christensen PB, Wermuth L, Hinge HH, Bomers K. Clinical course and long-term prognosis of acute transverse myelopathy. Acta Neurol Scand 1990;81:431–435.

5. Altrocchi PH. Acute Transverse Myelopathy. Arch Neurol 1963;9:21–29.

6. Misra UK, Kalita J, Kumar S. A clinical, MRI and neurophysiological study of acute transverse myelitis. J Neurol Sci 1996;138:150–156.

7. Lipton HL, Teasdall RD. Acute transverse myelopathy in adults. A follow-up study. Arch Neurol 1973;28:252–257.

8. Sakakibara R, Hattori T, Yasuda K, Yamanishi T. Micturition disturbance in acute transverse myelitis. Spinal Cord 1996;34:481–485.

9. Lucchinetti CF, Brueck W, Rodriguez M, Lassmann H. Multiple sclerosis: lessons from neuropathology. Semin Neurol 1998;18:337–349.

10. Ropper AH, Poskanzer DC. The prognosis of acute and subacute transverse myelopathy based on early signs and symptoms. Ann Neurol 1978;4:51–59.

11. Transverse Myelitis Consortium Working Group. Proposed diagnostic criteria and nosology of acute transverse myelitis. Neurology 2002;59:499–505.

12. Tippett DS, Fishman PS, Panitch HS. Relapsing transverse myelitis. Neurology 1991;41:703–706.

13. Pandit L, Rao S. Recurrent myelitis. J Neurol Neurosurg Psychiatry 1996;60:336–338.

14. Rudick RA, French CA, Breton D, Williams GW. Relative diagnostic value of cerebrospinal fluid kappa chains in MS: comparison with other immunoglobulin tests. Neurology 1989;39:964–968.

15. Hung KL, Chen WC, Huang CS. Diagnostic value of cerebrospinal fluid immunoglobulin G (IgG) in pediatric neurological diseases. J Formos Med Assoc 1991;90:1055–1059.

16. Jacobs LD, Beck RW, Simon JH, Kinkel RP, Brownscheidle CM, Murray TJ et al. Intramuscular interferon beta-1a therapy initiated during a first demyelinating event in multiple sclerosis. CHAMPS Study Group. N Engl J Med 2000;343:898–904.

17. Paine RS, Byers RK. Transverse myelopathy in childhood. AMA Am J Dis Child 1968;85:151–163.

18. Knebusch M, Strassburg HM, Reiners K. Acute transverse myelitis in childhood: nine cases and review of the literature. Dev Med Child Neurol 1998;40:631–639.

19. Dunne K, Hopkins IJ, Shield LK. Acute transverse myelopathy in childhood. Dev Med Child Neurol 1986;28:198–204.

20. Burns AS, Rivas DA, Ditunno JF. The management of neurogenic bladder and sexual dysfunction after spinal cord injury. Spine 2001;26(24 Suppl):S129–S136.

21. DasGupta R, Fowler CJ. Sexual and urological dysfunction in multiple sclerosis: better understanding and improved therapies. Curr Opin Neurol 2002;15:271–278.

22. Patten SB, Metz LM. Depression in multiple sclerosis. Psychother Psychosom 1997;66:286–292.

23. Scott TF, Bhagavatula K, Snyder PJ, Chieffe C. Transverse myelitis. Comparison with spinal cord presentations of multiple sclerosis. Neurology 1998;50:429–433.

24. al Deeb SM, Yaqub BA, Bruyn GW, Biary NM. Acute transverse myelitis. A localized form of postinfectious encephalomyelitis. Brain 1997;120(Pt 7):1115–1122.

25. Ferch RD, Morgan MK, Sears WR. Spinal arteriovenous malformations: a review with case illustrations. J Clin Neurosci 2001;8:299–304.

26. Moriarity JL, Clatterbuck RE, Rigamonti D. The natural history of cavernous malformations. Neurosurg Clin N Am 1999;10:411–417.

27. Wityk RJ. Dural arteriovenous fistula of the spinal cord: an uncommon cause of myelopathy. Semin Neurol 1996;16:27–32.

28. Schreck RI, Manion WL, Kambin P, Sohn M. Nucleus pulposus pulmonary embolism. A case report. Spine 1995;20:2463–2466.

29. Bots GT, Wattendorff AR, Buruma OJ, Roos RA, Endtz LJ. Acute myelopathy caused by fibrocartilaginous emboli. Neurology 1981;31:1250–1256.

30. Toro G, Roman GC, Navarro-Roman L, Cantillo J, Serrano B, Vergara I. Natural history of spinal cord infarction caused by nucleus pulposus embolism. Spine 1994;19:360–366.

31. Case records of the Massachusetts General Hospital. Weekly clinicopathological exercises. Case 5-1991. A 61-year-old woman with an abrupt onset of paralysis of the legs and impairment of the bladder and bowel function. N Engl J Med 1991;324:322–332.

32. Okada S, Okeda R. Pathology of radiation myelopathy. Neuropathology 2001;21:247–265.

33. Liu CY, Yim BT, Wozniak AJ. Anticoagulation therapy for radiation-induced myelopathy. Ann Pharmacother 2001; 35:188–191.

34. Glantz MJ, Burger PC, Friedman AH, Radtke RA, Massey EW, Schold SC Jr. Treatment of radiation-induced nervous system injury with heparin and warfarin. Neurology 1994;44:2020–2027.

35. Asamoto S, Sugiyama H, Doi H, Iida M, Nagao T, Matsumoto K. Hyperbaric oxygen (HBO) therapy for acute traumatic cervical spinal cord injury. Spinal Cord 2000;38:538–540.

36. Calabro F, Jinkins JR. MRI of radiation myelitis: a report of a case treated with hyperbaric oxygen. Eur Radiol 2000;10:1079–1084.

37. Angibaud G, Ducasse JL, Baille G, Clanet M. [Potential value of hyperbaric oxygenation in the treatment of post-radiation myelopathies]. Rev Neurol (Paris) 1995;151:661–666.

38. Hummers LK, Krishnan C, Casciola-Rosen L, et al. Recurrent transverse myelitis associates with anti-ro (SSA) autoantibodies. Neurology 2004;62:147–149.

39. Ford B, Tampieri D, Francis G. Long-term follow-up of acute partial transverse myelopathy. Neurology 1992;42:250–252.

40. de Seze J, Stojkovic T, Breteau G, et al. Acute myelopathies: clinical, laboratory, and outcome profiles in 79 cases. Brain 2001;124(Pt 8):1509–1521.

41. Miller DH, Ormerod IE, Rudge P, Kendall BE, Moseley IF, McDonald WI. The early risk of multiple sclerosis following isolated acute syndromes of the brainstem and spinal cord. Ann Neurol 1989;26:635–639.

42. Ungurean A, Palfi S, Dibo G, Tiszlavicz L, Vecsei L. Chronic recurrent transverse myelitis or multiple sclerosis. Funct Neurol 1996;11:209–214.

43. Bakshi R, Kinkel PR, Mechtler LL, et al. Magnetic resonance imaging findings in 22 cases of myelitis: comparison between patients with and without multiple sclerosis. Eur J Neurol 1998;5:35–48.

44. McDonald WI, Compston A, Edan G, et al. Recommended diagnostic criteria for multiple sclerosis: guidelines from the International Panel on the diagnosis of multiple sclerosis. Ann Neurol 2001;50:121–127.

45. O'Riordan JI, Losseff NA, Phatouros C, et al. Asymptomatic spinal cord lesions in clinically isolated optic nerve, brain stem, and spinal cord syndromes suggestive of demyelination. J Neurol Neurosurg Psychiatry 1998;64:353–357.

46. Nagaswami S, Kepes J, Foster DB, Twemlow SW. Necrotizing myelitis: a clinico-pathologic report of two cases associated with diplococcus pneumoniae and mycoplasma pneumoniae infections. Trans Am Neurol Assoc 1973;98:290–292.

47. Mirich DR, Kucharczyk W, Keller MA, Deck J. Subacute necrotizing myelopathy: MR imaging in four pathologically proved cases. AJNR Am J Neuroradiol 1991;12:1077–1083.

48. Katz JD, Ropper AH. Progressive necrotic myelopathy: clinical course in 9 patients. Arch Neurol 2000;57:355–361.

49. Krishnan C, Kaplin AI, Deshpande DM, Pardo CA, Kerr DA. Transverse myelitis: pathogenesis, diagnosis and treatment. Front Biosci 2004;9:1483–1499.

50. de Macedo DD, de Mattos JP, Borges TM. [Transverse myelopathy and systemic lupus erythematosus. Report of a case and review of the literature]. Arq Neuropsiquiatr 1979;37:76–84.

51. Kerr DA, Ayetey H. Immunopathogenesis of acute transverse myelitis. Curr Opin Neurol 2002;15:339–347.

52. Patja A, Paunio M, Kinnunen E, Junttila O, Hovi T, Peltola H. Risk of Guillain-Barre syndrome after measles-mumps-rubella vaccination. J Pediatr 2001;138:250–254.

53. Schonberger LB, Bregman DJ, Sullivan-Bolyai JZ, et al. Guillain-Barre syndrome following vaccination in the National Influenza Immunization Program, United States, 1976–1977. Am J Epidemiol 1979;110:105–123.

54. Langmuir AD, Bregman DJ, Kurland LT, Nathanson N, Victor M. An epidemiologic and clinical evaluation of Guillain-Barre syndrome reported in association with the administration of swine influenza vaccines. Am J Epidemiol 1984;119:841–879.

55. Merelli E, Casoni F. Prognostic factors in multiple sclerosis: role of intercurrent infections and vaccinations against influenza and hepatitis B. Neurol Sci 2000;21(4 Suppl 2):S853–S856.

56. Ascherio A, Zhang SM, Hernan MA, et al. Hepatitis B vaccination and the risk of multiple sclerosis. N Engl J Med 2001;344:327–332.

57. Confavreux C, Suissa S, Saddier P, Bourdes V, Vukusic S. Vaccinations and the risk of relapse in multiple sclerosis. Vaccines in Multiple Sclerosis Study Group. N Engl J Med 2001;344:319–326.

58. Moriabadi NF, Niewiesk S, Kruse N, et al. Influenza vaccination in MS: absence of T-cell response against white matter proteins. Neurology 2001;56:938–943.

59. Dowling PC, Cook SD. Role of infection in Guillain-Barre syndrome: laboratory confirmation of herpesviruses in 41 cases. Ann Neurol 1981 9 Suppl:44–55.

60. Sanders EA, Peters AC, Gratana JW, Hughes RA. Guillain-Barre syndrome after varicella-zoster infection. Report of two cases. J Neurol 1987;234:437–439.

61. Tsukada N, Koh CS, Inoue A, Yanagisawa N. Demyelinating neuropathy associated with hepatitis B virus infection. Detection of immune complexes composed of hepatitis B virus surface antigen. J Neurol Sci 1987;77:203–216.

62. Thornton CA, Latif AS, Emmanuel JC. Guillain-Barre syndrome associated with human immunodeficiency virus infection in Zimbabwe. Neurology 1991;41:812–815.

63. Rees JH, Soudain SE, Gregson NA, Hughes RA. Campylobacter jejuni infection and Guillain-Barre syndrome. N Engl J Med 1995;333:1374–1379.

64. Mishu B, Ilyas AA, Koski CL, et al. Serologic evidence of previous Campylobacter jejuni infection in patients with the Guillain-Barre syndrome. Ann Intern Med 1993;118:947–953.

65. Hariharan H, Naseema K, Kumaran C, Shanmugam J, Nair MD, Radhakrishnan K. Detection of Campylobacter jejuni/C. coli infection in patients with Guillain-Barre syndrome by serology and culture. New Microbiol 1996;19:267–271.

66. Jacobs BC, Endtz H, Van der Meche FG, Hazenberg MP, Achtereekte HA, Van Doorn PA. Serum anti-GQ1b IgG antibodies recognize surface epitopes on Campylobacter jejuni from patients with Miller Fisher syndrome. Ann Neurol 1995;37:260–264.

67. Kusunoki S, Shiina M, Kanazawa I. Anti-Gal-C antibodies in GBS subsequent to mycoplasma infection: evidence of molecular mimicry. Neurology 2001;57:736–738.

68. Jacobs BC, Endtz HP, Van der Meche FG, Hazenberg MP, de Klerk MA, Van Doorn PA. Humoral immune response against Campylobacter jejuni lipopolysaccharides in Guillain-Barre and Miller Fisher syndrome. J Neuroimmunol 1997;79:62–68.

69. Lee WM, Westrick MA, Macher BA. High-performance liquid chromatography of long-chain neutral glycosphingolipids and gangliosides. Biochim Biophys Acta 1982;712:498–504.

70. Moran AP, Rietschel ET, Kosunen TU, Zahringer U. Chemical characterization of Campylobacter jejuni lipopolysaccharides containing N-acetylneuraminic acid and 2,3-diamino-2,3-dideoxy-D-glucose. J Bacteriol 1991;173:618–626.

71. Gregson NA, Rees JH, Hughes RA. Reactivity of serum IgG anti-GM1 ganglioside antibodies with the lipopolysaccharide fractions of Campylobacter jejuni isolates from patients with Guillain-Barre syndrome (GBS). J Neuroimmunol 1997;73:28–36.

72. Jacobs BC, Hazenberg MP, Van Doorn PA, Endtz HP, Van der Meche FG. Cross-reactive antibodies against gangliosides and Campylobacter jejuni lipopolysaccharides in patients with Guillain-Barre or Miller Fisher syndrome. J Infect Dis 1997;175:729–733.

73. Hao Q, Saida T, Kuroki S, et al. Antibodies to gangliosides and galactocerebroside in patients with Guillain-Barre syndrome with preceding Campylobacter jejuni and other identified infections. J Neuroimmunol 1998;81:116–126.

74. Goodyear CS, O'Hanlon GM, Plomp JJ, et al. Monoclonal antibodies raised against Guillain-Barre syndrome-associated Campylobacter jejuni lipopolysaccharides react with neuronal gangliosides and paralyze muscle-nerve preparations. J Clin Invest 1999;104:697–708.

75. Plomp JJ, Molenaar PC, O'Hanlon GM, et al. Miller Fisher anti-GQ1b antibodies: alpha-latrotoxin-like effects on motor end plates. Ann Neurol 1999;45:189–199.

76. O'Hanlon GM, Paterson GJ, Veitch J, Wilson G, Willison HJ. Mapping immunoreactive epitopes in the human peripheral nervous system using human monoclonal anti-GM1 ganglioside antibodies. Acta Neuropathol (Berl) 1998;95:605–616.

77. Koga M, Yuki N, Kashiwase K, Tadokoro K, Juji T, Hirata K. Guillain-Barre and Fisher's syndromes subsequent to Campylobacter jejuni enteritis are associated with HLA-B54 and Cw1 independent of anti-ganglioside antibodies. J Neuroimmunol 1998;88:62–66.

78. Drulovic J, Dujmovic I, Stojsavlevic N, et al. Transverse myelopathy in the antiphospholipid antibody syndrome: pinworm infestation as a trigger? J Neurol Neurosurg Psychiatry 2000;68:249.

79. Bohach GA, Fast DJ, Nelson RD, Schlievert PM. Staphylococcal and streptococcal pyrogenic toxins involved in toxic shock syndrome and related illnesses. Crit Rev Microbiol 1990;17:251–272.

80. Bohach GA. Staphylococcal enterotoxins B and C. Structural requirements for superantigenic and entertoxigenic activities. Prep Biochem Biotechnol 1997;27:79–110.

81. Betley MJ, Borst DW, Regassa LB. Staphylococcal enterotoxins, toxic shock syndrome toxin and streptococcal pyrogenic exotoxins: a comparative study of their molecular biology. Chem Immunol 1992;55:1–35.

82. Zhang J, Vandevyver C, Stinissen P, Mertens N, Berg-Loonen E, Raus J. Activation and clonal expansion of human myelin basic protein-reactive T cells by bacterial superantigens. J Autoimmun 1995;8:615–632.

83. Kappler J, Kotzin B, Herron L, et al. V beta-specific stimulation of human T cells by staphylococcal toxins. Science 1989;244:811–813.

84. Hong SC, Waterbury G, Janeway CA, Jr. Different superantigens interact with distinct sites in the Vbeta domain of a single T cell receptor. J Exp Med 1996;183:1437–1446.

85. Webb SR, Gascoigne NR. T-cell activation by superantigens. Curr Opin Immunol 1994;6:467–475.

86. Acha-Orbea H, MacDonald HR. Superantigens of mouse mammary tumor virus. Annu Rev Immunol 1995;13:459–486.

87. Brocke S, Gaur A, Piercy C, et al. Induction of relapsing paralysis in experimental autoimmune encephalomyelitis by bacterial superantigen. Nature 1993;365:642–644.

88. Racke MK, Quigley L, Cannella B, Raine CS, McFarlin DE, Scott DE. Superantigen modulation of experimental allergic encephalomyelitis: activation of anergy determines outcome. J Immunol 1994;152:2051–2059.

89. Brocke S, Hausmann S, Steinman L, Wucherpfennig KW. Microbial peptides and superantigens in the pathogenesis of autoimmune diseases of the central nervous system. Semin Immunol 1998;10:57–67.

90. Kotzin BL, Leung DY, Kappler J, Marrack P. Superantigens and their potential role in human disease. Adv Immunol 1993;54:99–166.

91. Vanderlugt CL, Begolka WS, Neville KL, et al. The functional significance of epitope spreading and its regulation by co-stimulatory molecules. Immunol Rev 1998;164:63–72.

92. Fukazawa T, Hamada T, Kikuchi S, Sasaki H, Tashiro K, Maguchi S. Antineutrophil cytoplasmic antibodies and the optic-spinal form of multiple sclerosis in Japan. J Neurol Neurosurg Psychiatry 1996;61:203–204.

93. Leonardi A, Arata L, Farinelli M, et al. Cerebrospinal fluid and neuropathological study in Devic's syndrome. Evidence of intrathecal immune activation. J Neurol Sci 1987;82:281–290.

94. O'Riordan JI, Gallagher HL, Thompson AJ, et al. Clinical, CSF, and MRI findings in Devic's neuromyelitis optica. J Neurol Neurosurg Psychiatry 1996;60:382–387.

95. Reindl M, Linington C, Brehm U, et al. Antibodies against the myelin oligodendrocyte glycoprotein and the myelin basic protein in multiple sclerosis and other neurological diseases: a comparative study. Brain 1999;122(Pt 11):2047–2056.

96. Haase CG, Schmidt S. Detection of brain-specific autoantibodies to myelin oligodendrocyte glycoprotein, S100beta and myelin basic protein in patients with Devic's neuromyelitis optica. Neurosci Lett 2001;307:131–133.

97. Garcia-Merino A, Blasco MR. Recurrent transverse myelitis with unusual long-standing Gd-DTPA enhancement. J Neurol 2000;247:550–551.

98. Renard JL, Guillamo JS, Ramirez JM, Taillia H, Felten D, Buisson Y. [Acute transverse cervical myelitis following hepatitis B vaccination. Evolution of anti-HBs antibodies]. Presse Med 1999;28:1290–1292.

99. Matsui M, Kakigi R, Watanabe S, Kuroda Y. Recurrent demyelinating transverse myelitis in a high titer HBs-antigen carrier. J Neurol Sci 1996;139:235–237.

100. Kira J, Kawano Y, Yamasaki K, Tobimatsu S. Acute myelitis with hyperIgEaemia and mite antigen specific IgE: atopic myelitis. J Neurol Neurosurg Psychiatry 1998;64:676–679.

101. Kikuchi H, Osoegawa M, Ochi H, et al. Spinal cord lesions of myelitis with hyperIgEemia and mite antigen specific IgE (atopic myelitis) manifest eosinophilic inflammation. J Neurol Sci 2001;183:73–78.

102. Piper PG. Disseminated lupus erythematosus with involvement of the spinal cord. JAMA 1953;153:215–217.

103. Adrianakos AA, Duffy J, Suzuki M, Sharp JT. Transverse myelitis in systemic lupus erythematosus: report of three cases and review of the literature. Ann Intern Med 1975;83:616–624.

104. Nakano I, Mannen T, Mizutani T, Yokohari R. Peripheral white matter lesions of the spinal cord with changes in small arachnoid arteries in systemic lupus erythematosus. Clin Neuropathol 1989;8:102–108.

105. Sinkovics JG, Gyorkey F, Thoma GW. A rapidly fatal case of systemic lupus erythematosus: structure resembling viral nucleoprotein strands in the kidney and activities of lymphocytes in culture. Texas Rep Biol Med 1969;27: 887–908.

106. Weil MH. Disseminated lupus erythematosus with massive hemorrhagic manifestations and paraplegia. Lancet 1955;75:353–360.

107. Ayala L, Barber DB, Lomba MR, Able AC. Intramedullary sarcoidosis presenting as incomplete paraplegia: case report and literature review. J Spinal Cord Med 2000;23:96–99.

108. Garcia-Zozaya IA. Acute transverse myelitis in a 7-month-old boy. J Spinal Cord Med 2001;24:114–118.

109. Miller JA, Munro DD. Topical corticosteroids: clinical pharmacology and therapeutic use. Drugs 1980;19:119–134.

110. Hallam NF. The use and abuse of topical corticosteroids in dermatology. Scott Med J 1980;25:287–291.

111. Elovaara I, Lalla M, Spare E, Lehtimaki T, Dastidar P. Methylprednisolone reduces adhesion molecules in blood and cerebrospinal fluid in patients with MS. Neurology 1998;51:1703–1708.

112. Sellebjerg F, Christiansen M, Jensen J, Frederiksen JL. Immunological effects of oral high-dose methylprednisolone in acute optic neuritis and multiple sclerosis. Eur J Neurol 2000;7:281–289.

113. Williams CS, Butler E, Roman GC. Treatment of myelopathy in Sjogren syndrome with a combination of prednisone and cyclophosphamide. Arch Neurol 2001;58:815–819.

114. Dumas JL, Valeyre D, Chapelon-Abric C, et al. Central nervous system sarcoidosis: follow-up at MR imaging during steroid therapy. Radiology 2000;214:411–420.

115. Bracken MB, Shepard MJ, Collins WF, et al. A randomized, controlled trial of methylprednisolone or naloxone in the treatment of acute spinal-cord injury. Results of the Second National Acute Spinal Cord Injury Study. N Engl J Med 1990;322:1405–1411.

116. Defresne P, Meyer L, Tardieu M, et al. Efficacy of high dose steroid therapy in children with severe acute transverse myelitis. J Neurol Neurosurg Psychiatry 2001;71:272–274.

117. Lahat E, Pillar G, Ravid S, Barzilai A, Etzioni A, Shahar E. Rapid recovery from transverse myelopathy in children treated with methylprednisolone. Pediatr Neurol 1998;19:279–282.

118. Sebire G, Hollenberg H, Meyer L, Huault G, Landrieu P, Tardieu M. High dose methylprednisolone in severe acute transverse myelopathy. Arch Dis Child 1997;76:167–168.

119. Kennedy PG, Weir AI. Rapid recovery of acute transverse myelitis treated with steroids. Postgrad Med J 1988;64:384–385.

120. Kalita J, Misra UK. Is methyl prednisolone useful in acute transverse myelitis? Spinal Cord 2001;39:471–476.

121. Weinshenker BG. Plasma exchange for severe attacks of inflammatory demyelinating diseases of the central nervous system. J Clin Apheresis 2001;16:39–42.

122. Weinshenker BG. Therapeutic plasma exchange for acute inflammatory demyelinating syndromes of the central nervous system. J Clin Apheresis 1999;14:144–148.

123. Weinshenker BG, O'Brien PC, Petterson TM, et al. A randomized trial of plasma exchange in acute central nervous system inflammatory demyelinating disease. Ann Neurol 1999;46:878–886.

124. Keegan M, Pineda AA, McClelland RL, Darby CH, Rodriguez M, Weinshenker BG. Plasma exchange for severe attacks of CNS demyelination: predictors of response. Neurology 2002;58:143–146.

125. Wollinsky KH, Hulser PJ, Brinkmeier H, et al. CSF filtration is an effective treatment of Guillain-Barre syndrome: a randomized clinical trial. Neurology 2001;57:774–780.

126. Irani DN, Kerr DA. 14-3-3 protein in the cerebrospinal fluid of patients with acute transverse myelitis. Lancet 2000;355:901.

127. Robinson WH, Steinman L, Utz PJ. Protein arrays for autoantibody profiling and fine-specificity mapping. Proteomics 2003;3:2077–2084.

128. Robinson WH, Fontoura P, Lee BJ, et al. Protein microarrays guide tolerizing DNA vaccine treatment of autoimmune encephalomyelitis. Nat Biotechnol 2003;21:1033–1039.

129. Mohan N, Edwards ET, Cupps TR, et al. Demyelination occurring during anti-tumor necrosis factor alpha therapy for inflammatory arthritides. Arthritis Rheum 2001;44:2862–2869.

CME QUESTIONS

1. According to recently published criteria on the diagnosis of transverse myelitis (TM), which of the following would be inconsistent with this diagnosis?
   A. Progressive neurological symptoms progressing over a week
   B. Spinal fluid analysis of 17 WBCs and no oligoclonal bands
   C. Symptom progression to complete paraplegia in 2 h
   D. A gadolinium enhancing lesion at T7

2. Which of the following statements is unlikely to be associated with idiopathic TM?
   A. Bladder urgency
   B. Band-like dysesthesias in the torso or limbs
   C. Diplopia
   D. Hyperreflexia of the lower extremities

3. Which of the following would favor Guillain-Barré syndrome over TM in a patient with rapidly progressive weakness?
   A. Normal magnetic resonance imaging of the spinal cord
   B. Facial weakness on physical exam
   C. CSF analysis: 0 WBC, 0 RBCs, protein 115
   D. Sensory level of T7 with urinary retention
   E. A,B, C
   F. All of the above

4. Potential causes of TM include which of the following?
   A Direct microbial infection of the spinal cord
   B Molecular mimicry causing breakdown of immune tolerance
   C. Superantigen stimulation causing breakdown of immune tolerance
   D. Emboli from the descending aorta to the spinal cord
   E. A, B, C
   F. All of the above

12
Optic Neuritis
Pathogenesis, Immunology, Diagnosis and Clinical Management

Robert Zivadinov and Rohit Bakshi

1. EPIDEMIOLOGY AND CLINICAL MANIFESTATION

The incidence of optic neuritis (ON) is approximately three to five cases per 100,000 individuals per year in northern latitudes, where multiple sclerosis (MS) is common *(1–4)*. It affects women more often than men (female to male ratio 2:1) and is more common in younger age groups *(1)*. The age distribution is slightly different from that of MS, showing peaks in young (age group 15–25 yr) and old patients (age group 55–65 yr) of the distribution spectrum. Major histocompatibility complex (MHC) class II antigens are associated with ON, suggesting a genetic predisposition for specific immune responses *(5)*. In particular, the results of the Optic Neuritis Treatment Trial (ONTT) *(6)* showed that the human leukocyte antigen (HLA)-DR2 genotype predicted a higher susceptibility for conversion to clinically definite MS over 5 yr, especially in MS patients with signal abnormalities on brain magnetic resonance imaging (MRI). Usually, episodes of ON are more common at high latitudes *(1,2)*, in spring *(7)*, and in summer *(8)*, although one study showed that 43% of 42 patients who developed MS, had onset of ON between October and March *(9)*.

1.1. Loss of Vision

ON typically presents with relatively acute and rapidly progressive, unilateral loss of vision associated with pain in or behind the eye. Common symptoms and signs of ON are shown in Table 1. Usually, the loss of vision is monocular, but 19 to 50% of adults *(10,11)* present with bilateral loss, which can arise simultaneously or sequentially. Bilateral ON seems to be more common in people of Asian *(12)* and African *(13)* origin. Loss of visual acuity, especially of central vision, is the most common symptom reported in more than 90% of patients with ON. Some patients with normal visual acuity may complain of a loss of peripheral vision. Recovery of visual function typically occurs within 2 to 3 wk and resolution continues for several months. Complete recovery of visual acuity is common in the initial phase of the disease, even after near blindness. The degree of recovery relates to the resolution of acute inflammation and the conduction block in the optic nerve *(14)* and is related to remyelination and proliferation of sodium channels in demyelinated segments of the nerve *(15)*. The recovery may proceed for 2 yr or more *(16)*. Cortical reorganization has been reported after ON and may also function in recovery or represent an adaptive response *(17)*. The effects of demyelination and axonal degeneration on visual acuity become more evident with a higher occurrence of recurrent episodes of ON *(16)*.

From: *Current Clinical Neurology: Inflammatory Disorders of the Nervous System:*
Pathogenesis, Immunology, and Clinical Management
Edited by: A. Minagar and J. S. Alexander © Humana Press Inc., Totowa, NJ

Table 1
Common Symptoms and Signs in Optic Neuritis

Common symptoms
  Progressive monocular or (occasionally) bilateral visual loss over a few days to weeks
  Mild orbital pain above or behind the eye at rest or during eye movement
  Alteration of color vision, contrast, and depth perception
  Presence of light and fleeting flashes, Uthoff's phenomenon, visual blurring, and flight of colors
  Previous history of multiple sclerosis
  Spontaneous improvement in vision

Common signs
  Decreased visual acuity
  Altered color vision and contrast sensitivity
  Relative afferent papillary defect
  Visual field defects
  Temporal disc pallor
  Optic nerve atrophy

Atypical signs of demyelinating optic neuritis *(28)*
  Bilateral visual loss
  Painless visual disturbance
  Insidious onset
  Presence of systemic symptoms
  Normal brain MRI
  Atypical visual field abnormalities

MRI, magnetic resonance imaging.

The degree of visual loss in the acute phase is a poor predictor of the final visual outcome. Of 187 patients with visual acuity worse than 20/400 on admission to the ONTT, only 6% had this level of acuity or worse at 6 mo *(17)*. The visual function was reassessed more than 10 yr after the initial episode of ON in 319 patients enrolled in the ONTT *(18)*. In most patients, the affected eye was normal or only slightly abnormal after 9.9 to 13.7 yr. Visual acuity in the affected eye was less or equal to 20/20 in 74% of the patients, 20/25 to 20/40 in 18%, 20/40 to 20/200 in 5%, and less than 20/200 in 3%.

1.2. Pain

The patient usually experiences mild orbital or retro-orbital pain. In the ONTT, 92% of patients experienced ocular pain, and this pain worsened with eye movements in 87% *(4)*. The onset of pain may precede visual symptoms by several days. There is no correlation between the severity of the pain and the loss of visual acuity. Pain can be present at rest and may be aggravated by upward eye movement and may occasionally last for as long as several weeks *(19,20)*.

1.3. Other Vision Disturbances

Altered color perception, diminished contrast sensitivity, and relative afferent papillary defect are commonly noticed in the affected eye *(4)*. The alteration of color perception *(21)* and loss of contrast sensitivity *(4)* are sometimes worse than the loss of visual acuity. Light flashes are sometimes caused by eye movements and the mechanisms correspond to the Lhermitté sign characteristic for cervical cord lesions in MS *(22)*. Subclinical cases are frequent, in which patients may present with only Uthoff's phenomenon (visual deterioration provoked by heat or exercise) *(23)*. Other disturbances of vision may persist, even when acuity has returned to normal (e.g., visual blurring, *flight of colors, fleeting flashes*, altered depth perception).

1.4. Visual Field Defects

Patients who have acute ON can present with a variety of visual field defects, most frequently a central scotoma. Less common defects may include a superior or inferior scotoma, an arcuate and cecocentral scotoma, or unilateral and bilateral hemianoptic defect. This wide variety of visual field patterns has limited usefulness in differentiating ON of demyelinating origin from other optic nerve disorders *(21)*. Subclincial involvement in the contralateral eye, such as an alteration of the visual field, is not uncommon. In the ONTT, 48% of patients who had unilateral ON and no history of prior ON had an abnormal visual field in the asymptomatic eye *(11)*.

1.5. Fundus

Funduscopic findings help localize the site of optic nerve lesions. The fundus is often normal, especially when the inflammation is retrobulbar *(10)*. Papillitis with swelling of the optic nerve and peripheral hemorrhages may be present simultaneously with ON *(10)*. Vitritis, caused by infections or inflammation, is present in anterior ON and may be associated with MS as part of intermediate uveitis. Optic disc swelling and disc pallor are nonspecific findings in ON. Most patients with MS, regardless of the location of the lesion, will develop diffuse optic pallor, most commonly in the temporal region *(24)*, followed by optic nerve atrophy *(25,26)*.

2. PATHOGENESIS AND PATHOPHYSIOLOGY

The pathogenesis of ON is not completely known. ON is typically a primary immune-mediated inflammation of the optic nerve, although the specific mechanisms and target antigens are unclear. It may be associated with a variety inflammatory conditions, including demyelinating (acute and chronic ON in MS, Devic's disease, neuroretinitis, sarcoidosis and other demyelinating inflammatory optic neuropathies) *(27)* and nondemyelinating (viral and bacterial, ischemic, compressive or infiltrative, toxic, nutritional, and hereditary) *(28)*. Most of the postvaccination and postinfectious cases subsequently develop MS *(29)*. Patients with virus-specific oligoclonal immunoglobulin-G (IgG) antibodies in cerebrospinal fluid (CSF) are more likely to develop MS *(30–35)* than patients without the finding. The results from prospective studies raise the question of whether there is a real connection between ON and infectious antigens or whether ON is a nonspecific response to immune activation.

2.1. Immunologic Factors

During an attack of ON in MS, even before demyelination occurs, there is a disruption of the blood–brain barrier through inflammation of the vascular endothelium. Lymphocytes and monocytes infiltrate the optic nerve and immune cells directly damage myelin or indirectly cause dysfunction by secreting proteases and cytokines that interfere with nerve function *(36)*. In particular, cell-mediated cytotoxicity causes demyelination of optic nerves that results in conduction block. The demyelinating plaques show a perivenular cuffing of T and B cells, edema in the myelin sheaths, and subsequent myelin breakdown. The T cells are activated in both serum and CSF, as evidenced by increased levels of interleukin (IL)-6 and IL-2 receptors *(37)*. Serum interferon (IFN)-γ levels are sometimes increased in ON, although they do not reflect the degree of immune activation in the optic nerve. Adhesion molecules can be increased in CSF during the first attack of ON *(38)*. Frequently, MS patients with oligoclonal bands in CSF present myelin basic protein (MBP) antibodies. Antibodies to MBP have not been definitively proven to be the cause or consequence of ON; however, during an acute attack of ON, antibodies to MBP appear in the serum. MBP and phospholipid protein-reactive cells are increased in the CSF in ON *(39–41)*. The presence of MBP has been linked to a greater risk of developing clinically definite MS *(42,43)*. Moreover, increased CSF MBP-reactive B cells in patients with ON correlate with early myelin breakdown or restoration *(44)*. There are studies suggesting that anti-MBP and anti-PLP antibodies contribute to the pathophysiology of optic nerve damage *(41,45)*. Recently, Berger et al. *(45)* investigated whether the presence of serum antibodies against myelin oligo-dendrocyte glycoprotein (MOG) and MBP in patients with a clinically isolated syndrome pre-dicts conversion to clinically definite MS. Of 103 patients who participated in that study, patients with anti-MOG and anti-MBP antibodies had a higher risk of conversion to MS than patients without these antibodies. The authors proposed that antibodies against MOG and MBP in patients with a clinically isolated syndrome are a rapid, inexpensive, and precise method for the prediction of early conversion to clinically definite MS. Definitive conclusions regarding the prognostic value of anti-MOG or anti-MBP testing in patients with ON requires confirmation by other groups.

2.2. Genetic Factors

Several genes determine the susceptibility to MS, but environmental factors also have an important role. Evidence suggests that the MS population differs from local controls in their MHC. The most important confirmed genetic factor in MS has been identified and located in the HLA class II region on the short arm of chromosome 6. In particular, the combination of DRB1*1501-DQA1*0102-DQB1*0602 (DR15) in northern Europeans *(32,46–48)* and DRB1*0301-DQA1*0501-DQB1*0301 (DR3) in southern Europeans *(43,49,50)* increases the risk of MS three to four times; however, there may not be a single major susceptibility locus, but many genetic factors different than those related to the HLA region may be involved *(51)*.

Several studies examined the possible relationship between HLA status and MRI findings at disease onset, including ON *(6,52–56)*. The results drawn from these studies are consistent. They suggest that the presence and/or number of brain lesions on MRI is independent of HLA status at the first clinical event, but that HLA-DR2 and -DQ alleles are involved in susceptibility for the development of demyelinating lesions and the conversion to clinically definite MS in MRI-positive patients, especially those with isolated ON. In particular, the results of the ONTT *(47)* suggested that the HLA-DR2 genotype predicted a higher susceptibility for conversion from ON to clinically definite MS over 5 yr, especially in patients with abnormal brain MRI at baseline. Recently, it was reported that patients with opticospinal MS demonstrate a higher frequency of the HLA-DPB1*0501 allele *(57,58)*.

3. ETIOLOGY

3.1. Demyelinating Optic Neuropathies

3.1.1. Optic Neuritis in Multiple Sclerosis

MS is an inflammatory demyelinating autoimmune disease of the central nervous system (CNS). The association between ON and MS has been known for many years. Acute ON associ-ated with MS is clinically indistinguishable from acute idiopathic ON. The diagnosis may be made clinically by history and examination; however, only long-term follow-up will confirm the diagnosis in an individual patient with monosymptomatic ON.

3.1.2. Visual Recovery and Recurrence

The prognosis for visual recovery in ON is generally favorable, as has been reported in sev-eral short- *(17,59–61)* and long-term *(18,62,63)* follow-up studies of the ONTT group. Visual acuity at 12-mo follow-up was deteriorated in only 3% of the ONTT cohort. After 5 yr, the overall risk of recurrent ON in either eye was low (28%) *(63)*. At 10 yr, recurrent ON in either eye occurred in 35% of patients, and the recurrences were more frequent in patients with MS than in those without *(18)*. Moreover, the visual function was worse in patients who developed clinically definite MS than in those without MS. Bilateral ON has not been confirmed as a risk factor for development of MS *(64)*.

3.1.3. Development of Clinically Definite Multiple Sclerosis

No single clinical feature or diagnostic test is sufficient for the diagnosis of MS. A formal review of diagnostic criteria occurred in 1983, at which time degrees of diagnostic certainty were identified by categories ranging from clinically definite to laboratory-supported definite, clinically probable, and laboratory-supported probable MS *(65)*. Diagnostic criteria have recently been revised by an international panel, McDonald et al. *(66)*. The clinical diagnosis in MS is based on the dissemination of lesions in the CNS in time, and the occurrence of a second clinical episode at a different site in the CNS. Several studies have suggested that single or recurrent unilateral episodes of ON increase the risk of developing clinically definite MS *(9,30,32,35,62,63,67–71)*. The risk of MS after isolated ON increases with time *(25)*. The long-term epidemiological follow-up (1935–1991) of 159 patients with ON who experienced onset of the disease while residing in Olmsted County, Minnesota, showed that 39% of 95 patients with isolated ON in the incidence cohort had progressed to clinically definite MS by the 10-yr follow-up, 49% by the 20-yr, 54% by the 30-yr, and 60% by the 40-yr follow-up. There was no difference related to gender in the risk of MS.

The new McDonald criteria *(66)* allow MRI to be used to define dissemination in space *(72,73)* and, with a repeat MRI, in time. The McDonald criteria accept the occurrence of a new gadolinium(Gd)-enhancing lesion appearing after a minimum interval of 3 mo or a new T2 lesion after a minimum interval of 6 mo, as acceptable evidence for dissemination in time *(66,74)*. Recently, the McDonald criteria have been validated. One study showed that in adults ages 16 to 50 years presenting with a clinically isolated syndrome, the McDonald MRI criteria for dissemination in time should be expanded to include new T2 lesions seen on a 3-mo follow-up scan of symptom onset *(75)*. Recently, this evidence has been critically evaluated by the Therapeutics and Technology Assessment Subcommittee of the American Academy of Neurology, which recommended that the appearance of either new T2 lesion or Gd-enhanced lesion after 3 mo is highly predictive of the subsequent development of clinically definite MS in the near term *(76)*. According to these recommendations, MRI evidence of dissemination of CNS lesions in time and space is sufficient for the diagnosis of MS, even before clinical dissemination has occurred. In other words, this presumes that patients with isolated ON could be diagnosed as having MS, even in the absence of a second clinical episode. The minimum interval for MRI dissemination in time should be further validated. In addition, the optimal interval that provides the maximum yield in the most cost effective manner needs to be defined. Emerging data from serial MRI studies and clinical trials in patients with clinically isolated syndromes might provide additional information to make such recommendations *(77–79)*.

In 35 to 50% of cases, the first manifestation of MS is ON. The time between the first episode of ON and subsequent development of clinically definite MS, as well as the rate of accumulation of sustained neurological disability, is highly variable among patients. Baseline clinical and MRI findings are only moderately predictive of these subsequent occurrences. Baseline brain and spinal cord MRI at the time of presentation in patients with ON are useful for excluding other neurologic conditions and for stratifying patients with a high risk of developing MS (evidence of dissemination of lesions in time and space) (Figs. 1 and 2) *(66,72–79)*.

Several studies investigated the predictive value of MRI in patients with ON or other initial clinically isolated syndromes. In one study, 54% of 26 patients developed clinically definite MS after 8 yr *(80)*. The 5-yr risk for the development of clinically definite MS following ON in the ONTT was a strong predictor in patients with abnormal MRI at baseline, ranging from 51% in the 89 patients with three or more MRI lesions to 16% in the 202 patients with no MRI lesions *(63)*. Lack of pain, the presence of optic disk swelling, and mild visual acuity loss were features of ON associated with a low risk of clinically definite MS among the 189 patients who had no brain MRI lesions and no history of neurologic symptoms or ON in the affected eye *(63)*; however, even a normal brain MRI does not preclude the development of clinically definite MS. In another study *(69)*, MS occurred in 37 of 71 patients (52.1%) with one MRI lesion or more at baseline, whereas no patient with a normal

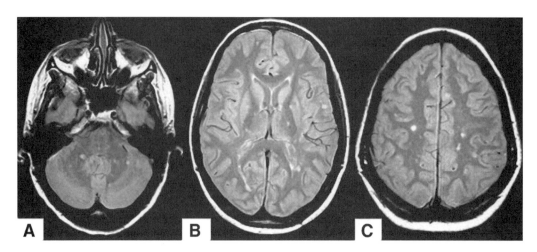

Fig. 1. Evidence of magnetic resonance imaging (MRI) dissemination in space on MRI. Axial proton density (PD) images of the brain in a 26-yr-old man with the first episode of optic neuritis showing several hyperintense lesions in the infratentorial (**A**) periventricular (**B**) and supratentorial (**C**) white and grey matter. The number and regional distribution of the lesions conform to the McDonald MRI criteria *(66)* for dissemination in space *(72,73)*.

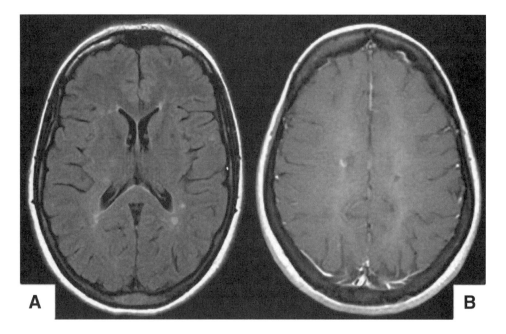

Fig. 2. Evidence of magnetic resonance imaging (MRI) dissemination in time on MRI. (**A**) Axial fast-FLAIR image in a 22-yr-old woman with a first episode of optic neuritis showing hyperintense lesions in the periventricular white matter. (**B**) Axial postcontrast T1-weighted conventional spin-echo image taken 3 mo later shows a new enhancing lesion in the juxtracortical part of the brain, sufficient to give a diagnosis of MS, according to McDonald criteria *(66)*.

MRI developed the disease after 10 yr. If asymptomatic spinal cord lesions are present at baseline in addition to brain lesions, the risk of developing a second attack of MS increases. Brex et al. *(81)* performed brain and spinal MRI on 60 patients after a first demyelinating event. After 1 yr, 26% of patients developed MS. The frequency of developing clinical MS was higher for those with both brain and spinal cord lesions at baseline (48%) than with brain lesions alone (18%).

Several studies investigated the progression of long-term disability in MS patients who presented with a first clinical attack in the form of ON. A systematic review study showed that patients with ON who develop clinically definite MS usually exhibited a more benign course of the disease (risk ratio 1.73, 95% C.I. 1.27–2.35) *(82)*. In the ONTT, only 17 of 105 patients who developed clinically definite MS (16.2%) had an Expanded Disability Status Scale (EDSS) rating of more than 3, and only 5 (4.7%) had an EDSS rating of more than 6 after 5 yr. Several longitudinal studies using conventional MRI demonstrated that the volume of T2 lesions in the brain in patients with ON and other clinically isolated syndromes was associated with a higher level of disability at long-term follow-up *(83–85)*.

3.1.4. Neuromyelitis Optica—Devic's Disease

Neuromyelitis optica (NMO) or Devic's disease is a multiphasic syndrome characterized by acute unilateral or bilateral simultaneous or sequential ON and severe transverse myelitis *(58,86)*. This disease is relatively more common in East Asian and South American populations than in other groups *(58)*. It is still controversial whether NMO is a variant of MS or a unique disease *(87)*. Distinct neuropathological characteristics and a fulminant clinical course argue in favor of NMO as a distinct disease. One of the major supportive criteria for the diagnosis of NMO is of the lack of clinical or MRI involvement of the CNS beyond the spinal cord or optic nerve *(86,88)*. Some patients may develop brain lesions on serial MRIs but rarely do these meet McDonald criteria for dissemination in space and in time *(66)*. In a retrospective study, 30 patients diagnosed with NMO were compared with 50 consecutive MS cases with ON or acute myelopathy *(87)*. MS patients were included only if a relapse occurred demonstrating dissemination in time and space. The two groups were compared in terms of clinical presentation, laboratory findings (MRI and CSF) and clinical outcome. The authors found that the CSF and MRI data were clearly different: oligoclonal bands were found in 23% of NMO cases and 88% of MS cases, abnormal brain MRI was observed in 10% of NMO cases and 66% of MS cases, and a large spinal cord lesion was observed in 67% of NMO cases and 7.4% of MS cases. Clinical outcome was more severe in the NMO group. Only two of the NMO patients met the criteria for MS, and one of the MS patients met criteria for NMO. Other studies found that patients with a relapsing NMO course usually have a worse prognosis, resulting in blindness and paraplegia, as well as respiratory failure during attacks of cervical myelitis *(89,90)*.

The immunopathological mechanisms responsible for the necrotizing and demyelinating spinal cord and optic nerve lesions in NMO are unknown. The extent of complement activation, eosinophilic infiltration, and vascular fibrosis observed in the NMO cases is more prominent than in prototypic MS and supports a role for humoral immunity *(91)*.

The combination of myelitis and ON may be associated with other inflammatory and infectious disorders *(58)*. This suggests that NMO can represent a syndrome caused by a variety of underlying disease states.

3.1.5. Other Inflammatory Demyelinating Optic Neuropathies

Several reports describe bulbar or retrobulbar ON of suspected inflammatory demyelinating origin *(27)*. Episodes of ON have been described in neuroretinitis, sarcoidosis, Reiter's syndrome, systemic lupus erythematosus [SLE], chronic inflammatory demyelinating polyneuropathy, Guillan-Barré syndrome, Bechet's disease, inflammatory bowel disease, and birdshot chorioretinopathy (*see ref. 27* for a systematic review). These optic neuropathies are characterized by moderate to severe visual loss that is usually followed by significant recovery. The long-term visual prognosis is generally excellent, although occasionally poor vision and optic atrophy can occur.

3.2. Non-Demyelinating Optic Neuropathies

3.2.1. Viral, Bacterial and Postvaccination Optic Neuropathies

ON may follow a large number of viral, or less often, bacterial infections by 1–3 wk *(92)* (Table 2). This usually is more common in children than in adults and may be unilateral but is

Table 2
Viral and Bacterial Infectious Optic Neuropathies

Viruses
   Adenovirus
   Coxsackievirus
   Cytomegalovirus
   Epstein-Barr virus
   Hepatitis A or B virus
   Human Immunodeficiency virus type I
   Measles virus
   Mumps virus
   Herpes zoster virus
   Herpes simplex virus
   Rubella virus
   Varicella zoster virus

Bacteria
   Anthrax
   Bartonella henselae (cat scratch disease)
   Beta-hemolytic streptococcal infection
   Borrelia burgdorferi (Lyme disease)
   Brucellosis
   Meningococcal infection
   Mycobacterium tuberculosis
   Pertussis
   Treponema pallidum
   Typhoid fever
   Whipple's disease

Fungi
   Cryptococcus
   Aspergillus

Parasites
   Toxoplasmosa gondii
   Toxocara canis
   Leptospira

Modified from ref. *28.*

more often bilateral *(93)*. The disease may affect only the optic nerve or may cause widespread CNS involvement, typically seen in acute disseminated encephalomyelitis. When neurologic manifestations are present, the CSF exam is usually abnormal.

Postvaccination ON is more frequently located in the anterior optic nerve *(94)*. The pathogenesis is similar to acute disseminated encephalomyelitis and may develop after vaccination with Bacillus Calmette-Guerin, hepatitis B, rabies virus, tetanus toxoid, variola virus, and influenza virus *(36)*. Visual function usually improves spontaneously, and the benefit of steroid treatment is unclear.

3.2.2. Ischemic Optic Neuropathy

Acute or subacute ON is commonly caused by ischemic vascular disease. In ischemic optic neuropathy (ION), the loss of vision is acute and characteristically involves the anterior optic nerve. Pain is much less common in ION (12%) than in ON of demyelinating origin (92%) *(95)*. The optic nerve is not swollen in ION, as it is in ON of demyelinating origin, and peripapillary hemorrhages are common. Severe and lasting visual loss is frequent. Usually, the CSF is normal. ION is caused by vascular insufficiency, leading to ischemia of the optic nerve head *(96)*, and the two most important diseases associated with ION are temporal arteritis and nonarteritic anterior ION.

Temporal arteritis is typically a disease of the elderly. In fewer than 5% of patients, onset occurs under age 50 *(97)*. The visual loss is complete, especially in older patients, and frequently accompanied by severe temporal pain. The disc is typically swollen and hemorrhages are more common than in ON. Fever, malaise, weight loss, and temporal headache are commonly associated symptoms characteristic of a systemic origin of the disease. The erythrocyte sedimentation rate is considerably elevated, and a temporal arterial biopsy can confirm the diagnosis.

Nonarteritic anterior ION is frequent in patients over age 50 and is characterized by sudden painless, unilateral or bilateral vision loss. The etiology of the disease remains unclear but is usually caused by microvascular occlusion of a branch of the posterior ciliary artery *(98)*. Most patients have one or more risk factors associated with small vessel cerebrovascular disease, including diabetes, hypertension, elevated cholesterol and triglyceride levels, or smoking.

Patients with CNS vasculitis can also experience visual disturbances that suggest an anterior or retrobulbar optic neuropathy. CNS vasculitis can be diagnosed using clinical and serological features. The term *autoimmune optic neuritis* has been suggested to identify cases with ON and serological evidence of vasculitis.

3.2.3. Toxic and Nutritional Optic Neuropathies

Toxic and nutritional optic neuropathies are caused by a variety of factors *(99)*. The visual symptoms are often bilateral at onset and painless. The loss of vision is partial, and the recovery is usually not complete. Optic nerve atrophy develops after a variable interval of time, especially in deficiency optic neuropathies. The ingestion of chloramphenicol, ethambutol, methanol, disulfiram, cyanide, isoniazid, phenothiazines, antineoplastic agents, ethylene glycol, trichloroethylene, tobacco, and toluene are the most common causes of toxic optic neuropathy *(28)*. Nutritional optic neuropathy includes deficiency of vitamins B_1, B_6, B_{12}, niacin, folic acid, or riboflavin. Typical tropical (Cuban and Tanzanian) epidemic optic neuropathies are probably also deficiency-related. The clinical manifestation of tobacco-alcohol amblyopia is similar to toxic and deficiency optic neuropathies. The etiology of tobacco-alcohol amblyopia is probably multifactorial: cyanide poisoning and concurrent malnutrition with vitamin B deficiency.

3.2.4. Compressive or Infiltrative Optic Neuropathies

Neoplastic (benign or malignant optic glioma, metastatic carcinoma, hemangioma, and lymphoreticular tumors), inflammatory (sarcoidosis, SLE, inflammatory bowel disease, idiopathic perioptic neuritis) or infectious (virus, bacteria, fungi) processes may infiltrate the optic nerves *(28,100–104)* (Fig. 3). Compressive or infiltrative optic neuropathies can occur anywhere in the optic nerves, including the portion of optic canals. The deterioration of visual acuity is slow but progressive and can be associated with diplopia *(103)*, proptosis, or optic disc swelling. Uthoff's phenomenon and pain can be triggered by a compressive lesion in the optic canal. There is no typical clinical or laboratory feature that permits a reliable differential diagnosis between ON of demyelinating origin and optic nerve compression or infiltration. Recently, orbital computed tomography (CT) and Gd-enhanced fat-suppressed MRI have increased the ability to visualize optic nerves and represent the most important tools to make a correct diagnosis (Fig. 3).

3.2.5. Hereditary Optic Neuropathy

Leber hereditary optic neuropathy (LHON) is a neuro-ophthalmic disorder of mitochondrial origin in which sequential attacks of ON are associated with MS-like symptoms and occasional MRI abnormalities *(105–111)*. Males between 15 and 35 yr are more commonly affected than are females *(107)*. The pattern of inheritance may be autosomal dominant or recessive, or maternal.

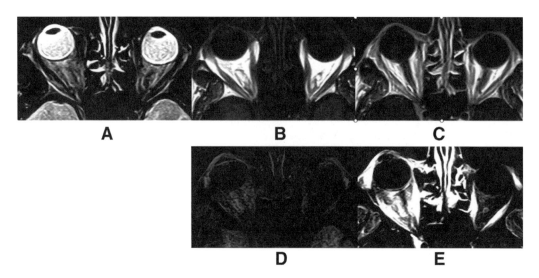

Fig. 3. Magnetic resonance imaging (MRI) of orbital pseudotumor and optic neuropathy caused by sarcoidosis. A 74-yr-old Caucasian man presented with 2 wk of headache, diplopia, orbital pain, ptosis, proptosis, redness, and epiphora of the right eye. The right pupil was slightly dilated and reacted poorly to light. Visual acuity was 20/70 OD and 20/20 OS. Conventional spin-echo 3-mm axial T2-weighted **(A)** and pre- **(B)** and postcontrast **(C)** T1-weighted images show no obvious intraconal abnormality, although fat-suppressed 3-mm axial slices pre- **(D)** and postcontrast **(E)** conventional spin-echo T1-weighted images show intraconal enlargement and abnormal intraconal enhancement of the right retrobulbar region. The right lacrimal gland shows mild enlargement. (Adapted from ref. *101*.)

The most frequent mitochondrial mutations are at 14484, 11778, and 3460. The variant of mitochondrial defect influences the visual prognosis, with the 11778 mutation carrying the worse prognosis *(112)*. The common symptoms of LHON include unilateral, painless, and acute or subacute central visual loss, which usually becomes bilateral several weeks or months after onset *(110,111)*. A small number of patients may have brain abnormalities indistinguishable from MS *(109,113)*. The use of nonconventional MRI techniques showed that microscopic brain damage occurs in LHON and is more severe in the MS-like form of the disease *(109,113)*.

4. DIAGNOSIS

ON of demyelinating origin can resemble other optic neuropathies and anterior segment, choroidal, or retinal diseases *(114)*. Generally, ON can be diagnosed on clinical grounds. Atypical features of ON (Table 1) are usually suggestive of alternative diagnoses and require prompt further investigation *(27,36,115,116)*. A complete neuro-ophthalmologic examination must be performed to differentiate optic nerve damage from diseases involving other ocular structures. Combined ophthalmological, neurological, imaging (Figs. 3 and 4), and laboratory exams are useful in improving diagnostic accuracy.

4.1. Magnetic Resonance Imaging

Acute optic nerve neuritis may be visualized using neuroimaging (Fig. 4). CT is one of the most frequently used imaging techniques for evaluation of the orbit *(117)*. It is optimal for the evaluation of the bony orbit, optic canal, and superior and inferior orbital fissures and allows for high contrast between bone, muscle, and orbital fat, although, in recent years, MRI has progressed technically to the point that it has become the imaging modality of choice for the imaging of optic nerves. Moreover, MRI is superior to CT in evaluating the optic chiasm and tracts, geniculate bodies, the optic radiations, and the occipital lobes *(117)*.

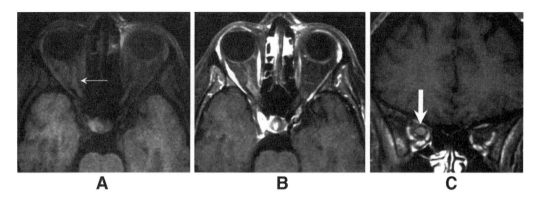

Fig. 4. MRI of acute ON. Fat-suppressed 3-mm axial slices pre- **(A)** and postcontrast **(B)** and 3-mm coronal postcontrast **(C)** conventional spin-echo T1-weighted images show swelling and enhancement of the right optic nerve 1 wk after the acute onset of painful visual loss in this 25-yr-old woman. (Adapted from ref. *157*.)

For evaluation of the optic nerve, thin-sliced (e.g., 3 mm) axial, coronal T1-weighted, and axial T2-weighted images are recommended (Fig. 4). Coronal short-δ inversion recovery (STIR) sequences are helpful for identifying abnormal signals in the optic nerves, as they traverse the intraconal fat (Fig. 5) *(117–119)*. Gd adds sensitivity to the diagnosis of orbital and optic nerve pathology and should be given routinely for the evaluation of patients with lesions suspected in these areas. Post-contrast T1-weighted images with fat saturation should be obtained in coronal and axial planes (Figs. 3 and 4). Edema within the inflamed optic nerve on T2-weighted and coronal STIR images manifests as a hyperintense signal within the nerve with or without the nerve swelling. Usually, Gd-enhancing lesions, showing inflammatory infiltrates, are solitary or multifocal and can be located centrally within the nerve or at its periphery *(120)*. It is important to note that similar lesions on T2-weighted, STIR, and postcontrast T1-weighted images can also be seen in patients with ischemic, infectious, or radiation-induced optic neuropathies and are not pathognomonic of the demyelination process *(117–119)*. Acute inflammatory changes, edema, demyelination, axonal loss, and chronic gliosis cannot usually be distinguished. Gd-enhancement is associated with decreased visual acuity and color vision, afferent papillary defect, and reduced P100 in the visual evoked potentials (VEP) *(119)*.

In chronic ON, the optic nerve is abnormal in most cases *(121)*. The long-term evolution of the lesions in the optic nerves is not completely clear but probably follows the pattern usually reported in MS *(25,122)*. The development of optic nerve atrophy in later stages of ON is a common feature (Fig. 5) *(25,26,123)*.

Although conventional MRI has substantially contributed to the diagnosis and prognosis of ON, the sensitivity and specificity of nonconventional MRI is limited. The hyperintense lesions on nonconventional MRI show pathologic nonspecificity and cannot distinguish inflammation, edema, demyelination, Wallerian degeneration, and axonal loss. More specific information about optic nerve damage has been acquired by magnetization transfer *(109,113,124–126)* and diffusion-weighted *(113,127)* and functional MRI *(128,129)*.

4.2. Visual Evoked Potentials

VEP are nearly always abnormal in the affected eye. They show prolonged latencies, even when vision has returned to normal. Three-dimensional VEP are more sensitive than conventional VEP in detecting postchiasmal lesions *(130)*. VEP might not be helpful in differentiating among causes of optic neuropathies in the acute phase *(131)* but are useful in determining whether the episode of

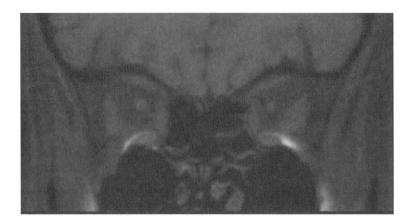

Fig. 5. Coronal short-τ fast-FLAIR image from a 39-yr-old woman with a 1-yr history of monosymptomatic left optic neuritis shows left optic nerve atrophy. At 1 yr, vision was 6/5 equivalent to approx 20/15, despite the optic nerve atrophy. (Courtesy of Dr. Simon J. Hickman and Dr. David H. Miller from the NMR Research Unit, Institute of Neurology, University College London, UK.)

visual loss involved a demyelinating process (characteristic delay and loss of amplitude of the P100 waveform) *(132)*. The combination of VEP with pattern electroretinography can be useful in differentiating macular from optic nerve disorders. The presence of a delayed but well preserved P100 wave in VEP is most useful in confirming a diagnosis of ON of demyelinating origin and in supporting a diagnosis of MS by showing dissemination in space *(133)*.

4.3. Laboratory Exams

The CSF in ON sometimes contains elevated protein, mild lymphocytosis, free κ-light chains, elevated IgG index, and oligoclonal bands *(30–35,67)*. CSF analysis adds little additional information to MRI results for predicting the 2- *(31)* or 5-yr development of clinically definite MS *(33)*; however, in one study, the patients who had abnormal MRI and elevated intrathecal IgG synthesis at baseline had a 46% increased risk of MS after 4 yr, compared with 33% in patients who had only an abnormal MRI but no presence of intrathecal IgG synthesis *(134)*. Based on the ONTT *(59)*, ancillary laboratory testing in patients who have ON typically does not yield any clinically useful information. These additional tests include routine blood tests, antiphospholipid and fluorscein treponemal antibodies, and chest x-ray. Of 457 patients enrolled in the ONTT, three were subsequently diagnosed as having anterior ischemic optic neuropathy, two had compressive lesions, and two had connective tissue diseases *(4,59)*. In another study *(135)*, 17 of 102 patients enrolled were later excluded because of misdiagnosis.

5. TREATMENT

5.1. Corticosteroid Therapy

Prior to the publication of the ONTT, a survey of general ophthalmologists indicated that almost 70% treated ON with corticosteroids *(136,137)*. Patients were treated with various regimens of corticosteroids but usually a high dose of intravenous methylprednisolone (IVMP) followed a low dose of oral corticosteroids. Early observational studies used corticotrophin *(138,139)*, but these studies produced conflicting results. Subsequently, placebo-controlled trials *(18,59–61,63,122,140–143)* confirmed that high-dose IVMP hastens recovery in ON and, in the short term, increases the likelihood of clinical improvement. A meta-analysis of these trials showed that corticosteroids had a beneficial effect on acute attacks but did not result in long-term improvement of visual outcome *(144)*. The use of corticosteroids for the treatment of ON was reviewed in 2000 by the Quality Standard Subcommittee of the American Academy of Neurology *(145)*. The committee confirmed that there is no evidence to recommend the use of low-dose oral prednisolone (1 mg/kg/d) for the treatment of acute ON, although the committee stated that higher doses of oral methylprednisolone or IVMP may hasten and improve the degree of recovery. IVMP 1 g/d for 3 d has become the preferred option *(146)*. An abrupt discontinuation of corticosteroids may precipitate attacks of ON, and high doses of IVMP should be tapered with oral prednisone for 2 to 3 wk. An oral taper is also prudent with respect to homeostasis of the hypothalamic–pituitary–adrenal axis *(147)*.

There is no long-term evidence of benefit to visual function in patients who have been treated with corticosteroids. In the ONTT trial, rapid visual recovery was associated with the use of IVMP in the first 2 to 3 wk after onset of visual symptoms *(59)*. However, after 1 mo, the recovery rate was similar in treated and placebo patients. Some further improvement has been reported from 6 mo to 1 yr *(148)*. The IVMP-treated group had better contrast sensitivity and visual color function than the placebo group did, although after 1 yr, there was no difference of visual function in patients who were treated with IVMP, oral prednisone, or placebo *(60,61)*.

In patients with acute ON, treatment with a 3-d course of high-dose IVMP (followed by a short course of prednisone) reduces the rate of development of MS over a 2-yr period, especially in those with baseline brain MRI abnormalities *(60)*. The ONTT showed that definite MS developed within the first 2 yr in 7.5% of the IVMP group (134 patients), 14.7% of the oral prednisone group (129 patients), and 16.7 % of the placebo group (126 patients). The adjusted RR for the development of definite MS within 2 yr in the IVMP group was 0.34 compared with the placebo group and 0.38 compared with the oral prednisone group. Treatment with oral prednisone increased the risk of a new attack in either eye. Of the 150 patients who were treated with corticosteroids and had two or more lesions on baseline MRI scan, 36% developed clinically definite MS within 2 yr. The beneficial effect of treatment was lost within 3 yr, with a cumulative incidence of clinically definite MS of 17.3% in the IVMP group, 24.7% in the oral prednisone group, and 21.3% in the placebo group *(140)*.

Despite some criticism (the findings of the ONTT were based on a retrospective analysis, using an open-label treatment with only a small number of patients developing clinically definite MS), the ONTT is considered a hallmark for a well-controlled prospective clinical trial on the evaluation and treatment of ON. The ONTT generated considerable controversy because its results were not anticipated in advance. Also, it was unclear whether the ONTT results could be generalized to clinically isolated syndromes other than ON or to patients with relapsing–remitting MS (RRMS). Recently, we demonstrated in a randomized, controlled, single-blind, phase II clinical trial in patients with RRMS that prolonged treatment with pulsed IVMP slowed development of destructive lesions and delayed the rate of brain atrophy and disability progression *(149)*. In our opinion, IVMP should be given in ON when there is a high probability of developing clinically definite MS (evidence of MRI dissemination in space and time, according to McDonald criteria). Further studies are needed to establish definitively whether single or pulse cycles of IVMP may prevent or delay the development of clinically definite MS.

5.2. *Interferon-β Therapy*

Two randomized, placebo-controlled trials have recently addressed whether IFN-β therapy can slow the progression of clinically isolated syndromes to clinically definite MS *(150,151)*. Based on recent results of the Controlled High-Risk Subjects Avonex Multiple Sclerosis Prevention Study (CHAMPS) *(150)*, patients who received weekly intramuscular IFN-β1a at the time of the first demyelinating event, such as ON, had a significantly lower cumulative probability of developing clinically definite MS over 3 yr of follow-up (RR, 0.56; 95% confidence interval, 0.38–0.81; $p = 0.002$). The trial was stopped after a preplanned interim efficacy analysis. As compared with the patients in the placebo group, patients in the IFN-β1a group had a relative reduction in the volume of brain lesions, fewer new or enlarging T2 lesions, and fewer Gd-enhancing lesions at 18 mo. In the extended analysis of the CHAMPS study, Beck et al. *(152)* reported that a beneficial effect of treatment occurred in all clinical subgroups of patients, regardless of type of presenting event (ON, brainstem-cerebellar syndromes, and spinal cord syndromes). Adjusted rate ratios for the development of clinically definite MS in patients with ON treated with IFN-β1a was 0.58 and, for the development of the combined clinically definite MS/MRI, the outcome was 0.50. Based on the results of the CHAMPS trial, the Food and Drug Adminitration has approved IFN-β1a for treating patients with a first demyelinating event, such as ON, when there is a high probability of developing clinically definite MS (evidence of MRI dissemination in space and time, according to McDonald criteria).

In the Early Treatment of MS Study (ETOMS) *(151)*, the effect of once weekly subcutaneous IFN-β1a on the occurrence of relapses was assessed in patients after the first presentation with a neurological event who were at high risk of conversion to clinically definite MS. Fewer patients developed clinically definite MS in the IFN-treated group than in the placebo group (34 vs 45%; $p = 0.047$). The time to the development of clinically definite MS was significantly delayed in the IFN group vs the placebo group (mean 569 vs 252 d). The annual relapse rate was significantly lower (0.33 vs 0.43) in the IFN group. The number of new T2-weighted MRI lesions and the increase in lesion burden were significantly lower with treatment than with placebo. The results of validation of the modified McDonald criteria in the ETOMS study *(79)* suggested that meeting the criteria increased the odds of conversion to clinically definite MS; thus, the number of patients requiring treatment to prevent one patient from converting to clinically definite MS within 2 yr decreased from 50 with two or fewer positive criteria to 5.6 with four positive criteria. On the other hand, the effect of once weekly IFN-β1a therapy seems to be stronger in patients with a high number of positive criteria than in those with a low number of positive criteria.

5.3. Intravenous Immunoglobulin

Intravenous immunoglobulin (IVIg) has been reported to improve visual acuity in patients with MS who developed ON, but no definite conclusions for treatment guidelines could be reached from the two trials *(153,154)*. An early report suggested that IVIg could promote remyelination and improve vision in ON. Another trial evaluated whether IVIg reversed chronic visual impairment in MS patients with ON. Fifty-five patients with persistent loss of visual acuity after ON were randomized to receive either 0.4 g/kg IVIg daily for 5 d, followed by three infusions monthly for 3 mo, or placebo. The trial, which had enrolled 55 of the 60 patients originally planned, was terminated in advance because of negative results. The authors found that the IVIg administration did not reverse persistent visual loss from ON to a degree that merited general use.

5.4. Treatment of Ischemic Decompression Neuropathy

There is no effective treatment for nonarteritic ION. Surgical optic nerve decompression initially seemed to improve vision in some patients; however, the results of the Ischemic Optic Neuropathy Decompression Trial *(98,155)* ultimately showed that the decompression surgery did not improve visual outcome and may have been harmful. Of concern, patients who received optic nerve decompression had a lower rate of visual recovery and a higher rate of visual loss at the 3-mo follow-up than patients who did not have the procedure. A 24-mo follow-up *(156)* confirmed no benefit of surgery.

ACKNOWLEDGMENTS

We thank Eve Salczynski and Jitendra Sharma for technical support. We are grateful to Dr. Simon J. Hickman and Dr. David H. Miller of NMR Research Unit, Institute of Neurology, University College London, UK, for providing us the illustrated case of optic nerve atrophy. This work was supported in part by a research grant to R. Bakshi from the National Institutes of Health (NIH-NINDS 1 K23 NS42379-01).

REFERENCES

1. Jin YP, de Pedro-Cuesta J, Soderstrom M, Stawiarz L, Link H. Incidence of optic neuritis in Stockholm, Sweden 1990-1995: I. Age, sex, birth and ethnic-group related patterns. J Neurol Sci 1998;159:107–114.
2. Rodriguez M, Siva A, Cross SA, O'Brien PC, Kurland LT. Optic neuritis: a population-based study in Olmsted County, Minnesota. Neurology 1995;45:244–250.
3. MacDonald BK, Cockerell OC, Sander JW, Shorvon SD. The incidence and lifetime prevalence of neurological disorders in a prospective community-based study in the UK. Brain 2000;123(Pt 4):665–676.
4. The clinical profile of optic neuritis. Experience of the Optic Neuritis Treatment Trial. Optic Neuritis Study Group. Arch Ophthalmol 1991;109:1673–1678.
5. Kinnunen E, Konttinen YT, Bergroth V, Kemppinen P. Immunological studies on patients with optic neuritis without evidence of multiple sclerosis. J Neurol Sci 1989;90:43–52.
6. Hauser SL, Oksenberg JR, Lincoln R, et al. Interaction between HLA-DR2 and abnormal brain MRI in optic neuritis and early MS. Optic Neuritis Study Group. Neurology 2000;54:1859–1861.
7. Jin YP, de Pedro-Cuesta J, Soderstrom M, Link H. Incidence of optic neuritis in Stockholm, Sweden, 1990-1995: II. Time and space patterns. Arch Neurol 1999;56:975–980.
8. Farris BK, Pickard DJ. Bilateral postinfectious optic neuritis and intravenous steroid therapy in children. Ophthalmology 1990;97:339–345.
9. Sandberg-Wollheim M, Bynke H, Cronqvist S, Holtas S, Platz P, Ryder LP. A long-term prospective study of optic neuritis: evaluation of risk factors. Ann Neurol 1990;27:386–393.
10. Hutchinson WM. Acute optic neuritis and the prognosis for multiple sclerosis. J Neurol Neurosurg Psychiatry 1976;39:283–289.
11. Beck RW, Kupersmith MJ, Cleary PA, Katz B. Fellow eye abnormalities in acute unilateral optic neuritis. Experience of the Optic Neuritis Treatment Trial. Ophthalmology 1993;100:691–697, discussion 697–698.
12. Hwang JM, Lee YJ, Kim MK. Optic neuritis in Asian children. J Pediatr Ophthalmol Strabismus 2002;39:26–32.
13. Pokroy R, Modi G, Saffer D. Optic neuritis in an urban black African community. Eye 2001;15(Pt 4):469–473.
14. Youl BD, Turano G, Miller DH, et al. The pathophysiology of acute optic neuritis. An association of gadolinium leakage with clinical and electrophysiological deficits. Brain 1991;114(Pt 6):2437–2450.
15. Smith KJ, McDonald WI. The pathophysiology of multiple sclerosis: the mechanisms underlying the production of symptoms and the natural history of the disease. Philos Trans R Soc Lond B Biol Sci 1999;354:1649–1673.
16. Brusa A, Jones SJ, Plant GT. Long-term remyelination after optic neuritis: a 2-year visual evoked potential and psychophysical serial study. Brain 2001;124(Pt 3):468–479.
17. Beck RW, Cleary PA. Recovery from severe visual loss in optic neuritis. Arch Ophthalmol 1993;111:300.
18. Beck RW, Gal RL, Bhatti MT, Brodsky MC, Buckley EG, Chrousos GA, et al. Visual function more than 10 years after optic neuritis. Experience of the Optic Neuritis Treatment Trial. Am J Ophthalmol 2004;137:77–83.
19. Lepore FE. The origin of pain in optic neuritis. Determinants of pain in 101 eyes with optic neuritis. Arch Neurol 1991;48:748–749.
20. Cantore WA. Optic neuritis. Pa Med 1996;99(Suppl):96–98.
21. Keltner JL, Johnson CA, Spurr JO, Beck RW. Baseline visual field profile of optic neuritis. The experience of the Optic Neuritis Treatment Trial. Optic Neuritis Study Group. Arch Ophthalmol 1993;111:231–234.
22. Davis FA, Bergen D, Schauf C, McDonald I, Deutsch W. Movement phosphenes in optic neuritis: a new clinical sign. Neurology 1976;26:1100–1104.
23. Selhorst JB, Saul RF. Uhthoff and his symptom. J Neuroophthalmol 1995;15:63–69.
24. Beck RW. Optic Neuritis. In: Miller NR, Newman NJ, eds. The Essentials: Walsh & Hoyt's Clinical Neuro-ophtalmology. Baltimore, Williams & Wilkins, 1999;599–648.
25. Hickman SJ, Brierley CM, Brex PA, et al. Continuing optic nerve atrophy following optic neuritis: a serial MRI study. Mult Scler 2002;8:339–342.
26. Hickman SJ, Kapoor R, Jones SJ, Altmann DR, Plant GT, Miller DH. Corticosteroids do not prevent optic nerve atrophy following optic neuritis. J Neurol Neurosurg Psychiatry 2003;74:1139–1141.
27. Eggenberger ER. Inflammatory optic neuropathies. Ophthalmol Clin North Am 2001;14:73–82.
28. Martinelli V, Bianchi Marzoli S. Non-demyelinating optic neuropathy: clinical entities. Neurol Sci 2001;22(Suppl 2): S55–59.
29. Riikonen R, Donner M, Erkkila H. Optic neuritis in children and its relationship to multiple sclerosis: a clinical study of 21 children. Dev Med Child Neurol 1988;30:349–359.
30. Stendahl-Brodin L, Link H. Optic neuritis: oligoclonal bands increase the risk of multiple sclerosis. Acta Neurol Scand 1983;67:301–304.
31. Rolak LA, Beck RW, Paty DW, Tourtellotte WW, Whitaker JN, Rudick RA. Cerebrospinal fluid in acute optic neuritis: experience of the Optic Neuritis Treatment Trial. Neurology 1996;46:368–372.

32. Soderstrom M, Ya-Ping J, Hillert J, Link H. Optic neuritis: prognosis for multiple sclerosis from MRI, CSF, and HLA findings. Neurology 1998;50:708–714.

33. Cole SR, Beck RW, Moke PS, Kaufman DI, Tourtellotte WW. The predictive value of CSF oligoclonal banding for MS 5 years after optic neuritis. Optic Neuritis Study Group. Neurology 1998;51:885–887.

34. Sastre-Garriga J, Tintore M, Rovira A, et al. Conversion to multiple sclerosis after a clinically isolated syndrome of the brainstem: cranial magnetic resonance imaging, cerebrospinal fluid and neurophysiological findings. Mult Scler 2003;9:39–43.

35. Jin YP, de Pedro-Cuesta J, Huang YH, Soderstrom M. Predicting multiple sclerosis at optic neuritis onset. Mult Scler 2003;9:135–141.

36. Chan JW. Optic neuritis in multiple sclerosis. Ocul Immunol Inflamm 2002;10:161–186.

37. Deckert-Schluter M, Schluter D, Schwendemann G. Evaluation of IL-2, sIL2R, IL-6, TNF-alpha, and IL-1 beta levels in serum and CSF of patients with optic neuritis. J Neurol Sci 1992;113:50–54.

38. Petersen AA, Sellebjerg F, Frederiksen J, Olesen J, Vejlsgaard GL. Soluble ICAM-1, demyelination, and inflammation in multiple sclerosis and acute optic neuritis. J Neuroimmunol 1998;88:120–127.

39. Soderstrom M, Link H, Sun JB, et al. T cells recognizing multiple peptides of myelin basic protein are found in blood and enriched in cerebrospinal fluid in optic neuritis and multiple sclerosis. Scand J Immunol 1993;37:355–368.

40. Navikas V, Link H. Review: cytokines and the pathogenesis of multiple sclerosis. J Neurosci Res 1996;45:322–333.

41. Potter NT, Bigazzi PE. Acute optic neuritis associated with immunization with the CNS myelin proteolipid protein. Invest Ophthalmol Vis Sci 1992;33:1717–1722.

42. Sellebjerg F, Christiansen M, Nielsen PM, Frederiksen JL. Cerebrospinal fluid measures of disease activity in patients with multiple sclerosis. Mult Scler 1998;4:475–479.

43. Soderstrom M. Clues to the immunopathogenesis of multiple sclerosis by investigating untreated patients during the very early stage of disease. Neurol Sci 2001;22:145–149.

44. Soderstrom M, Link H, Xu Z, Fredriksson S. Optic neuritis and multiple sclerosis: anti-MBP and anti-MBP peptide antibody-secreting cells are accumulated in CSF. Neurology 1993;43:1215–1222.

45. Berger T, Rubner P, Schautzer F, et al. Antimyelin antibodies as a predictor of clinically definite multiple sclerosis after a first demyelinating event. N Engl J Med 2003;349:139–145.

46. Compston DA, Batchelor JR, McDonald WI. B-lymphocyte alloantigens associated with multiple sclerosis. Lancet 1976;2:1261–1265.

47. Haines JL, Terwedow HA, Burgess K, et al. Linkage of the MHC to familial multiple sclerosis suggests genetic heterogeneity. The Multiple Sclerosis Genetics Group. Hum Mol Genet 1998;7:1229–1234.

48. Hillert J, Kall T, Olerup O, Soderstrom M. Distribution of HLA-Dw2 in optic neuritis and multiple sclerosis indicates heterogeneity. Acta Neurol Scand 1996;94:161–166.

49. Marrosu MG, Murru MR, Costa G, Murru R, Muntoni F, Cucca F. DRB1-DQA1-DQB1 loci and multiple sclerosis predisposition in the Sardinian population. Hum Mol Genet 1998;7:1235–1237.

50. Saruhan-Direskeneli G, Esin S, Baykan-Kurt B, Ornek I, Vaughan R, Eraksoy M. HLA-DR and -DQ associations with multiple sclerosis in Turkey. Hum Immunol 1997;55:59–65.

51. Kantarci OH, de Andrade M, Weinshenker BG. Identifying disease modifying genes in multiple sclerosis. J Neuroimmunol 2002;123:144–159.

52. Frederiksen JL, Madsen HO, Ryder LP, Larsson HB, Morling N, Svejgaard A. HLA typing in acute optic neuritis. Relation to multiple sclerosis and magnetic resonance imaging findings. Arch Neurol 1997;54:76–80.

53. Kelly MA, Cavan DA, Penny MA, et al. The influence of HLA-DR and -DQ alleles on progression to multiple sclerosis following a clinically isolated syndrome. Hum Immunol 1993;37:185–191.

54. Morrissey SP, Miller DH, Kendall BE, et al. The significance of brain magnetic resonance imaging abnormalities at presentation with clinically isolated syndromes suggestive of multiple sclerosis. A 5-year follow-up study. Brain 1993;116(Pt 1):135–146.

55. Soderstrom M, Lindqvist M, Hillert J, Kall TB, Link H. Optic neuritis: findings on MRI, CSF examination and HLA class II typing in 60 patients and results of a short-term follow-up. J Neurol 1994;241:391–397.

56. Zivadinov R, Uxa L, Zacchi T, et al. HLA genotypes and disease severity assessed by magnetic resonance imaging findings in patients with multiple sclerosis. J Neurol 2003;250:1099–1106.

57. Yamasaki K, Horiuchi I, Minohara M, et al. HLA-DPB1*0501-associated opticospinal multiple sclerosis: clinical, neuroimaging and immunogenetic studies. Brain 1999;122(Pt 9):1689–1696.

58. Cree BA, Goodin DS, Hauser SL. Neuromyelitis optica. Semin Neurol 2002;22:105–122.

59. Beck RW, Cleary PA, Anderson MM Jr, et al. A randomized, controlled trial of corticosteroids in the treatment of acute optic neuritis. The Optic Neuritis Study Group. N Engl J Med 1992;326:581–588.

60. Beck RW, Cleary PA, Trobe JD, et al. The effect of corticosteroids for acute optic neuritis on the subsequent development of multiple sclerosis. The Optic Neuritis Study Group. N Engl J Med 1993;329:1764–1769.

61. Beck RW, Cleary PA. Optic neuritis treatment trial. One-year follow-up results. Arch Ophthalmol 1993;111:773–775.

62. Beck RW, Trobe JD. The Optic Neuritis Treatment Trial. Putting the results in perspective. The Optic Neuritis Study Group. J Neuroophthalmol 1995;15:131–135.

63. The 5-year risk of MS after optic neuritis. Experience of the optic neuritis treatment trial. Optic Neuritis Study Group. Neurology 1997;49:1404–1413.

64. Morrissey SP, Borruat FX, Miller DH, et al. Bilateral simultaneous optic neuropathy in adults: clinical, imaging, serological, and genetic studies. J Neurol Neurosurg Psychiatry 1995;58:70–74.

65. Poser CM, Paty DW, Scheinberg L, et al. New diagnostic criteria for multiple sclerosis: guidelines for research protocols. Ann Neurol 1983;13:227–231.

66. McDonald WI, Compston A, Edan G, et al. Recommended diagnostic criteria for multiple sclerosis: guidelines from the International Panel on the diagnosis of multiple sclerosis. Ann Neurol 2001;50:121–127.

67. Frederiksen JL, Petrera J, Larsson HB, Stigsby B, Olesen J. Serial MRI, VEP, SEP and biotesiometry in acute optic neuritis: value of baseline results to predict the development of new lesions at one year follow up. Acta Neurol Scand 1996;93:246–252.

68. Jacobs LD, Kaba SE, Miller CM, Priore RL, Brownscheidle CM. Correlation of clinical, magnetic resonance imaging, and cerebrospinal fluid findings in optic neuritis. Ann Neurol 1997;41:392–398.

69. Ghezzi A, Martinelli V, Torri V, et al. Long-term follow-up of isolated optic neuritis: the risk of developing multiple sclerosis, its outcome, and the prognostic role of paraclinical tests. J Neurol 1999;246:770–775.

70. Interferon beta-1a for optic neuritis patients at high risk for multiple sclerosis. Am J Ophthalmol 2001;132:463–471.

71. Ghezzi A, Martinelli V, Rodegher M, Zaffaroni M, Comi G. The prognosis of idiopathic optic neuritis. Neurol Sci 2000;21(4 Suppl 2):S865–869.

72. Barkhof F, Filippi M, Miller DH, et al. Comparison of MRI criteria at first presentation to predict conversion to clinically definite multiple sclerosis. Brain 1997;120(Pt 11):2059–2069.

73. Tintore M, Rovira A, Martinez MJ, et al. Isolated demyelinating syndromes: comparison of different MR imaging criteria to predict conversion to clinically definite multiple sclerosis. AJNR Am J Neuroradiol 2000;21:702–706.

74. Dalton CM, Brex PA, Miszkiel KA, et al. Application of the new McDonald criteria to patients with clinically isolated syndromes suggestive of multiple sclerosis. Ann Neurol 2002;52:47–53.

75. Dalton CM, Brex PA, Miszkiel KA, et al. New T2 lesions enable an earlier diagnosis of multiple sclerosis in clinically isolated syndromes. Ann Neurol 2003;53:673–676.

76. Frohman EM, Goodin DS, Calabresi PA, et al. The utility of MRI in suspected MS: report of the Therapeutics and Technology Assessment Subcommittee of the American Academy of Neurology. Neurology 2003;61:602–611.

77. MRI predictors of early conversion to clinically definite MS in the CHAMPS placebo group. Neurology 2002;59:998–1005.

78. Tintore M, Rovira A, Rio J, et al. New diagnostic criteria for multiple sclerosis: application in first demyelinating episode. Neurology 2003;60:27–30.

79. Barkhof F, Rocca M, Francis G, et al. Validation of diagnostic magnetic resonance imaging criteria for multiple sclerosis and response to interferon beta1a. Ann Neurol 2003;53:718–724.

80. Miller DH, Ormerod IE, McDonald WI, et al. The early risk of multiple sclerosis after optic neuritis. J Neurol Neurosurg Psychiatry 1988;51:1569–1571.

81. Brex PA, O'Riordan JI, Miszkiel KA, et al. Multisequence MRI in clinically isolated syndromes and the early development of MS. Neurology 1999;53:1184–1190.

82. Ramsaransing G, Maurits N, Zwanikken C, De Keyser J. Early prediction of a benign course of multiple sclerosis on clinical grounds: a systematic review. Mult Scler 2001;7:345–347.

83. Filippi M, Horsfield MA, Morrissey SP, et al. Quantitative brain MRI lesion load predicts the course of clinically isolated syndromes suggestive of multiple sclerosis. Neurology 1994;44:635–641.

84. Sailer M, O'Riordan JI, Thompson AJ, et al. Quantitative MRI in patients with clinically isolated syndromes suggestive of demyelination. Neurology 1999;52:599–606.

85. Brex PA, Ciccarelli O, O'Riordan JI, Sailer M, Thompson AJ, Miller DH. A longitudinal study of abnormalities on MRI and disability from multiple sclerosis. N Engl J Med 2002;346:158–164.

86. Wingerchuk DM, Hogancamp WF, O'Brien PC, Weinshenker BG. The clinical course of neuromyelitis optica (Devic's syndrome). Neurology 1999;53:1107–1114.

87. de Seze J, Lebrun C, Stojkovic T, Ferriby D, Chatel M, Vermersch P. Is Devic's neuromyelitis optica a separate disease? A comparative study with multiple sclerosis. Mult Scler 2003;9:521–525.

88. de Seze J, Stojkovic T, Ferriby D, et al. Devic's neuromyelitis optica: clinical, laboratory, MRI and outcome profile. J Neurol Sci 2002;197:57–61.

89. Baudoin D, Gambarelli D, Gayraud D, et al. Devic's neuromyelitis optica: a clinicopathological review of the literature in connection with a case showing fatal dysautonomia. Clin Neuropathol 1998;17:175–183.

90. Wingerchuk DM, Weinshenker BG. Neuromyelitis optica: clinical predictors of a relapsing course and survival. Neurology 2003;60:848–853.

91. Lucchinetti CF, Mandler RN, McGavern D, et al. A role for humoral mechanisms in the pathogenesis of Devic's neuromyelitis optica. Brain 2002;125(Pt 7):1450–1461.

92. Selbst RG, Selhorst JB, Harbison JW, Myer EC. Parainfectious optic neuritis. Report and review following varicella. Arch Neurol 1983;40:347–350.

93. Milla E, Zografos L, Piguet B. Bilateral optic papillitis following mycoplasma pneumoniae pneumonia. Ophthalmologica 1998;212:344–346.

94. Semba RD. The ocular complications of smallpox and smallpox immunization. Arch Ophthalmol 2003;121:715–719.

95. Swartz NG, Beck RW, Savino PJ, et al. Pain in anterior ischemic optic neuropathy. J Neuroophthalmol 1995;15:9–10.

96. Rizzo JF 3rd, Lessell S. Optic neuritis and ischemic optic neuropathy. Overlapping clinical profiles. Arch Ophthalmol 1991;109:1668–1672.

97. Keltner JL. Giant-cell arteritis. Signs and symptoms. Ophthalmology 1982;89:1101–1110.

98. Optic nerve decompression surgery for nonarteritic anterior ischemic optic neuropathy (NAION) is not effective and may be harmful. The Ischemic Optic Neuropathy Decompression Trial Research Group. JAMA 1995;273:625–632.

99. Kesler A, Pianka P. Toxic optic neuropathy. Curr Neurol Neurosci Rep 2003;3:410–414.

100. Balcer LJ. Optic nerve disorders. Curr Opin Ophthalmol 1997;8:3–8.

101. Shaikh ZA, Bakshi R, Greenberg SJ, Fine EJ, Shatla A, Lincoff NS. Orbital involvement as the initial manifestation of sarcoidosis: magnetic resonance imaging findings. J Neuroimaging 2000;10:180–183.

102. Purvin VA. Optic neuropathies for the neurologist. Semin Neurol 2000;20:97–110.

103. Loong SC. The eye in neurology: evaluation of sudden visual loss and diplopia—diagnostic pointers and pitfalls. Ann Acad Med Singapore 2001;30:143–147.

104. Jacobs D, Galetta S. Diagnosis and management of orbital pseudotumor. Curr Opin Ophthalmol 2002;13:347–351.

105. Lessell S, Gise RL, Krohel GB. Bilateral optic neuropathy with remission in young men. Variation on a theme by Leber? Arch Neurol 1983;40:2–6.

106. Harding AE, Sweeney MG, Miller DH, et al. Occurrence of a multiple sclerosis-like illness in women who have a Leber's hereditary optic neuropathy mitochondrial DNA mutation. Brain 1992;115(Pt 4):979–989.

107. Cock H, Mandler R, Ahmed W, Schapira AH. Neuromyelitis optica (Devic's syndrome): no association with the primary mitochondrial DNA mutations found in Leber hereditary optic neuropathy. J Neurol Neurosurg Psychiatry 1997;62:85–87.

108. Tran M, Bhargava R, MacDonald IM. Leber hereditary optic neuropathy, progressive visual loss, and multiple-sclerosis-like symptoms. Am J Ophthalmol 2001;132:591–593.

109. Inglese M, Ghezzi A, Bianchi S, et al. Irreversible disability and tissue loss in multiple sclerosis: a conventional and magnetization transfer magnetic resonance imaging study of the optic nerves. Arch Neurol 2002;59:250–255.

110. Man PY, Turnbull DM, Chinnery PF. Leber hereditary optic neuropathy. J Med Genet 2002;39:162–169.

111. Howell N. LHON and other optic nerve atrophies: the mitochondrial connection. Dev Ophthalmol 2003;37:94–108.

112. Brown MD, Torroni A, Reckord CL, Wallace DC. Phylogenetic analysis of Leber's hereditary optic neuropathy mitochondrial DNA's indicates multiple independent occurrences of the common mutations. Hum Mutat 1995;6:311–325.

113. Inglese M, Rovaris M, Bianchi S, et al. Magnetic resonance imaging, magnetisation transfer imaging, and diffusion weighted imaging correlates of optic nerve, brain, and cervical cord damage in Leber's hereditary optic neuropathy. J Neurol Neurosurg Psychiatry 2001;70:444–449.

114. Bianchi Marzoli S, Martinelli V. Optic neuritis: differential diagnosis. Neurol Sci 2001;22(Suppl 2):S52–54.

115. Lee AG, Lin DJ, Kaufman M, Golnik KC, Vaphiades MS, Eggenberger E. Atypical features prompting neuroimaging in acute optic neuropathy in adults. Can J Ophthalmol 2000;35:325–330.

116. Hickman SJ, Dalton CM, Miller DH, Plant GT. Management of acute optic neuritis. Lancet 2002;360:1953–1962.

117. Smith MM, Strottmann JM. Imaging of the optic nerve and visual pathways. Semin Ultrasound CT MR 2001;22:473–487.

118. Gass A, Moseley IF. The contribution of magnetic resonance imaging in the differential diagnosis of optic nerve damage. J Neurol Sci 2000;172(Suppl 1):S17–22.

119. Simon JH, McDonald WI. Assessment of optic nerve damage in multiple sclerosis using magnetic resonance imaging. J Neurol Sci 2000;172(Suppl 1):S23–26.

120. Miller DH, Mac Manus DG, Bartlett PA, Kapoor R, Morrissey SP, Moseley IF. Detection of optic nerve lesions in optic neuritis using frequency-selective fat-saturation sequences. Neuroradiology 1993;35:156–158.

121. Davies MB, Williams R, Haq N, Pelosi L, Hawkins CP. MRI of optic nerve and postchiasmal visual pathways and visual evoked potentials in secondary progressive multiple sclerosis. Neuroradiology 1998;40:765–770.

122. Kapoor R, Miller DH, Jones SJ, et al. Effects of intravenous methylprednisolone on outcome in MRI-based prognostic subgroups in acute optic neuritis. Neurology 1998;50:230–237.

123. Youl BD, Turano G, Towell AD, et al. Optic neuritis: swelling and atrophy. Electroencephalogr Clin Neurophysiol Suppl 1996;46:173–179.

124. Boorstein JM, Moonis G, Boorstein SM, Patel YP, Culler AS. Optic neuritis: imaging with magnetization transfer. AJR Am J Roentgenol 1997;169:1709–1712.

125. Filippi M, Rocca MA, Moiola L, et al. MRI and magnetization transfer imaging changes in the brain and cervical cord of patients with Devic's neuromyelitis optica. Neurology 1999;53:1705–1710.

126. Hickman SJ, Toosy AT, Jones SJ, et al. Serial magnetization transfer imaging in acute optic neuritis. Brain 2004;127:692–700.

127. Iwasawa T, Matoba H, Ogi A, et al. Diffusion-weighted imaging of the human optic nerve: a new approach to evaluate optic neuritis in multiple sclerosis. Magn Reson Med 1997;38:484–491.

128. Rombouts SA, Lazeron RH, Scheltens P, et al. Visual activation patterns in patients with optic neuritis: an fMRI pilot study. Neurology 1998;50:1896–1899.

129. Gareau PJ, Gati JS, Menon RS, et al. Reduced visual evoked responses in multiple sclerosis patients with optic neuritis: comparison of functional magnetic resonance imaging and visual evoked potentials. Mult Scler 1999;5:161–164.

130. Towle VL, Witt JC, Nader SH, Reder AT, Foust R, Spire JP. Three-dimensional human pattern visual evoked potentials. II. Multiple sclerosis patients. Electroencephalogr Clin Neurophysiol 1991;80:339–346.

131. Acheson J. Optic nerve and chiasmal disease. J Neurol 2000;247:587–596.

132. Andersson T, Siden A. An analysis of VEP components in optic neuritis. Electromyogr Clin Neurophysiol 1995; 35:77–85.

133. Halliday AM, McDonald WI, Mushin J. Visual evoked response in diagnosis of multiple sclerosis. Br Med J 1973;4: 661–664.

134. Ghezzi A, Torri V, Zaffaroni M. Isolated optic neuritis and its prognosis for multiple sclerosis: a clinical and para-clinical study with evoked potentials. CSF examination and brain MRI. Ital J Neurol Sci 1996;17:325–332.

135. Wakakura M, Minei-Higa R, Oono S, et al. Baseline features of idiopathic optic neuritis as determined by a multi-center treatment trial in Japan. Optic Neuritis Treatment Trial Multicenter Cooperative Research Group (ONMRG). Jpn J Ophthalmol 1999;43:127–132.

136. Beck RW. The Optic Neuritis Treatment Trial. Arch Ophthalmol 1988;106:1051–1053.

137. Foroozan R, Buono LM, Savino PJ, Sergott RC. Acute demyelinating optic neuritis. Curr Opin Ophthalmol 2002; 13:375–380.

138. Rawson MD, Liversedge LA, Goldfarb G. Treatment of acute retrobulbar neuritis with corticotrophin. Lancet 1966; 2:1044–1046.

139. Bowden AN, Bowden PM, Friedmann AI, Perkin GD, Rose FC. A trial of corticotrophin gelatin injection in acute optic neuritis. J Neurol Neurosurg Psychiatry 1974;37:869–873.

140. Beck RW. The optic neuritis treatment trial: three-year follow-up results. Arch Ophthalmol 1995;113:136–137.

141. Sellebjerg F, Nielsen HS, Frederiksen JL, Olesen J. A randomized, controlled trial of oral high-dose methylprednisolone in acute optic neuritis. Neurology 1999;52:1479–1484.

142. Wakakura M, Mashimo K, Oono S, et al. Multicenter clinical trial for evaluating methylprednisolone pulse treatment of idiopathic optic neuritis in Japan. Optic Neuritis Treatment Trial Multicenter Cooperative Research Group (ONMRG). Jpn J Ophthalmol 1999;43:133–138.

143. Beck RW, Trobe JD, Moke PS, et al. High- and low-risk profiles for the development of multiple sclerosis within 10 years after optic neuritis: experience of the optic neuritis treatment trial. Arch Ophthalmol 2003;121:944–949.

144. Brusaferri F, Candelise L. Steroids for multiple sclerosis and optic neuritis: a meta-analysis of randomized controlled clinical trials. J Neurol 2000;247:435–442.

145. Kaufman DI, Trobe JD, Eggenberger ER, Whitaker JN. Practice parameter: the role of corticosteroids in the manage-ment of acute monosymptomatic optic neuritis. Report of the Quality Standards Subcommittee of the American Academy of Neurology. Neurology 2000;54:2039–2044.

146. Trobe JD, Sieving PC, Guire KE, Fendrick AM. The impact of the optic neuritis treatment trial on the practices of ophthalmologists and neurologists. Ophthalmology 1999;106:2047–2053.

147. Wenning GK, Wietholter H, Schnauder G, Muller PH, Kanduth S, Renn W. Recovery of the hypothalamic-pituitary-adrenal axis from suppression by short-term, high-dose intravenous prednisolone therapy in patients with MS. Acta Neurol Scand 1994;89:270–273.

148. Beck RW, Cleary PA, Backlund JC. The course of visual recovery after optic neuritis. Experience of the Optic Neuritis Treatment Trial. Ophthalmology 1994;101:1771–1778.

149. Zivadinov R, Rudick RA, De Masi R, et al. Effects of IV methylprednisolone on brain atrophy in relapsing-remitting MS. Neurology 2001;57:1239–1247.

150. Jacobs LD, Beck RW, Simon JH, et al. Intramuscular interferon beta-1a therapy initiated during a first demyelinating event in multiple sclerosis. CHAMPS Study Group. N Engl J Med 2000;343:898–904.

151. Comi G, Filippi M, Barkhof F, et al. Effect of early interferon treatment on conversion to definite multiple sclerosis: a randomised study. Lancet 2001;357:1576–1582.

152. Beck RW, Chandler DL, Cole SR, et al. Interferon beta-1a for early multiple sclerosis: CHAMPS trial subgroup analyses. Ann Neurol 2002;51:481–490.

153. van Engelen BG, Hommes OR, Pinckers A, Cruysberg JR, Barkhof F, Rodriguez M. Improved vision after intra-venous immunoglobulin in stable demyelinating optic neuritis. Ann Neurol 1992;32:834–835.

154. Noseworthy JH, O'Brien PC, Petterson TM, et al. A randomized trial of intravenous immunoglobulin in inflammatory demyelinating optic neuritis. Neurology 2001;56:1514–1522.

155. Characteristics of patients with nonarteritic anterior ischemic optic neuropathy eligible for the Ischemic Optic Neuropathy Decompression Trial. Arch Ophthalmol 1996;114:1366–1374.

156. Ischemic Optic Neuropathy Decompression Trial: twenty-four-month update. Arch Ophthalmol 2000;118:793–798.

157. Bakshi R, Ketonen L. MRI of the brain in clinical neurology. In: Joynt RJ, Griggs RC, eds. Baker and Joynt's Clinical Neurology on CD-ROM. Philadelphia, PA: Lippincott, Williams & Wilkins, 2004.

CME QUESTIONS

1. According to the guidelines of Quality Standard Subcommittee of the American Academy of Neurology, the standard treatment for acute optic neuritis is:
   A. Low-dose oral prednisolone
   B. High-dose oral or intravenous methylprednisolone
   C. Interferon-β therapy
   D. Intravenous immunoglobulin therapy

2. Which of the following statements is *false*?
   A. Optic neuritis is always associated with the development of clinically definite multiple sclerosis
   B. The prognosis for visual recovery in optic neuritis is generally good
   C. Acute optic neuritis associated with multiple sclerosis is clinically indistinguishable from acute idiopathic optic neuritis
   D. Only long-term follow-up will confirm the diagnosis in an individual patient with monosymptomatic optic neuritis

3. According to the Optic Neuritis Treatment Trial, the 5-yr risk for clinically definite multiple following optic neuritis was a strong predictor in patients with:
   A. Normal magnetic resonance imaging (MRI)
   B. Abnormal MRI
   C. One spinal cord lesion on MRI
   D. Three or more lesions on brain MRI

4. According to the recommendation of the Therapeutics and Technology Assessment Subcommittee of the American Academy of Neurology, the appearance of either new T2 lesion or gadolinium-enhancement lesions after 3 mo following optic neuritis confirms:
   A. Dissemination in space and time on MRI
   B. Dissemination in space on MRI
   C. Possible diagnosis of MS, even before clinical dissemination has occurred
   D. Clinically definite diagnosis of MS

13

Central Nervous System Vasculitis
Pathogenesis, Immunology, and Clinical Management

Shariq Mumtaz, Marjorie R. Fowler, Eduardo Gonzales-Toledo, and Roger E. Kelley

1. INTRODUCTION

The vasculitides are a heterogenous group of multisystemic disorders that are pathologically characterized by inflammation of the blood vessels, structural damage to vessels, and usually vascular necrosis. Because involvement of blood vessels can result from inflammation of any type, vasculitis may be a presentation of diverse disorders. Vasculitis can occur either as a primary vasculitic disease or secondarily to another underlying pathology *(1–3)*. Vasculitis of the nervous system is both a diagnostic and management challenge for clinicians. Both the central nervous system (CNS) and peripheral nervous system (PNS) may be involved in the vasculitic process.

Vasculitis of the CNS is a rare entity that may result from numerous causes responsible for the presence of inflammatory lesions at the vascular wall. These inflammatory lesions may occasionally be associated with necrosis. Cerebral vessels of all sizes can be affected, and the clinical manifestations are highly variable, ranging from focal neurological signs to diffuse manifestations with an acute to chronic evolution. Vasculitic disorders of the CNS consist of primary angiitis of the CNS, giant cell arteritis, Takayasu's arteritis (TA), Wegner's granulomatosis, Churg-Strauss syndrome, Kawasaki's disease, CNS vasculitis associated with connective tissue disorders, vasculitis associated with Behcet's disease, and sarcoidosis, as well as infectious and neoplastic diseases.

The pathogenesis of most vasculitic syndromes affecting the nervous system remains largely unknown. Various immunological mechanisms that share the final pathway of vascular inflammation lead to upregulation of adhesion molecules on activated endothelium, increased adhesion of activated leukocytes to the endothelial layer, and transendothelial migration of leukocytes, particularly T lymphocytes and granuloma formation. Additionally, these mechanisms lead to generation and release of various chemokines and cytokines, generation of auto-antibodies (particularly anti-neutrophilic auto-antibodies), and formation and/or deposition of immune complexes.

Delayed hypersensitivity and cell-mediated immune responses, as reflected in the neuropathology of granulomatous vasculitis, have significant roles in vessel damage in vasculitides. When endothelial cells are stimulated by proinflammatory cytokines, particularly by interferon-γ, they activated and behave similar to antigen-presenting cells. The activated endothelial cells express human leukocyte antigen (HLA) class II molecules, which in turn, enable them to participate in immunological processes involving CD4$^+$ T lymphocytes. Endothelial cells release interleukin (IL)-1, which further activates T lymphocytes and initiates or promotes *in situ* immunologic reactions within

From: *Current Clinical Neurology: Inflammatory Disorders of the Nervous System:*
Pathogenesis, Immunology, and Clinical Management
Edited by: A. Minagar and J. S. Alexander © Humana Press Inc., Totowa, NJ

the blood vessel. Tumor necrosis factor (TNF)-α, another potent proinflammatory cytokine, induces upregulation of adhesion molecules by both endothelial cells and activated leukocytes. This promotes leukocyte-endothelium adhesion and the transendothelial migration of leukocytes into the CNS.

Antineutrophil cytoplasmic antibodies (ANCA) are directed against certain proteins in the cytoplasm of neutrophils and are present in a large number of patients with systemic vasculitis, particularly those with Wegener's granulomatosis. Two major groups of ANCA have been identified: cytoplasmic ANCA (cANCA) and perinuclear ANCA (pANCA). Proteinase-3, a 29-kDa neutral serine proteinase, exists in neutrophil azorophilic granules and is the most significant cANCA antigen. The enzyme myeloperoxidase is the major target for pANCA. The pathophysiological process for generating these particular types of auto-antibodies in vasculitides has not been established.

Formation of immune complexes and their deposition in vessel walls has long been implicated as an inciting mechanism of vascular inflammation and injury. Detection of complement and immunoglobulin (Ig) in human vasculitic lesions by immunofluorescent or immunohistochemical methods provides circumstantial evidence of an immune complex mediation of vasculitides. The mechanisms of tissue injury in immune complex-mediated vasculitis are similar to those described in serum sickness. Immune complexes (caused by antigen–antibody interactions) are formed in antigen excess and are deposited within the vascular walls. Deposition of immune complexes results in further activation of the complement components, particularly C5a, which is chemotactic for neutrophils. These cells invade the vascular wall, phagocytize the immune complexes, and release their intracytoplasmic enzymes, resulting in injury to the vessel wall.

2. PRIMARY ANGIITIS OF THE CNS

Primary aniitis of the CNS (PACNS) affects males and females of all age groups, with a mean age of 46 yr. Clinical manifestations of PACNS are restricted to the nervous system and can include headache, encephalopathy, stroke, coma, cranial neuropathies, and myelopathy. The most frequent early manifestations of primary CNS angiitis are headache and alteration of mental status. The headache may be severe and without any characterizing features. Nearly three-fourths of patients initially present with altered mental status. Of interest, clinical and laboratory evidence of systemic inflammation (e.g., malaise, leukocytosis, low-grade fever) is absent in the majority of patients.

The inflammatory process of PACNS characteristically involves small and medium-sized arterioles of the meninges and cortex of the brain and only rarely affects the veins and venules *(2,4–9)*. Pathologically, PACNS is characterized by segmental granulomatous angiitis limited to the CNS. The inflammatory infiltrate of PACNS mainly consists of lymphocytes, particularly T cells with a variable number of plasma cells, histiocytes, neutrophils, and eosinophils. The presence of intimal fibrosis within a lesion indicates that it has healed.

Examination of the cerebrospinal fluid (CSF) reveals abnormalities in 80 to 90% of patients. CSF may reveal elevated protein, lymphocytic pleocytosis, increased IgG synthesis, and the presence of oligoclonal bands. Magnetic resonance imaging (MRI) of the brain with contrast is abnormal in 50 to 100% of these patients *(10)*, which reveals abnormal signals indicative of ischemia. Conventional cerebral angiography is a sensitive diagnostic procedure for PACNS and can reveal single or multiple areas of segmental narrowing and dilatation along the affected vessels, vascular occlusion, hazy vascular margins, and/or the formation of collateral vessels. A prolonged circulation time may be found in the involved vascular territories. Many of these patients have only small vessel involvement, resulting in a negative cerebral angiogram. MRI abnormalities of PACNS are usually supratentorial and bilateral (Fig. 1) *(10–13)*, although brainstem and cerebellar lesions have also been described. Some of the parenchymal lesions caused by PACNS enhance following contrast (gadolinium-DTPA) infusion and may mimic the demyelinating lesions of multiple sclerosis (MS). Meningeal enhancement also may be present. In certain cases, mass lesions similar to low-grade gliomas have been reported *(11,12)*.

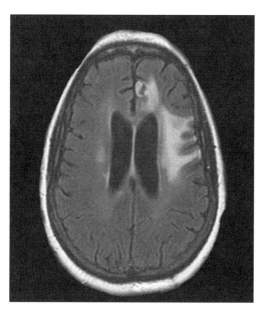

Fig. 1. A 22-yr-old female with PACNS. Fluid attenuation inverse recovery MRI, axial images of the brain shows multiple cortical and subcortical abnormal hyperintense signals.

A definite diagnosis of PACNS rests on brain biopsy, which can serve as a reliable tool to exclude other disorders imitating PACNS, such as MS, vasculopathy secondary to hypertension and atherosclerosis, cytomegalovirus infection, herpes simplex infection, and progressive multifocal leukoencephalopathy. The biopsy location is chosen based on the abnormalities on the MRI and performance of the biopsy on the contrast-enhancing lesions improves sensitivity. To increase the diagnostic accuracy, the biopsied specimen should include leptomeninges, along with cortical and subcortical tissue.

3. INFECTIOUS VASCULITIS

Various pathogenic mechanisms have been proposed for vasculitis in the context of infection. Normally, blood vessels are relatively resistant to infection; however, certain pathogens, such as varicella zoster virus (VZV), can directly invade the vascular wall and cause damage. Other pathogenic agents (Table 1) can cause vasculitis indirectly through immune or toxic mechanisms. Immune-mediated mechanisms of infectious vasculitis consist of a generation of cross-reacting auto-antibodies, cellular immune responses with granuloma formation, and deposition of immune complexes with activation of complement. These immune-mediated responses may indicate a direct invasion of the vascular antigens, a crossreactive attack mediated by molecular mimicry or an indirect bystander effect. Activation of the host immune system during the infectious vasculitis process can result in generation of factors with potential toxicity for vascular structures. For example, antibodies against neutrophil cytoplasmic antigens are formed in response to parasitic and fungal infections *(13)*. Cryoglobulins triggered by hepatitis virus infection or streptococcus have been associated with vascular damage, probably resulting from immune complex formation.

VZV causes a spectrum of neurological disorders involving both the central and peripheral nervous system. Encephalopathy caused by VZV is a vasculopathy that involves large or small vessels *(14)*. The large-vessel (granulomatous) encephalitis caused by VZV manifests with stroke-like acute focal neurological deficits. This type of large-vessel encephalitis generally occurs in immunocompetent patients, whereas small-vessel vasculitis is more likely to affect immunocompromised patients. Clinically, small-vessel VZV-vasculitis manifests with a progressive encephalopathy of acute or

Table 1
Classification of CNS Vasculitis

1. Primary angiitis of the central nervous system

2. Infectious vasculitis
   Varicella zoster virus
   Human immunodeficiency virus
   Syphilis
   Fungal infections
   Other bacterial infections

3. Necrotizing vasculitis
   Wegner's granulomatosis
   Churg–Strauss syndrome
   Polyarteritis nodosa

4. Vasculitis associated with collagen vascular disorders
   Systemic lupus erythematosus
   Sjogren syndrome
   Rheumatoid arteritis
   Polyarteritis nodosa

5. Giant cell arteritis
   Giant cell arteritis
   Takayasu's arteritis

6. Hypersensitivity vasculitis
   Drug-induced
   Toxin-induced

7. Vasculitis associated with systemic disorders
   Sarcoidosis
   Behcet's disease

8. Miscellaneous
   Vasculitis associated with neoplasia
   Kawasaki's disease
   Cogan syndrome

subacute onset, along with headache, fever, seizures, and focal neurological deficits. Most patients with large-vessel arteritis demonstrate pleocytosis (usually less than 100 cells/mm^3, predominantly mononuclear cells), oligoclonal bands, and elevated levels of IgG in their CSF examination. Cerebral angiography shows focal constriction and segmental stenosis, mainly in middle and anterior cerebral arteries, as well as in internal carotid arteries. Neuropathologic examination shows arterial inflammation with the presence of multinucleated giant cells, VZV antigen, Cowdry A inclusions, and herpes virus particles *(15)*. More recently, polymerase chain reaction (PCR) has detected VZV DNA in affected large cerebral arteries of affected patients. In small-vessel VZV-vasculitis, intraparenchymal arterioles demonstrate intramural and perivascular inflammatory cell infiltration, demyelinated areas, and necrosis at the grey–white matter junction *(16)*. Diagnosis of VZV infection depends on PCR analysis and antibody testing of the CSF for VZV DNA.

Human immunodeficiency virus (HIV) infection can affect both the CNS and PNS *(17,18)*. Vasculitis of the CNS in the context of HIV infection, if not related to opportunistic infections or lymphoproliferative disorders, is a rare event. In addition, necrotizing vasculitis of the CNS is extremely uncommon. CNS manifestations of the HIV-induced vasculitic syndrome include encephalitis, lymphocytic meningitis, stroke, and myelopathy. The neuropathology of CNS vasculitis in patients with acquired immunodeficiency disease (AIDS) is heterogeneous, and the various patterns can include granulomatous angiitis, eosinophilic vasculitis, or necrotizing vasculitis *(17,18)*, as well as vascular inflammation with transmural infiltration *(3)*.

A number of hypotheses have been offered to explain the development of vasculitis in patients with AIDS. HIV infection shares similarities with certain autoimmune disorders, and in patients with AIDS, polyclonal B-cell expansion and activation, with an increased incidence of positive antinuclear antibodies, have been reported *(19)*. Immune complex formation and their deposition in blood vessels may account for necrotizing vasculitis, and HIV antigens have been identified within vessels in a number of patients with necrotizing vasculitis *(20)*. In addition, HIV infection, at least initially, is associated with a massive immune activation characterized by high levels of proinflammatory cytokines and activated $CD4^+$ and $CD8^+$ T lymphocytes *(21)*. This massive inflammatory cascade of HIV infection may cause autoimmune tissue damage. Other proposed mechanisms include direct infection of endothelial cells by HIV or other organisms and impaired regulation of cytokines and adhesion molecules. Diagnosis of HIV-induced CNS vasculitis mainly depends of the exclusion of other causes of vasculitis (i.e., infective and neoplastic causes) in this patient population. The diagnosis should be considered in patients with AIDS who develop acute or subacute recurrent focal neurological deficits or those with diffuse neurological dysfunction, particularly when CSF and MRI abnormalities coexist. Cerebral angiography and brain biopsy can help confirm the diagnosis.

4. WEGNER'S GRANULOMATOSIS

Wegner's granulomatosis is a multisystemic inflammatory disorder characterized by necrotizing granulomatous vasculitis involving the upper and lower respiratory tracts, with or without focal segmental glomerulonephritis. Additionally, variable degrees of systemic vasculitis involving both small- and medium-sized arteries, as well as veins, may develop. Wegner's granulomatosis is an uncommon disorder, which affects males and females equally and rarely affects blacks. It can occur at any age, and the mean age of onset is 40 yr. In large series, involvement of both the CNS and PNS has been reported in 22 to 54% of cases *(22,23)*. Manifestations can include exophthalmos, cranial neuropathies, optic nerve or optic chiasm involvement, involvement of the base of the brain and meninges, and cerebrovascular events (e.g., ischemic stroke, venous thrombosis, intracerebral bleeding, cerebritis, seizures, peripheral neuropathy, mononeuritis multiplex, myopathy) *(22,23)*.

The etiology of Wegner's granulomatosis remains unknown, although cANCA along with intercurrent infections have been implicated in its development. It has been proposed that an infectious process triggers the production and release of cytokines, such as IL-1, IL-8, and TNF-α, which in turn causes neutrophils to express adhesion molecules, adhere to the endothelial layer, and express other proteins that are targets for cANCA (proteinase 3 and myeloperoxidase). Binding of circulating cANCA to these antigens leads to degranulation of neutrophils, generation of oxidative stress, and injury to the endothelial layer. The presence of ANCA, regardless of the underlying pathology, is strongly associated with a certain HLA allele, DQB*0301.24.

5. CHURG-STRAUSS SYNDROME

Churg-Strauss syndrome is an allergic and granulomatous cANCA-associated vasculitis, which is characterized by pulmonary and systemic necrotizing vasculitis (involving small- and medium-sized muscular arteries, capillaries, veins, and venules), extravascular granulomas, and hypereosinophilia, in association with asthma and allergic rhinitis. Pathologically, the Churg-Strauss syndrome is recognized by angiitis and extravascular necrotizing granulomas with eosinophilic infiltrates. Churg-Strauss can occur at any age, with a mean age of onset of 44 yr and a male to female ratio of 1.3:1. Neurological involvement is frequent, with 60 to 70% of patients developing peripheral neuropathies, either mononeuritis multiplex or polyneuropathy, and 25% of patients developing CNS complications. Patients may present with cranial neuropathies, encephalopathy, stroke-like manifestations, ischemic optic neuropathy, facial nerve paresis, or hearing loss.

6. VASCULITIS ASSOCIATED WITH COLLAGEN VASCULAR DISORDERS

The CNS and/or PNS can be involved in the vasculitic process that occurs in patients with systemic lupus erythematosus (SLE), Sjogren syndrome, rheumatoid arthritis, scleroderma, Polyarteritis nodosa, and dermatomyositis. CNS involvement has been reported in 25 to 75% of patients *(25)*, 30% of whom do not have inflammation and only 12.5% have true vasculitis. SLE uncommonly can cause CNS vasculitis. Clinical manifestations of SLE-induced CNS vasculitis include headache, fever, neck rigidity, altered mental status, or coma. Focal neurological deficits may occur secondary to thromboembolic disease, intracranial bleeding, or infection. Examination of CSF is necessary to exclude infections. Other CSF studies, such as cell count, total protein, and oligoclonal bands, are neither reliable nor specific markers of CNS vasculitis. MRI of the brain may reveal nonspecific abnormal signal intensity or areas of infarction in the distribution of involved small or large vessels. Cerebral angiography may reveal extracranial and intracranial vessel stenosis.

7. GIANT CELL ARTERITIS

There are two significant giant cell arteritides: giant cell arteritis (temporal arteritis) and Takayasu's arteritis. Despite sharing similar histopathological features, these vasculitic disorders affect individuals of different ethnic backgrounds and at opposite ends of the age spectrum.

Giant cell arteritis is a granulomatous panarteritis with preferential involvement of the aorta and its large primary branches, including the carotid and vertebral arteries, which supply the brain and eyes. Giant cell arteritis almost exclusively affects individuals older than 50 yr (persons ages 75–85 yr have the highest risk) *(26)*. Increased susceptibility to giant cell arteritis has been reported in patients of northern European descent, and women comprise two-thirds of the affected individuals. Giant cell arteritis typically affects the extracranial branches of the aorta and spares the intracranial vessels. Transmural inflammation of the affected arteries causes luminal occlusion through intimal hyperplasia, and clinical manifestations are indicators of end-organ ischemia *(27–29)*. In two-thirds of the cases, giant cell arteritis presents with polymyalgia rheumatica. External and internal carotid arteries and their branches are particularly involved in the vasculitic process of giant cell arteritis and clinically manifest with new-onset headache or dramatic changes in the pattern of long-standing headaches in elderly patients. It can be associated with scalp tenderness, visual loss, or jaw claudication. Indeed, abrupt and irreversible visual loss is the most dramatic manifestation of giant cell arteritis, whereas transient ischemic attacks (TIAs) and stroke are rare and involve the vertebrobasilar territory. Vasculitis of the vertebral arteries can cause stroke, TIAs, vertigo, and dizziness.

The diagnostic work-up of patients suspected of giant cell arteritis includes erythrocyte sedimentation rate, C-reactive protein, plasma electrophoresis, and temporal artery biopsy. A marked elevation of the erythrocyte sedimentation rate is the most characteristic laboratory feature of giant cell arteritis. Mild anemia is commonly found, as are varying degrees of leukocytosis, sometimes with a left shift. Serum protein electrophoresis often reveals a rise of acute-phase reactants (α- and β-globulins) in the early stages and elevated γ-globulin in the more chronic phases; both of these will elevate the erythrocyte sedimentation rate. Demonstration of inflammatory granulomatous lesions involving the temporal artery has made the temporal artery biopsy a specific diagnostic procedure, but its sensitivity is limited by *skip* lesions. The typical lesion consists of a granulomatous inflammatory reaction concentrated at the innermost part of the vascular media near zones of fragmented and reduplicated internal elastic lamina with adjacent intimal proliferation, sometimes to the point of occluding the lumen. Multinucleated giant cells are classically present but are not necessary for the diagnosis (Fig. 2).

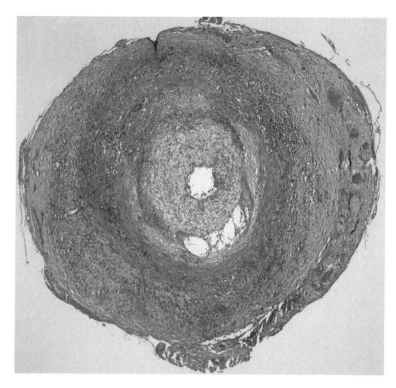

Fig. 2. Temporal arteritis with granulomatous angiitis showing fragmentation of the elastic lamina and granulomaouts inflammation of the intima and media. (Hematoxylin and eosin, original magnification × 100.)

8. TAKAYASU'S ARTERITIS

TA, also known as *pulseless disease*, is a chronic inflammatory disorder that affects the aorta and its major branches and, less frequently, pulmonary and coronary arteries. The inflammatory cascade in TA results in post-inflammatory stenosis of the aorta and its proximal branches. The stenosis of the involved vessels, caused by the inflammatory cascade, surpasses the pace of development of collateral circulation and, in turn, this leads to hypoperfusion of the affected organ.

The clinical manifestations of TA may be divided into a systemic stage and an occlusive stage. The systemic manifestations include fever, nocturnal sweats, malaise, arthralgias, headaches, generalized pain, and weight loss. Clinical features of the occlusive stage depend on the distribution of the lesions and may include ischemic symptoms caused by carotid and vertebrobasilar involvement. The involvement of these vessels can result in TIAs or stroke. Patients may also present with syncopal attacks or visual obscurations *(30)*. Funduscopic abnormalities are frequent. Patients with TA can present with nonspecific neurological manifestations, such as headache, visual disturbance, or cognitive abnormalities.

Common laboratory abnormalities in patients with TA include a normochromic normocytic anemia, leukocytosis, elevated erythrocyte sedimentation rate, and hypergammaglobulinemia.

9. DRUG-INDUCED VASCULITIS

Illicit drugs cause psychological dependence and physical dependence and can be associated with occlusive and hemorrhagic strokes. The proposed mechanisms for these drug-associated strokes include endocarditis, meningitis, foreign body embolism, accelerated atherosclerosis, abnormalities of platelet and coagulation factors, hypertension, cerebral vasospasm, and immune-mediated vasculitis. Major categories of illicit drugs include opioids, psychostimulants, hypnotics and seda-

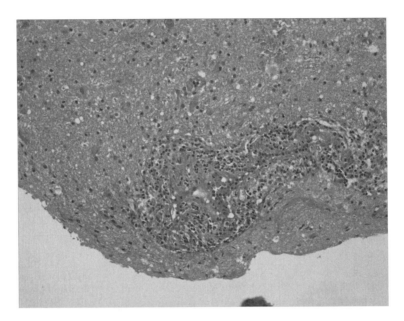

Fig. 3. Behcet's syndrome involving a small cerebral blood vessel with vascular necrosis and an infiltrate of mononuclear cells in and around the vessel wall. (Hematoxylin and eosin, original magnification × 200.)

tives, marijuana, hallucinogens, inhalants, phencyclidine and anticholinergics, as well as ethanol and tobacco. Of these drugs, cocaine, a prototype of psychostimulants, is discussed in more detail.

Cocaine, a major psychostimulant and sympathomimetic amine, blocks reuptake of norepinephrine and dopamine at synaptic nerve endings. Cocaine is either sniffed or injected parenterally. Cocaine abuse has been associated with both occlusive/ischemic and hemorrhagic strokes. Cocaine-induced cerebral ischemia consists of TIAs or complete infarction of cerebrum, thalamus, brainstem, spinal cord, or retina. Intracranial hemorrhagic strokes are frequently associated with an underlying saccular aneurysm or vascular malformation. Either type of stroke may be linked to cocaine-associated cerebral vasculitis.

10. BEHCET'S DISEASE

Behcet's disease is a chronic relapsing multisystem disorder of unknown etiology. It can present with a variety of skin and mucosal lesions, uveitis, CNS abnormalities, major vessels involvement, musculoskeletal problems, and gastrointestinal abnormalities. The diagnosis of Behcet's disease is clinical and, according to the work of the International Study Group, the major diagnostic criteria for Behcet disease include oral ulcers recurring at least three times a year, genital ulcers or scars, eye involvement, skin lesions (erythema nodosum, folliculitis, acneiform lesions), and pathergy skin test observed by a physician.

Minor diagnostic criteria include arthritis or arthralgia, deep venous thromboses, subcutaneous thrombophlebitis, epididymitis, family history, and gastrointestinal, CNS, or vascular involvement. The CNS is involved in 4 to 49% of cases, usually during active disease. In 5% of cases, CNS manifestations are the presenting syndrome. CNS involvement can have an acute or chronic onset. About 75% of patients with CNS involvement develop parenchymal lesions, and the remainder has dural sinus thrombi presenting as headaches. Paranchymal lesions develop most frequently in the brainstem, followed by the spinal cord, cerebrum, and cerebellum. Patients can have pyramidal motor signs, as well as cerebellar and sensory symptoms. The major histopathological feature in Behcet's disease is vasculitis (Fig. 3). Mucocutaneous lesions consist of dermal, epidermal, and perivascular mononuclear cell infiltration. Foci of perivascular inflammation in the meninges and necrosis and gliosis in the gray and white matter, as well as demyelination, have been observed in CNS lesions.

MRI examination reveals extensive lesions involving the brainstem and basal ganglia or the pontobulbar junction. Chronic neurological disease may cause brainstem atrophy. Enhancement with gadolinium is observed in acute parenchymal or meningeal involvement. Gliosis or hemosiderin deposition may be observed in older lesions. Cranial sinus thromboses are often visible on MRI; cerebral angiography is rarely needed.

11. CENTRAL NERVOUS SYSTEM VASCULITIS ASSOCIATED WITH NEOPLASIA

Certain neoplastic disorders, such as Hodgkin's disease, non-Hodgkin's lymphoma, and angioimmunolymphoproliferative lesions (AIL), can be associated with CNS vasculitis *(11)*. Interestingly, the anatomic focus of the lymphoproliferative disease may be inside or outside the CNS. The clinical picture of neoplasia-associated CNS vasculitis may be similar to PACNS and may include mass lesions, myelopathy, and CNS hemorrhage *(11)*. It is important to recognize that the histopathological examination of the mass lesions within the CNS may reveal only angiitis without evidence of the malignancy itself. On the other hand, a lymphocytic angiitis may be the hallmark lesion of AIL, and a diagnosis can be established by T-cell receptor analysis, immunohistochemistry, and B-cell immunoglobulin studies.

12. KAWASAKI'S DISEASE

Kawasaki's disease, also known as *mucocutaneous lymph node syndrome*, is an uncommon acute febrile vasculitis that involves medium-sized arteries but may also affect large and small arteries. The etiology of Kawasaki's disease remains unknown; however, its occurrence in epidemic forms indicates an apparent infectious etiology. Interestingly, it is unresponsive to antibiotics. Kawasaki's disease manifests with nonsuppurative cervical adenitis and abnormalities of skin and mucous membranes (e.g., edema; congestion of conjunctivae; redness of the oral cavity, lips, and palms; and desquamation of the skin of the fingertips). Coronary artery aneurysm is a serious complication of Kawasaki's disease and occurs in almost 25% of patients between the third and fourth wk of the illness, which is the convalescent period. Infants and young children are typically affected and, in most cases, Kawasaki's disease is benign and self-limiting. It is possible that immune-mediated insult to the endothelial cells participates in pathogenesis of Kawasaki's disease. Massive immune activation characterized by elevated numbers of activated helper T lymphocytes, increased serum-soluble IL-2 receptor levels, increased levels of IL-1 generation by peripheral mononuclear cells, and elevated titers of antiendothelial cell antibodies have been reported in these patients. Neurologic manifestations can include seizures, facial nerve palsy, encephalopathy, and uncommonly strokes. CSF examination reveals pleocytosis.

13. COGAN SYNDROME

Cogan syndrome is an uncommon inflammatory disease, which is identified by an acute phase of ocular (interstitial keratitis) and aural involvement (vestibular dysfunction and sensorineural hearing loss) lasting months to years, followed by a chronic phase of relatively low disease activity. Although ocular and aural symptoms predominate in Cogan syndrome, some patients develop systemic vasculitis, including aortitis and mesentric arteritis. The disease may occur at any age and in both sexes. Neurologic manifestations involving the CNS occur in 7% of patients with Cogan syndrome and can consist of seizures, electroencephalogram abnormalities, lateral medullary infarcts, thalamic lacunar infarcts, ataxia, hyperreflexia, facial diplegia, ophthalmoplegia, trigeminal neuralgia, transverse myelitis, or cerebral sinus thrombosis. Cerebellar ataxia with multiple cerebellar lesions on neuroimaging studies and elevated CSF protein have also been described *(31)*. Histopathological examination of corneal and vestibule-auditory organs reveals infiltration of lymphocytes and plasma cells, demyelination of the eight nerve, and degeneration of the organ of Corti, cochlea, and vestibular apparatus *(32)*.

14. CLINICAL MANAGEMENT

Once CNS vasculitis is diagnosed, a decision regarding treatment strategy must be made. Because CNS vasculitic syndromes are potentially lethal conditions, therapy should be initiated immediately. Immunosuppression remains the main mode of treatment for CNS vasculitis.

Primary angiitis of the CNS should be treated with intravenous 1000 mg methylprednisolone sodium succinate daily for 3 to 5 d, followed by high-dose daily prednisone (typically 80 mg) and cyclophosphamide (2 mg/kg/d). Later, the prednisolone can be reduced to alternate-day therapy, the cyclophosphamide should be maintained *(6)*. Corticosteroids alone are not sufficient and should be combined with other immunosuppressive agents.

Infectious vasculitis secondary to VSV should be treated with intravenous acyclovir (10–15 mg/kg of body weight, three times daily for 7–10 d) to destroy persistent virus and then a short course of a corticosteroid (60 to 80 mg prednisone daily for 3–5 d) to reduce inflammation *(15)*.

Treatment of CNS vasculitis in the context of HIV infection is a clinical challenge, since cytotoxic/immunosuppressive agents, which are commonly used in the treatment of vasculitis, are contraindicated in immunocompromised patients with AIDS. Dramatic improvement following corticosteroid therapy alone has been reported *(20)*. Successful treatment of HIV vasculitis using plasmapheresis followed by AZT has also been reported *(33)*.

Wegner's granulomatosis is most effectively controlled with 2 mg/kg/d oral cyclophosphamide in combination with corticosteroids. The leukocyte count should be monitored closely during treatment and kept above 3000 μL. With careful monitoring of the leukocyte count, clinical remission can be induced without causing leucopenia or predisposing patients to infections. Cyclophosphamide therapy should be continued for 12 mo and, following the induction of immunosuppression and complete remission, gradually tapered and stopped.

Churg-Strauss syndrome is treated with glucocorticoids (prednisone), which, in up to half of patients, improves survival by more than 50%. In Churg-Strauss syndrome, it is frequently impossible to discontinue glucocorticoids because of residual asthma. In cases of glucocorticoid failure or in patients with fulminant systemic disease, the treatment should include a combination of cyclophosphamide and alternate-day prednisone.

Oral corticosteroids are the mainstay of treatment of giant cell arteritis because the disease's clinical manifestations are very sensitive to steroid therapy. Treatment begins with 40–80 mg/d oral prednisone for 1 mo, followed by a gradual tapering to a maintenance dose of 7.5–10 mg/d. The corticosteroid therapy should be continued for at least for 2 yr, since the disease may recur. The erythrocyte sedimentation rate (ESR) can serve as a marker of inflammatory activity and assist physicians in monitoring response to immunosuppressive therapy.

Treatment of TA begins with 1 mg/kg/d oral prednisone, with close monitoring of clinical manifestations and ESR, although the effect of this treatment regimen on improving patients' survival rate is unknown. The combination of prednisone with surgical and angioplastic procedures to open the stenosed vessels has improved survival and has decreased morbidity associated with TA. Doses of up to 25 mg/wk of methotrexate may be used in patients who are refractory to glucocorticoids.

Treatment of Behcet's disease mainly involves immunosuppression. For acute CNS involvement, 20–100 mg/day oral prednisolone for 1–3 wk or 1000 mg/d intravenous methylprednisolone for 3 d is prescribed. Following induction of remission, treatment involves tapering doses of prednisone (5–10 mg/d) and cyclophosphamide, chlorambucil, or methotrexate for 12 mo. The full dose of prednisone should be resumed if new relapses develop. Low-dose weekly methotrexate has been recommended for progressive neurologic symptoms that are resistant to treatment *(34)*.

Management of neoplasia-associated CNS vasculitis should focus on the underlying malignancy and generally consists of chemotherapy or irradiation.

Kawasaki's disease, in most cases, carries an excellent prognosis with an uneventful recovery. High-dose intravenous immunoglobulin (2 g/kg as a single infusion) combined with aspirin

(100 mg/kg/d) for 14 d, followed by 3–5 mg/kg/d for several weeks is effective in decreasing the prevalence of coronary artery abnormalities, if applied early in the course of the disease.

REFERENCES

1. Calabrese LH. Clinical management issues in vasculitis. Angiographically defined angiitis of the central nervous system: diagnostic and therapeutic dilemmas. Clin Exp Rheumatol 2003;21(6 Suppl 32):S127–130.
2. Kelley RE. CNS vasculitis. Front Biosci 2004;9:946–955.
3. Siva A. Vasculitis of the nervous system. J Neurol. 2001 Jun;248(6):451–468.
4. Lie JT. Primary (granulomatous) angiitis of the central nervous system: a clinicopathologic analysis of 15 new cases and a review of the literature. Hum Pathol 1992;23:164–171.
5. Parisi JE, Moore PM. The role of biopsy in vasculitis of the central nervous system. Semin Neurol 1994;14:341–348.
6. Cupps TR, Moore PM, Fauci AS. Isolated angiitis of the central nervous system: prospective diagnostic and therapeutic experience. Am J Med 1983;74:97–105.
7. Moore PM. Immune mechanisms in the primary and secondary vasculitides. J Neurol Sci 1989;93:129–145.
8. Jellinger K. Giant cell granulomatous angiitis of the central nervous system. J Neurol 1977;215:175–190.
9. Crane R, Kerr LD, Spiera H. Clinical analysis of isolated angiitis of the central nervous system. A report of 11 cases. Arch Intern Med 1991;151:2290–2294.
10. Calabrese LH. Vasculitis of the central nervous system. Rheum Dis Clin North Am 1995;21:1059–1076.
11. Calabrese LH, Duna GF, Lie JT. Vasculitis in the central nervous system. Arthritis Rheum 1997;40:1189–1201.
12. Greenan TJ, Grossman RI, Goldberg HI. Cerebral vasculitis: MR imaging and angiographic correlation. Radiology 1992;182:65–72.
13. Wenisch C, Wenisch H, Bankl HC, et al. Detection of anti-neutrophil cytoplasmic antibodies after acute Plasmodium falciparum malaria. Clin Diagn Lab Immunol 1996;3:132–134.
14. McKelvie PA, Collins S, Thyagarajan D, Trost N, Sheorey H, Byrne E. Meningoencephalomyelitis with vasculitis due to varicella zoster virus: a case report and review of the literature. Pathology 2002;34:88–93.
15. Gilden DH, Kleinschmidt-DeMasters BK, LaGuardia JJ, Mahalingam R, Cohrs RJ. Neurologic complications of the reactivation of varicella-zoster virus. N Engl J Med 2000;342:635–645.
16. Kleinschmidt-DeMasters BK, Amlie-Lefond C, Gilden DH. The patterns of varicella zoster virus encephalitis. Hum Pathol 1996;27:927–938.
17. Nogueras C, Sala M, Sasal M, et al. Recurrent stroke as a manifestation of primary angiitis of the central nervous system in a patient infected with human immunodeficiency virus. Arch Neurol 2002;59:468–473.
18. Garcia-Garcia JA, Macias J, Castellanos V, et al. Necrotizing granulomatous vasculitis in advanced HIV infection. J Infect 2003;47:333–335.
19. Savige JA, Chang L, Horn S, Crowe SM. Anti-nuclear, anti-neutrophil cytoplasmic and anti-glomerular basement membrane antibodies in HIV-infected individuals. Autoimmunity 1994;18:205–11.
20. Valeriano-Marcet J, Ravichandran L, Kerr LD. HIV associated systemic necrotizing vasculitis. J Rheumatol 1990; 17:1091–1093.
21. Lawn SD, Butera ST, Folks TM. Contribution of immune activation to the pathogenesis and transmission of human immunodeficiency virus type 1 infection. Clin Microbiol Rev 2001;14:753–777.
22. Drachman DA. Neurological complications of Wegner's granulomatosis. Arch Neurol 1963;8:145–155.
23. Nishino H, Rubino FA, DeRemee RA, Swanson JW, Parisi JE. Neurological involvement in Wegener's granulomatosis: an analysis of 324 consecutive patients at the Mayo Clinic. Ann Neurol 1993;33:4–9.
24. Arnett FC. Histocompatibility typing in the rheumatic diseases. Diagnostic and prognostic implications. Rheum Dis Clin North Am 1994;20:371–390.
25. Johnson RT, Richardson EP. The neurological manifestations of systemic lupus erythematosus. Medicine (Baltimore) 1968;47:337–369.
26. Hunder GG. Epidemiology of giant-cell arteritis. Cleve Clin J Med 2002;69(Suppl 2):SII79–82.
27. Salvarani C, Cantini F, Boiardi L, Hunder GG. Polymyalgia rheumatica and giant-cell arteritis. N Engl J Med 2002; 347:261–271.
28. Smetana GW, Shmerling RH. Does this patient have giant cell arteritis? JAMA 2002;287:92–101.
29. Ghanchi FD, Dutton GN. Current concepts in giant cell (temporal) arteritis. Surv Ophthalmol 1997;42:99–123.
30. Minagar A, Ghaemmaghami AM. Central nervous system vasculitis. Advances Clin Neurosci 2001;11:299–313.
31. Manto MU, Jacquy J. Cerebellar ataxia in Cogan syndrome. J Neurol Sci 1996;136:189–191.
32. Schuknecht HF, Nadol JB. Temporal bone pathology in a case of Cogan's syndrome. Laryngoscope 1994;104: 1135–1142.
33. Gisselbrecht M, Cohen P, Lortholary O, et al. HIV-related vasculitis: clinical presentation and therapeutic approach on six patients. AIDS 1997;11:121–123.
34. Hirohata S, Suda H, Hashimoto T. Low-dose weekly methotrexate for progressive neuropsychiatric manifestations in Behcet's disease. J Neurol Sci 1998;159:181–185.

CME QUESTIONS

1. Which statement is correct about central nervous system (CNS) vasculitis?
   A. CNS vasculitis is a heterogeneous group of inflammatory disorders, which affect blood vessels of different types and sizes and cause inflammation and necrosis of affected blood vessels
   B. CNS vasculitis affects only women
   C. CNS vasculitis is a neurodegenerative syndrome and is unresponsive to treatment with immunosuppressive agents
   D. CNS vasculitis affects only the brain

2. Which of the following syndromes is *not* a manifestation of human immunodeficiency virus-induced CNS vasculitic syndrome?
   A. Encephalitis
   B. Lymphocytic meningitis
   C. Stroke
   D. Vertigo

3. Which statement about giant cell arteritis is *incorrect*?
   A. It affects mainly individuals younger than age 50 yr
   B. If untreated, it can potentially lead to blindness
   C. An elevated erythrocyte sedimentation rate is a frequent finding in patients with giant cell arteritis
   D. Histopathology examination of affected vessels may show skip lesions and multinucleated giant cells

4. Which procedure is *not* usually used for diagnosis of CNS vasculitis?
   A. Examination of cerebrospinal fluid
   B. Cerebral angiography
   C. Brain biopsy
   D. Magnetic resonance imaging of brain and spinal cord
   E. Electromyography

14

Neurosarcoidosis

Pathogenesis, Immunology, and Clinical Management

Dakshinamurty Gullapalli and Lawrence H. Phillips, II

1. INTRODUCTION

Among the inflammatory disorders, sarcoidosis is one of the most intriguing. It is a complex disorder with unknown etiology. New insights regarding epidemiology, immunology, and pathogenesis have expanded our knowledge of this disease in the last one to two decades. More novel therapeutic applications from the knowledge of immunopathogensis will hopefully improve our treatment armamentarium against this disorder.

Sarcoidosis is a systemic disorder with the propensity to involve multiple organs. Though initially described as a skin disorder, it generally involves lungs and lymph nodes. Pathologically, sarcoidosis is characterized by noncaseating granuloma formation. Pathological changes do not always manifest disease symptoms, as many patients may be asymptomatic. Sarcoidosis occurs all over the world. Although it affects all races, there are some ethnic and racial predispositions. It also affects a wide range of ages.

The nervous system is affected generally as a part of the systemic disease, but nervous system manifestations occasionally can be the presenting or sole symptoms of the disease. Neurosarcoidosis is associated with serious manifestations and a poor outcome. The epidemiological features, immunopathogenesis, and effects of immunomodulatory therapy of neurosarcoidosis do not differ from the systemic disease. Hence, it is imperative to review systemic sarcoidosis before discussing neurosarcoidosis.

2. HISTORY

Sarcoidosis was first described in 1877. It derives its name from *sarkoid*, a name coined by Caeser Boeck, who noticed histological resemblance of the skin lesions to sarcoma *(1,2)*. Subsequently, Ansgar Kveim and Louis Siltzbach developed cutaneous tests for diagnosis of the disease. The first neurological manifestation of sarcoidosis (i.e., cranial neuropathies along with uveoparotid fever) was described by Heerfordt in 1909, followed by a report by Colover in 1948 of a large case series of patients with nervous system involvement in sarcoidosis *(3)*. A detailed historical description of the sequence of events in our understanding of sarcoidosis was reviewed recently *(1,4)*.

3. EPIDEMIOLOGY

Although sarcoidosis affects all age groups, it has a prediliction for middle-aged adults *(5,6)*. In the United States, women have a slightly higher disease rate than men do. The lifetime risk and prevalence in black men is significantly higher than in whites *(7,8)*. The highest rates of the

From: *Current Clinical Neurology: Inflammatory Disorders of the Nervous System:*
Pathogenesis, Immunology, and Clinical Management
Edited by: A. Minagar and J. S. Alexander © Humana Press Inc., Totowa, NJ

disease were reported among Swedes, Danes, and US blacks *(9)*. It is recognized less frequently in certain regions of the world, partly because of a lack of screening programs and coexistence of other granulomatous disorders with higher prevalence in the populations. Among reported cases of sarcoidosis, one- to two-thirds of patients are asymptomatic and are only diagnosed because of health screening chest x-rays *(10)*. The mortality rate from sarcoidosis ranges from 1 to 5%. Death is generally caused by respiratory complications because the lungs are the most commonly involved organs *(6,11)*, although death is more commonly caused by cardiac failure in some countries *(4)*.

Although the cardiac and nervous systems are less frequently involved than the lungs, diseases in these organ systems have more severe manifestations and greater mortality. Precise epidemiological studies have not been performed; nevertheless, several interesting observations help further our understanding of the disease process. There is some epidemiological evidence to indicate a role for a transmissible agent, which we discuss in detail later in the chapter. Similarly, there is also familial clustering and a human leukocyte antigen (HLA) association of cases, which suggests a genetic predisposition.

4. IMMUNOPATHOGENESIS

The histological hallmark of sarcoidosis is the noncaseating granuloma (Fig. 1). Precise knowledge about the etiology of the disease is lacking. Several factors, including transmissible microorganisms, occupational exposure to nonorganic substances, and genetic predisposition are implicated in the pathogenesis.

Since Mitchell and Rees suggested the possibility of a transmissible agent in sarcoidosis in 1969, there has been active interest in this area *(12)*. Multiple lines of evidence implicate a transmissible agent. One excellent study reported an outbreak of several cases of sarcoidosis on the Isle of Man among patients who lived within 100 m of each other *(13,14)*. Seasonal clustering of cases has also been reported in several countries *(15–17)*. Occupational clustering of cases has been reported among health care workers, naval aircraft service people, and firefighters *(18–20)*, which suggests a possible link to an occupational exposure independent of an infectious agent. Based on these observations, several studies have attempted to find an infecting agent responsible for the disease. A recent review has summarized the available evidence that implicates microorganisms in the pathogenesis of sarcoidosis *(21)*. Among the infecting agents, propionibacteria and mycobacteria emerge as the most likely organisms. The evidence for the role of mycobacteria is stronger compared to that for other organisms and is based on histopathological studies of lesions, coincidental mycobacterial infections, disease transmission in passage experiments in animals, antimycobacterial antibodies, and molecular studies. The lack of caseation, rarity of organism isolation, and failure of response to antimycobacterial therapy argue against this theory. One can argue that mycobacteria merely act as a trigger by causing formation of granulomas caused by chronic exposure to a poorly degradable and persistent antigen.

Some authors argue that propionibacteria should be considered a more likely pathogen than mycobacteria, because genetic material of this bacteria is detected more frequently in sarcoid lesions *(22)*. Noninfectious environmental agents, such as aluminum, beryllium, and zirconium are also possible triggers for the disease owing to their ability to induce a granulomatous response *(4)*.

Contrary to earlier views of suppressed immunity, there is now evidence to suggest that sarcoidosis is associated with heightened immunity that is mediated primarily by CD4$^+$ helper cells and macrophages *(24)*. The immunology of sarcoidosis is associated with a dichotomy of depressed systemic cellular immunity and heightened T-lymphocyte activity locally in affected organs *(25,26)*.

The inflammatory response in sarcoidosis is associated with the release of several proinflammatory cytokines and chemokines at disease sites *(23)*. Knowledge of the cytokine network has improved our understanding of the immunopathogenesis of sarcoidosis. Because granuloma formation requires an antigen as a trigger, it is believed that an unknown stimulus activates quiescent

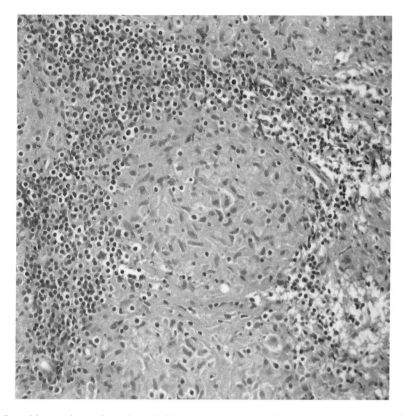

Fig. 1. Sarcoid granuloma. Lymph node biopsy specimen showing a noncaseating epithelioid granuloma. (Hematoxylin and eosin stain).

T cells and macrophages, leading to cytokine release. Cytokines, in turn, generate a further inflammatory response by activating and proliferating mononuclear cells. This results in formation of a granuloma.

Granuloma formation involves a series of steps (Fig. 2). Mononuclear phagocytic antigen-presenting cells initially internalize poorly soluble antigen, which is then processed by protein degradation into peptide fragments. The peptide fragments are then bound within α-helices of major histocompatibility complex (MHC) class II molecules and transported to the cell surface for analysis by CD4+ T cells (27). Alveolar T cells, following exposure to antigen in the presence of HLA complex, release T helper (Th)1 cytokines. They in turn release interleukin (IL)-2, interferon (IFN)-γ, and lymphotoxin (28,29). IL-12, which is secreted by alveolar macrophages, is an important cytokine involved in the induction of Th1 cells. Increased levels of this cytokine in bronchioalveolar lavage (BAL) fluid has been associated with a poorer prognosis (30).

The early sarcoid reaction in the lung is characterized by the accumulation of activated T cells and macrophages at sites of inflammation. These T cells spontaneously release IFN-γ, IL-2 and other cytokines (29,31). T cells, apart from releasing cytokines, also attract mononuclear cells to the alveoli. Sarcoid alveolar macrophages further release a variety of cytokines, including tumor necrosis factor (TNF)-α, IL-12, IL-15, and growth factors (32,33). Various studies indicate that IL-2 acts as a local growth factor for T lymphocytes by infiltrating the lung parenchyma and other involved sarcoid tissues (28).

It is hypothesized that CD4+ T helper cells are required for granuloma formation in sarcoidosis. This is exemplified further in the coexistence of sarcoidosis and human immunodeficiency virus infection only in patients with CD4+ cell counts of more than 200/μL (34). The finding of increased

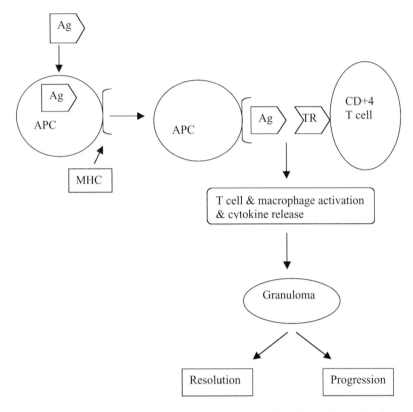

Fig. 2. Immunopathogenesis of sarcoidosis. An unknown sarcoid antigen (Ag) is first internalized by an antigen-presenting cell, followed by degradation into peptide fragments, and then is bound within major histocompatibility complex (MHC) class II molecules, which are then transported to the cell surface. Interaction of MHC and Ag with the T-cell receptor results in activation of T cells and further immunologic cascade resulting in granuloma formation.

IL-2 levels along with lymphocytic alveolitis suggests a poor prognosis *(35)*. Serum levels of soluble IL-2 receptor are associated with a higher risk of disease progression and a poor prognosis *(36,37)*. On the other hand, increased transforming growth factor-β in alveolar macrophages is associated with spontaneous remission *(38)*. It has also been shown that increased proinflammatory mediator release is seen more commonly in newly diagnosed and progressive sarcoidosis patients rather than in those with stable, chronic disease *(39)*. The CD25 and HLA-DR expression were increased on CD4+ lymphocytes from BAL and peripheral blood at disease onset but not in patients with clinically resolved disease or controls. Analysis of these activation markers could be useful in determining disease activity in sarcoidosis *(40)*.

IFN-γ was hypothesized to function in the persistence of inflammation by inhibiting apoptosis in macrophages through increased expression of p21 (Waf 1) in sarcoid granulomas *(41)*. More recently, in neutrophilic alveolitis, other cytokines including IL-18, have been shown to possibly have an important role in the immunopathogenesis of sarcoidosis *(42)*. In a recent review of the correlation of BAL fluid and serum parameters with disease severity, Ziegenhagen et al. studied newly diagnosed pulmonary sarcoidosis patients. They found increased percentages of neutrophils (>3%) and eosinophils (>1%) in BAL fluid and elevated serum levels of soluble IL-2 receptor and neopterin. This finding was associated with a significantly higher likelihood of need for steroid therapy *(43)*. It is suggested that helpful markers of progressive disease may include the total BAL fluid cell count, the percentage of alveolar lymphocytes, and lymphocyte CD4/CD8 ratio; however, these markers have not been shown to be useful predictors of outcome. It is recognized that only alveolar T cells, not peripheral blood T cells, secrete IL-2; thus, the initiating event likely occurs in the lung *(44)*.

TNF-α, which has an important role in granuloma formation, likely also has a key role in the pathogenesis of sarcoidosis. Among cytokines, it is the most extensively studied, exemplifying its key role in the immunopathogenesis of sarcoidosis. TNF-α release is higher in patients with active disease than in those not exhibiting symptoms *(45)*. Increased macrophage TNF-α release also has been associated with a higher risk of disease progression in 6 mo, even in those patients who lack clinical indications for steroid therapy *(36)*. Higher alveolar macrophage TNF-α release has been shown in patients with active sarcoidosis who are not on corticosteriod therapy as well as in patients with corticosteroid-resistant disease when they are compared with controls and patients who have stable or inactive disease *(43)*. To explain resistance to corticosteroids in autoimmune/inflammatory disorders, Franchimont et al. have shown that corticosteroids differentially modulate TNF-α and IL-10 secretion by human monocytes. The sensitivity of these cells to glucocorticoids is altered by TNF-α or IL-10 pretreatment. TNF-α blocks their effects, whereas IL-10 acts synergistically with glucocorticoids *(46)*; thus, the presence of high TNF-α levels, caused by the inability of the immune system to downregulate the inflammatory process, may result in corticosteroid resistance. This hypothesis is the basis of strategies that use anti-TNF-α to treat steroid-resistant cases.

None of the above-discussed cytokine markers may be used for diagnosis, since they are nonspecific. In established cases of sarcoidosis, monitoring their levels can be a means to follow or predict disease progression. Since the natural clinical course of the disease is unpredictable in a given patient, these factors are essential for following the disease process.

Along with the cytokine network, the HLA complex has an important role in the immunopathogenesis of sarcoidosis. The MHC antigen presents antigen to Th cells. Genetic polymorphisms lead to interindividual differences in cytokine production and disease severity. The genetic influence in the pathogenesis of sarcoidosis is shown by the different incidence and prevalence rates in certain ethnic and racial populations. For example, there is familial clustering and linkage to chromosome 6 in some German families *(47)*. Similarly, several studies have shown associations between MHC class II alleles and sarcoidosis *(42,48)*. These studies suggest the presence of multiple alleles that either confer susceptibility or are protective. It seems, from all the available evidence, that multiple gene loci, rather than a single gene locus, are likely involved in the disease process.

Despite the extensive research in the immunopathogenesis of sarcoidosis, it is still unclear why the disease persists or progresses actively in some patients and why it is quiescent and/or asymptomtomatic in others. Specific triggering factors are unknown, and a single factor cannot be identified as the cause of the disease. The available evidence suggests that the interaction of environmental factors in a genetically susceptible individual is likely to be responsible for induction of the disease process. It appears that the chronic nature of the sarcoid lesions is caused by persistence of an antigenic stimulus and/or an intrinsic dysregulation of the immune system *(49)*. Multinucleated giant cells may provide a cellular reservoir for the antigen. There is an ongoing National Institutes of Health-funded multicenter case study that is designed to investigate the etiologic mechanisms of sarcoidosis *(50)*.

5. PATHOLOGY

The diagnostic histopathological lesion of sarcoidosis is a discrete, compact, noncaseating epitheloid cell granuloma (Fig. 1). Epithelioid cell granulomas consist of highly differentiated mononuclear phagocytes (epithelioid cells and giant cells) surrounded by lymphocytes. Langhans'-type multinucleated giant cells are frequently present. The central portion of the granuloma consists of predominantly CD4$^+$ lymphocytes, whereas CD8$^+$ lymphocytes are present in the peripheral zone *(51,52)*.

The inflammatory process is similar in all organs affected by sarcoidosis, including the nervous system. Granulomas resolve spontaneously or with treatment. With progression, fibrotic changes occur in the granuloma, with deposition of collagen and proteoglycans that form a diffuse network around the granulomas and cause irreversible tissue damage *(25)*.

Occasionally, there is focal coagulative necrosis in granulomas, and these lesions are thought to be variants of sarcoidosis *(51,52)*. About 20% of granulomatous lesions have an undetermined etiology. These clinical syndromes are grouped under the rubric Granulomatous Lesions of Unknown Significance or *GLUS (53)*. The clinical presentation of sarcoidosis varies with the specific organ involved. The lungs are involved in 90% of patients with sarcoidosis, and the severity ranges from asymptomatic to severe interstitial lung pathology. Other common organ involvement includes lymph nodes (33%), liver (histopathological abnormalities occur in 50 to 80% of biopsy specimens), skin (25%), eyes (11–83%), musculoskeletal system (25–39%), and endocrine glands (2–10%) *(4)*. In children, sarcoidosis is more common in whites than in blacks. The distribution of organ involvement is similar to that of adults, and children usually have a better prognosis than adults *(54)*. Sarcoidosis does not usually affect pregnancy, but the disease may worsen after delivery.

Because histopathological findings by themselves are not specific, it is essential to exclude other etiologies that cause similar pathological findings, including foreign bodies and microorganisms. Special stains and cultures of biopsy specimens should be done for acid-fast bacilli and fungi.

The differential diagnosis of granulomatous involvement of blood vessels includes granulomatous angiitis, which presents with sudden multifocal stroke-like episodes and vasculitic changes on angiogram. Wegener's granulomatosis is another granulomatous disease, but it presents with clinical features that are distinguishable from sarcoidosis.

Despite a lack of specific research into the immunopathology of neurosarcoidosis, inflammatory processes similar to those seen in the lung are considered to be responsible for the neurologic manifestations. Neurosarcoidosis occurs primarily as a result of infiltration of the meninges by inflammatory cells that cause pachymeningitis with cranial neuropathies, hydrocephalus, encephalopathy, and hypothalamic dysfunction *(55)*. Any part of the central nervous system (CNS) or peripheral nervous system (PNS) can be involved by the inflammatory response. Following the primary meningeal involvement, extension of inflammatory exudates from the subarachnoid space along Virchow-Robin spaces occurs. This leads to involvement of the brain parenchyma *(56,57)*. The predilection of sarcoid lesions for the basal leptomeninges with frequent involvement of the hypothalamus, third ventricle, and optic and other cranial nerves can be explained by the fact that the Virchow-Robin spaces are especially large at the base of the brain *(58)*. Spreading via Virchow-Robin spaces has been demonstrated histologically and can be visualized radiologically on magnetic resonance imaging (MRI) *(56,57)*.

The inflammatory process can be either diffuse or localized. Primary inflammation of blood vessels is not common, although blood vessels may be involved in the general inflammatory process *(55,59)*. The severity of the inflammatory reaction correlates with the clinical picture. Irreversible neurologic damage can occur once the inflammation becomes chronic and causes fibrosis.

In the PNS, the epineurium and perineurium are involved primarily by the granulomatous process, but the endoneurium often has mononuclear cell accumulation. Epineurial and perineurial granulomas, combined with granulomatous vasculitis, cause axonal damage rather than demyelination. This is a common histological finding in nerve biopsies of patients with sarcoid neuropathy. In teased nerve fiber preparations, axonopathy that spares unmyelinated fibers is a more prominent feature than is compressive injury from granulomas *(60)*. Muscle involvement is common, but it is mostly asymptomatic. About 50% of all sarcoidosis patients have granulomatous changes on muscle biopsy *(61)*.

The natural history and prognosis of the disease vary with the specific organs involved and the extent of their involvement. Spontaneous remissions occur in about two-thirds of cases. The majority of remissions occur within the first 2 yr *(50)*. About 10 to 20% of patients with sarcoidosis develop a chronic form of the disease. Most functional disability is caused by cardiac, ocular, neurological, or pulmonary disease *(4)*. Serious extrapulmonary disease is found in 4 to 7% of patients at presentation. Most patients with systemic sarcoidosis improve or stabilize with or without treatment, but relapse occurs in 16 to 74%. The mortality rate varies from 1 to 5%, and death is mainly linked to severe pulmonary, cardiac, and neurological disease *(4,62)*.

Despite the wide range of organ involvement and diverse patterns of presentation and progression, some generalizations about natural history can be made. These include spontaneous waxing and waning of symptoms or changes in symptoms in response to treatment, spontaneous clinical and radiological remissions in a significant number of patients, and high mortality associated with progressive respiratory, cardiac, or neurological involvement *(4,10)*. Age greater than 40 yr, lupus pernio, nasal mucosal involvement, chronic uveitis, hypercalcemia, nephrocalcinosis, progressive pulmonary function decline, cystic bone lesions, and neurological or cardiac sarcoidosis are associated with a poorer prognosis. Patients with normal chest x-rays or only hilar lymphadenopathy, as well as those with an acute presentation (Lofgren syndrome), have a benign prognosis. Nonspecific constitutional symptoms, such as fever, fatigue, malaise, and weight loss, may occur in about one-third of patients *(4)*.

6. CLINICAL MANIFESTATIONS OF NEUROSARCOIDOSIS

6.1. General Overview

Neurosarcoidosis is an uncommon but serious manifestation of sarcoidosis. Our view of the disease is biased toward the more severe manifestations of the disease. Minor neurologic manifestations in systemic sarcoidosis may go unrecognized or unpublished.

Neurological involvement is generally reported to occur in 5 to 10% of sarcoidosis patients *(4,55,63–66)*. A higher rate of neurological involvement (up to 14%) is reported in autopsy studies; thus, many of the neurological lesions are asymptomatic *(67–69)*. In one study, up to one-third of patients with systemic sarcoidosis had neurological symptoms at presentation *(66)*. In the absence of systemic disease, the diagnosis of neurosarcoidosis can be difficult. There are occasional reports of isolated neurosarcoidosis *(50,63)*, but it is estimated to occur at a rate of less than 0.2 per 100,000 Caucasians *(58)*.

Sarcoidosis is thought to involve the meninges preferentially, especially over the base of the brain, but any part of the nervous system can be involved in the inflammatory process. In view of the predilection for the base of the brain, cranial nerve and hypothalamic–pituitary axis involvement commonly occur. Although emphasis is given generally to CNS sarcoidosis, the PNS is also reportedly involved with a similar frequency *(55)*. As with systemic disease, the clinical presentation depends on where the nervous system is involved. In about 50% of patients with neurosarcoidosis, neurological symptoms are the presenting features *(64,66,70,71)*. Patients with systemic sarcoidosis who have minor neurological involvement may not present for neurological evaluation; thus, case series of neurosarcoidosis reported by neurologists are primarily a reflection of more severe nervous system involvement.

Neurosarcoidosis tends to occur at a slightly later age than extraneurological sarcoidosis *(69,70)*. This is also true for involvement of other organs such as the heart and kidney. In most patients, neurological manifestations appear within the first 2 yr of presentation of sarcoidosis *(66,71,72)*. The majority of neurosarcoidosis patients also have evidence of disease in other organ systems *(55,66,70,73)*. This necessitates a search for involvement of other organs. In many cases, this can complicate diagnosis because obtaining tissue from the nervous system is difficult.

Certain presentations of neurosarcoidosis are more common. Patients with an acute presentation tend to have isolated cranial neuropathies or aseptic meningitis, and patients with a chronic onset usually present with parenchymal involvement, hydrocephalus, multiple cranial neuropathies, or PNS manifestations *(73)*. Cranial neuropathies tend to occur early and respond

Table 1
Clinical Manifestations of Neurosarcoidosis in Case Series (%)

	Delaney ($n = 23$)	Chapelon ($n = 30$)	Stern ($n = 33$)	Oksanen ($n = 50$)	Sharma ($n = 37$)	Lower ($n = 71$)	Zajicek ($n = 68$)
Facial neuropathy	—[a]	31	—	30	30	55	19
Cranial neuropathy	48	37	73	42	21	—	72
Aseptic meningitis	26	37	18	—	16	40	37
Neuroendocrine	26	8	15	—	—	8	3
Other CNS lesions	—	—	—	78	19	—	21
Mass lesions	35	—	—	—	—	—	—
Encephalopathy	48	—	—	—	8	—	10
Seizures	22	14	—	—	5	7	—
Myelopathy	9	—	6	—	3	—	28
Peripheral neuropathy	4	40	6	18	30	3	—
Myopathy	9	26	12	10	—	—	—

[a] = no data reported
CNS, central nervous system.

favorably to treatment *(74)*. Sarcoid granulomas within the CNS can occur and disappear at various intracranial locations and thus mimic the clinical and radiological picture of multiple sclerosis (MS) *(75,76)*.

6.2. Cranial Neuropathy

Neurological manifestations reported in different series are summarized in Table 1. As mentioned above, cranial neuropathy, the most common manifestation of neurosarcoidosis, occurs in up to 75% of patients *(55,58,66,70)*. More than one cranial nerve commonly is involved. The cranial nerve most frequently affected is the facial nerve. Facial neuropathy occurs in 25 to 50% of neurosarcoidosis, making it the most common neurologic manifestation of the disease *(69)*. Unilateral facial palsy is most common, but bilateral lesions occur simultaneously or sequentially in about one-third of patients *(3,70)*. The risk of bilateral facial nerve palsy caused by sarcoidosis is rare *(77)*; thus, one should also consider other diagnoses, such as neuroborreliosis and Guillain-Barre syndrome. In unilateral facial neuropathy, idiopathic facial palsy (Bell's palsy) is far more common than facial palsy caused by sarcoidosis. In isolated facial palsy caused by neurosarcoidosis, the cerebrospinal fluid (CSF) can be normal, but when the disease is associated with other neurologic involvement, the CSF is more likely to be abnormal. Isolated facial paresis in neurosarcoidosis has a good prognosis with or without treatment *(66,68,73)*.

Other cranial neuropathies, including olfactory, optic, oculomotor, and vestibulocochlear mononeuropathies occur in about 10 to 20% of cases *(3,66,69,70)*. When multiple cranial nerves at the base of the brain are involved simultaneously, one should exclude basal meningitis secondary to chronic infectious meningitis, other inflammatory disorders, or neoplastic processes. Tuberculous, fungal, and carcinomatous meningitis, in particular, share a predilection for the basal meninges. Olfactory nerve dysfunction can present as anosmia or hyposmia in 2 to 17% of patients and is caused by subfrontal meningitis or nasal mucosal involvement by sarcoid lesions *(3,55,62)*. Nasal mucosal biopsy for evidence of nasal sarcoidosis should be considered in patients who have olfactory dysfunction. Optic neuropathy is a serious manifestation that presents as either acute or chronic visual loss that may be painful *(78)*. In a recent series, involvement of the optic nerve was reported in 26 out of 68 patients with neurosarcoidosis *(79)*. Optic nerve involvement is generally caused by either local granulomatous invasion of the optic nerve or to extraneural compression by a granulomatous mass. It may be associated with papilledema or optic atrophy *(80)*. Differentiation from optic nerve glioma and meningioma is difficult *(81)*. Electrophysiologic studies of cranial nerves frequently show abnormalities, even in the absence of clinical symptoms *(82)*.

6.3. Meningeal Involvement

Meningeal involvement has been found in 64 to 100% of patients in pathologic studies *(55,66,70)*. It can be asymptomatic or can present as an aseptic meningitis. When asymptomatic, it is either detected at autopsy or as meningeal enhancement on imaging studies *(55,83)*. Occasionally, it presents as a mass lesion. There are multiple reports of meningeal sarcoid mass lesions that are mistaken for meningiomas *(84–86)*, and there are cases in which the true diagnosis of neurosarcoidosis was made only during surgery *(87)*. The CSF shows a mononuclear pleocytosis with increased protein and occasional hypoglycorrhachia. The course of meningitis can vary from an acute monophasic illness to recurrent episodes. Rarely, it can become chronic, in which case, it is generally associated with multiple cranial neuropathies. The presence of meningeal enhancement on MRI suggests active inflammation. This serves as a good prognostic sign, because there is an increased likelihood of response to corticosteroids. On the other hand, a lack of meningeal enhancement may suggest chronicity and fibrosis *(62)*.

Hydrocephalus, either the communicating or obstructive type, occurs in 6 to 30% of patients with neurosarcoidosis *(55,66,70)*. Mechanisms of hydrocephalus include chronic basilar meningitis with obliteration of CSF flow, granulomatous obstruction of the venticular system, and compression of the cerebral acqueduct *(66)*.

6.4. Neuroendocrine Dysfunction

Hypothalamic dysfunction is the most common manifestation of parenchymal lesions. It can result in impairment of the neuroendocrine system *(69,88–90)*, and it is correlated with a high prevalence of subependymal granulomata in the anterior portion of the third ventricle. The endocrine manifestations of neurosarcoidosis range from hypothalamic dysfunction to diabetes insipidus, pituitary failure, amenorrhea-galactorrhea, or various combinations of these symptoms. There are less frequent reports of inappropriate antidiuretic hormone secretion, isolated secondary hypothyroidism, adrenal insufficiency, or altered counter-regulation of glucose homeostasis. Thus, a search for thyroid, adrenal, and sexual dysfunction is necessary in patients with neurosarcoidosis. In addition, hypothalamic dysfunction can affect vegetative functions such as fluid and electrolyte balance, appetite, temperature, sleep, and libido. Pituitary and hypothalamic involvement should be differentiated from other lesions of these structures, such as pituitary adenoma, craniopharyngioma, or Rathke's cleft cyst *(91)*. Simultaneous involvement of both the anterior and posterior pituitary, along with diabetes insipidus, does not occur generally in pituitary tumors. The discovery of such involvement may be a clue for neurosarcoidosis *(92)*.

6.5. Other CNS Lesions

Granulomas within brain parenchyma can present as intracerebral mass lesions. They are often asymptomatic *(93)*, but they may present with focal cerebral dysfunction or raised intracranial pressure. They may appear as isolated or multiple nodules or as subdural *en plaque* lesions *(66)*. Cerebral sarcoid granulomas are also responsible for seizures in some patients. Neurosarcoid mass lesions can be mistaken for meningiomas, intraventricular tumors, cerebellopontine angle tumors, or *en plaque* subdural lesions that are indistinguishable from meningiomas. Biopsy may be necessary to make a secure histological diagnosis *(63,94)*.

Diffuse encephalopathy secondary to sarcoidosis generally presents as delirium, a psychiatric disorder, memory loss, cognitive impairment, or multifocal relapsing encephalopathy. There is associated diffuse enhancement of meninges with contrast studies and increased signal intensity on T2-weighted MRI. Encephalopathy can also occur secondary to metabolic disturbances and endocrine dysfunction associated with systemic sarcoidosis *(55)*. Psychiatric manifestations, either in isolation or as part of an encephalopathy, occur in 9 to 48% of cases, but they are not usually the presenting symptoms *(69)*.

Granulomatous arteritis, in addition to meningeal involvement, can be seen in pathological specimens from neurosarcoid patients with encephalopathy *(59)*. Because this is a small vessel vasculitis, vasculitic changes are rarely observed on cerebral angiography *(95)*. Occasionally, transient ischemic attack and ischemic stroke-like events result from arteritis, external compression of arteries by inflammatory mass lesions, or from cardiogenic emboli caused by myocardial invovement *(59,86,95)*. The coexistence of granulomatous vasculitis with granulomata in the leptomeninges suggests the presence of neurosarcoidosis. On the other hand, granulomas are confined only to blood vessels.

Seizures have been reported in up to 20% of patients with neurosarcoidosis *(50)*. They reflect CNS parenchymal lesions, such as cerebral mass lesions, encephalitis, or vasculopathy, as well as hypercalcemia. Seizures are generally associated with a poorer prognosis owing to the underlying parenchymal involvement *(55)*. Although spinal cord involvement was considered rare in neurosarcoidosis in the past, there are several case reports of myelopathy *(79,96)*. Symptomatic myelopathy can be secondary to lesions in intramedullary, extramedullary, intradural, or extradural sites *(97)*.

6.6. PNS Involvement

The PNS can be involved in sarcoidosis with the same frequency as the CNS; however, many patients with PNS disease are asymptomatic and escape detection *(98)*. Peripheral neuropathy is reported in 15 to 18% of neurosarcoidosis patients *(66,69,70)*. Symmetric axonal sensorimotor neuropathy is the most common type of neuropathy. Other rare presentations include mononeuritis multiplex, polyradiculopathy, and Guillain-Barre syndrome *(50,96,99)*.

Sarcoid myopathy is common but is usually asymptomatic. Sarcoid granulomas are found in 25 to 75% of muscle biopsy specimens *(69,50)*. Symptomatic muscle involvement occurs about 1% of patients with systemic sarcodosis and has a higher incidence in those with primary neurological disease *(69,70)*. The modes of presentation of muscle involvement include acute to chronic myopathy, myositis, palpable nodules and, rarely, psudohypertrophy. Differentiation from other inflammatory myopathies can be difficult. The creatine kinase is sometimes elevated. Muscle involvement is more common in women than in men, with a ratio of 4:1 to 8:1. Sarcoid myopathy is more frequent in postmenopausal women than in premenopausal women; this suggests that sex hormones have a role in the etiology of the disease *(69,70)*.

7. DIAGNOSIS

7.1. Systemic Sarcoidosis

The diagnosis of neurosarcoidosis may be relatively apparent if neurologic symptoms occur in an individual with a known diagnosis of systemic sarcoidosis. In this scenario, neurosarcoidosis is identified when the clinical features and imaging findings are compatible and typical. On the other hand, diagnosis may be more challenging in a case of isolated neurosarcoidosis or one in which the neurologic features are atypical in a patient with known systemic sarcoidosis. This is especially true, since obtaining neural tissue for biopsy is difficult in most cases. Exclusion of other conditions that mimic neurosarcoidosis is also important. In addition to histopathological confirmation, the diagnostic process should also encompass assessment of the extent, severity, and stability of the disease.

The diagnosis of sarcoidosis requires a tissue diagnosis that shows noncaseating granulomata, along with a compatible clinical picture that excludes other known etiologies that can have similar clinical or histological features *(69)*. An expert panel with representatives from the American Thoracic Society, the European Respiratory Society, and the World Association of Sarcoidosis and Other Granulomatous Disorders proposed standard diagnostic criteria for sarcoidosis to help guide clinical evaluation and standardize research *(4)*. The criteria include the presence of typical clinical and radiological findings, histological evidence of noncaseating granulomata, and exclusion of other known granulomatous disorders. Clinical, biochemical, and imaging markers of disease activity were also suggested. Additionally, it is important to determine the extent and severity of the disease and to exclude critical organ involvement. The sites that commonly undergo biopsy are the skin, lungs, and lymph nodes.

In the presence of a compatible clinical picture, determination of the site for biopsy should be the initial step. If the lungs are clinically involved, transbronchial biopsy is the recommended procedure. Common alternative sites for biopsy include skin, superficial lymph nodes, and lips. Biopsy by mediastinoscopy is recommended if abnormal mediastinal lymph nodes are identified on computed tomography *(100)*. If lung biopsy is refused or contraindicated in a patient with suspected pulmonary sarcoidosis, the clinical and radiological features alone may be diagnostic for patients in the early stages of the disease *(101)*. The finding of a granuloma is not specific for sarcoidosis, since many other conditions can cause granulomas *(4,102)*.

Developments in diagnostic tools such as fiberoptic bronchoscopy, BAL, and imaging studies have made the diagnostic process more effective and and linked to lower morbidity. According to one study, a CD4/CD8 ratio greater than 3.5 has a sensitivity of 53%, a specificity of 94%, a positive predictive value of 76%, and a negative predictive value of 85% *(103)*. Chest x-rays have a very high yield for pulmonary sarcoidosis and are useful for staging the disease radiologically *(4)*. The initial radiological staging system described by Wurm et al. has been adopted and is used as both a prognostic guide for clinicians and a means to stratify patients for clinical trials *(104)*.

Gallium-67 scanning can show increased uptake at sites of inflammation. It can be used to select sites for biopsy, even when there are asymptomatic lesions. Although this test can be positive at any site of inflammation, certain patterns on Gallium-67 scintigraphy in the lungs strongly suggest a diagnosis of sarcoidosis. The appearance of a *Panda* pattern combined with a *Lambda* pattern on a total body Gallium 76 scan may obviate the need for invasive diagnostic procedures *(105)*.

The serum angiotensin-converting (ACE) enzyme is a product of epitheloid cells in granulomas. Elevated levels are seen in 70 to 80% of patients with systemic sarcoidosis *(106)*. Mild elevations of ACE are less useful for diagnostic purposes because they have poor specificity *(107)*. Elevations of more than two times the upper limit of normal are more specific if tuberculosis, Gaucher's disease, and hypothyroidism can be excluded. Levels may correlate with disease activity, and they may help in monitoring treatment effects *(108)*. Occasionally, familial elevation of serum ACE levels occur in some patients *(109)*.

The Kveim-Slitzbach test, which is an intradermal test, was reportedly very sensitive (67–92%) and specific *(69)*. Other routine tests for systemic sarcoidosis include chest x-ray, complete blood count, serum chemistries, electrocardiogram, abdominal ultrasound, BAL for CD4/CD8 ratio, pulmonary function tests, and ophthalmological evaluation *(106)*. Hypercalcemia and hypercalciuria, which are often seen in systemic sarcoidosis, are caused by secretion of 1,25-dihydroxyvitamin D by the epitheloid cells of the sarcoid granuloma. When they occur, this is an indication of disease activity *(4)*. Cutaneous anergy to tuberculin injection is thought to be caused by alteration of the systemic T-cell population *(106)*.

7.2. Neurosarcoidosis

Recently, Zajicek et al. *(79)* proposed criteria for the diagnosis of neurosarcoidosis. All patients require the presence of compatible clinical features for neurosarcoidosis and exclusion of other diagnoses that can share similar signs and symptoms. The definitive diagnosis requires demonstration of noncaseating granulomata from a neural tissue. A probable diagnosis is considered when there is laboratory evidence of inflammation within the nervous system (e.g., CSF abnormalities) and/or compatible MRI findings on a background of evidence for systemic sarcoidosis. In the absence of the above criteria, only a possible diagnosis can be considered.

In the clinical setting of systemic sarcoidosis and additional neurological symptoms, the diagnosis of intracranial neurosarcoidosis can be relatively straightforward; however, none of the available diagnostic modalities, including cerebral imaging, CSF examination, or serum markers, provide information specific enough for diagnosis. One must rely on tissue evidence or the presence of confirmed systemic sarcoidosis in association with typical neurological findings to make the diagnosis. Multiple systemic and CNS diseases can mimic neurosarcoidosis and hence should be excluded.

MRI is a highly sensitive tool for the diagnosis of neurosarcoidosis, but it is less specific. The common MRI findings include diffuse meningeal enhancement, white-matter lesions, and focal parenchymal lesions *(67,79,110)*. Because of the wide range of neuroradiological findings, some findings may mimic neoplastic lesions such as meningioma *(111)*, glioma *(110)*, intrasellar tumors *(91)*, or CNS infections *(112,113)*. T1-weighted imaging using gadolinium is especially useful for demonstrating both meningeal- and parenchymal-enhancing lesions, and it also aids in the identification of a region for biopsy. Large sarcoid masses within the brain parenchyma are isointense on T1-weighted images and hyperintense on T2-weighted images *(75,113–115)*. Smaller parenchymatous lesions usually require intravenous administration of gadolinium for visualization. Enhancement patterns of intraparenchymal lesions may vary from homogenous to more irregular patterns *(57,75)*. MRI is not only useful for narrowing the differential diagnosis but also can be helpful for monitoring the response to immunomodulatory therapy.

Lymphoma preferentially involves the basal leptomeninges and periventricular white matter, as does sarcoid. Lymphoma, however, appears hypointense to the surrounding edema on T2-weighted MRI. Primary CNS lymphoma has an affinity for subcortical white matter, especially periventricular brain parenchyma, whereas secondary intracranial lymphoma with multiorgan distribution preferentially involves the leptomeninges. CSF analysis for malignant lymphocytes, chest radiography, abdominal ultrasonography, and bone marrow aspiration are additional tests for distinguishing between the two entities *(58)*. Periventricular and diffuse white-matter lesions, which are characteristic of MS, are also commonly seen in neurosarcoidosis *(75)*.

Sarcoid lesions within the spinal cord can be radiologically indistinguishable from true neoplasms. Because they may sometimes have an associated syrinx and enhancement, they may resemble spinal cord astrocytomas *(116)*. Junger et al. *(97)* proposed an MRI classification of spinal cord sarcoidosis in four stages that correlate with clinical stages of the disease. They proposed that linear enhancement along the leptomeninges that corresponds to early inflammation be designated as stage 1. Stage 2 disease occurs as parenchymal involvement that results in a diffusely enhancing lesion. In stage 3 disease, the inflammation decreases, and the enlarged spinal cord tends to return to a normal size, with focal or multifocal intramedullary lesions. Finally, stage 4 disease has features of spinal cord atrophy. Stages 2 and 3 may be radiologically indistinguishable from intramedullary spinal cord tumors, and a tissue diagnosis by means of a spinal cord biopsy may be necessary.

Abnormal CSF is seen in about 80% of cases. The most common abnormalities are increased cell counts (10–200 cells/μL) and elevated protein levels *(55,64,65,96)*. Other abnormal CSF findings may include oligoclonal bands, increased immunoglobulins, and reduced glucose levels. Despite the initial importance attributed to serum and CSF ACE levels, their use has fallen out of vogue owing to nonspecificity. Elevated CSF ACE levels are seen in about 55% of patients with neurosarcoidosis, 5% of those with systemic sarcoidosis, and up to 13% of patients with other inflammatory, infective, or neoplastic conditions of the nervous system *(117–119)*. Serum and CSF ACE levels may be used to monitor disease activity after immunomodulatory treatment.

If an obvious intracranial lesion is not detected, gallium-67 scintigraphy can be used to find systemic inflammatory lesions *(79)*. Recently, gallium-67 scintigraphy was used to detect asymptomatic muscle disease *(120)*. Once a lesion is found, whether in the lungs, lymph node, skin, liver, or other

Table 2
Differential Diagnosis of Neurosarcoidosis

1. Multiple sclerosis
2. Lyme disease
3. Tuberculosis
4. Granulomatous angiitis
5. Wegener's granulomatosis
6. Systemic lupus erythematosis
7. Carcinomatous meningitis
8. Lymphoma

organs, biopsy should be undertaken for histopathological diagnosis. Similarly, whole-body fluorodeoxyglucose positron emission tomography is useful in detecting sarcoid lesions for biopsy *(121)*.

The Kveim-Slitzbach intradermal test, although used often in the past, is no longer generally available, except in a few centers. In one study, 41 out of 48 neurosarcoid patients (85%) had a positive Kveim test *(79)*. The test can produce false positives in about 3% of patients, and it produces false-negatives in patients taking corticosteroids *(79)*.

When confronted with a patient who has an isolated inflammatory lesion suspected to be caused by neurosarcoidosis, the only option available for diagnosis is biopsy of the lesion. If there is a discrete lesion, especially in an inaccessible location, stereotactic biopsy is a possibility. For a large lesion that is unresponsive to corticosteroids and is associated with raised intracranial pressure, with or without hydrocephalus, open biopsy is indicated to exclude neoplastic, infectious, and other inflammatory lesions.

7.3. Differential Diagnosis

In systemic sarcoidosis patients who have neurological findings suspicious for neurosarcoidosis, other neurological disorders that mimic neurosarcoidosis should be excluded (Table 2). In patients with isolated neurosarcoidosis, one should look for evidence of systemic sarcoidosis or other systemic inflammatory disorders that might involve the nervous system. In some instances, treatment modalities might mimic the disease process; both methotrexate and diphenylhydantoin can cause hilar and mediastinal lymphadenopathy that is indistinguishable from sarcoidosis *(122)*. A detailed occupational history is important to avoid making a misdiagnosis of granulomatous disease resulting from occupational exposure *(123)*.

8. TREATMENT

8.1. Current Strategies

The wide variety of manifestations, unpredictable natural course of the disease, and comorbidity associated with drug therapy challenge the clinician who treats patients with sarcoidosis. Despite advances in our understanding of the immunopathogenesis of this disorder, drug selection, until recently, has been more or less empirical and based on observational studies, although knowledge of disease pathogenesis hopefully can facilitate future therapies.

Along with cardiac and pulmonary involvment, neurosarcoidosis is associated with significant mortality. It is generally associated with a poor outcome with few exceptions. Unlike the practice in pulmonary sarcoidosis, in which treatment is withheld for mild and asymptomatic cases *(124,125)*, the presence of nervous system involvement almost always necessitates treatment. Much of the current knowledge and recommendations in the therapy of neurosarcoidosis is obtained from case reports, neurosarcoidosis case series *(65,69,72,126)*, and clinical trials in pulmonary sarcoidosis. Randomized studies are not available to show the effect of therapeutic agents because of the rarity

Table 3
Strategic Mechanisms for Drug Treatment

1. Inhibition of antigen deposition:
    antibiotics
2. Inhibition of antigen presentation:
    antimalarial drugs
3. Suppression of granuloma formation:
    corticosteroids
    immunosuppressive agents
    anti-TNF agents
4. Antigen clearance enhancement:
    Peptide-based therapy (future)
5. Inhibition of fibrosis:
    corticosteroids
    immunosuppressive agents
    anti-TNF agents

TNF, tumor necrosis factor.

and wide diversity of clinical manifestations. It is time for a multicenter trial with international collaboration to assess diagnostic techniques and therapeutic agents.

As mentioned in earlier sections, the formation of sarcoid granulomata determines the clinical expression of the disease. Suppression of granuloma formation results in organ function preservation and a better clinical outcome. Drugs used in sarcoidosis act at different levels of the pathogenetic process (Table 3) *(27)*. Antibiotics active against propionibacteria and mycobacteria have been used successfully in a subset of patients with sarcoidosis. Their use has been based on evidence that links these organisms to the disease process *(127)*. The success of treatment is limited to only a few cases, possibly because viable microbial agents may no longer be present or necessary for granuloma formation.

Since corticosteroids were first used in 1951 *(128)*, they have been the cornerstone of treatment of sarcoidosis *(72,129,130)*, despite the lack of well-controlled trials that show improvement in the long-term outcome of the disease *(21)*. Significant morbidity is associated with the use of corticosteroids, but they have been associated with impressive therapeutic responses *(70,74,131,132)*. In contrast, some studies show that as many as 70% of patients with neurosarcoidosis discontinued steroids because of intolerable side effects or lack of efficacy *(68,79)*. In many of the patients who have responded initially, symptoms recur when the prednisone dose is tapered below 20 and 25mg/d, making steroid discontinuation impossible. Higher doses and longer treatment duration often result in intolerable side effects. Concomitant anticonvulsant therapy, which induces hepatic microsomal enzymes, may reduce prednisone concentration and efficacy and make even higher doses necessary *(79)*.

Treatment with prednisone should begin with doses in the range of 40 to 80 mg/d. The duration of treatment is necessarily long, since the disease is chronic. Unresponsive cases and patients with severe parenchymal disease may require higher doses and pulse therapy. After a clinical response is obtained, the dose is gradually tapered in a fashion similar to the protocols used in other inflammatory conditions *(69,73)*. Complete withdrawal can be attempted if the clinical course permits. In case of relapse, repeat high-dose steroid treatment is warranted, and tapering can be attempted at a later date. Patients should be monitored for complications and treated appropriately. Some authors suggest that the use of bolus pulsed intravenous methylprednisone may prevent long-term side effects and effect a better outcome *(79,107,133)*, but experience with this method is limited. One suggested regimen is 1 g/d intravenous methylprednisone for 3 d, followed by once-weekly dosing, along with 25mg/d oral prednisone *(79)*. Corticosteroid therapy should be individualized for dosing and duration of treatment.

The mechanisms of corticosteroids are broad. They include inhibition of lymphocyte and mononuclear phagocytic activity, inhibition of transcription of proinflammatory cytokines, downregulation of important cellular receptors, and interference with collagen synthesis. Thus, steroids have a biological rationale for their use in sarcoidosis, although there is no evidence that they change the natural history and long-term course of the illness. The main goal of treatment is to salvage tissue function and prevent progression of the disease process, especially fibrosis and ischemic changes. It is important to reduce the morbidity of treatment and thus avoid discontinuation because of side effects *(68,72)*.

Much less is known about alternative medications for treatment of neurosarcoidosis. Indications for their use include contraindications to corticosteroids, serious drug-related side effects, and refractoriness of the disease to treatment. Most of the alternative drugs have been used as adjuncts to steroid treatment, rather than as primary therapies, and they can help reduce steroid use to about 15 to 30% of the stabilizing dose *(134)*. The steroid-sparing therapies include cyclosporine, azathioprine, methotrexate, cyclophosphamide, chlorambucil, chloroquine, hydroxychloroquine, and radiotherapy *(72,74,134–141)*.

Most of these drugs have been used only sporadically; hence, reliable conclusions about their efficacy cannot be drawn. Among these drugs, the greatest experience is with cyclosporine. It is a T-cell inhibitor. Although available information suggests that this drug may have low penetrance into lung tissue *(143)*, it might be used successfully in neurosarcoidosis, even in patients who do not respond to steroid treatment *(69,72,134)*. It can be initiated at 4 mg/kg/d in two divided doses, given 12 h apart. Trough levels should be monitored monthly to maintain a therapeutic range and avoid side effects.

Methotrexate, a folate analogue, inhibits purine metabolism and polyamine synthesis. At high doses, it is antiproliferative. At low doses, it has anti-inflammatory actions owing to enhanced adenosine release, inhibition of TNF-α, and release of other cytokines. It is generally well tolerated, but it can potentially cause liver, bone marrow, and lung toxicity. The usual dose is 10 mg/wk, along with folic acid (1 mg/d) used to offset gastrointestinal toxicity. The cumulative dose should not exceed 1 g, beyond which liver biopsies are required *(68,136,140)*.

Azathioprine, which is a purine analogue, is an immunosuppressant. It produces greater suppression of cellular immunity than humoral immunity. It is generally reserved for progressive disease that does not respond to safer alternative drugs. Toxicities include bone marrow suppression, gastrointestinal effects, hepatitis, and late oncogenic potential. The usual dose is 50 to 200 mg/d, with initiation at lower doses followed by gradual upward titration if blood counts and hepatic functions are normal.

Antimalarial drugs have established benefit in sarcoidosis of the skin and mucosa. Since their unique mode of action inhibits antigen presentation, they are likely to be useful in most cases of sarcoidosis in which multidrug regimens are considered *(27)*. They have been used with beneficial effects in small case series of neurosarcoidosis *(74)*. Their use is limited by retinal toxicity.

There are a few reports of radiation therapy in neurosarcoidosis, especially in patients with diffuse encephalopathy and vasculopathy *(69,137,144)*. Either total nodal or craniospinal irradiation is used. Surgical treatment may be required for patients who have large parenchymal lesions that cause hydrocephalus or raised intracranial pressure. Radiation should be considered a last resort because it is rarely curative *(66)*.

Patients refractory to immunosuppressive therapy have a poor prognosis, but combination immunosuppressive therapy might be helpful because it targets different limbs of the immune system *(145)*.

The response to therapy is not uniform in all cases of neurosarcoidosis. Cranial neuropathies generally respond better than other forms of the disease. Patients with isolated cranial nerve involvement can be treated with lower doses and shorter courses of steroids, compared to other patients *(62)*, although patients who have optic and vestibulocochlear nerve involvement may require prolonged and aggressive therapy *(62)*. Similarly, aseptic meningitis responds well to therapy, but complete normalization of CSF need not be attempted. Mild hydrocephalus might require only monitoring, but when progressive hydrocephalus ensues, a ventriculoperitoneal shunt should be considered. Some researchers advise the use of pulse intravenous methylprednisone treatments (20 mg/kg/d for 3d) to provide clinical stabilization prior to surgical intervention *(62)*. Neuroendocrine involvement requires early initiation of treatment *(55)*. Parenchymal involvement is associated with a poorer prognosis, and high-dose steroid treatment is recommended *(69)*. Seizures are also associated with a poorer prognosis resulting from parenchymal involvement, but they respond well to antiepileptic therapy, once the parenchymal disease is under control *(69,70)*. Patients with peripheral neuropathy and myopathy should be treated like patients with brain parenchymal involvement *(69)*. Critically ill patients should be treated with boluses of pulsed intravenous methylprednisone therapy, followed by high-dose oral prednisone.

8.2. Newer Treatments

Novel therapies for sarcoidosis are emerging because of a better understanding of the immunopathogenesis of the disease. Several new immunomodulating agents have been shown to be beneficial in neurosarcoidosis. Mycophenolate mofetil is a relatively new drug that acts by inducing death of activated T cells. Koub et al. successfully used it in five sarcoidosis patients, and they found that the prednisone dose could be reduced from 60 mg/d to 10 mg/d *(146)*. Rapamycin, is another theoretically promising new drug. It acts by blocking cytokine responses and lymphocyte proliferation.

TNF-α is released by macrophages and other cells during granuloma formation, and it is believed to have a major role in the disease process. Because TNF-α has been hypothesized to interfere with responsiveness to steroid therapy, inhibition of TNF-α is a very appealing and sensible concept. Some anti-TNF-α drugs have shown promise in the treatment of other chronic inflammatory diseases, such as rheumatoid disease.

Pentoxyfylline, a nonselective phosphodiesterase inhibitor, inhibits TNF-α, but it had only limited benefit in a clinical trial for treatment of mild sarcoidosis *(147)*. Infliximab is a chimeric monoclonal human-murine antibody directed against TNF-α. It binds to TNF-α and blocks its interactions with the TNF receptor. Although pentoxyfylline has been shown effective in chronic inflammatory disorders, this drug generates antimurine antibody reactions that limit therapy. After Serio reviewed the available literature on the use of infliximab, he concluded that the limited evidence indicates that the drug shows promise for the treatment of sarcoidosis *(148)*. Pettersen et al. reported a dramatic response to infliximab in a patient with systemic and CNS parenchymal neurosarcoidosis. The disease was refractory to radiation therapy, corticosteroids, cyclosporine, methotrexate, azathioprine, chloroquine, and hydroxychloroquine *(149)*. On the other hand, etanercept, a dimeric fusion protein that binds specifically to TNF-α and renders it biologically inactive, has been effective in rheumatoid arthritis. Unfortunately, it has been reported to be not beneficial in sarcoidosis *(150)*.

Thalidomide, another TNF-α inhibitor, has some benefit in some cases of cutaneous sarcoidosis but not in pulmonary disease *(27)*. A refractory case of sarcoid myopathy has been shown to improve following a course of 50 mg/d thalidomide *(151)*. Toxicities include teratogenicity, peripheral neuropathy, and sedation.

Although the concept of blocking TNF-α is very attractive, none of the available TNF inhibitors have demonstrated potential therapeutic benefit in sarcoidosis. Given their theoretical promise, further experience is needed.

8.3. Future Strategies

Future strategies in the treatment of sarcoidosis include prevention of initial deposition of antigen, enhancement of antigen clearance, facilitation of remission by modification of antigen presentation to T cells, increase in anti-inflammatory cytokines such as IL-10, and targeting of cytokines and their receptors. Such therapies should be less toxic, since they provide for targeted immunosuppression.

9. PROGNOSIS

Neurosarcoidosis, along with cardiac and severe pulmonary disease, is associated with a poor prognosis and higher mortality, but there are exceptions to this general rule. Aseptic meningitis and cranial neuropathy, especially facial palsy, have a better prognosis *(69,70)*. Neurosarcoid involvement of the spinal cord, optic nerve, and brain parenchyma with associated epilepsy may carry a poor prognosis *(79)*. Aseptic meningitis, cranial neuropathies, and peripheral neuropathy and myopathy generally have a protracted course, but they are not associated with fatality *(152)*.

Among the PNS manifestations, polyradiculitis and acute myopathy tend to respond well to steroids in contrast with more slowly progressive peripheral neuropathy and myopathy *(70)*. In a study, 27 patients with neurosarcoidosis who had CNS lesions but not PNS manifestations had a poor outcome over a mean follow-up period of 6.6 yr *(152)*.

In some series, better outcomes were reported in as many as 35–50% of neurosarcoidosis patients *(69,70)*. This is attributed to early initiation and aggressive treatment, including adjunctive immunosuppression and radiation therapy. On the other hand, a significant number of patients with neurosarcoidosis worsened despite treatment in other studies *(68,72,74,79)*. As with systemic sarcoidosis, acute and subacute presentations of neurosarcoidosis have a better outcome than chronic forms *(73)*. In a more recent prospective study of 32 patients with neurosarcoidosis, 84% of treated and 38% of untreated patients improved. One-third of those treated with prednisone required additional pulse intravenous methylprednisone therapy *(107)*.

10. CONCLUSION

Neurosarcoidosis is associated with increased mortality and morbidity and warrants an aggressive management approach. Most basic concepts of neurosarcoidosis are derived from systemic sarcoidosis. Remarkable progress has been made in understanding the immunopathogenesis of this multifaceted and intricate disease, and this has paved the way for improved treatment strategies; however, knowledge of the underlying etiology is still obscure. There is a need for better understanding of predictors for disease persistence and progression. Despite the promise of newer therapeutic agents, corticosteroids still remain the mainstay of treatment of this disorder.

REFERENCES

1. Burns TM. Neurosarcoidosis. Arch Neurol 2003;60:1166–1168.
2. Hosoda Y, Odaka M. History of sarcoidosis. Semin Respir Med 1992;13:359–367.
3. Colover J: Sarcoidosis with involvement of the nervous system. Brain 1948;71:451–475.
4. Hunninghake GW, Costabel U, Ando M, et al. ATS Statement on sarcoidosis. Am J Respir Crit Care Med 1999;160:736–755.
5. Gordis, L. In: Sarcoidosis: Epidemiology of Chronic Lung Diseases in Children. Baltimore, The John Hopkins University Press, 1973;53–78.
6. Newman LS, Rose CS, Maier LA. Medical progress: sarcoidosis. N Engl J Med 1997;336:1224–1234.
7. Henke, CE, Henke G, Elveback LR, Beard CM, Ballard DJ, Kurland LT. The epidemiology of sarcoidosis in Rochester, Minnesota: a population-based study of incidence and survival. Am J Epidemiol 1986;123:840–845.
8. Rybicki BA, Major M, Popovich J Jr, Maliarik MJ, Iannuzzi MC. Racial differences in sarcoidosis incidence: a 5-year study in a health maintenance organization. Am J Epidemiol 1997;145:234–241.
9. James GD (ed.). In: Sarcoidosis and Other Granulomatous Disorders. New York, Marcel Dekker, 1994.
10. Thomas KW, Hunninghake GW. Sarcoidosis. JAMA 2003;289:3300–3303.
11. Gideon NM, Mannino DM. Sarcoidosis mortality in the United States 1979-1991: an analysis of multiple-cause mortality data. Am J Med 1996;100:423–427.
12. Mitchell, DN, Rees RJ.A transmissible agent from sarcoid tissue. Lancet 1969;2:81–84.
13. Hills SE, Parkes SA, Baker SB. Epidemiology of sarcoidosis in the Isle of Man–2: evidence for space-time clustering. Thorax 1987;42:427–430.
14. Parkes SA, Baker SB, Bourdillon RE, Murray CR, Rakshit M. Epidemiology of sarcoidosis in the Isle of Man–1: a case controlled study. Thorax 1987;42:420–426.
15. Panayeas S, Theodorakopoulos P, Bouras A, Constantopoulos S. Seasonal occurrence of sarcoidosis in Greece. Lancet 1991;338:510–511.

16. Bardinas F, Morera J, Fite E, Plasencia A. Seasonal clustering of sarcoidosis. Lancet 1989;2:455–456.

17. Hosoda Y, Hiraga Y, Odaka M, et al. A cooperative study of sarcoidosis in Asia and Africa: analytic epidemiology. Ann N Y Acad Sci 1976;278:355–367.

18. Edmondstone WM. Sarcoidosis in nurses: is there an association? Thorax 1988;43:342–343.

19. Sarcoidosis among US Navy enlisted men, 1965–1993. Morb Mortal Wkly Rep 1997;46:539–543.

20. Prezant DJ, Dhala A, Goldstein A, et al. The incidence, prevalence, and severity of sarcoidosis in New York City firefighters. Chest 1999;116:1183–1193.

21. du Bois RM. Corticosteroids in sarcoidosis: friend or foe? Eur Respir J 1994;7:1203–1209.

22. Ishige I, Usui Y, Takemura T, Eishi Y. Quantitative PCR of mycobacterial and propionibacterial DNA in lymph nodes of Japanese patients with sarcoidosis. Lancet 1999;35:4120–4123.

23. Muller-Quernheim J. Sarcoidosis: immunopathogenetic concepts and their clinical application. Eur Respir J 1998;12:716–738.

24. Hunninghake GW, Crystal RG. Pulmonary sarcoidosis: a disorder mediated by excess helper T-lymphocyte activity at sites of disease activity. N Engl J Med 1981;305:429–434.

25. Newman LS, Rose CS, Maier LA. Medical progress: sarcoidosis. N Engl J Med 1997;336:1224–1234.

26. Kataria YP. Chlorambucil in sarcoidosis. Chest 1980;78:36–43.

27. Moller DR. Treatment of sarcoidosis – from a basic science point of view. J Intern Med 2003;253:31–40.

28. Pinkston P, Bitterman PB, Crystal RG. Spontaneuous release of interleukin-2 by lung T-lymphocytes in active pulmonary sarcoidosis. N Engl J Med 1983;308:793–800.

29. Robinson BW, McLemore T, Crystal RG. Gamma-interferon is spontaneously released by alveolar macrophages and lung T-lymphocytes in patients with pulmonary sarcoidosis. J Clin Invest 1985;75:1488–1495.

30. Kim DS, Jeon YG, Shim TS et al. The value of interleukin-12 as an active marker of pulmonary sarcoidosis. Sarcoidosis Vasc Diffuse Lung Dis 2000;17:271–276.

31. Konishi K, Moller DR, Saltini C, Kirby M, Crystal RG. Spontaneous expression of the interleukin 2 receptor gene and presence of functional interleukin 2 receptors on T lymphocytes in the blood of individuals with active pulmonary sarcoidosis. J Clin Invest 1988;82:775–781.

32. Baughman, RP, Strohofer SA, Buchsbaum J, Lower EE. Release of tumor necrosis factor by alveolar macrophages of patients with sarcoidosis. J Lab Clin Med 1990;115:36–42.

33. Kreipe H, Radzun HJ, Heidorn K, et al. Proliferation, macrophage colony-stimulating factor, and macrophage colony-stimulating factor-receptor expression of alveolar macrophages in active sarcoidosis. Lab Invest 1990;62:697–703.

34. Morris DG, Jasmer RM, Huang L, Gotway MB, Nishimura S, King TE Jr. Sarcoidosis following HIV infection: evidence for CD4$^+$ lymphocyte dependence. Chest 2003;124:929–935.

35. Muller-Quernheim J, Pfeifer S, Kienast K, Zissel G. Spontaneous interleukin 2 release of bronchoalveolar lavage cells in sarcoidosis is a codeterminator of prognosis. Lung 1996;174:243–253.

36. Ziegenhagen MW, Benner UK, Zissel G, Zabel P, Schlaak M, Muller-Quernheim J. Sarcoidosis: TNF-alpha release from alveolar macrophages and serum level of sIL-2R are prognostic markers. Am J Respir Crit Care Med 1997;156:1586–1592.

37. Grutters JC, Fellrath JM, Mulder L, Janssen R, van den Bosch JM, van Velzen-Blad H. Serum soluble interleukin-2 receptor measurement in patients with sarcoidosis: a clinical evaluation. Chest 2003;124:186–195.

38. Zissel G, Homolka J, Schlaak J, Schlaak M, Muller-Quernheim J. Anti-inflammatory cytokine release by alveolar macrophages in pulmonary sarcoidosis. Am J Respir Crit Care Med 1996;154:713–719.

39. Ziegenhagen MW, Schrum S, Zissel G, Zipfel PF, Schlaak M, Muller-Quernheim J. Increased expression of proinflammatory chemokines in bronchoalveolar lavage cells of patients with progressing idiopathic pulmonary fibrosis and sarcoidosis. J Invest Med 1998;46:223–231.

40. Planck A, Katchar K, Eklund A, Gripenback S, Grunewald J. T-lymphocyte activity in HLA-DR17 positive patients with active and clinically recovered sarcoidosis. Sarcoidosis Vasc Diffuse Lung Dis 2003;20:110–117.

41. Xaus J, Besalduch N, Comalada M, et al. High expression of p21 Waf1 in sarcoid granulomas: a putative role for long-lasting inflammation. J Leukocyte Biol 2003;74:295–301.

42. Ziegenhagen MW, Muller-Quernheim J. The cytokine network in sarcoidosis and its clinical relevance. J Intern Med 2003;253:18–30.

43. Ziegenhagen MW, Rothe ME, Schlaak M, Muller-Quernheim J. Bronchoalveolar and serological parameters reflecting the severity of sarcoidosis. Eur Respir J 2003;21:407–413.

44. Muller-Quernheim J, Saltini C, Sondermeyer P, Crystal RG. Compartmentalized activation of the interleukin-2 gene by lung T-lymphocytes in active pulmonary sarcoidosis. J Immunol 1986;137:3475–3483.

45. Muller-Quernheim J, Pfeifer S, Mannel D, Strausz J, Ferlinz R. Lung restricted activation of the alveolar macrophage/monocyte system in pulmonary sarcoidosis. Am Rev Respir Dis 1992;145:187–192.

46. Franchimont D, Martens H, Hagelstein M, et al. Tumor necrosis factor alpha decreases, and interleukin-10 increases, the sensitivity of human monocytes to dexamethasone: potential regulation of the glucocorticoid receptor. J Clin Endocrinol Metab1999;84:2834–2839.

47. Schürmann M, Lympany PA, Reichel P, et al. Familial sarcoidosis is linked to the major histocompatibility complex region. Am J Respir Crit Care Med 2000;162:861–864.

48. Baughman RP, Lower EE, du Bois RM. Sarcoidosis. Lancet 2003;361:1111–1118.

49. Mangiapan G, Hance AJ. Mycobacteria and sarcoidosis: an overview and summary of recent molecular biological data. Sarcoidosis 1995;12:20–37.

50. Gullapalli D, Phillips L. Neurologic manifestations of sarcoidosis. Neurol Clin 2002;20:59–83.

51. Rosen Y. Sarcoidosis. In: Dail DH, Hammer SP, eds. Pulmonary Pathology, 2nd ed. New York, Springer-Verlag, 1994;13–645.

52. Colby TV. Interstitial lung diseases. In: Thurlbeck W, Churg A, eds. Pathology of the Lung, 2nd ed. New York, Thieme Medical Publishers, 1995:589–737.

53. Brincker H. Granulomatous lesions of unknown significance: the GLUS syndrome. In: James D, ed. Sarcoidosis and Other Granulomatous Disorders. New York, Marcel Dekkar, 1994:69–86.

54. Kendig EL Jr. The clinical picture of sarcoidosis in children. Pediatrics 1974;54:289–292.

55. Delaney P. Neurological manifestations in sarcoidosis: review of the literature, with report of 23 cases. Ann Intern Med 1977;87:336–345.

56. Mirfakhraee M, Crofford MJ, Guinto FC, Nauta HJW, Weedon VW. Virchow-Robin space: a path of spread in neurosarcoidosis. Radiology 1986;158:715–720.

57. Williams DW, Elster AD, Kramer SI. Neurosarcoidosis: gadolinium-enhanced MR imaging. J Comput Assist Tomogr 1990;14:704–707.

58. Nowak DA, Widenka DC. Neurosarcoidosis: a review of its intracranial manifestation. J Neurol 2001;248:363–372.

59. Caplan L, Corbett J, Goodwin J, et al. Neuro-ophthalmologic signs in the angiitic form of neurosarcoidosis. Neurology 1983;33:1130–1135.

60. Vital C, Aubertin J, Ragnault JM, et al. Sarcoidosis of the peripheral nerve: a histologic and ultrastructural study of two cases. Acta Neuropathol (Berl) 1982;58:111–114.

61. Stjernberg N, Cajander S, Truedsson H. Muscle involvement in sarcoidosis. Acta Med Scand 1981;209:213–216.

62. Krumholz A, Stern BJ. Neurological manifestations of sarcoidosis. In: Aminoff MJ, Goetz, eds. Handbook of Clinical Neurology, Vol 27, Systemic Diseases, Part III. St. Louis, MO, Elsevier Science, 1998;463–499.

63. Cahill DW, Salcman M. Sarcoidosis: a review of the rarer manifestations. Surg Neurol 1981;15:204–211.

64. Chen RC, McLeod JG. Neurological complications of sarcoidosis. Clin Exp Neurol 1989;26:99–112.

65. Sharma OP, Sharma AM. Sarcoidosis of the nervous system: a clinical approach. Arch Intern Med 1991;151:1317–1321.

66. Stern BJ, Krumholz A, Johns C, Scott P, Nissim J. Sarcoidosis and its neurological manifestations. Arch Neurol 1985;42:909–917.

67. Ricker W, Clark M. Sarcoidosis: a clinical pathologic review of 300 cases. Am J Clin Pathol 1949;19:725–749.

68. Lower EE, Broderick JP, Brott TG, et al: Diagnosis and management of neurological sarcoidosis. Arch Intern Med 1997;157:1864–1868.

69. Chapelon C, Ziza JM, Piette JC, et al. Neurosarcoidosis: signs, course and treatment in 35 confirmed cases. Medicine (Baltimore) 1990;69:261–276.

70. Oksanen V. Neurosarcoidosis: clinical presentation and course in 50 patients. Acta Neurol Scand 1986;73:283–290.

71. Oksanen V, Gronhagen-Riska C, Fyhrquist F, et al. Systemic manifestations and enzyme studies in sarcoidosis with neurologic involvement. Acta Med Scand 1985;218:123–127.

72. Agobogu BN, Stern BJ, Sewell C. Therapeutic considerations in patients with refractory neurosarcoidosis. Arch Neurol 1995;52:875–879.

73. Luke RA, Stern BJ, Krumholz A, et al. Neurosarcoidosis: the long-term clinical course. Neurology 1987;37:461–463.

74. Sharma OP. Neurosarcoidosis. A personal prospective based on the study of 37 patients. Chest 1997;112:220–228.

75. Lexa FJ,Grossman RI. MR of sarcoidosis in the head and spine: spectrum of manifestation and radiographic response to steroid therapy. Am J Neuroradiol 1994;15:973–982.

76. Miller DH, Kendall BE, Barter S, et al. Magnetic resonance imaging in central nervous system sarcoidosis. Neurology 1988;38:378–383.

77. Keane JR. Bilateral seventh nerve palsy: analysis of 43 cases and review of literature. Neurology 1994;44:1198–1202.

78. Graham EM, Ellis CJK, Sanders MD. Optic neuropathy in sarcoidosis. J Neurol Neurosurg Psychiatry 1986;49:756–763.

79. Zajicek JP, Scolding NJ, Foster O, et al. Central nervous system sarcoidosis—diagnosis and management. Q J Med 1999;92:103–117.

80. Blain JG, Logothetis J. Optic nerve manifestations of sarcoidosis. Arch Neurol 1965;13:307–309.

81. Gudeman SK, Selhorst JB, Susac JO, et al. Sarcoid optic neuropathy. Neurology 1982;32:597–603.

82. Oksanen V, Salmi T. Visual and auditory evoked potentials in the early diagnosis and follow-up of neurosarcoidosis. Acta Neurol Scand 1986;74:38–42.

83. Herring AB, Ulrich H. Sarcoidosis of the central nervous system. J Neurol Sci 1969;9:405–422.

84. Israel HL. Diagnostic value of the Kveim reaction. In: Fanburg BL, ed. Sarcoidosis and Other Granulomatous Diseases of the Lung. New York, Marcel Dekkar, 1983;273–286.

85. Osenbach RK, Blumenkoff B, Ramirez H Jr, et al. Meningeal neurosarcoidosis mimicking convexity en-plaque menigioma. Surg Neurol 1986;26:387–390.

86. Sethi KD, El Gammal T, Patel BR, et al. Dural sarcoidosis presenting with transient neurologic symptoms. Arch. Neurol 1986;43:595–597.

87. Tobias S, Prayson RA, Lee JH. Necrotizing neurosarcoidosis of the cranial base resembling an en plaque sphenoid wing meningioma: case report. Neurosurgery 2002;51:1290–1294.

88. Stuart CA, Neelon FA, Lobovitz HE. Hypothalamic insufficiency: the cause of hypopituitarism in sarcoidosis. Ann Intern Med 1978;88:589–594.

89. Ismail F, Miller JL, Kahn SE. Hypothalamic-pituitary sarcoidosis. S Afr Med J 1985;97:139–142.

90. Murialdo G, Tamagno G. Endocrine aspects of neurosarcoidosis. J Endocrin Invest 2002;25:650–662.

91. Sato N, Gordon S, Jung HK. Cystic pituitary mass in neurosarcoidosis. Am J Neuroradiol 1997;18:1182–1185.

92. Bullmann C, Faust M, Hoffmann A, et al. Five cases with central diabetes insipidus and hypogonadism as first presentation of neurosarcoidosis. Eur J Endocrinol 2000;142:365–372.

93. Brooks BS, El Gammal T, Hungerford GD. Radiologic evaluation of neurosarcoidosis: role of computed tomography. Am J Neuro Radiol 1982;3:513–521.

94. Clark WC, Acker JD, Dohan FC, Robertson JH. Presentation of central nervous system sarcoidosis as intracranial tumours. Surg Neurol 1981;63:851–856.

95. Brown MM, Thomson AJ, Wedzicha JA, et al. Sarcoidosis presenting with stroke. Stroke 1989;20:400–405.

96. Scott TF. Neurosarcoidosis: progress and clinical aspects.Neurology 1993;43:8–12.

97. Junger SS, Stern BJ, Levine SR, Sipos E, Marti-Masso JF. Intramedullary spinal cord sarcoidosis: clinical and magnetic resonance imaging characteristics. Neurology 1993;43:333–337.

98. Challenor YB, Felton CP, Brust JCM. Peripheral nerve involvement in sarcoidosis: an electrodiagnostic study. J Neurol Neurusurg Psychiatry 1984;47:1219–1222.

99. Koffman, B, Junck L, Elias SB, Feit HW, Levine SR. Polyradiculopathy in sarcoidosis. Muscle Nerve 1999;22:608–613.

100. Gossot, D, Toledo L, Fritsch S, Celerier M. Mediastinoscopy vs thoracoscopy for mediastinal biopsy: results of a prospective nonrandomized study. Chest 1996;110:1328–1331.

101. Hiraga, Y, Hosoda Y. Acceptability of epidemiological diagnostic criteria for sarcoidosis without histological confirmation. In: Mikami R, Mikami Y, Hosoda Y, eds. Sarcoidosis. Tokyo, University of Tokyo Press, 1981;373–377.

102. Popper HH. Epithelioid cell granulomatosis of the lung: new insights and concepts. Sarcoidosis Vasc Diffuse Lung Dis 1999;16:32–46.

103. Costabel, U. Sensitivity and specificity of BAL findings in sarcoidosis. Sarcoidosis 1992;9(Suppl. 1):211–214.

104. Wurm, K, Reindell H, Heilmeyer L. In: Der Lungenboeck in Röntgenbild. Germany, Thieme, 1958.

105. Sulavik, SB, Spencer RP, Weed DA, Shapiro HR, Shiue ST, Castriotta RJ. Recognition of distinctive patterns of gallium-67 distribution in sarcoidosis. J Nucl Med 1990;31:1909–1914.

106. Crystal RG. Sarcoidosis. In:Wilson JD, Braunwald E, Isselbacher KJ, et al., eds. Harrison's Principles of Internal Medicine, 12th ed., Vol 2. New York, McGraw-Hill, 1991;1463–1469.

107. Allen RK. A review of angiotensin converting enzyme in health and disease. Sarcoidosis 1991;8:95–100.

108. Consensus conference. Activity of sarcoidosis. Eur Respir J 1994;7:624–627.

109. Kramers C, Deinum J. Increased serum activity of angiotensin-converting enzyme (ACE): indication of sarcoidosis? A 'Bayesian' approach. Nederlands Tijdschrift voor Geneeskunde 2003;147:473–476.

110. Powers WJ, Miller EW. Sarcoidosis mimicking glioma: case report and review of intracranial sarcoid mass lesions. Neurology 1981;31:907–910.

111. Nowak DA, Gumprecht H, Widenka DC, Stölzle A, Lumenta CB. Solitary sarcoid granulomatosis mimicking meningioma. J Neurosurg 2000;93:897.

112. Mayer SA, Yim GK, Onesti ST, Lynch T, Faust PL, Marder K. Biopsy proven isolated sarcoid meningitis. Case report. J Neurosurg 1993;78:994–996.

113. Pickuth D, Spielmann RP, Heywang-Kobrunner SH. Role of radiology in the diagnosis of neurosarcoidosis. Eur Radiol 2000;10:941–944.

114. Christoforidis GA, Spickler EM, Recio MV, Metha BM. MR of CNS sarcoidosis: correlation of imaging features to clinical symptoms and response to treatment. Am J Neuroradiol 1999;20:655–669.

115. Seltzer S, Mark AS, Atlas SW. CNS sarcoidosis: evaluation with contrast-enhanced MR imaging. Am J Neuroradiol 1991;12:1227–1233.

116. Vinas FC, Rengachary S. Diagnosis and management of neurosarcoidosis. J Clin NeuroSci 2001;8:505–513.

117. Oksanen V. New cerebrospinal fluid, neurophysiological and neuroradiological examinations in the diagnosis and follow–up of neurosarcoidosis. Sarcoidosis 1987;4:105–110.

118. Oksanen V, Fyhrquist F, Sommer H, Gronhagen-Riska C. Angiotensin converting enzyme in cerebrospinal fluid: a new assay. Neurology 1985;35:1220–1223.

119. Dale JC, O'Brien JF. Determination of angiotensin-converting enzyme levels in cerebrospinal fluid is not a useful test for the diagnosis of neurosarcoidosis. Mayo Clin Proc 1999;74:535.

120. Suehiro S, Shiokawa S, Taniguchi S, et al. Gallium-67 scintigraphy in the diagnosis and management of chronic sarcoid myopathy. Clinical Rheumatology 2003;22:146–148.

121. Dubey N, Miletich RS, Wasay M, Mechtler LL, Bakshi R. Role of fluorodeoxyglucose positron emission tomography in the diagnosis of neurosarcoidosis. J Neurol Sci 2002;205:77–81.

122. Sharma OP, Kalkat G. Drug-induced clinical syndromes mimicking sarcoidosis. Sarcoidosis 1991;8:3–5.

123. Fireman E, Haimsky E, Noiderfer M, Priel I, Lerman Y. Misdiagnosis of sarcoidosis in patients with chronic beryllium disease. Sarcoidosis Vasc Diffuse Lung Dis 2003;20:144–148.

124. Hunninghake GW, Gilbert S, Pueringer R, et al. Outcome of the treatment of sarcoidosis. Am J Respir Care Med 1994;149:893–898.

125. Baughman RP, Lynch JP. Difficult treatment issues in sarcoidosis. J Int Med 2003;253:41–45.

126. Oksanen V. Neurosarcoidosis. In: James DG, ed. Sarcoidosis and Other Granulomatous Disorders, New York, Marcel Dekker, 1994;285–309.

127. Bachelez H, Senet P, Cadranel J, Kaoukhov A, Dubertret L. The use of tetracyclines for the treatment of sarcoidosis. Arch Dermatol 2001;137:69–73.

128. Sones, M, Israel HL, Dratman MB, Frank JH. Effect of cortisone in sarcoidosis. N Engl J Med 1951;244:209–213.

129. Sharma OP. Pulmonary sarcoidosis and corticosteroids. Am Rev Respir Dis 1993;147:1598–1600.

130. Paramothayan S, Jones PW. Corticosteroid therapy in pulmonary sarcoidosis: a systematic review. JAMA 2002; 287:1301–1307.

131. Ried LD, Abbas S, Markivee CR. Neurosarcoidosis responding to steroids. AJR 1986;146:819–821.

132. Martin CA, Murali R, Trash SS. Spinal cord sarcoidosis. Case report. J Neurosurg 1984;61:981–982.

133. Molina A, Mana J, Villabona C, Fernandez-Castaner M, Soler J. Hypothalamic-pituitary sarcoidosis with hypopituitarism. Long-term remission with methylprednisolone pulse therapy. Pituitary 2002;5:33–36.

134. Stern BJ, Schonfeld SA, Sewell C, Krumholz A, Scott P, Belendiuk G. The treatment of neurosarcoidosis with cyclosporine. Arch Neurol 1992;49:1065–1072.

135. Winget D, O'Brien GM, Laver EE, et al. Bell's palsy as an unrecognized presentation for sarcoidosis. Sarcoidosis 1994;11(suppl 1):368–370.

136. Kaye O, Palazzo E, Grossin M, et al. Low dose methotrexate: an effective corticosteroids-sparing agent in the musculoskeletal manifestations of sarcoidosis. Br J Rhematol 1995;34:642–44.

137. Stelzer KJ, Thomas CR Jr, Berger MS, et al. Radiation therapy for sarcoid of the thalamus/posterior third ventricle: case report. Neurosurgery 1995;36:1188–1191.

138. Ahmad K, Kim YH, Spitzer AP, et al. Total nodal radiation in progressive sarcoidosis. Am J Clin Oncol 1992;15:311–313.

139. Zuber M, Defer G, Cesaro P. Efficacy of cyclophosphamide in sarcoid radiculomyelitis. J Neurol Neurosurg Psychiatry 1992;55:166–167.

140. Lower EE, Baughman RP. The use of low dose methotrexate in refractory sarcoidosis. Am J Med Sci 1990; 299:153–157.

141. Soriano FG, Caramelli P, Nitrini R, Rocha AS. Neurosarcoidosis: therapeutic success with methotrexate. Postgrad Med J 1990;66:142–143.

142. Cunnah D, Chew S, Wass J. Cyclosporin for central nervous system sarcoidosis. Am J Med 1988;85:580–581.

143. Wyser CP, van Schalkwyk EM, Alheit B, et al. Treatment of progressive pulmonary sarcoidosis with cyclosporin A: a randomized controlled trial. Am J Respir Crit Care Med 1997;1556:1371–1376.

144. Kang S, Suh JH. Radiation therapy for neurosarcoidosis: report of three cases from a single institution. Radia Oncol Invest 1999;7:309–312.

145. Pia G, Pascalis L, Aresu G, et al. Evaluation of the efficacy and toxicity of the cyclosporine A-flucortolone-methotrexate combination in the treatment of sarcoidosis. Sarcoidosis Vasc Diffuse Lung Dis 1996;13:146–152.

146. Kouba DJ, Mimouni D, Rencic A, Nousari HC. Mycophenolate mofetil may serve as a steroid-sparing agent for sarcoidosis. Br J Dermatol 2003;148:147–148.

147. Zabel P, Entzian P, Dalhoff K, Schlaak M. Pentoxyfylline in treatment of sarcoidosis. Am J Respir Crit Care Med 1997;155:1665–1669.

148. Serio RN. Infliximab treatment of sarcoidosis. Ann Pharmacother 2003;37:577–81.

149. Pettersen JA, Zochodne DW, Bell RB, Martin L, Hill MD. Refractory neurosarcoidosis responding to infliximab. Neurol 2002;59:1660–1661.

150. Utz JP, Limper AH, Kalra S, et al. Etanercept for the treatment of stage II and III progressive pulmonary sarcoidosis. Chest 2003;124:177–185.

151. Walter MC, Lochmuller H, Schlotter-Weigel B, Meindl T, Muller-Felber W. Successful treatment of muscle sarcoidosis with thalidomide. Acta Myologica 2003;22:22–25.

152. Ferriby D, de Seze J, Stojkovic T, Hachulla E, Wallaert B, Destee A, Hatron PY, Vermersch P. Long-term follow-up of neurosarcoidosis. Neurology 2001;57:927–929.

CME QUESTIONS

1. Which of the following participates in antigen presentation in the pathogenesis of sarcoidosis?
   A. Major histocompatibility complex
   B. Interleukin-2
   C. Tumor necrosis factor-α
   D. Interferon-γ

2. Which of the following neurologic manifestations of sarcoidosis is associated with a relatively better prognosis?
   A. Cerebral parenchymal granuloma
   B. Epilepsy
   C. Optic neuropathy
   D. Facial neuropathy

3. Which of the following is the most important test in the diagnosis of neurosarcoidosis?
   A. Magnetic resonance imaging
   B. Tissue biopsy of the lesion
   C. Cerebrospinal fluid exam with angiotensin-converting enzyme levels
   D. Gallium-67 scintigraphy

4. Which of the following is suspected to be an etiological agent in the pathogenesis of sarcoidosis?
   A. Mycobacteria
   B. Borrelia
   C. Viral agents
   D. Beryllium exposure

15
Neuropsychiatric SLE
Pathogenesis, Immunology, and Clinical Management

Deborah Aleman-Hoey and Robin L. Brey

1. BACKGROUND

Systemic lupus erythematosus (SLE) is a chronic autoimmune disease affecting multiple organ systems. The incidence of SLE is 5.6 per 100,000, with an estimated prevalence of 130 per 100,000 people in the United States *(1)*. Thus, about 380,000 Americans have SLE. Women are affected nine times more frequently than men *(2)*. African Americans and Hispanics are affected much more frequently than Euro-Americans and have more disease morbidity *(2–6)*. Although SLE-related morbidity remains high, the prognosis for survival has improved in recent years, from a 5-yr survival of 51% in the 1950s to more than 90% in recent studies *(3)*. A bimodal pattern of mortality, in which early deaths are caused by SLE disease activity or infections and later deaths are owing primarily to vascular causes *(7–9)* has been described. Because of this greater survival, emphasis has shifted towards improving health status and quality of life.

Neuropsychiatric systemic lupus erythematosus (NPSLE) has been recognized since Kaposi first described the pathological entity in the late 19th century *(10)*. Seizures and psychosis are well-recognized NPSLE manifestations; however, within the past 15 yr, it has become clear that the nervous system is much more widely affected than previously thought. The American College of Rheumatology (ACR) established the first set of case definitions and diagnostic criteria for 19 central nervous system (CNS) and peripheral nervous system (PNS) syndromes associated with SLE in 1999 *(11)*. The term *lupus cerebritis* does not appear in these case definitions. For decades, *lupus cerebritis* and *cerebral vasculitis* were perpetuated as misnomers for the broad spectrum of nervous system involvement in patients with SLE. Although vasculitis is seen in the PNS and other systemic organs, vasculitis in the brain is rare *(12)*.

2. IMMUNOPATHOLOGY

SLE is the *sine qua non* of an immune system gone awry. The aberrant interaction of genetic, environmental, hormonal, and immune factors triggers the development of autoantibodies to self-antigens, cellular dysfunction, and/or apoptosis *(13)*. Serum anti-DNA antibodies, an SLE hallmark, appear to correlate best with disease activity. They crossreact with bacterial polysaccharides, protein antigens, non-nucleic-acid auto-antigens, cellular membranes, and extracellular matrix components *(14,15)*.

Neuropathological studies in SLE patients have frequently found a small vessel vasculopathy consisting of proliferative changes of the intima, vascular hyalinization, and perivascular lymphocytosis.

From: *Current Clinical Neurology: Inflammatory Disorders of the Nervous System:*
Pathogenesis, Immunology, and Clinical Management
Edited by: A. Minagar and J. S. Alexander © Humana Press Inc., Totowa, NJ

This small-vessel vasculopathy has been seen in SLE patients with only psychiatric symptoms as well as those with focal nervous system manifestations *(16)*.

Histopathological studies reveal a wide range of brain abnormalities caused by multifocal microinfarcts, cortical atrophy, gross infarcts, hemorrhage, ischemic demyelination, and patchy multiple sclerosis-like demyelination *(16,17)*, but these findings are not diagnostic for NPSLE *(18)*. Bland microvasculopathy (characterized by vessel tortuosity, cuffing of small vessels, vascular hyalinisation, endothelial proliferation, and perivascular gliosis), formerly attributed to deposition of immune complexes but now suspected to arise from activation of complement, appears to be the most common microscopic finding *(17,19)*; however, this too is a nonspecific finding, as patients without NPSLE also show these changes *(16)*. A histologically normal brain with no specific pathognomic brain lesions is not uncommon in patients with NPSLE *(19)*.

Interestingly, single photon emission computed tomography (SPECT) and magnetic resonance spectroscopy (MRS) studies suggest that both cerebral atrophy and cognitive decline in SLE patients may be related to chronic cerebral ischemia *(18,20,21)*. It is possible that SPECT and MRS studies represent a functional image correlate for cerebral vasculopathic change.

Auto-antibody production has been implicated in vasculopathic and auto-antibody-mediated neuronal injury mechanisms. Anti-ribosomal P antibodies (anti-P) have been linked to diffuse CNS involvement in NPSLE *(22,23)*. Antiphospholipid (aPL) autoantibodies, detected by immunoreactivity to anticardiolipin (aCL) assays and/or their ability to prolong phospholipid-dependent coagulation assays (lupus anticoagulant [LA]), are implicated in the microvascular thrombo/embolitic and endothelial damage found in the brains of patients with NPSLE *(18)*. More about these mechanisms can be found in the sections that follow.

The brain has relative protection from systemic immune responses because of the blood–brain barrier (BBB). In patients with SLE, the permeability of the BBB is increased for a variety of reasons, including cytokine and antibody effects *(24)*. There are also CNS-derived cells that can serve immune functions. Brain microglial cells have the ability to phagocytize apoptotic T cells and can contribute to T-cell mediated neuroinflammatory disease *(25)*. Moreover, treatment of adult human CNS-derived microglia with supernatants from allo-antigen or myelin basic protein T helper (Th)1 cell lines, leads to the upregulation of major histocompatability complex class II, CD80, CD86, CD45, and CD54 on the T-cell surface; this favors the microglia's antigen-presenting capacity and increases tumor necrosis factor-α and interleukin (IL)-6 production *(26)*. Supernatant-treated Th1 lymphocytes also upregulate intracellular adhesion molecule (ICAM)-1 and vascular adhesion molecule (VCAM)-1 molecules on endothelial cells *(27)*. All of these factors contribute to the initiation and perpetuation of an immune response within the CNS.

2.1. Cytokines and Systemic Lupus Erythematosus

Cytokines appear to have regulatory roles in mediating SLE-disease activity and inflammation in target organs *(28,29)*. Recent work has highlighted the importance of SLE monocytes in the generation of potentially pathogenic cytokines, particularly IL-6 and IL-10 *(30)*. The balance between proinflammatory and anti-inflammatory cytokines and the degree and extent of inflammation appear to profoundly influence SLE-mediated disease manifestations *(28)*.

Several, largely cross-sectional, studies in SLE have suggested that IL-6 is a marker of disease activity *(31–33)*. There are multiple other mechanisms that contibute to patients with SLE possibly having higher IL-6 levels than in patients without SLE. The C5b-9 complex stimulates IL-6 *(34)*. Diabetes, which is increased in SLE patients taking prednisone, is associated with higher IL-6 levels *(35,36)*. Homocysteine, which is elevated in 30% of SLE patients, also leads to higher IL-6 levels *(37)*. More than 33% of SLE patients are morbidly obese, another associate of increased IL-6 levels *(38)*. Finally, dehydroepiandrosterone sulphate (DHEA) is low in SLE, and a low level of DHEA could increase IL-6 secretion *(39,40)*.

Few studies have investigated the role of cytokine abnormalities in patients with NPSLE. IL-1 and IL-6 levels are increased in the cerebrospinal fluid (CSF) of patients with SLE who have CNS involvement, compared with non-SLE neurological controls *(30,31)*. Both serum and CSF IL-6 levels are elevated in NPSLE patients vs non-NPSLE patients or healthy controls *(30,31)*, although one study found no difference in serum IL-6 levels between NPSLE patients and CNS-infection control patients *(30)*. In another study, CSF IL-6 activity consistently paralleled NPSLE disease activity *(32)*. In a study of 15 patients with SLE who did not have overt CNS disease (comparing them to patients with rheumatoid arthritis [RA] and healthy controls), regression analysis showed that serum DHEA and IL-6 accounted for unique portions of the variance in measures of learning and attention, after controlling for depression and corticosteroid treatment *(41)*.

2.2. Adhesion Molecules and Systemic Lupus Erythematosus

Other processes leading to immune-mediated brain dysfunction in SLE probably involve abnormal endothelial–white blood cell interactions that allow proteins or cells access to the CNS. The expression of adhesion proteins on endothelial cells appears to be upregulated in SLE and facilitates lymphocyte entry in CNS disease *(25,27,42–45)*. Shedding of the active form of these molecules occurs, and soluble levels can be measured in both serum and CSF *(45)*.

Studies of circulating soluble adhesion molecules in SLE have yielded contradictory results *(46,47)*. In addition, there is disagreement as to whether soluble adhesion molecules are an accurate reflection of membrane-bound proteins. Elevated levels of ICAM-1, VCAM-1, and E-selectin were detected in a cohort of predominantly Hispanic SLE patients, compared to normal control values in the San Antonio Lupus Study of Neuropsychiatric Disease (SALUD) *(48)*. High levels of all soluble adhesion molecule levels were found in Hispanic lupus patients, compared with African-American and Euro-American lupus patients and Hispanic control subjects. This suggests that the upregulation of adhesion molecules in Hispanic lupus patients may account for some of the ethnic differences in disease expression that have been previously described *(5)*.

Soluble serum levels of ICAM-1 increase with systemic disease activity in patients with SLE *(49,50)*. Elevated soluble serum levels of VCAM-1 have been demonstrated in patients with rheumatoid arthritis and SLE, compared to normal controls *(51)*. In two studies of soluble serum levels of ICAM-1, VCAM-1, and E-Selectin in SLE, soluble VCAM-1 levels were elevated during active disease and normalized with remission *(52,53)*. There was no difference in mean ICAM-1 levels between patients with SLE, patients with RA, and normal controls in another study *(53)*; however, within the patient groups, soluble serum ICAM-1 levels correlated with other markers of disease activity, for example sedimentation rates and clinical findings.

The SALUD study systematically evaluated the relationship between soluble VCAM-1, ICAM-1, and E-selectin molecule levels and nervous system manifestations outlined by the ACR NPSLE case definitions, in addition to evaluating their importance in acute SLE activity and SLE-related damage *(48)*. An abnormal level of soluble VCAM-1 (sVCAM-1) at the first study visit was associated with a history of stroke and the presence of one or more psychiatric manifestations in this cohort. These findings support two other small studies that found a relationship between soluble adhesion molecule levels and neurological disease *(52,54)*.

A relationship between both sVCAM-1 and sICAM-1 levels and levels of auto-antibodies that have been associated with NPSLE manifestations, namely aPL, were also seen in the SALUD study *(48)*. Antiphospholipid antibodies can activate endothelial cells, leading to the upregulation of adhesion molecules and adherence of leukocytes *(55)*. There is also evidence from animal knock-out models that aPL may require the upregulation of adhesion molecules to cause thrombosis and possibly other NPSLE manifestations *(56)*. Elevated levels of soluble adhesion molecules (ICAM-1, VCAM-1 and E-selectin) were found in patients with primary antiphospholipid syndrome (APS) and SLE with APS in comparison to control patients with thrombosis unrelated to

APS and healthy control subjects *(57)*. When patients with primary APS and SLE with APS were divided into two groups based on severity and frequency of thrombosis, sVCAM-1 levels were increased in the groups with greater severity and more frequent thromboses. Patients in the primary APS group who had cerebral arterial thrombosis, fetal loss, or renal vein thrombosis had increased sVCAM-1 levels when compared to primary APS patients without these manifestations. This study did not evaluate the association between soluble adhesion molecule levels and other neurological manifestations.

2.3. Anti-Ribosomal P Antibodies and Systemic Lupus Erythematosus

Anti-P antibodies have been correlated with psychosis, depression, and other CNS abnormalities in SLE patients in some *(58–64)*, but not all *(65,66)*, studies. This lack of concordance has been explained by differences in diagnostic criteria, ethnic make-up of the study population, and differences in purity of the ribosomal P antigen used in the immunological assays *(62)*. Anti-P antibodies occur in approximately 17% of SLE patients, although the prevalence varies greatly among ethnic groups *(60)*. Arnett and colleagues studied 394 patients with SLE who were of different ethnicities and found that between 13–20% of Euro-American, African Americans, Hispanics, and Greeks studied had positive anti-P antibody values, although only 6% of Bulgarians and as many as 36% of Chinese-Americans had positive values *(60)*. Interestingly, although serum levels of anti-P antibody correlate with psychosis and depression in SLE, CSF levels do not *(61,62)*. One possible explanation for this is that anti-P antibodies may be taken up by neuronal cells, which leads to cellular injury. In several studies that have evaluated serum anti-P antibody levels serially, anti-P antibody levels peak at the time of psychiatric symptoms and decreased in parallel with resolution of symptoms *(61,62)*. Isshi and Hirohata found that a combination of antineuronal antibodies and anti-P antibodies both contributed to SLE-related psychosis *(62)*. These investigators put forth the interesting notion that the "cooperation" of multiple antibodies may be required to achieve a pathological effect. The mechanism by which anti-P antibodies could lead to CNS symptoms is not known for certain. These antibodies have been shown to bind to a 38 Kd protein on the surface of neuroblastoma cell lines *(67)* and also on the surfaces of other cells *(68)*. There is good evidence that P protein is present on neuronal cells in an immunologically accessible way *(67)*. Furthermore, in vitro studies demonstrated the cellular penetration of anti-P antibodies in culture and the inhibition of protein synthesis with cellular penetration *(69)*.

2.4. Anti-NR2 Glutamate Receptor Antibodies in SLE

Diamond and colleagues demonstrated that a subset of lupus anti-DNA antibodies crossreacts with the NR2 glutamate receptor in patients with SLE *(70)*. Her group has also shown that the penta-peptide Asp/Glu-Trp-Asp/Glu-Tyr-Ser/Gly is a molecular mimic of double-stranded DNA *(71)*. This sequence is also present in the extracellular domain of the murine and human *N*-methyl-D-aspartate receptor subunits NR2a and NR2b. This group showed that the NR2 receptor is recognized by both murine and human anti-DNA antibodies and that these antibodies mediate apoptotic cell death of neurons in vitro and in vivo. CSF obtained from a single patient with SLE containing these antibodies also mediated cell death through an apoptotic pathway *(70)*. NR2 receptors bind the neurotransmitter glutamate and are present on neurons *(72–78)*. Mice with a targeted disruption of the gene encoding NR2a display a defect in hippocampal long-term potentiation *(79)*. Patients with psychosis may have altered glutamate-receptor expression, and excitotoxic neuron death can occur with over stimulation of NR2 *(80–83)*. Omdal and colleagues recently reported an association between anti-NR-glutamate-receptor antibodies and both cognitive dysfunction and depression in a group of 57 patients with SLE who were from Norway *(84)*. More work is needed to further elicit the relationship between this autoantibody and cognitive dysfunction and psychiatric disease in SLE.

2.5. *Antiphospholipid Antibodies in NPSLE*

aPLs are associated with the APS (recurrent thrombosis, recurrent fetal loss, and thrombocytopenia) *(85)*. APS may be primary or secondary, if it is associated to other connective tissue diseases, particularly SLE. aPLs are a family of antibodies directed against plasma proteins bound to negatively charged phospholipids that lead to hypercoaguability through effects on the Protein C/Protein S system, platelets, endothelial cells, and complement activation *(85,86)*. aPLs, defined as LA, aCL, and anti-β_2 glycoprotein 1 (anti-β2GP1), are strongly associated with localized NPSLE manifestations *(87)*. LAs are detected using several types of phospholipid coagulation assays and are an indirect way of measuring aPLs, whereas aCL and anti-β2GP1 are detected directly using enzyme-linked immunosorbant assays. It is important to perform assays for all of these aPLs, as their concordance is no greater than 70% *(85)*.

Multiple studies have shown an association between aPLs and cognitive dysfunction in SLE *(88–92)*. In a study of the prospective association between neuropsychological functioning and antiphospholipid antibodies in SLE patients without NPSLE manifestation, significant differences between LA-positive and LA-negative groups (but not aCL-positive and aCL-negative groups) were observed in several domains *(92)*. LA-negative patients performed better than LA-positive patients in all cases. Antibody positivity was associated with impairment on cognitive tests assessing attention, concentration and visuospacial searching. These results persisted after controlling for the influence of depression.

3. MURINE NEUROBEHAVIORAL SLE

All of the inbred autoimmune strains develop a variety of clinical and serological features that are similar to disease manifestations seen in patients with SLE, RA, or Sjögrens syndrome *(93,94)*. Although the time-course and particular expression of disease varies between strains, these strains have been studied most widely as models for autoimmune renal disease associated with high-serum anti-DNA antibody levels and immune complex formation. Only recently have these strains been investigated more intensively for the development of neurological disease.

Lampert and Oldstone described immune complexes in the choroids plexus of (NZB × NZW) F1 mice *(95)*. Neuropathological changes in MRL-lpr and MRL/++ mice *(96)* and (NZB × NZW) F1 mice *(97)* have been described. Although brain inflammation in (NZB × NZW) F1 mice increased steadily with age, it was not consistently present until 14 mo *(97)*. Neither study systematically evaluated neurobehavioral dysfunction associated with these neuropathological findings.

(NZB × NZW) F1, MRL-lpr, and BXSB mice develop a variety of autoantibodies, including those that are reactive with brain antigens *(98–106)*. In addition, learning, behavioral, and sensorimotor abnormalities have been noted in all autoimmune strains. These increase with age and are associated with increases in serum levels of brain-reactive and other antibodies and the magnitude of brain inflammation over time *(107)*. Many of the less subtle features of neurological dysfunction in all of the autoimmune murine strains appear late in the disease course when many other abnormalities that could affect neurological functioning are present, including renal failure, hemolytic anemia, systemic vasculitis, arthritis, and high levels of many auto-antibodies.

For auto-antibodies to be causally associated with neurological dysfunction, they must first gain access through the BBB. This has been demonstrated using a sensitive immunohistochemical technique in MRL/lpr mice *(107)*. There was an age-related increase in the frequency of both CNS inflammation, composed predominantly of CD4+ cells, and perivascular leakage immunoglobulin-G around brain vessels of MRL/lpr mice. Both aCL and brain-reactive antibody-producing monocytes from whole-brain homogenates of individual 18-wk-old MRL/lpr mice have also been demonstrated *(108)*. Taken together, these data suggest that antibodies reactive to important brain antigens can gain access to the CNS. The BBB in these models appears to be disrupted early on and thus could have a key role in SLE-related neurologic dysfunction, especially if antibodies or other systemic mediators of inflammation (e.g., cytokines) are causally related to disease manifestations.

Several studies *(109–111)* raise the possibility that, in addition to any deleterious effects of autoantibodies, an even earlier immune-mediated event may be the trigger of some behavioral defects in MRL/lpr mice. MRL/lpr mice exhibit some signs of behavioral dysfunction at a young age, before CNS inflammation or even serologic auto-antibodies are present, in comparison to congenic MRL/++ controls *(109)*. This antedates other lupus-related manifestations and worsens with age. One interpretation of these results is that the onset of autoimmune disease in MRL/lpr mice is associated with alterations in emotional and motivational aspects of behavior *(110,111)*. This hypothesis has also been recently supported by findings in NZB autoimmune mice *(112)*.

One limitation to using autoimmune-prone mouse strains for studying nervous system dysfunction is that often there are other systemic disease manifestations that could affect nervous system function, as is the case in human lupus patients. Therefore, another approach has been to induce autoimmune disease in permissive animal strains or to accelerate disease in strains that have mild autoimmune disease that develops later in life. Some of these have been associated with nervous system manifestations *(113,114)*.

4. CLINICAL MANIFESTATIONS

NPSLE occurs in 50 to 91% of patients with SLE *(11,115–123)*, depending on the sampling procedures and diagnostic criteria used, and is a major source of morbidity and decreased quality of life. Given the estimated prevalence of SLE, this means that as many as 342,000 Americans with SLE have NPSLE manifestations. A cross-sectional, population-based study of people with definite SLE in Finland compared with matched controls using the ACR NPSLE case definitions and found that 91% of SLE patients had at least one NPSLE manifestation, for an odds ratio of 9.5 (CI 2.2–40.8) *(121)*. Cognitive dysfunction occurred most frequently and was found in 80% of patients (mild, 57%; moderate, 15%; severe, 9%). This experience is comparable to data from the initial study visit of subjects enrolled in SALUD, which comprised predominantly Hispanic SLE patients *(122)*.

The neurologic and psychiatric syndromes recognized by the ACR NPSLE case definitions are listed in Table 1. It is important to remember that patients with SLE are immune-compromised hosts and the diagnosis of infection should always be considered when evaluating NPSLE manifestations *(124)*. Focal neurological signs, severe headache, seizures, or psychosis with or without fever require the search for infection and active SLE involvement in other organ systems. Pertinent cultures, CSF analysis, electroencephalogram, and imaging studies should also be performed. If the patient is taking steroids or other immunosuppressive agents, a clear-cut diagnosis should be established to increase steroid dosage if symptoms are caused by SLE activity or quickly taper them and begin antibiotic treatment should the syndrome be owing to an associated infectious process.

Patients with SLE frequently report cognitive and memory problems *(87)*, and the study of SLE-related cognitive dysfunction has been the topic of recent research efforts. Many studies have documented significant cognitive deficits with traditional neuropsychological test batteries *(88–92,118–123)*. Most find cognitive deficits on tests measuring attention, mental flexibility, free recall memory, and speed of information processing, suggesting a subcortical cognitive syndrome, which sometimes reaches the dementia severity range *(90,92)*. Longitudinal studies using these tests have found that the rates of impairment in SLE vary greatly over time for individual patients and may not support the hypothesis of a steady decline into dementia *(89,119,123)*.

A major challenge for both SLE clinical care and research is to distinguish between SLE-mediated brain dysfunction, medication side effects, depression, and other co-morbid conditions (e.g., fibromyalgia) as the cause of NPSLE manifestations. Furthermore, it is not known whether some of these, for example, mild cognitive dysfunction, are harbingers of increased SLE-related morbidity, as has been reported for other more severe nervous system involvement *(125)*.

Table 1
Neuropsychiatric Syndromes Associated With Systemic Lupus Erythematosus

NPSLE Associated With the CNS
- Aseptic meningitis
- Cerebrovascular disease
    Stroke
    Transient ischemic attack
    Cerebral venous sinus thrombosis
- Cognitive disorders
    Delirium (acute confusional state)
    Dementia
    Mild cognitive impairment
- Demyelinating syndromes
- Headaches
    Tension headaches
    Migraine headaches
- Movement disorders (chorea)
- Psychiatric disorders
    Psychosis
    Mood disorders
    Anxiety disorders
- Seizure disorders
- Transverse myelopathy

NPSLE Associated with the PNS
- Autonomic neuropathy
- Myasthenia gravis
- Peripheral neuropathy
- Sensorineural hearing loss
    Sudden onset
    Progressive
- Cranial neuropathy

Modified from the American College of Rheumatology ad hoc committee *(11)*. NSPLE, neuropsychiatric systemic lupus erythematosus; CNS, central nervous system.

There have been no prospective treatment trials for any of the NPSLE manifestations. Thus, treatment remains empiric. Many NPSLE manifestations need to be treated symptomatically, sometimes in combination with immunomodulatory therapy. In Table 2, we suggest treatment options for some of the NPSLE manifestations based on empirical evidence and our own clinical experience.

5. SUMMARY

NPSLE manifestations are common and occur in up to 91% of SLE patients. It can be difficult to distinguish primary SLE-mediated nervous system manifestations from secondary effects of medications, infection, or other SLE-mediated non-nervous system involvement. It is always important to search diligently for infection as a potential cause of CNS manifestations in patients with SLE. The mechanisms of SLE-mediated nervous system manifestations are multiple and include abnormalities in cytokine production, soluble adhesion molecule upregulation, complement, immune complex deposition, and auto-antibodies. Some nervous system manifestations may also be caused by brain ischemia related to vasculopathic changes in brain blood vessels and a prothrombotic state owing to aPLs. Animal models have provided some insight into unique mechanisms for some NPSLE manifestations but remain sufficiently imperfect, which limits their

Table 2
Treatment of Various Manifestation of Neuropsychiatric Systemic Lupus Erythematosus

Neuropsychiatric manifestations	Symptomatic treatment[a]	Immune-modulating treatment
Aseptic meningitis	Withdrawal and avoidance of offending drugs	Corticosteroids
Autonomic neuropathy	Mineralocorticoids	Azathiaprine, corticosteroids
Cerebrovascular disease	Anticoagulation, antiplatelet agents	High-dose corticosteroids, cytotoxic immunosuppressives, or both
Cognitive dysfunction	None	Treatment of extraneural disease activity
Demyelinating syndromes		
Lupoid sclerosis	Physical therapy	None
Optic neuritis	None	Corticosteroids
		Pulse cytoxan (monthly)
		Plasmaphoresis
Transverse myelitis	None	High-dose corticosteroids
		Cytotoxic immunosuppressives
		Combination of both
Delirium	None	Treatment of extraneural disease activity
Headaches	Migraine treatments, antiplatelet agents	Treatment of extraneural disease activity
Idiopathic pseudotumor cerebri	Carbonic anhydrase inhibitors Repeated lumbar punctures Optic nerve decompression	High-dose corticosteroids
Movement disorders	Dopamine antagonists	High-dose corticosteroids, anticoagulation therapy, if disorder is related to antiphospholipid antibodies
Myasthenia gravis	Oral anticholinesterase inhibitors	Corticosteroids, plasmaphoresis, IVIG, thymectomy
Peripheral or cranial neuropathy	Tricyclic antidepressants, gabapentin	Corticosteroids
Psychiatric disorders		
Anxiety and depression	Psychotherapy Cognitive-behavior therapy Supportive-type therapy Biofeedback Antidepressive agents Anxiolytics	Effective treatment of extraneural disease activity
Psychosis	Antipsychotic agents	Withdraw corticosteroids if due to medication side effects, high-dose corticosteroids if due to SLE.
Seizures	Antiepileptic therapy	High-dose corticosteroids or effective treatment of extraneural disease activity

[a]Includes treatment of secondary causes, such as drugs, infections, and metabolic problems related to kidney and liver dysfunction and electrolyte disturbances. IVIG, intravenous immunoglobulin; SLE, systemic lupus erythematosus.

utility in evaluating potential therapy. Treatment options for presumed SLE-mediated NPSLE manifestations remain empirically based. Current treatment strategies include both symptomatic and immunomodulatory therapies.

REFERENCES

1. Uramoto KM, Michet CJ, Thumboo J Jr, et al. Trends in the incidence and mortality of systemic lupus erythematosus, 1950–1992. Arthritis Rheum 1999;42:46–50.
2. Fessel WJ. Systemic lupus erythematosus in the community: incidence, prevalence, outcome, and first symptoms; the high prevalence in black women. Arch Intern Med 1974;134:1027–1035.
3. Bresnihan B. Outcome and survival in systemic lupus erythematosus. Ann Rheum Dis 1989;48:443–445.
4. Rivest C, Lew R, Welsing P, et al. Association between clinical factors, socio-economic status, and organ damage in recent onset systemic lupus erythematosus. J Rheumatol 2000;27:680–684.
5. Alarcon GS, Friedman AW, Straaton KV, et al. Systemic lupus erythematosus in three ethnic groups: III. A comparison of characteristics early in the natural history of the LUMINA cohort. Lupus in minority populations: nature vs nurture. Lupus 1999;8:197–209.
6. Alarcon GS, Roseman JM, Bartolucci AA, et al. Systemic lupus erythematosus in three ethnic groups: II. Features predictive of disease activity early in its course. LUMINA Study Group. Lupus in minority populations: nature vs nurture. Arthritis Rheum 1998;41:1173–1180.
7. Urowitz MB, Bookman AAM, Koehler BE, Gordon DA, Smythe HA, Ogryzlo MA. The bimodal mortality pattern of systemic lupus erythematosus. Am J Med 1976;60:221–225.
8. Roman MJ, Shanker BA, Davis A, et. al. Prevalence and correlates of accelerated atherosclerosis in system lupus erythematosus. N Engl J Med 2003;349:2399–2406.
9. Asanuma Y, Oeser A, Shintani AK, et al. Premature coronary-artery atherosclerosis in systemic lupus erythematosus. N Engl J Med 2003;349:2407–2415.
10. Kaposi MK. Neue Beitrage zur Kenntniss des. Lupus erythematosus. Arch Dermatol Syph 1872;4:36–78.
11. American College of Rheumatology (ACR) ad hoc committee on neuropsychiatric lupus. The American College of Rheumatology nomenclature and case definitions for neuropsychiatric lupus syndrome. Arthritis Rheumatism 1999;42:599–608.
12. Drenkard C, Villa AR, Reyes E, et al. Vasculitis in systemic lupus erythematosus. Lupus 1997;6:235–242.
13. Emlen W, Neibur J, Kadera R. Accelerated in vitro apoptosis of lymphocytes from patients with systemic lupus erythematosus. J Immunol 1994;152:3685–92.
14. Chan TM, Yu PM, Tsang KL, Cheng IK. Endothelial cell binding by human polyclonal anti-DNA antibodies: relationship to disease activity and endothelial functional alterations. Clin Exp Immunol 1995;100:506–513.
15. Hahn BH. Antibodies to DNA. N Engl J M 1998;338:1359–68.
16. Hanly JG. Evaluation of patients with CNS involvement in SLE. Baillieres Clinical Rheumatology. 1998; 12(3):415–31.
17. Hanly JG, Walsh NMG, Sangalang V. Brain pathology in systemic lupus erythematosus. J Rheumatol 1992;19: 732–741.
18. Sibbitt WL, Sibbitt RR, Brooks WM. Neuroimaging in neuropsychiatric systemic lupus erythematosus. Arthritis Rheum 1999;42:2026–2038.
19. Belmont HM, Abramson SB, Lie JT. Pathology and pathogenesis of vascular injury in systemic lupus erythematosus: interactions of inflammatory cells and activated endothelium. Arthritis Rheum 1996;39:9–22.
20. Karassa F, Ioannidis JP, Boki K, et al. Predictors of clinical outcome and radiologic progression in patients with neuropsychiatric manifestations of systemic lupus erythematosus. Am J Med 2000;109:628–634.
21. Gonzalez-Crespo MR, Blanco FJ, Ramos A, et al. Magnetic resonance of the brain in systemic lupus erythematosus. Br J Rheumatol 1995;34:1055–1060.
22. Isshi K, Hirihata S. Association of anti-ribosomal P protein antibodies with neuropsychiatric systemic lupus erythematosus. Arthritis Rheum 1996;39:1483–1490.
23. Isshi K, Hirohata S. Differential roles of the anti-ribosomal P antibody and antineuronal antibody in the pathogenesis of central nervous system involvement in systemic lupus erythematosus. Arthritis Rheum 1998;41:1819–27.
24. Alter A, Duddy M, Hebert S, et al. Determinants of human B cell migration across brain endothelial cells. J Immunol 2003;170:4497–4505.
25. Chan A, Seguin R, Magnus T, et al. Phagocytosis of apoptotic inflammatory cells by microglia and its therapeutic implications: termination of central nervous system autoimmune inflammation and modulation by IFN-beta. Glia 2003;43:231–242.
26. Seguin R, Biernacki K, Prat A, et al. Differential effects of Th1 and Th2 lymphocyte supernatants on human microglia. Glia 2003;42:36–45.
27. Biernacki K, Prat A, Blain M, Antel JP. Regulation of Th1 and Th2 lymphocyte migration by human adult brain endothelial cells. J Neuropathol Exp Neurol 2001;60:1127–1136.
28. Kelley VR, Wuthrich RP. Cytokines in the pathogenesis of systemic lupus erythematosus. Sem Nephrol 1999;19:57–66.
29. Kirou KA, Crow MK. New pieces to the SLE cytokine puzzle. Clin Immunol 1999;91:1–5.
30. Jara LJ, Irigoyen L, Ortiz MJ, Zazueta B, Bravo G, Espinoza LR. Prolactin and interleukin 6 in neuropsychiatric lupus erythematosus. Clin Rheumatol 1998;17:110–114.

31. Alcocer-Varela J, Aleman-Hoey D, Alarcon-Segovia D. Interleukin-1 and interleukin-6 activities are increased in the cerebrospinal fluid of patients with CNS lupus erythematosus and correlate with local late T-cell activation markers. Lupus 1992;1:111–7.

32. Tesar V, Jirsa M, Masek Z, et al. Soluble cytokinin receptors in renal vasculitis and lupus nephritis. Cas Lek Cesk 1998;137:271–275.

33. Waszczykowska E, Robak E, Wozniacka A, Narbutt J, Torzecka JD, Sysa-Jedrzejowska A. Estimation of SLE activity based on the serum level of chosen cytokines and superoxide radical generation. Mediators Inflamm 1999;8: 93–100.

34. Viedt C, Hansch GM, Brandes RP, Kubler W, Kreuzer J. The terminal complement complex C5b-9 stimulates inter-leukin-6 production in human smooth muscle cells through activation of transcription factors NF-κB and AP-1. Faseb J. 2000;14:2370–2372.

35. Shikano M, Sobajima H, Yoshikawa H, et al. Usefulness of a highly sensitive urinary and serum IL-6 assay in patients with diabetic nephropathy. Nephron 2000;85:81–85.

36. Kado S, Nagase T, Nagata N. Circulating levels of interleukin-6, its soluble receptor and interleukin-6/interleukin-6 receptor complexes in patients with type 2 diabetes mellitus. Acta Diabetol 1999;36:67–72.

37. van Aken BE, Jansen J, van Deventer SJ, Reitsma PH. Elevated levels of homocysteine increase IL-6 production in monocytic Mono Mac 6 cells. Blood Coagul Fibrinolysis 2000;11:159–164.

38. Yudkin JS, Kumari M, Humphries SE, Mohamed-Ali V. Inflammation, obesity, stress and coronary heart disease: is interleukin-6 the link? Atherosclerosis 2000;148:209–214.

39. Young DG, Skibinski G, Mason JI, James K. The influence of age and gender on serum dehydroepiandrosterone sulphate (DHEA-S), IL-6, IL-6 soluble receptor (IL-6 sR) and transforming growth factor beta 1 (TGF-beta1) levels in normal healthy blood donors. Clin Exp Immunol 1999;117:476–481.

40. Straub RH, Konecna L, Hrach S, et al. Serum dehydroepiandrosterone (DHEA) and DHEA sulfate are negatively correlated with serum interleukin-6 (IL-6), and DHEA inhibits IL-6 secretion from mononuclear cells in man in vitro: possible link between endocrinosenescence and immunosenescence. J Clin Endocrinol Metab 1998;83: 2012–2017.

41. Kozora E, Laudenslager M, Lemieux A, West SG. Inflammatory and hormonal measures predict neuropsychological functioning in systemic lupus erythematosus and rheumatoid arthritis patients. J Int Neuropsychol Soc 2001;7: 745–754.

42. Hickey WF. T-lymphocyte entry into the central nervous system. J Neurosci Res 1991;28:254–260.

43. Zabry Z, Waldschmidt MM, Hendrickson D, et al. Adhesion molecules on murine brain microvascular endothelial cells: expression and regulation of ICAM-1 and Lgp 55. J Neuroimmunol 1992;36:1–11.

44. Belmont HM, Buyon J, Giorno R, Abramson S. Upregulation of endothelial cell adhesion molecules characterized disease activity in systemic lupus erythematosus. Arthritis Rheum 1994;37:376–383.

45. Janssen BA, Luqmani RA, Gordon C, et al. Correlation of blood levels of soluble vascular cell adhesion molecule-1 with disease activity in systemic lupus erythematosus and vasculitis. Br J Rheumatol 1994;33:1112–1116.

46. Egerer K, Feist E, Rohr U, Pruss A, Burmester GR, Dörner T. Increased serum soluble CD14, ICAM-1 and E-selectin correlate with disease activity and prognosis in systemic lupus erythematosus. Lupus 2000;9:614–621.

47. Barcellini W, Rizzardi GP, Borghi MO, et al. In vitro type-1 and type-2 cytokine production in systemic lupus erythematosus: lack of relationship with clinical disease activity. Lupus 1996;5:139–145.

48. Zaccagni H, Fried J, Cornell J, Padilla P, Brey RL. Soluble adhesion molecule levels, neuropsychiatric lupus and lupus-related damage. Front Biosci 2004,9:1654–1659.

49. Sfikakis PP, Charalambopoulos D, Vayoipoulos G, Oglesby RPS, Tsokos GC. Increased levels of intercellular adhe-sion molecule-1 in the serum of patients with SLE. Clin Exp Rheumatol 1994;12:5–9.

50. Matsuda J, Gohchi K, Gotoh M, Tsukamoto M, Saitoh N. Circulation intercellular adhesion molecule-1 and soluble interleukin 2-receptor in patients with systemic lupus erythematosus. Eur J Haematol 1994;52:302–303.

51. Wellicome SM, Kapahi P, Mason JC, Lebranchu Y, Yarwood H, Haskard DO. Detection of a circulating form of vas-cular cell adhesion molecule-1: raised levels in rheumatoid arthritis and systemic lupus erythematosus. Clin Exp Immunol 1993;92:412–418.

52. Spronk PE, Bootsma H, Huitema MG, et al. Levels of soluble VCAM-1, ICAM-1 and E-selectin during disease exacerbations in patients with SLE. Clin Exp Immunol 1994;97:439–444.

53. Machold KP, Kiener HP, Graninger W, et al. Soluble ICAM-1 in patients with rheumatoid arthritis and SLE. Clin Immunol Immunopathol 1993;68:74–78.

54. Baraczka K, Pozsonyi T, Szongoth M, et al. A study of increased levels of soluble vascular cell adhesion molecule-1 in the cerebrospinal fluid of patients with multiple sclerosis and systemic lupus erythematosus. Acta Neurol. Scand 1999;99:95–99.

55. Del Papa N, Guidali L, Sala A, et al. Endothelial cells as target for antiphospholipid antibodies. Arthritis Rheum 1997;40:551–561.

56. Pierangeli SS, Espinola RG, Liu X, Harris EN. Thrombogenic effects of antiphospholipid antibodies are mediated by intercellular cell adhesion molecule-1, vascular cell adhesion molecule-1, and P-selectin. Circ Res 2001;88: 245–50.

57. Kaplanski G, Cacoub P, Farnarier C, et al. Increased soluble vascular cell adhesion molecule-1 concentrations in patients with primary or systemic lupus erythematosus-related antiphospholipid syndrome: correlations with the severity of thrombosis. Arthritis Rheum 2000;43:55–60.

58. Reichlin M. Ribosomal P antibodies and CNS Lupus. Lupus 2003;12:916–918.

59. Nojima Y, Minota S, Yamada A, Aosuka S, Yokohari R. Correlation of antibodies to ribosomal P protein with psychosis in patients with systemic lupus erythematosus. J Rheum Dis 1992;51:1053–1055.

60. Arnett FC, Reveille JD, Moutsopoulos HM, Georgescu L, Elkon KB. Ribosomal P autoantibodies in systemic lupus eruthematosus. Arthritis Rheum 1996;39:1833–1839.

61. Press J, Palayew K, Laxer RM, et al. Antiribosomal P antibodies in pediatric patients with systemic lupus erythematosus and psychosis. Arthritis Rheum 1996;39:671–676.

62. Isshi K, Hirohata S. Association of anti-ribosomal P protein antibodies with neuropsychiatric systemic lupus erythematosus. Arthritis Rheum 1996;39:1483–1490.

63. Bonfa E, Golombek SJ, Kaufman LD, et al. Association between lupus psychosis and anti-ribosomal P protein antibodies. N Engl J Med 1987;317:265–271.

64. Schneebaum AB, Singleton JD, West SG, et al. Associations of psychiatric manifestations with antibodies to ribosomal P proteins in systemic lupus erythematosus. Am J Med 1991;90:54–62.

65. Van Dam A, Nossent H, de Jong J, et al. Diagnostic value of antibodies against ribisimal phosphoproteins: a cross sectional and longitudinal study. J Rheumatol 1991;18:1026–1034.

66. Isenberg DA. Antiribosomal P protein antibodies in systemic lupus erythematosus: a reappraisal. Arthritis Rheum 1994;37:307–315.

67. Isshi K, Hirohata S. Differential roles of the anti-ribosmal P antibody and anti-neuronal antibody in the pathogenesis of central nervous system involvement in systemic lupus erythematosus. Arthritis Rheum 1998;41:1819–1827

68. Koren E, Reichlin MW, Koscec M, Fugate RD, Reichlin M. Autoantibodies to the ribosomal P proteins react with a plasma membrane related target on human cells. J Clin Invest 1992;89:1236–1241.

69. Koscec M, Koren E, Reichlin MW, et al. Autoantibodies to the ribosomal P proteins penetrate into live hepatocytes and cause cellular dysfunction in culture. J Immunol 1997;159:2033–2041.

70. DeGiorgio LA, Konstantinov KN, Lee SC, Hardin JA, Volpe BT, Diamond B. A sub-set of lupus anti-DNA antibodies cross-reacts with the NR2 glutamate receptor in systemic lupus erythematosus. Nature Medicine 2001;7: 1189–1193.

71. Gaynor B, Putterman C, Valadon P, Spatz L, Scharff MD, Diamond B. Peptide inhibition of glomerular deposition of a pathogenic anti-DNA antibody: implications for therapy. Proc Natl Acad Sci USA 1997;94:1955–1960.

72. Standaert DG, Testa CM, Penney JB, Young AB. Organization of *N*-methyl-D-aspartate glutamate receptor gene expression in the basal ganglia of the rat. J Comp Neurol 1994;343:1–16.

73. Scherzer CR, Landwehrmeyer GB, Kerner JA, et al. Expression of *N*-methyl-1-D-aspartate receptor subunit mRNAs in the human brain: hippocampus and cortex. J. Comp. Neurol 1998;390:75–90.

74. Counihan TJ, Landwehrmeyer GB, Standaert DG, et al. Expression of *N*-methyl-D-aspartate receptor subunit mRNAs in the human brain: striatum and globus pallidus. J Comp Neurol 1998;390:63–74.

75. Kuppenbender KD, Standaert DG, Feuerstein TJ, Penney JB Jr, Young AB, Landwehrmeyer GB. Expression of NMDA receptor subunit mRNAs in neurochemically identified projection and interneurons in the human striatum. J Comp Neurol 2000;419:407–421.

76. Lu J, Goula D, Sousa N, Almeida OF. Ionotropic and metabotropic glutamate receptor mediation of glucocorticoid-induced apoptosis in hippocampal cells and the neuroprotective role of synaptic *N*-methyl-D-aspartate receptors. Neuroscience 2003;121:123–31.

77. Ozawa S, Kamiya H, Tsuzuki K. Glutamate receptors in the mammalian central nervous system. Prog Neurobiol 1998;54:581–618.

78. Sakimura K, Kutsuwada T, Ito I, et al. Reduced hippocampal LTP and spatial learning in mice lacking NMDA receptor, 1 subunit. Nature 1995;373:151–155.

79. Morris RG, Anderson E, Lynch GS, Baudry M. Selective impairment of learning and blockade of long-term potentiation by an *N*-methyl-D-aspartate receptor antagonist, AP5. Nature 1986;319:774–776.

80. Choi DW, Rothman SM. The role of glutamate neurotoxicity in hypoxicischemic neuronal death. Annu Rev Neurosci 1990;13:171–182.

81. Mattson MP, LaFerla FM, Chan SL, Leissring MA, Shepel PN, Geiger JD. Calcium signaling in the ER: its role in neuronal plasticity and neurodegenerative disorders. Trends Neurosci 2000;23:222–229.

82. Akbarian S, Sucher NJ, Bradley D, et al. Selective alterations in gene expression for NMDA receptor subunits in prefrontal cortex of schizophrenics. J Neurosci 1996;16:19–30.

83. Volpe BT. Delayed neuronal degeneration results from endogenous glutamate excess: Possible role in "Neuro-SLE". Ann N Y Acad Sci 1997;280:614–620.

84. Omdal R, Brokstad K, Waterloo K, Koldingsnes W, Jonsson R, Mellgren SI. Anti-DNA antibodies crossreacting with the NR2 glutamate receptor are associated with psychological and cognitive disturbances in human SLE. Arthritis Rheum 2003;48:404.

85. Roubey RA. Immunology of the antiphospholipid antibody syndrome. Arthritis Rheum 1996;39:1444–1454.

86. Holers VM, Girardi G, Mo L, et al. Complement C3 activation is required for antiphospholipid antibody-induced fetal loss. J Exp Med 2002;195:211–220.

87. Brey RL, Escalante A. Neurological manifestations of antiphospholipid antibody syndrome. Lupus 1998;7 (Suppl 2):S67–74.

88. Menon S, Jameson-Shortall E, Newman SP, Hall-Craggs MR, Chinn R, Isenberg DA. A longitudinal study of anticardiolipin antibody levels and cognitive functioning in systemic lupus erythematosus. Arthritis Rheum 1999;42:735–741.

89. Hanly JG, Hong C, Smith S, Fisk JD. A prospective analysis of cognitive function and anticardiolipin antibodies in systemic lupus erythematosus. Arthritis Rheum 1999;42:728–734.

90. Denburg SD, Carbotte RM, Ginsberg JS, Denburg JA. The relationship of antiphospholipid antibodies to cognitive function in patients with systemic lupus erythematosus. J Int Neuropsychol Soc 1997;3:377–386.

91. Lai NS, Lan JL. Evaluation of cerebrospinal anticardiolipin antibodies in lupus patients with neuropsychiatric manifestations. Lupus 2000;9:353–357.

92. Leritz E, Brandt J, Minor M, Reis-Jensen F, Petri M. Neuropsychological functioning and its relationship to antiphospholipid antibodies in patients with systemic lupus erythematosus. J Clin Exp Neuropsych 2002;24:527–533.

93. Theofilopoulos AN. Murine models of lupus. In: Lahita RG. Systemic Lupus Erythematosus. New York, Churchill Livingstone, 1992;121–194.

94. Klinman DM, Steinberg AD. Inquiry into murine and human lupus. Immunol Rev 1995;144:157–193.

95. Lampert P, Oldstone MB. Host immunoglobulin IgG and complement deposits in the choroids plexus during spontaneous immune complex disease. Science 1973;180:408–410.

96. Alexander EL, Murphy ED, Roths JB, Alexander GE. Congenic autoimmune murine models of central nervous system disease in connective tissue disorders. Ann Neurol 1983;14:242–248.

97. Rudick RA, Eskin TA. Neuropathological features of a lupus-like disorder in autoimmune mice. Ann Neurol 1983;14:325–332.

98. Hoffman SA, Arbogast DN, Ford PM, Shucard DW, Harbeck RJ. Brain-reactive autoantibody levels in the sera of aging autoimmune mice. Clin Exp Immunol 1987;70:74–83.

99. Nandy K, Lal H, Bennett M, Bennett D. Correlation between a learning disorder and elevated brain-reactive antibodies in aged C57BL/6 and young NZB mice. Life Sci 1983;33:1499–1503.

100. Khin NA, Hoffman ST. Brain reactive monoclonal auto-antibodies: production and characterization. J Neuroimmunol 1993;44:137–148.

101. Hess DC, Taormina M, Thompson J, et al. Cognitive and neurologic deficits in the MRL/lpr mouse: a clinicopathologic study. J Rheumatol 1993;20:610–617.

102. Sakic B, Szechtman H, Stead R, Denburg JA. Joint pathology and behavioral performance in autoimmune MRL-lpr mice. Physiol Behav 1996;60:901–905.

103. Schrott LM, Morrison L, Wimer R, Wimer C, Behan PO, Denenberg VH. Autoimmunity and avoidance learning in NXRF recombinant inbred strains. Brain Behav Immun 1994;8:100–110.

104. Sakic B, Szechtman H, Denburg SD, Carbotte RM, Denburg JA. Brain-reactive antibodies and behavior of autoimmune MRL-lpr mice. Physiol Behav 1993;54:1025–1029.

105. Shoenfeld Y, Nahum A, Korczyn AD, et al. Neuronal-binding antibodies from patients with antiphospholipid syndrome induced cognitive deficits following intrathecal passive transfer. Lupus 2003;12:436–442.

106. Keir AB. Clinical neurology and brain histopathology I NZB/NZW F1 lupus mice. J Comparative Pathol 1990; 102:165–177.

107. Vogelweid CM, Hohnson GC, Besch-Williford CL, Basler J, Walker SE. Inflammatory central nervous system disease in lupus-prone MRL/lpr mice: comparative histologic and immunohistochemical findings. J Neuroimmunol 1991;35:89–97.

108. Brey RL, Cote S, Teale JM. Neurological dysfunction and autoantibody producing B cells from brain in a lupus-prone mouse strain. Neurology 1993;43:420.

109. Sakic B, Szechtman H, Stead R, Denburg JA. Joint pathology and behavioral performance in autoimmune MRL-lpr mice. Physiol Behav 1996;60:901–905.

110. Sakic B, Szechtman H, Talangbayan H, Denburg SD, Carbotte RM, Denburg JA. Disturbed emotionality in autoimmune MRL-lpr mice. Physiol Behav 1994;56:609–617.

111. Sakic B, Denburg JA, Denburg SA, Szechtman H. Blunted sensitivity to sucrose reward in autoimmune MRL-lpr mice: A curve-shift study. Brain Res Bull 1996;41:305–311.

112. Crnic LS, Schrott LM. Increased anxiety behaviors in autoimmune mice. Behav Neurosci 1996;110:492–502.

113. Ziporen L, Eilam D, Goldberg I, et al. Neurological dysfunctions associated with antiphospholipid antibodies: animal model. Lupus 1996;5:533.

114. Aron AL, Cuellar ML, Brey RL, Gharavi AE, Shoenfeld Y. Early onset of autoimmunity in MRL/++ mice following immunization with Beta-2-glycoprotein 1. Clin Exp Rheum Immunol 1995;101:78–81.

115. Kaell AT, Shetty M, Lee BCP, Lockshin MD. The diversity of neurologic events in systemic lupus erythematosus. Arch Neurol 1986;43:273–276.

116. McNicholl J, Glynn D, Mongey A, Hutchinson M, Bresnihan B. A prospective study of neurophysiologic, neurologic and immunologic abnormalities in systemic lupus erythematosus. J Rheumatol 1994;21:1061–1066.

117. West SG, Emlen W, Wener MH, Kotzin BL. Neuropsychiatric lupus erythematosus: a 10-year prospective study on the value of diagnostic tests. Am J Med 1995;99:153–163.

118. Carbotte RM, Denburg SD, Denburg JA. Cognitive dysfunction in systemic lupus erythematosus is independent of active disease. J. Rheumatol 1995;22:863–867.

119. Hay EM, Huddy A, Black D, et al. A prospective study of psychiatric disorder and cognitive impairment in systemic lupus erythematosus. Ann Rheum Dis 1994;53:298–303.

120. Ginsburg KS, Wright EA, Larson MG, et al. A controlled study of the prevalence of cognitive dysfunction in randomly selected patients with systemic lupus erythematosus. Arthritis Rheum 1992;35:776–782.

121. Ainiala H, Loukkola J, Peltola J, Korpela M, Hietaharju A. The prevalence of neuropsychiatric syndromes in systemic lupus erythematosus. Neurology 2001;57:496–499.

122. Brey RL, Holliday SL, Saklad AR, et al. Neuropsychiatric syndromes in SLE: prevalence using standardized definitions in the San Antonio Study of Neuropsychiatric Disease Cohort. Neurology 2002;58:1214–1220.

123. Carlomagno S, Migliaresi S, Ambroxone L, Sannino M, Sanges G, Di Ioro G. Cognitive impairment in systemic lupus erythematosus: a follow up study. J Neurol 2000;247:273–279.

124. Iliopoulos AG, Tsokos GC. Immunopathogenesis and spectrum of infections in systemic lupus erythematosus. Semin Arthritis Rheum 1996;25:318–36.

125. Rivest C, Lew R, Welsing P, et al. Association between clinical factors, socio-economic status, and organ damage in recent onset systemic lupus erythematosus. j Rheumatol 2000;27:680–684.

CME QUESTIONS

1. Which of the following are part of the diagnostic criteria for systemic lupus erythematosus, according to the American College of Rheumatology?
   A. Seizures and psychosis
   B. Seizures and stroke
   C. Psychosis and stroke
   D. Stroke and cognitive dysfunction

2. Which of the following is the most common histopathologic finding in the brain of patients with neuropsychiatric lupus manifestations?
   A. Vasculitis
   B. Vasculopathy
   C. Abscess
   D. Thrombosis

3. Which of the following is *not* thought to be a potential disease mechanism in neuropsychiatric lupus?
   A. Cytokine production
   B. Adhesion molecule upregulation
   C. Autoantibodies
   D. β-Amyloid production

4. Which of the following is the most common neuropsychiatric lupus manifestation, according to studies published since the 1999 American College of Rheumatology case definitions have been established?
   A. Seizures
   B. Psychosis
   C. Cognitive dysfunction
   D. Depression

16

Gene Expression in HIV-Associated Dementia

Paul Shapshak, Alireza Minagar, Elda M. Duran, Fabiana Ziegler, Wade Davis, Raman Seth, and Toni Kazic

1. INTRODUCTION

In past decades, the prime methods used for the study of genes and their respective products were Northern blots, Western blots, *in situ* hybridization, and immunocytochemistry. The applicability of these methods was restricted to the study of single genes or a few simultaneously *(1,2)*.

With the development of gene expression and bioinformatics technology, we can finally easily identify crucial interactions between viral proteins and the cellular proteins responsible for the establishment and perpetuation of the human immunodeficiency virus (HIV) life cycle, particularly in the brain. DNA and protein microarrays, gene chips, or biochips hold great promise for discovery of novel molecular and cellular mechanisms of neurological disease because they allow the simultaneous rapid and parallel assessment of thousands of genes *(2,3)*. Gene expression uses microscopic amounts of DNA, oligonucleotide, or antibody probes arranged in very small grid-like organization. The instruments that handle samples (including automated robotics) read the reporter molecule intensities (scanning). In addition, methods to analyze the data (bioinformatics and statistics) are in progress. These technologies are revolutionizing gene expression analysis by providing hybridization-based RNA and protein monitoring, polymorphism detection, and phenotyping on a genomic scale. Microarray technology is being extensively developed and applied to study gene expression in several neurological and psychiatric disorders *(2,4)*. We review gene expression studies of HIV-1 associated dementia (HAD), as well as the need for improved bioinformatics methods.

2. HIV-ASSOCIATED DEMENTIA

The determination of the basic mechanisms of the pathogenesis of HAD remains unsolved. HIV-1 infection is the cause of HAD, which presents with progressive encephalopathy. HAD also presents in the absence of detectable primary effects of other pathogenic agents or conditions, including opportunistic infections and lymphoma, but with HIV-related impairment of normal cerebral function. HAD affects 20 to 50% of patients with acquired immunodeficiency syndrome (AIDS) who are not taking therapy and 5 to 10% of patients with AIDS are taking highly active antiretroviral therapy *(5–8)*.

Torres-Munoz et al. *(9)* demonstrated cytopathic effects of HIV-1 on neurons using laser capture microdissected neurons in the hippocampus consistent with latent infection by HIV-1. Thus, neuronal

From: *Current Clinical Neurology: Inflammatory Disorders of the Nervous System:*
Pathogenesis, Immunology, and Clinical Management
Edited by: A. Minagar and J. S. Alexander © Humana Press Inc., Totowa, NJ

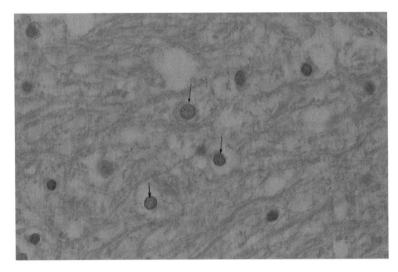

Fig. 1. Formalin-fixed paraffin-embedded (FFPE) section from white matter associated with Globus Pallidus from male Caucasian patient, age 50 yr, HIV-1 seropositive, homosexual, without HIV-associated dementia (HAD), and without HIV encephalitis (HIVE). Five micron thickness, original magnification × 220, Hematoxylin and Eosin. Arrows: oligodendrocytes.

infection may contribute to pathology because of the vulnerability of neurons to HIV-1 infection. Neuronal HIV infection could contribute to neuronal injury and death and may be mediated through cytokine and chemokine production *(10)*.

The basic mechanisms of pathogenesis involving brain cells remain largely unknown. Perhaps events external to the central nervous system (CNS) that activate moncytes initiate a priming process that leads to HAD *(11)*. Certainly, there is a compartmentalization of HIV evolution in the brain *(7,12,13)*, and HIV recombination occurs frequently in the brain *(14)*. Brain tissue is an HIV infection reservoir and compartment. Furthermore, data suggests that HIV-1-associated neurological disease is related to the level of viral infection in activated macrophages in humans and in a mouse model *(15–17)*. As examples of studies in the human brain, we show recently stained brain tissue from subjects who were HIV-1 infected (Figs. 1–3).

Astrocytes may have a major role in the pathogenesis of HAD and recently were studied in the context of AIDS by Galey et al *(18)*. Microarray analysis and ribonuclease protection assays were used following HIV infection or treatment with gp120. 1,153 oligonucleotides were used on an immune-based array and found 108 genes (53 upregulated, 55 downregulated) changed by gp120 treatment and 82 genes (32 upregulated, 50 downregulated) changed by HIV infection. Of the 1153 oligonucleotides on the neurobased array, 58 genes (25 upregulated, 33 downregulated) were altered by gp120 treatment and 47 genes (17 upregulated, 30 downregulated) were altered by HIV infection.

Gp120 treatment downregulated tumor necrosis factor (TNF)-receptor-associated factor 3, and HIV-1 infection downregulated expression of TNF-ligand and interleukin (IL)-1b but induced expression of IL-15. The decreased importance for the TNF system in HIV infection reported by Galey et al. *(18)* is consistent with results in brains of patients with AIDS *(19,20)*. Progeny HIV-1 virions affect neuronal signal transduction and apoptosis through the CXCR4 receptor, independent of CD4 binding *(21)*. Apoptosis via BCL2-associated X protein (BAX) expression is a well-described pathway. Intracellular HIV protein expression might promote apoptosis via transcription of BAX, and extracellular treatment of astrocytes with gp120 downregulates BAX in astrocytes *(18)*. Table 1 shows a summary selection of genes from Gayley et al. *(18)*.

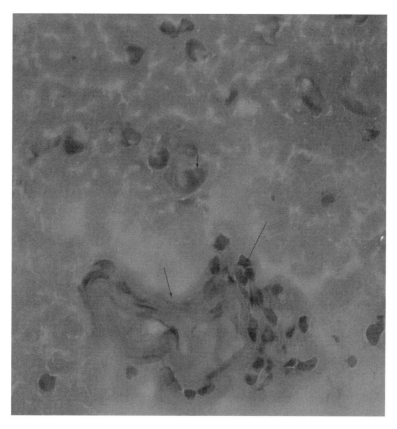

Fig. 2. Cryosection from Globus Pallidus from HIV-1 seropositive patient with HIV-associated dementia and HIV encephalitis, age 47 yr. Perivascular inflammation and neurons are shown. Five micron thickness, original magnification × 220, Hematoxylin and Eosin. Small arrow: neuron; medium arrow: blood vessel; large arrow: macrophage/monocyte.

HIV-1-host interaction studies commenced recently using microarrays. Geiss et al. *(22)* performed early HIV-1 infection-related quantitative analyses of host gene expression during HIV-1 infection of the CEM-CCRF CD4[+] T-cell line. They identified 20 cellular mRNAs using 1506 cDNAs. Pathways for T-cell receptor-mediated signaling, subcellular trafficking, transcriptional regulation, host-cell defense, facilitation of the viral life cycle, and a variety of cellular metabolic pathways were pinpointed, based on differential gene expression. Table 2 shows a summary selection of genes from the Geiss et al. study *(22)*.

At the Fox laboratory, HIV-related hypotheses were developed and tested by Roberts *(23)* using an SIVmac182 and Rhesus macaque animal model to characterize brain gene expression 70 to 110 d postinfection. CNS abnormalities and neuropathology occurred in all the infected monkeys. Sophisticated methods of immunohistochemistry and *in situ* hybridization in monkey brain sections evaluated genes that changed in expression using human Affymetrix arrays and genes *(23)*. A selection of genes in the Roberts et al. *(23)* study is summarized in Table 3. One gene is exemplified in each category (out of 98 genes).

In a related study in the brain of macaques with simian HIV (SHIV)-encephalitis, Sui et al. *(24)* performed microarray analysis of chemokine and cytokine genes in reference to HIV encephalitis, including macrophage/microglia activation, astrocytosis, neuronal dysfunction, and death. They produced gene-expression profiles in SHIV 89.6P-infected macaques. Of 277 genes

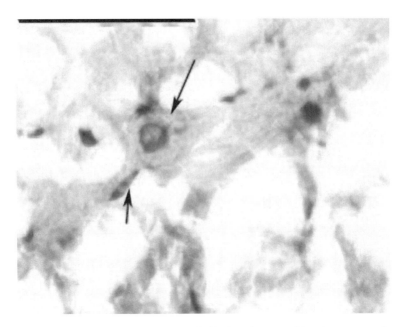

Fig. 3. Cryosection of Globus Pallidus from female black patient, age 64 yr, intravenous drug user, HIV-1 seropositive, with HIV-associated dementia, and without HIV encephalitis. Large arrow: neuron; small arrow: macrophage/microglia. Five μ thickness, original magnification × 300, Nissl stain. The neuron cytoplasm is less visible because the section was stained for only 60 s. The section was then used for laser capture microdissection.

screened in the encephalitic brains, several proinflammatory genes were upregulated: monocyte chemoattractant protein-1, interferon-inducible peptide IP-10, and IL-4, which are genes that promote virus replication, macrophage infiltration, and activation. Nonetheless, there was downregulation of neurotrophic function-related genes, including brain-derived neurotrophic factor, although apoptosis genes were up- or downregulated. Gene expression in the SHIV-macaque model results in dystrophic changes in neurons and enhanced virus replication in brain macrophages, according to Sui et al. A selection of results from Sui et al. is shown in Table 4 *(24)*.

Another animal study also produced information in regard to neuroAIDS using peripheral blood mononuclear cells (PBMNCs) from Rhesus macaques infected with SIVmac251.25. Gene expression in PBMNCs was analyzed in infected animals exhibiting rapid, typical, or slow rates of disease progression. They used fold change, Z score, and Self Organizing Map (SOM) data analysis. Among the three progession groups, gene expression showed different patterns involving fold change, variation between groups, and temporal coordination of gene expression. Immune response and cytoskeleton genes were elevated in the typically vs rapidly progressing group. Rapid course of disease was associated with some increase in but a lack of coordination of gene expression. Rapid and typical groups showed minimal differences in categories and numbers of genes expressed; however, differences between the rapid and slow groups were more distinct. Typical group gene expression demonstrated the largest numbers of gene expression changes in expression and some coordination of their expression, although typical and slow groups showed less distinct differences than the rapid and slow groups did. The slow group showed the lowest degree of gene-expression change and the maximum coordinated gene expression. Possibly, the authors conclude, the changes are indicative of gene expression specific for each type of disease progression and also for gene expression specific to a drive for survival of the postinfection host.

Table 1
Astrocyte Culture Gene Expression Changes[a]

Accession number	Gene ID	p value	Z ratio
Upregulated by gp120 treatment			
AA284528	Protease, Serine, 2 (Trypsin 2)	2.22E-16	2.14
NM_001028	Ribosomal protein S25	5.29E-05	1.91
NM_007315	STAT 1	4.83 E-04	1.56
NM_000484	APP	9.7E-4	1.56
Upregulated by HIV-1 infection			
NM_004324	BAX	1.04E-11	2.30
NM_002545	Opioid binding protein	0	3.67
NM_001225	Caspase 4	1.31E-13	2.83
NM000416	IFNGR1	5.54E-4	2.03
Downregulated by gp120 treatment			
NM_004324	BAX	0	−1.73
NM_002545	Opioid-binding protein	0	−3.12
AA069414	GFAP	0	−3.09
R98851	Membrane metalloendopeptidase (enkephalinase)	0	−2.93
NM_003300	TRAF3	0	−3.75
Downregulated by HIV-1 infection			
AA284528	Protease, Serine, 2 (Trypsin 2)	0	−2.79
NM_001028	Ribosomal protein S25	3.2E-4	−3.07
AA069414	GFAP	0	−6.73
R98851	Membrane metalloendopeptidase (enkephalinase)	2.05E-5	−2.00
NM_000576	IL-1b	4.69E-5	−1.94
NM_003807	TNF (ligand) superfamily, member 14	1.24E-4	−1.92

STAT 1, signal transducer and activator of transcription 1; APP, amyloid β (A4) precursor protein; BAX, BCL2-associated X protein; IFNGR1, interferon-γ receptor 1; GFAP, glial fibrillary acidic protein; TRAF3, TNF receptor-associated factor 3.

[a]Methods for p-value and Z-ratio calculations are described in Galey et al. *(18)*.

A preliminary study comparing brains with AIDS and normal brains was done to test hypotheses related to known genes involved in neuroAIDS and for gene discovery for related genes, as well as for unanticipated genes. These are important issues in the neuroAIDS field because hypothesis-driven research is considered its cornerstone. Changes are occurring in this field because of the tremendous advantage of the new microarray technology and its attendant development of bioinformatics. Initial assessments of gene expression in brain tissue from patients with AIDS vs control (HIV-negative) patients indicated a wide range of unanticipated changes in gene expression, including cell-signaling, Notch 3, and homeobox gene changes, as well as anticipated inflammation-related genes *(4,26,27)*. Genes identified by taking ratios of gene expression (whose significance was confirmed by Mann-Whitney analysis) between AIDS and controls were different from those identified by K-means cluster analysis *(27)*. A few examples are shown in Tables 5 and 6. (It should be noted that gene expression identification was performed through the NetAffx Analysis Center of Affymetrix Corp *[28]*.) This suggested to us that additional studies are required to compare significance among various bioinformatics approaches. We discuss this in the next section.

Table 2
Peripheral Blood Mononuclear Cell Culture Gene Expression Changes

Accession number	Gene ID	Fold change	
		Day 2 PI	Day 3 PI
Upregulated			
AA427491	T-cell receptor α-chain, c region	1.19 ± 0.14	3.13 ± 0.77
AA443584	CD8-α precursor	0.99 ± 0.14	1.63 ± 0.24
AA455278	Human neurogranin	1.02 ± 0.07	1.68 ± 0.24
AA458503	RIP140	0.84 ± 0.10	1.74 ± 0.17
AA457123	Transfer valyl-tRNA synthetase	0.89 ± 0.13	1.68 ± 0.14
AA457118	HTOM34 translocase	1.03 ± 0.13	1.82 ± 0.12
AA290698	Image ID 700414	1.21 ± 0.14	2.23 ± 0.27
H47026	Image ID 178468	0.93 ± 0.16	1.52 ± 0.11
AA455695	Image ID 813990	1.10 ± 0.09	1.66 ± 0.25
Downregulated			
AA455931	Adenylosuccinate lyase	1.00 ± 0.21	0.65 ± 0.02
M26708	Prothymosin-α	0.81 ± 0.14	0.48 ± 0.04
L00160	Phosphoglycerate kinase	1.17 ± 0.21	0.58 ± 0.13
AA401111	Glucose phosphate isomerase	1.04 ± 0.07	0.51 ± 0.04
AA621300	P18 protein mRNA/stathmin	0.95 ± 0.12	0.60 ± 0.10
AA463631	Signal recognition particle 72	0.66 ± 0.16	ND[a]
AA399473	PP5	ND*	0.67 ± 0.09
AA504327	Type IVA protein tyrosine phosphatase	0.83 ± 0.13	0.57 ± 0.06
U34379	Txk kinase	0.65 ± 0.15	ND
AF038953	E25 mRNA clone 1	1.21 ± 0.13	0.57 ± 0.04
	E25 mRNA clone 2	1.15 ± 0.08	0.61 ± 0.06

[a]ND, not determined because of insufficient signal above background. PI, postinfection; RIP140, receptor-interacting protein 140; PP5, placental protein 5. (From ref. *22*.)

Table 3
Rhesus Macaque Brain Gene Expression

Upregulated category (no. of genes in category)	Accession number	Gene ID	Fold change
Monocyte migration (10)	AF052124	Osteopontin	3.4
Inflammation and disease (17)	X68733	α1-antichymotrypsin	2.6
Antigen presentation (18)	M32578	HLA-DRβ1	4.4
Lysozomal (7)	U51240	LAPTM-5	2.9
Interferon inducible (13)	U22970	G1P3	8.4
Antiviral (3)	X79448	Adenosine deaminase	2.6
Transcriptional regulation (11)	X52560	NF-IL6	2.5
Cell cycle (7)	M92287	Cyclin D3	2.1
Growth, differentiation, signaling (8)	X66945	FGFR1	2.5
Cytoskeleton (6)	X53587	Integrin β 4	2.1
Immune system	AI142565	Ribonuclease K6	2.6

There were seven additional genes detected not in the above categories. Similar changes in several of these genes were also detected in other brain regions analyzed. (From ref. *23*.)

Table 4
Some Changes in Gene Expression by Ratio of Encephalitic vs Nonencephalitic SHIV-Positive Brain Tissue

Category	Gene name	Ratio of expression change
Interleukins and interferons		
	IL-4	3.05
	IL-1 receptor 1A	0.64
Chemokines		
	Leukocyte IP-10	8.4
	MIP-1A receptor	1.62
	RANTES receptor	1.62
Neurotropic growth factors		
	BDNF	0.22
	Neuromodulin	0.53
	GDNPF	0.66
Protein kinase		
	ERBB-3 protein protein-tyrosine kinase	0.69
Apoptosis-related protein		
	CD27BP (Siva)	2.79
	TNF-R	1.86
	CD30L	0.64
	CD40L	0.29

IL, interleukin; IP, interferon-inducible peptide; TNF, tumor necrosis factor.

Table 5
Genes Indicated by K-Means Cluster Analysis[a]

3AL031670: ferritin, light polypeptide-like 1
M13577: myelin basic protein (MBP)
D29675: inducible nitric oxide synthase gene
M54927: myelin proteolipid protein
U12022: calmodulin (CALM1)
U48437: amyloid precursor-like protein 1
L20941: ferritin heavy chain
L13266: *N*-methyl-D-aspartate receptor (NR1-1)
M58378: synapsin I (SYN 1) gene
M33210: colony stimulating factor 1 receptor
M21121: T cell-specific protein (RANTES)
M29273: myelin-associated glycoprotein (MAG)
X86809: major astrocytic phosphoprotein PEA-15
L13268: *N*-methyl-D-aspartate receptor (NR1-3)
U97669: Notch 3
U22970: interferon-inducible peptide (6-16) gene
D31815: senescence marker protein-30
AF039555: visinin-like protein 1 (VSNL1)
AB015202: gene for hippocalcin
D88799: cadherin, partial cds
AL022326: Synaptogyrin 1A
U31767: neuronatin α & β genes

These genes were in different cluster groups when comparisons were made between AIDS and HIV-negative controls brains. (From ref. *27*.)

Table 6
Genes Ranked by Ratios of HIV+/HIV-[a]

Gene Description	Ratio	Ratio rank
AF062739: GSK-3 binding protein FRAT2	0.140941	1
M61156: activator protein 2B (AP-2B)	0.142538	2
D00096: prealbumin, (26,469)	0.143123	3
D78514 ubiquitin-conjugating enzyme	0.155713	4
J04131: γ-glutamyl transpeptidase (GGT) protein	0.158651	5
AF030107: regulator of G protein signaling (RGS13)	0.165479	6
L23805 CATENINα1(E)-catenin	0.168352	7
AF082558: truncated TRF1-interacting ankyrin-related	0.168513	8
ADP-ribose polymerase TT7		
U40572: β2-syntrophin (SNT B2)	7.2271	12569
AL031652: dJ1119D9.1 (PAK1-like serine/threonine-protein kinase)	7.595604	12571
M63438: Ig rearranged γ chain, V-J-C region and (0,1049)	8.058278	12572
M27504 TOPIIX topoisomerase type II (Topo II)	8.585115	12574
U06632: p80-coilin	8.685422	12575
AJ223948: putative RNA helicase	9.021651	12576
D86864: acetyl LDL receptor	9.109537	12577
X97324: adipophilin	9.171688	12578
Y14737: immunoglobulin λ heavy chain	9.224281	12579
L10717 TKTCST cell-specific tyrosine kinase	9.260073	12581

[a]Ratios of gene expression intensity were produced for this examination and confirmed by Mann-Whitney analysis. Ig, immunoglobulin; LDL, low-density lipoprotein.

3. BIOINFORMATICS FOR HIV-ASSOCIATED DEMENTIA

The previously discussed studies *(18,22–25,27)* demonstrate the power of gene expression analysis in the study HAD but also illustrate the need for improved bioinformatics tools. This need is not unique to HAD—this need pervades genomic research. The demand for mature bioinformatics tools has never been greater, and innovation must continue in order to keep pace with evolving technology.

The credibility of results obtained using state-of-the-art gene expression is only as good as the design of the experiment and the statistical methods employed to analyze such daedal data. Kerr et al. *(29)* emphasize that the structure of the data, the number of possible analyses, and the quality of the results are determined by the experimental design. Furthey, they prove that a commonly used design for cDNA array experiments is inefficient and may introduce confounded effects, and they propose a superior design.

Another factor critical to the analysis is the allocation of samples to microarrays with respect to the type and level of replication. Given the high cost of gene chips and the scarcity of tissue samples, the need for efficient resource allocation is essential. Zien et al. *(30)* provide some practical advice in this regard via interactive Monte Carlo simulations.

The challenging aspects of analyzing gene expression data are caused its high dimensionality. The latest human chip sets can target more than 33,000 genes but rarely more than 60 observations (chips) are collected in an experiment and, in fact, the typical number is less than 20 chips. Traditional classification algorithms cannot cope with such a large number of variables (genes) and so few observations; thus, modifications of existing procedures or the development of new methods are needed to address these issues. One solution is to use dimension-reduction techniques. Existing-dimension reduction techniques, such as principal components analysis, partial least squares, and singular value decomposition, have been used in analyzing microarray data *(31–33)*.

These methods have been implemented in conjunction with pattern recognition algorithms to classify disease states based on gene expression *(32)*.

Cluster analysis is popular a bioinformatics tool for identifying gene expression profiles associated with different diseases or disease states *(25,27,34)*. Although cluster analysis traces its roots back to the sixties and early seventies, it has received a great deal of attention in the literature since Eisen et al. *(34)* popularized its use in bioinformatics circles. Shapshak et al. *(27)* used K-means clustering to study gene expression in brain tissue from patients with AIDS vs control (HIV-negative) patients, whereas Vahey et al. *(25)* used SOM clusters to examine patterns of gene expression associated with the rate of disease progression in Rhesus macaques infected with SIVmac251. It is important to note that clustering is an exploratory tool rather than a confirmatory tool, and statistical inference cannot be drawn from the application of such methods; however, cluster analysis is a powerful instrument for the exploration of gene-expression analysis.

Careful hypothesis testing is necessary to draw valid statistical inferences from properly designed microarray experiments. The primary aim of most studies is to identify which genes exhibit upregulation or downregulation owing to pathogenesis. A myriad of inferential procedures have been proposed for determining these differentially expressed genes, many of which are modifications of basic statistical methods, such as the *t*-test or analysis of variance. Before any tests are conducted, careful preprocessing is recommended, especially when dealing with cDNA arrays *(35)*. Recent work by Giles and Kipling *(36)* suggests that Affymetrix data may not need as much preprocessing as had been previous thought. Following preprocessing, the level of significance for each individual test must be adjusted to account for large number of genes being tested. Otherwise, the family-wise error rate becomes unacceptable. Multiple correction procedures are used to compute this adjustment, and recent methods have focused on controlling the false discovery rate. Tusher et al. *(37)* propose the significance analysis of microarrays as one method for achieving this. This is an active area of research and will continue to receive attention in the bioinformatics literature.

Bioinformatics for neuroAIDS poses three types of challenges. The first type is related specifically to microarray experiments, rather than to neurological or viral diseases. The second type revolves around the explosive growth in images, atlases, and databases of neurobiological information in the last 15 yr. The third type is truly global: how to let these different resources *talk sensibly* with each other, so that people can use this cornucopia and input it into algorithms to understand and treat diseases. We briefly discuss each of these in turn.

First, the microarray-specific problems involve the acquisition of the experimental data and their processing and analysis (a good introduction is found in ref. *38*). Systems for acquiring and storing microarray data take two forms: laboratory information management systems (LIMS) and publicly accessible repositories of information. In addition to recording the experimental data, fully functional LIMS support experimental design, protocols, and tracking; recording information on sample sources, preparation, and usage; and inventory control, quality control, and appropriate data security. Although a number of different open source systems have been developed, each support some but not all of these *desiderata* (e.g., see refs. *39–42*). For example, BioArray Software Environment (BASE) makes no attempt to handle process-related information or inventory; Stanford Microarray Database (SMD) and its descendant Longhorn Array Database (LAD) concentrate mainly on the intensity data and descriptions of protocols, and samples are relatively weak and buried in textual comments. SMD is used to support a publicly accessible repository of microarray data, and several other groups have developed repositories and portals that similarly support a variety of queries via websites *(43–49)*. We have already discussed some of the issues involved in processing the acquired data; indeed, an analytical pipeline that permits the use of a variety of algorithms and the incorporation of new ones has been developed for just this reason *(50)*.

The second type of challenge is to build useful models of brain function that incorporate what we know and stimulate discovery. In the last 15 yr, the neuroscience community has seen an explosion of information about the brain and immediately understood that databases of this information would be absolutely vital. Images, functional magnetic resonance imaging data, anatomical connections, cortical surfaces, and computational models are just a few of many of types of data electronically available *(51–55)*. Understanding how the brain works and the etiology of neurological diseases, such as HAD, necessarily draws on all this information. It is difficult to fit the pieces together into a partial model that explains the mechanism of the phenotype well enough to be worth pursuing but leaves ample room to expose gaps in both the data and the model. For example, suppose gene X is identified in a microarray experiment as being upregulated in HAD from post mortem brain tissue. Does this gene contribute to the dementia, or is the elevation of its expression incidental to the disease? In evaluating these possibilities, an investigator might consider information on the histological and cytological localization of the gene's product in normal brains and similarities in brain images from patients with late-stage HAD or Alzheimer's disease. Finding these data in a targeted search is a significant challenge; uncovering data that may be relevant but that are unknown to the investigator is even more difficult, and being able to recognize if information on whether gene product copurifies with neurofibrillary tangles is missing is even more difficult. When the amount of data is small, the models are compact enough to evaluate on the back of an envelope, although with our present embarrassment of riches, the models and the techniques for discovering the important positive and negative relationships, as well as nonrelationships, among the data will require computation.

The third challenge is generic to many problems, systems, and databases: how to can databases talk sensibly with each other to allow algorithmically pursuit of questions from many different sources (*semantic interoperability*). This is distinct from the second challenge of building models because, in this case, the data for stocking the model is available. Humans can converse indefinitely until each person understands what the other means by a particular word or phrase, but computers obviously cannot yet rely on natural language processing to interpret terms. Some investigators have avoided the problems of interoperability by manually translating schema and semantics of different databases into an integrated warehouse or cluster of databases *(39,43,48,54)*. The difficulty with this approach is that it does not scale, both as a function of the number of databases and their complexity. Thus, methods of achieving semantic interoperability have been the focus of intensive work for several years. There are two main approaches to achieving interoperability: the suggestion of standard terms and notions and the development of formal methods to declare and interconvert the semantics of complex ideas. Regarding the first suggestion, there have been substantial efforts in the microarray, bioinformatics, and the neuroinformatics communities. In the microarray community, a set of minimal descriptors and a basic schema for microarray databases have been suggested to facilitate data exchange (minimum information about a microarray experiment [MIAME] and microarray gene expression [MAGE], respectively; see references 56–60). SMD and LAD predate the MIAME and MAGE proposals, and BASE does not strictly follow MAGE *(39–41)*. The Gene Ontology seeks to develop a classification of terms, along with definitions, that can be used to denote cellular structures, physiological processes, and molecular functions and will be broadly useful in databases of molecular and some organismal information *(61–62)*. In its earliest days, the neuroinformatics community has understood interoperability to be a central challenge *(63–65)*. Proposed solutions range from standardized schemata *(66–65)* and anatomical nomenclature *(67–69)* to automatic generation of databases using the same schema *(70)*.

As yet, no standards have been uniformly adopted by the relevant databases. Indeed, there are significant practical problems in retrofitting new standards to existing databases, since usage and the organization of concepts varies so widely among databases; retrofitting is necessarily a manual operation that often involves restructuring the entire database. The usage of a term in a database may not correspond to its new definition or its definition may be vague. Databases that evolve with a standardized set of ideas obviously do not need retrofitting, but they do need to conform closely to the standards if interoperability is to be preserved. For these reasons, an alternative approach that uses formal methods to declare semantics remains of interest *(71–73)*. If successful, such methods would provide an abstract semantic layer that databases could use to translate each other's ideas into their own, eliminating the need for retrofitting or compliance with a fixed view of biology.

4. CONCLUSION

Absolute and conclusive logic would be premature at this point because previous studies were on different types of cells and tissues, used different analytic algorithms, and were not prospectively designed. Future reviews will address these issues as data becomes available. Despite problems with previous studies, noteworthy parallels have been found in the disparate studies that are both enigmatic and suggestive of future direction. Thus, this chapter indicates direction taken by prior studies in their analysis of neuroAIDS-related gene expression.

ACKNOWLEDGMENTS

We thank Carol K. Petito, MD for neuropathology discussions. We gratefully acknowledge the NIH National NeuroAIDS Tissue Consortium for providing brain tissue. This work was supported in part by NIH grants DA 14533, DA 12580, DA 07909, DA 04787, and AG 19952 (to P.S.) and GM-56529 (to T.K. and P.S.)

REFERENCES

1. Geschwind DH. DNA microarrays: translation of the genome from laboratory to clinic. Lancet Neurol 2003; 2:275–282.
2. Minagar A, Shapshak P, Duran EM, et al. Gene expression in HIV-associated dementia, Alzheimer's disease, multiple sclerosis, and schizophrenia. Under review, 2004.
3. Marcotte ER, Srivastava LK, Quirion R. cDNA microarray and proteomic approaches in the study of brain diseases: focus on schizophrenia and Alzheimer's disease. Pharmacol Ther 2003;100:63–74.
4. Shapshak P, Stengel R. Discovering brain mechanisms and the rules of molecular biology. 6th World Multiconference on Systemics, Cybernetics and Informatics. Orlando, FL, July 14–18, 2002. Available from: www.iiis. org/sci2002/.
5. Goodkin K, Wilkie FL, Concha M, et al. Subtle neuropsychologic impairment and minor cognitive-motor disorder in HIV-1 infection. Neuroimaging of AIDS II. Neuroimaging Clin N Am, 1997;7:561–579.
6. Goodkin K, Shapshak P, Wilkie FL, et al. Immune function, brain, and HIV-1 infection. In Goodkin K, Visser A, eds. Psychoneuroimmunology: Stress, Mental Disorders & Health. Washington, DC, American Psychiatric Association, 1999.
7. Goodkin K, Baldewicz TT, Wilkie FL, Tyll MD, Shapshak P. HIV-1 infection of brain: a region-specific approach to its neuropathophysiology and therapeutic prospects. Psychiatric Annals 2001;31:182–192.
8. Sperber K, Shao L. Neurologic consequences of HIV infection in the ERA of HAART. AIDS Patient Care STDs. 2003;17:509–518.
9. Torres-Munoz J, Stockton P, Tacoronte N, Roberts B, Maronpot RR, Petito CK. Detection of HIV-1 gene sequences in hippocampal neurons isolated from postmortem AIDS brains by laser capture microdissection. J Neuropathol Exp Neurol 2001;60:885–892.
10. Hesselgesser J, Halks-Miller M, DelVecchio V, et al. CD4-independent association between HIV-1 gp120 and CXCR4: functional chemokine receptors are expressed in human neurons. Curr Biol 1997;7:112–121.
11. Fischer-Smith T, Croul S, Sverstiuk AE, et al. CNS invasion by CD14+/CD16+ peripheral blood-derived monocytes in HIV dementia: perivascular accumulation and reservoir of HIV infection. J Neurovirol. 2001;7:528–541.
12. Ohagen A, Devitt A, Kunstman KJ, et al. Genetic and functional analysis of full-length human immunodeficiency virus type 1 env genes derived from brain and blood of patients with AIDS. J Virol 2003;77:12,336–12,345.
13. Shapshak P, Segal DM, Crandall KA, et al. Independent evolution of HIV type I in different brain regions. AIDS Res Hum Retroviruses 1999;15:811–820.
14. Morris A, Marsden M, Halcrow K, et al. Mosaic structure of the HIV-1 genome infecting lymphoid cells and the brain: evidence for frequent in vivo recombination events in the evolution of region populations. J Virol 1999;73:720–731.

15. Eilbott DJ, Peress N, Burger H, et al. Human immunodeficiency virus type 1 in spinal cords of acquired immunodeficiency syndrome patients with myelopathy: expression and replication in macrophages. Proc Natl Acad Sci USA 1989;86:3337–3341.

16. Yoshioka M, Shapshak P, Sun NCJ, et al. Ferritin immunoreactivity in microglial nodules in AIDS brain, Acta Neuropathologica 1992;84:297–306.

17. Nukuna A, Gendelman HE, Limoges J, et al. Levels of HIV replicaton in macrophages determines the severity of murine HIV-1 encephalitis. J Neurovirol 2004;10(Suppl 1):82–90.

18. Galey D, Becker K, Haughey N, et al. Differential transcriptional regulation by human immunodeficiency virus type 1 and gp120 in human astrocytes. J Neurovirol 2003;9:358–371.

19. Shapshak P, Duncan D, Minagar D, Rodriguez de la Vega P, Stewart R, Petito CK. Elevated expression of IFN-γ in the HIV-1 infected brain. Front Biosci 2004;9:1073–1081.

20. Vitkovic L, J Bockaert, C Jacque. Inflammatory cytokines: neuromodulators in normal brain? J Neurochem 2000;74:457–471.

21. Zeng J, Ghorpade A, Niemann D, et al. Lymphotropic virions affect chemokine receptor-mediated neural signaling and apoptosis: implications for HIV-1 associated dementia. J Virol 1999;73:8256–8267.

22. Geiss GK, Bumgarner RE, An MC, et al Large-scale monitoring of host cell gene expression during HIV-1 infection using cDNA microarrays. Virology 2000;266:8–16.

23. Roberts ES, Zandonatti MA, Watry DD, Madden LJ, Henriksen MA, Fox HS. Induction of pathogenic sets of genes in macrophages and neurons in NeuroAIDS. Am J Pathol 2003;162;2041–2057.

24. Sui Y, Potula R, Pinson D, et al. Microarray analysis of cytokine and chemokine genes in the brains of macaques with SHIV-encephalitis, J Med Primatol 2003;32:229–239.

25. Vahey MT, Nau ME, Taubman M, Yalley-Ogunro J, Silvera P, Lewis MG. Patterns of gene expression in PBMNCs of rhesus macaques infected with SIVmac251 and exhibiting differential rates of disease progression. AIDS Res Hum Retrov 2003;19:369–387.

26. Shapshak P, Torres-Munos J, Petito CK. Bioinformatics in neurodegenerative diseases. Proc Virt Conf Genom Bioinf. North Dakota State University, 2001. Available from: www.ndsu/virtual-genomics.

27. Shapshak, P, Duncan, R, Torres-Munoz JE, Duran EM, Minagar A, Petito CK. Analytic approaches to differential gene expression in AIDS vs. control brains. Front Biosci 2004;9:2935–2946.

28. Liu G, Loraine AE, Shigeta R, et al. NetAffx: affymetrix probesets and annotations. Nucleic Acids Res 2003;31:82–86.

29. Kerr MK, Churchill GA. Bootstrapping cluster analysis: assessing the reliability of conclusions from microarray experiments. Proc Natl Acad Sci USA 2001;98:8961–8965.

30. Zien A, Fluck J, Zimmer R, Lengauer T. Microarrays: how many do you need? J Comp Biol 2003;10:653–667.

31. Alter O, Brown PO, Botstein D. Singular value decomposition for genome-wide expression data processing and modeling. Proc Natl Acad Sci USA 2000;97:10,101–10,106.

32. Bicciato S, Luchini A, Di Bello C. PCA disjoint models for multiclass cancer analysis using gene expression data. Bioinformatics 2003;19:571–578.

33. Nguyen DV, Rocke DM. Tumor classification by partial least squares using Microarray gene expression data. Bioinformatics 2002;8:39–50.

34. Eisen MB, Spellman PT, Brown PO, Botstein D. Cluster analysis and display of genome-wide expression patterns. Proc Natl Acad Sci USA 1998;95:14,863–14,868.

35. Huber W, Von Heydebreck A, Sultmann H, Poustka A, Vingron M. Variance stabilization applied to microarray data calibration and to the quantification of differential expression. Bioinformatics 2002;18(Suppl 1):S96–S104.

36. Giles PJ, Kipling D. Normality of oligonucleotide microarray data and implications for parametric statistical analyses. Bioinformatics 2003;19:2254–2262.

37. Tusher VG, Tibshirani R, Chu G. Significance analysis of microarrays applied to the ionizing radiation response. Proc Natl Acad Sci U S A 2001;98:5116–5121.

38. Geschwind DH, Gregg JP. Microarrays for the Neurosciences. Cambridge, MA, MIT Press, 2002.

39. Sherlock G, Hernandez-Boussard T, Kasarskis A, et al. The Stanford Microarray Database. Nucleic Acids Res 2001;29:152–155.

40. Killon PJ, Sherlock G, IyerVR. The Longhorn Array Database (LAD): an open-source, MIAME compliant implementation of the Stanford Microarray Database (SMD). BMC Bioinfo 2003;4:32–38.

41. Saal LH, Troein C, Vallon-Christersson J, Gruvberger S, Borg A, Peterson C. BioArray Software Environment (BASE): a platform for comprehensive management and analysis of microarray data. Genome Biol: software0003.1–software 0003.6,2002.

42. Ermolaeva O, Rastogi M, Pruitt KD, et al. Data management and analysis for gene expression arrays. Nature Genet 1998;20:19–23.

43. Brazma A, Parkinson H, Sarkans U, et al. ArrayExpress-a public repository for microarray gene expression data at the EBI. Nucleic Acids Res 2003;31:68–71.

44. Gollub J, Ball CA, Binkley G, et al. The Stanford Microarray Database: data access and quality assessment tools. Nucleic Acids Res 2003;31:94–96.

45. Cornell M, Paton NW, Hedeler C, et al. GIMS: an integrated data storage and analysis environment for genomic and. Yeast 2003;20:1291–1306.

46. Aach J, Rindone W, Church G. Systematic management and analysis of yeast gene expression data. Genome Res 2000;10:431–445.

47. Dennis G Jr, Sherman BT, Hosack DA, et al. David: Database for Annotation, Visualization, and Integrated Discovery. Genome Biol 2003;4:P3.

48. Chen J, Zhao P, Massaro D, et al. The PEPR GeneChip data warehouse, and implementation of a dynamic time series query tool (SGQT) with graphical interface. Nucleic Acids Res 2004;32:D578–D581.

49. Kasprzyk A, Keefe D, Smedley D, et al. Ensmart: a generic system for fast and flexible access to biological data. Genome Res 2004;14:160–169.

50. Grant JD, Somers LA, Zhang Y, Manion FJ, Bidaut G, Ochs MF. Fgdp: functional genomics data pipeline for automated, multiple microarray data analyses. Bioinformatics 2004;20:282–283.

51. Toga AW. Imaging databases and neuroscience. Neuroscientist 2002;8:423–436.

52. Van Horn JD, Grethe JS, Kostelec P, et al. The functional magnetic resonance imaging data center (FMRIDC): the challenges and rewards of large-scale databasing of neuroimaging studies. Phil Trans Roy Soc (London) B 2001;356:1323–1339.

53. Dickson J, Drury H, van Essen D. 'The surface management system' (SUMS) database: a surface-based database to aid cortical surface reconstruction, visualization and analysis. Phil Trans Roy Soc (London) B 2001;356:1277–1292.

54. Peterson BE, Healy MD, Nadkarni PM, Miller PL, Shepherd GM. Modeldb: an environment for running and storing computational models and their results applied to neuroscience. J Am Med Inform Assoc 1996;3: 389–398.

55. Bota M, Arbib MA. Integrating databases and expert systems for the analysis of brain structures: connections, similarities, and homologies. Neuroinformatics 2004;2:19–58.

56. Brazma A, Hingamp P, Quackenbush J, et al. Minimum information about a microarray experiment (miame)—toward standards for microarray data. Nature Genet 2001;29:365–371.

57. MAGE-OM Working Group. MAGE-OM. MGED Society. 2003–present. Available from: www.mged.org/Workgroups/MAGE/mage-om.html.

58. MIAME Working Group. Minimum information about a microarray experiment ~ MIAME. MGED Society. 2003–present. Available from: www.mged.org/-Workgroups/MIAME/miame.html.

59. MIAME Working Group. Minimum information about a microarray experiment, MIAME. MGED Society. 2003–present.

60. Spellman PT, Miller M, Stewart J, et al. Design and implementation of microarray gene expression markup language (MAGE-ML). Genome Biol 2002;3:RESEARCH 0046.1–0046.9.

61. Ashburner M, Ball CA, Blake JA, et al. Gene Ontology: tool for the unification of biology. Nature Genet 2000;25:25–29.

62. EMAGE Editorial Office (2003–present). EMAGE gene expression database. Available from: http://genex.hgu.mrc. ac.uk/Emage/database/-emageIntro.html/.

63. Amari SI, Beltrame F, Bjaalie JG, et al. Neuroinformatics: the integration of shared databases and tools towards integrative neuroscience. J Integ Neurosci 2002;1:117–128.

64. Dashti AE, Ghandeharizadeh S, Stone J, Swanson LW, Thompson RH. Database challenges and solutions in neuroscientific applications. Neuroimage 1997;5:97–115.

65. Gardner D, Knuth K, Abato M, et al. Common data model for neuroscience data and data model exchange. J Am Med Inform Assoc 2001;8:17–33.

66. Gorin F, Hogarth M, Gertz M. The challenges and rewards of integrating diverse neuroscience. Neuroscientist 2001;7:18–27.

67. Bowden DM, Martin RF. Neuronames brain hierarchy. Neuroimage 1995;2:63–83. Available from: www.mged.org/Workgroups/MIAME/miame.html.

68. Hole W, Srinivasan S. Adding NeuroNames to the UMLS Metathesaurus. Neuroinformatics 2003;1:61–63.

69. Bowden D, Dubach M. Neuronames 2002. Neuroinformatics 2003;1:43

70. Roland P, Svensson G, Lindeberg T, et al. A database generator for human brain imaging. Trends Neurosci 2001;24:562–564.

71. Kazic T. Semiotes a semantics for sharing. Bioinformatics 16:1129–1144. Available from: www.biocheminfo.org/repository/semiotes.ps.

72. Wiederhold G, Jannink J. Composing diverse ontologies. Stanford University. Available from: www.db.stanford.edu/SKC/publications/ifip99.html.

73. Chilukuri P, Kazic T. Semantic interoperability of heterogeneous systems. University of Missouri Bioinformatics Technical Report, 2004-01. Available from: www.biocheminfo.org/repository/parser.ps.

CME QUESTIONS

1. Which statement about human immunodeficiency virus (HIV)-associated dementia (HAD) is correct?
   A. HAD presents with a progressive encephalopathy with impairment of normal cerebral function, and despite major advances in our understanding of the pathogenesis of HAD, the basic mechanisms of the pathological and direct involvement of essential cells, such as neurons, astrocytes, and invading macrophages still remain largely unknown
   B. HAD occurs only as a late manifestation of acquired immunodeficiency disease
   C. HAD presents initially with apraxia and aphasia
   D. HAD affects males more often than females

2. Which statement about microarray gene expression analysis is correct?
   A. It allows us to examine the expression of thousands of genes at once
   B. It allows us to look at the expression of only hundreds of proteins
   C. It has never been used in the study of HAD
   D. It allows us to calculate the molecular weight of gene products, particularly proteins

3. Which of these cells has a role in the pathogenesis of HAD?
   A. Astrocytes
   B. Microglia/macrophages
   C. Neurons
   D. All of the above

17

Human T-Lymphotropic Virus-Associated Neurological Disorders

Pathogenesis, Immunology, and Clinical Management

Michael D. Lairmore, Bindhu Michael, Lee Silverman, and Amrithraj Nair

1. INTRODUCTION

Human T-cell lymphotropic virus type 1 (HTLV-1), the first human retrovirus discovered, has a tropism for T lymphocytes and has been established as the causative agent of adult T-cell leukemia/lymphoma (ATLL), an aggressive CD4 T-cell malignancy *(1–4)*. HTLV-2 was subsequently isolated and found to share approximately 60% nucleotide sequence homology with HTLV-1 *(5)*. In the mid-1980s, HTLV-1 began to be associated through epidemiologic studies as a contributing factor in chronic neurodegenerative disorders. These clinical syndromes were first reported in Japan and Martinique (French West Indies), both regions that were endemic for HTLV-1 infection *(6,7)*. Through important international cooperative studies, both syndromes were revealed to be identical in clinical presentation and are now known collectively as HTLV-1-associated myelopathy/tropical spastic paraparesis (HAM/TSP). HTLV-2 has been sporadically associated with lymphoproliferative diseases and recently has been implicated in isolated case reports of neurological disease *(8,9)*.

Currently, a total of 10 to 20 million people worldwide are estimated to be infected with HTLV-1, and HTLV-1 is considered endemic in southwestern Japan, the Caribbean basin, Central and West Africa, the Middle East, Melanesia, and South America *(10)*. It is also a serious public health problem among the at-risk groups in Europe and North America and therefore is a target of intervention policies, including blood-donor screening *(10–16)*. Although the majority of the infected persons (~95%) remain lifelong asymptomatic carriers of the virus, 2 to 3% of those infected develop ATLL, and another 2 to 3% develop chronic inflammatory diseases, such as HAM/TSP *(11,17,18)*. Natural transmission of HTLV-1 and HTLV-2 occurs through cell-associated transmission by three primary routes: orally via breast milk from infected mothers to children, via sexual contact (predominantly from male to female), and by exposure to infected blood or whole-cell blood products (e.g., transfusion, use of contaminated needles) *(9,10,19)*.

Although the molecular events of virus replication are beginning to be unraveled and knowledge about HTLV-1- and HTLV-2-associated diseases has increased, many questions regarding the pathogenesis of neurologic diseases associated these retroviruses remain. For example, it is unclear why some HTLV-1-infected subjects develop ATLL or HAM/TSP, whereas the majority remains

From: *Current Clinical Neurology: Inflammatory Disorders of the Nervous System:*
Pathogenesis, Immunology, and Clinical Management
Edited by: A. Minagar and J. S. Alexander © Humana Press Inc., Totowa, NJ

Table 1
Summary of HTLV-1- and HTLV-2-Associated Inflammatory Neurological Diseases

Viral etiology	Associated neurological diseases	Typical presenting symptoms	Treatments	Host factors associated with disease
HTLV-1	HAM/TSP	Spasticity in the lower extremities, hyperreflexia, muscle weakness, sphincter disorders (urinary bladder and intestines), and less frequently, cerebellar syndrome with ataxia and intention tremor	Corticosteroids, plasmapheresis, interferon, and antiretroviral drugs. Experimentally, BPHA inhibitors of MMP-2 and MMP-9	Certain patient HLA haplotypes (HLA-A*02 and Cw*08) lead to a lower risk of HAM/TSP, whereas HLA-B*5401 and DRB1*0101 are associated with an elevated risk of HAM/TSP
HTLV-2	Isolated cases of spastic pararesis and ataxia	Spastic ataxia	Corticosteroids and symptomatic support	Unknown

HTLV, human T-lymphotropic virus; HAM/TSP, HTLV-1-associated myelopathy/tropical spastic paraparesis; BPHA, *N*-biphenyl sulphonyl-phenylalanine hydroxamic acid; MMP, matrix metalloproteinase.

asymptomatic. What factors contribute to the pathogenesis of these two widely divergent clinical disorders? In HAM/TSP patients, why is there preferential damage to the thoracic spinal cord? What is the mechanism of viral persistence in the face of a strong immune response? What is the nature of the cell-mediated immune response to HTLV-1 infection, and is this response protective or could it lead to lymphocyte-mediated lesion development if it is uncontrolled? In this chapter, we focus on the pathogenesis of HAM/TSP in terms of its clinical features, pathologic lesions, patient susceptibility factors, and immune responses and review the proposed mechanisms for the development of this chronic neurological disorder.

2. CLINICAL FEATURES OF HAM/TSP

In evaluation of the clinical presentation of HTLV-associated neurological disorders, it is important to understand that HTLV-1 has been associated not only with HAM/TSP but also with several inflammatory diseases, such as alveolitis, polymyositis, arthritis, uveitis, and peripheral myopathy *(11,18)*. HAM/TSP is strongly associated with HTLV-1 infection and is characterized as a progressive chronic myelopathy, with preferential damage of the thoracic spinal cord *(11,20–23)*. In affected patients, the myelopathy presents as paraparesis with spasticity in the lower extremities, hyperreflexia, muscle weakness, and sphincter disorders, including dysfunction of the urinary bladder and intestines (Table 1). Less frequently, it may precede or give rise to a cerebellar syndrome with ataxia and intention tremor *(24)*. Some HAM/TSP patients exhibit a predominance of sympathetic nervous system dysfunction *(25)*. HAM/TSP patients may exhibit prolonged central motor conduction time (CMCT) in all the limbs and central sensory conduction time in lower limbs, with CMCT in upper limbs correlating with the clinical severity of HAM/TSP *(26,27)*. Magnetic resonance imaging (MRI) of HAM/TSP patients reveals the presence of multiple white-matter lesions in both the spinal cord and the brain, involving perivascular demyelination and axonal degeneration *(28–31)*. In addition, recent studies show that the carriers and patients with HAM/TSP exhibit mild cognitive impairments in verbal and visual memory, attention, and visuomotor abilities *(32)*.

3. SPINAL CORD AND BRAIN PATHOLOGY ASSOCIATED WITH HAM/TSP

In patients with HAM/TSP, the primary site of lesion development is the spinal cord; lesions are particularly severe in the middle to lower thoracic regions *(11,33,34)*. This lesion distribution is consistent with neurological symptoms, such as spastic paraparesis of the lower limbs. Brain lesions less commonly may occur simultaneously with spinal cord involvement and may be detected using MRI, which reveals abnormal-intensity lesions in the brain (white matter) of patients with HAM/TSP *(28,29,31,35)*. Within the spinal cord, regions mainly affected are the so-called *watershed* zones, suggesting a nonrandom distribution *(36)*. These include degenerative lesions in the lateral corticospinal tract and spinocerebellar or spinothalamic tract of the lateral column. Damage to the anterior and posterior columns is less extensive and more variable than that of the lateral column, in correlation with the clinical findings. In addition, there is also perivascular and parenchymal cellular infiltration, consisting of mainly T cells (both CD4+ and CD8+ T cells), macrophages, astrocytes, and glial cells *(33)*. Similar perivascular inflammatory infiltration is also present in the brain, particularly in the deep white matter and the marginal area of the cortex and white matter *(33)*. Interestingly, the nature of perivascular-infiltrate and cytokine expression varies depending on the duration of the disease. Patients with short duration of illness, extending from 2.5 to 4.5 yr, exhibit distribution of CD4+ cells, CD8+ cells, and macrophages with the presence of proinflammatory cytokines, such as interleukin (IL)-1β, tumor necrosis factor (TNF)-α, and interferon (IFN)-γ *(37,38)*, whereas in those with more prolonged duration of illness, extending from 8 to 10 yr, there are greater numbers of CD8+ cells compared to CD4+ cells, with fewer proinflammatory cytokines *(33,39)*. The distribution of macrophages and microglia varies depending on the duration of illness *(40)*. Intriguingly, patients with shorter duration of spinal cord lesions and with a predominance of CD4+ cells appear to contain more HTLV-1 *pX* and *pol* DNA than do those with longer duration of illness who exhibit fewer CD4+ cells *(41)*. HTLV-1 *tax* RNA is also found in infiltrating CD4+ T lymphocytes in active central nervous system (CNS) lesions in patients with HAM/TSP *(42)*, particularly within astrocytes, but not in perivascular infiltrating cells *(43)*. These reports collectively suggest that viral proteins may elicit the early inflammatory lesions associated with HAM/TSP, but subsequent lesions may develop as a result of secondary injury caused by cytokines and other inflammatory mediators from infiltrating leukocytes.

Within the myelopathy, widespread loss of myelin and axons has been observed *(33,44)*. β-Amyloid precursor protein (APP), an early axonal damage marker, is more intensively expressed in areas of active-inflammatory lesions than in those of inactive-chronic lesions, suggesting that axonal damage is closely associated with inflammation in active-chronic lesions *(34)*. Additionally, the presence of APP+ axons without relation to inflammatory cells in inactive-chronic lesions suggests that soluble neurotoxic factors might induce the axonal changes *(34)*. This same study reported that myelinated fibers in the anterior and posterior spinal roots in lower thoracic to lumbar levels had occasional APP+ axons, suggesting that spinal nerve roots can be affected in HAM/TSP, especially in lower thoracic to lumbar levels.

4. ANIMAL MODELS OF HAM/TSP

A variety of animal models of HTLV-1 infection have been reported, although the virus consistently infects only rabbits *(45,46)*, some nonhuman primates *(47,48)* and, to a lesser extent, rats *(49,50)*. Viral transmission in mice using typical methods of infection produces inconsistent infections and limited virus expression in tissues *(51–55)*. Nonhuman primates have been infected with HTLV-1, and certain species have a natural infection with simian T-lymphotropic virus infection type 1 *(56–62)*. The squirrel monkey has been successfully infected with HTLV-1 and offers an attractive nonhuman primate model of HTLV-1 for vaccine testing *(63–66)*. Rats have been infected with HTLV-1 cell lines and offer a model of the neurological disease associated with the viral infection *(67–70)*. In addition, rats have been successfully used to test the role of cell-mediated immunity to the infection *(71–73)*, although controversy exists regarding the reproducibility of the viral infection in rats *(50)*.

The WKA strain of rat appears to be uniquely susceptible to an inflammatory neurological disease resembling HAM/TSP when is infected with HTLV-1-infected cell lines via inoculation *(74)*. This strain appears susceptible to the infection with approximately 80% infection efficiency when rats are exposed at 16 wk of age with HTLV-1 cell lines derived from rat, human, or rabbit cells *(74–76)*. In this model, affected rats develop spastic paraparesis of the hind legs with lesions confined primarily to the lateral and anterior funiculi of the spinal cord. Lesions include extensive symmetrical white-matter degeneration characterized by loss of myelin, axon damage, vacuolar degeneration, infiltration with foamy macrophages, and astrocytic gliosis, most severe within the thoracic cord and continuing from the cervical to the lumbar area with degeneration of nerve roots and peripheral nerves *(70,75)*. Electron microscopic studies of these lesions indicated symmetrical alterations mainly confined to the marginal areas of white matter with distribution in the anterior and the lateral columns. Additional ultrastructural features included separation of myelin lamellae and vacuolation of myelin sheaths with debris and the presence of both demyelinated and remyelinated axons, occasionally with tubuloreticular inclusions *(74,75)*. Ultrastructural alterations in the peripheral nerve were similar to those of the spinal cord with the addition of apoptosis of oligodendrocytes and Schwann cells. Similar to the human infection virus, particles were absent in either the spinal cord or peripheral nerve lesions *(75)*. Antibodies against HTLV-1 antigens were demonstrated in the plasma and cerebrospinal fluid (CSF) of these rats, whereas HTLV-1 provirus was less frequently detected from the peripheral blood mononuclear cells (PBMCs) and spinal cords of these rats; however, many other strains of rats do not develop inflammatory neurological lesions under the same conditions, suggesting that the development of the lesions in rats is under strict genetic restriction *(69)*. Although the clinical and neuropathological features of the WKA rat model of HAM/TSP generally mimic those of HAM/TSP in humans, the inflammatory cell infiltration is generally reduced or absent in the affected rat spinal cord lesions, unlike the disease in humans *(77)*.

Using a variety of promoters and enhancers to drive gene expression, transgenic mouse models of HTLV-1-associated diseases have provided new tools to understand the role of *tax* and envelope proteins in the pathogenesis of HTLV-1-associated lesions. Nerenberg et al. *(78,79)* produced neurofibromas associated with peripheral nerves in *tax* transgenic mice by 8 mo of age. These mice also exhibit skeletal lesions similar to that in patients with neurofibromatosis who have a mutation in the *NF-1* gene. Dysregulation of cytokines, in particular granulocyte-macrophage colony-stimulating factor (GM-CSF), may have resulted in the infiltration of neutrophils associated with these lesions *(80)*. Kitajima and Nerenberg *(81)* decreased the size of these neurofibroma tumors with antisense inhibition of NF-κB, directly demonstrating the importance of this transcription factor in the development of the tumors. A limitation of this line using mice as a model of HTLV-1 is the lack of reports associating the virus with lesions of peripheral nerves. Seeking to understand how the virus targets nervous system tissue, Coscoy and Ozden et al. *(82)* demonstrated that the HTLV-1 promoter directs the expression of lacZ markers in choroid plexus cells, ependymal cells and, occasionally, in neurons. Some lines of *tax* transgenic mice have increased nerve growth factor-, GM-CSF-, and IL-2-receptor expression in their tissues *(83,84)*. The wide array of inflammatory lesions associated with HTLV-1 have long been hypothesized to be mediated by autoimmune reactions triggered by the virus *(78,85–87)*.

5. VIRAL AND HOST FACTORS THAT CONTRIBUTE TO HAM/TSP

For carriers in Japan, the lifetime risk of HAM/TSP is estimated to be 0.23%, based on multiple risk factors *(88)*. Significant progress has been made in the understanding of the risk factors that contribute to the development of HAM/TSP. These studies collectively indicated that the disease is influenced by a complex interplay between host factors, in particular the immune response of infected subjects and viral properties that allow HTLV-1 and HTLV-2 to persist in the presence of a vigorous immune response.

5.1. Human T-Cell Lymphotropic Virus Proviral Load and Patient Gender

Among the factors that have been linked to a higher risk of HAM/TSP is a high HTLV-1 proviral load *(51,89–92)*. PBMCs of HAM/TSP patients have ~16-fold more proviral DNA than do asymptomatic carriers *(93,94)*. Patients with proviral loads representing more than 1% of the total PBMC may have a significantly higher risk of HAM/TSP, suggesting that increased viral loads contribute to the development of lesions *(11)*. In patients with HAM/TSP, the anti-HTLV-1 antibody titer, which parallels the number of viral-infected PBMC, is a useful correlate to predict HAM/TSP in HTLV-1 carriers *(89,91)*.

5.2. Host Genetic Factors

Host genetic factors have been demonstrated to clearly have a role in the development of HTLV-1-associated diseases, including HAM/TSP. Asymptomatic carriers from families of patients with HAM/TSP were found to have elevated proviral loads, compared to unrelated asymptomatic carriers *(95)*, suggesting the role of inherited traits in the control of HTLV-1 proviral loads. Certain human leukocyte antigen (HLA) alleles have been associated with a lower risk of developing HAM/TSP, whereas other HLA alleles have been linked to a higher risk of developing ATLL *(96–98)*. HLA-A*02 and Cw*08 are associated with lower patient HTLV-1 proviral loads and a reduced risk of developing HAM/TSP, whereas HLA-B*5401 is associated with higher proviral loads and an elevated risk of developing HAM/TSP *(96,97)*. Additionally, HLA-DRB1*0101 was linked to a higher risk of HAM/TSP *(99)*, which was later demonstrated to be only in the absence of the protective effect linked to HLA-A*02 *(96)*. Intriguingly, those individuals with major histocompatibility complex (MHC) class I molecules linked to a higher risk of ATLL, such as HLA-A*26, HLAB*4002, HLA-B*4006, and HLA-B*4801, have anchoring regions, unable to bind to 69 different HTLV-1 *tax* peptides and are thus predicted to be unable to produce efficient *tax*-specific cytotoxic T lymphocytes (CTL) responses, characteristic of HAM/TSP *(98)*. On the other hand, MHC class I molecules predisposing to persons to HAM/TSP likely have a strong affinity through anchoring regions for binding *tax* peptides and thus are able to generate a strong CTL response against HTLV-1-infected cells and also against resident CNS cells, leading to HAM/TSP. In support of this contention, patients with HAM/TSP exhibit elevated HTLV-1-specific CTL activity, whereas patients with ATLL have been found in some studies to have lower HTLV-1-specific CTL activity *(100,101)*; however, these findings and theories are not unequivocal. For example, the frequency of HLA-A*02 allele considered to be protective in HAM/TSP *(96)* is similar in some studies of asymptomatic carriers and patients with HAM/TSP *(98)*. Moreover, this allele is also found in patients with ATLL. In addition, stromal cell-derived factor 1 +801A 3' untranslated region, and IL-15 191C alleles have been recently linked to a lower risk for developing HAM/TSP, whereas the promoter TNF-863A allele was associated with higher risk for developing HAM/TSP *(102)*.

5.3. Strain Variations in HTLV-1

There have been several studies attempting to identify viral strains that are uniquely neuropathogenic or leukemogenic; however to date, unique viral strains associated with neurologic disease have not been conclusively identified *(89,103–107)*. Most of these studies focused on variation in the HTLV-1 *tax* gene. In addition to being recognized by HTLV-1-specific CD8[+] T cells, *tax* is a strong transactivator of many host genes, such as inflammatory cytokines and their receptors. The role of *tax* in the pathogenesis of HAM/TSP is not completely understood; however, it is thought that a variation of HTLV-1 *tax* could cause changes in host immune functions and disease progression.

Based on the high frequency of defective proviruses carrying only part of the *tax* gene in the CNS of patients with HAM/TSP, *tax* was suggested to have a role in the development of the disease *(108)*.

Sequence analysis of HTLV-1 *tax* in patients with HAM/TSP and asymptomatic carriers revealed that four nucleotide substitutions in the *tax* gene increase the risk of HAM/TSP *(109)*. Another study of monozygotic twins and their infected mothers and brothers who also had HAM/TSP indicated that three infected individuals had the consensus *tax* sequence, whereas the asymptomatic twin carried sequence variations in five nucleotide positions, including four substitutions resulting in amino acid changes *(110)*. Some patients with ATLL had cells containing HTLV-1 proviral mutants with large deletions of *tax* or premature stop codons in the 5´ half of *tax* *(111)*. Renjifo et al. *(112)* also reported that amino acid substitutions in *tax* are associated with HAM/TSP, but Mahieux et al. *(113)* refuted this, reporting that HAM/TSP is simply linked to the cosmopolitan genotype.

Other viral proteins are also thought to contribute to the diversity in diseases caused by HTLV-1. HTLV-1 accessory protein p12^I, which is a product of the pX open reading frame I (ORF-I), is associated with immature forms of the MHC class I, interferes with the interaction of MHC class I with β_2-microglobulin, decreases the surface expression of transfected MHC-I, directs its degradation in the proteasome, and is coexpressed in Hela-Tat cells *(114,115)*. These results suggest that p12^I might help the virus escape immune surveillance by downregulating MHC class I surface expression. Interestingly, proteasome destabilization of viral proteins is considered to be an intracellular defense mechanism against viral infection *(116,117)*. Lysine is a known target for covalent binding of ubiquitin *(118)*, and the metabolic instability of p12^I is mediated in part by ubiquitylation at a single lysine residue at position 88 and subsequent proteasomal degradation, as well as by destabilizing residues at its amino terminus *(119)*.

Interestingly, earlier analysis of p12^I ORF in 21 HTLV-1 strains from different geographical areas *(120)* had demonstrated that the p12^I amino acid sequence is highly conserved and that an arginine residue is found more frequently at position 88, whereas the less frequent lysine-carrying allele was found only in some HAM/TSP cases. Trovato et al. *(119)* extended this information by studying an additional 32 ex vivo samples from healthy carriers, patients with HAM/TSP or ATLL, and families in which both diseases occur, and confirmed that the lysine residue is found only in patients with TSP/HAM, regardless of geographical locations, suggesting that a selective pressure over p12^I might occur in the host; however, lysine residue at position 88 in p12^I was not found in all patients with HAM/TSP. It is hypothesized that the reduced stability of p12^I in patients with HAM/TSP caused by this sequence variation may facilitate generation of a viral-specific CTL response, since degradation of p12^I would alleviate the reduction of MHC class I molecules at the cell surface. This lysine residue at position 88 of p12^I did not appear to be a universal diagnostic marker for HTLV-1-associated neurological disease, since this phenotype was found not only in patients with HAM/TSP patients but also in asymptomatic HTLV-1 carriers who did not develop neurologic signs *(121)*. A limitation of most studies is the analysis of samples from individuals who were born in the same geographic region, and thus, these findings might simply represent a particular HTLV-1 carrier population in which the selective pressure on the p12^I sequence would not occur. Therefore, the significance of natural p12^I alleles is unclear, and it is possible that the lysine at position 88 of p12^I might have a significant effect on the biological effects of the protein in the host, including giving a possible selective advantage in individuals with a certain MHC class I. Thus, to date the role of HTLV-1 sequence variation does not appear to be a significant factor in the pathogenesis of HAM/TSP, and most evidence indicates host immunologic factors are more important determinants of HTLV-1-associated neurological disease.

5.4. Route of Infection

HTLV-1 and HTLV-2 are highly cell-associated viruses and are transmitted by routes that favor preservation of infected cells. Consequently, these viruses are transmitted by exposure to whole blood or blood products that contain intact cells, intravenous drug use, sexual transmission (predominantly from male seminal fluid), and breastfeeding *(90,122)*. Exposure to HTLV-1 via blood transfusion has been associated with the development of HAM/TSP *(123)*, whereas mucosal exposure has been linked to the development of ATLL *(122,124)*. In a rat model of HTLV-1 infection, oral inoculation of HTLV-1-infected cells resulted in immune unresponsiveness in spite of persistent HTLV-1 infection *(125)*. Oral vs intravenous routes of infection in rats has revealed differences in levels of anti-HTLV-1 antibodies and proliferative T-cell response against the virus, indicating that oral exposure may result in a reduced antiviral immune response *(73)*. From these data, investigators have hypothesized that the absence of an effective T-cell response in subjects exposed via mucosal or oral routes might lead to survival and subsequent transformation of the infected cell population, resulting in ATLL. On the other hand, intravenous inoculation may result in a vigorous immune response that, in the process of elimination of cells infected with HTLV-1, may promote inflammation in the CNS typical of HAM/TSP *(33)*. Collectively, these studies suggest that the route of infection, in particular intravenous inoculation of HTLV-1-infected cells, influences the immune response generated against the virus and contributes to the incidence of HAM/TSP in patients exposed by this route.

5.5. *The Host Immune Response to HTLV-1*

Patients with HAM/TSP exhibit 10 to 100-fold increases in proviral DNA in their peripheral blood, compared to asymptomatic, but infected, subjects *(90,126)*. Furthermore, when an infected subject's proviral load is more than 1% of PBMCs, there is higher risk of HAM/TSP *(11)*, although HAM/TSP occurs in some patients with a low proviral DNA load, indicating that a high proviral DNA load by itself is not a conclusive predictor for the development of HAM/TSP *(11)*. Most studies support the hypothesis that the progression to HAM/TSP is influenced by an interaction of host factors, including the immune response, viral factors, and high proviral DNA load. Typically, T-cell transformation is a feature of ATLL, whereas cellular destruction and inflammation are a feature of HAM/TSP. These distinctive characteristics might account for the fact that there are very few patients with both ATLL and HAM/TSP. Similarly, these diseases differ in various immunologic parameters related to HTLV-1 infection. Although CD4$^+$ T cells, CD8$^+$ T cells, and activated macrophages are present within white-matter lesions of patients with HAM/ TSP *(127)*, leukemic cells in ATLL are mostly CD4$^+$ T cells and occasionally are CD4/CD8 double-positive *(17,18)*. Peripheral blood and the CSF of patients with HAM/TSP have high levels of proinflammatory cytokines, such as IFN-γ, TNF-α, IL-1, and IL-6, suggesting the importance of these proinflammatory cytokines in HAM/TSP *(128–131)*. Additionally, CSF of these patients contains activated lymphocytes, suggesting that activated lymphocytes and macrophages also have a role in the development of HAM/TSP *(127)*.

Patients with HAM/TSP develop a vigorous expansion of CD8$^+$ T cells, compared to asymptomatic carriers *(132)* and HTLV-1 *tax*-specific CTLs are readily demonstrated in the CSF of these patients *(133)*. In fact, patients with HAM/TSP have about 40 to 280-fold more *tax*-specific precursor CTLs than do asymptomatic carriers, consistent with an increase in virus-specific CD8$^+$ CTL response in these patients. Additionally, patients with HAM/TSP have high levels of anti-HTLV-1 antibodies in serum and CSF *(134)*. Studies of peripheral blood and CSF from the same patient with HAM/TSP have revealed *tax*-specific CTLs to be about twofold higher in the CSF, suggesting the possible role of *tax*-specific CTLs in the cellular destruction and inflammation in the CNS of these patients *(133)*. Activated CTLs are present in active inflammatory lesions in the spinal cords of patients with HAM/TSP *(92,135)*. The mechanism of cell destruction by *tax*-specific CTLs is not elucidated; however, it is proposed that CTLs could directly kill not only HTLV-1-infected cells expressing *tax* but also CNS cells expressing a crossreactive cellular determinant and neighboring uninfected neuronal cells by apoptosis mediated via the toxic inflammatory cytokines *(18)*.

6. VIRAL ENTRY INTO THE CENTRAL NERVOUS SYSTEM

HTLV-1-infected cells are present in the CNS of patients with HAM/TSP. These patients also have higher HTLV-1 proviral loads in the CSF than in their PBMCs *(136)*. The HTLV-1 integration site in the cellular DNA of HTLV-1-infected lymphocytes was the same in the CSF and peripheral blood of these patients, indicating that HTLV-1-infected cells in peripheral blood migrate to the CNS and accumulate in lesions in patients with HAM/TSP *(137,138)*. The mechanism of selective migration of HTLV-1-infected cells to the CNS of these patients is not clear. CD4$^+$ T cells from patients with HAM/TSP have an enhanced ability to attach and transmigrate through reconstituted basement membranes in vitro and endothelial cells, compared with CD4$^+$ T cells from asymptomatic carriers *(139,140)*, indicating that these cells likely have more ability to migrate into the CNS across the blood–brain barrier (BBB). Additionally, close contact between brain endothelial cells and HTLV-1-infected CD4$^+$ T cells causes increased production of TNF-α, likely increasing the paracellular permeability of the brain endothelial monolayer and transmigration of activated T cells and monocytes across the BBB. Romero et al. *(141)* demonstrated that viral particles were taken up into vesicles by brain endothelial cells and released from the basolateral surface, whereas HTLV-1-infected T cells fuse to brain endothelial cells. Based on these observations, mechanisms proposed for the entry of HTLV-1 into the CNS of patients with HAM/TSP include paracellular transmigration of virus-infected cells through the BBB, absorption and release of viral particles from vesicles within brain endothelial cells, and direct infection of brain endothelial cells *(127)*. Adhesion molecules are considered critical for this migration, correlating with the increased expression of vascular cell adhesion molecule-1 expression in spinal cord lesions *(142)* and very late antigen-4 (VLA-4), as well as monocyte chemoattractant protein-1 in perivascular inflammatory infiltrates and matrix metalloproteinase (MMP)-2 and MMP-9 in infiltrating mononuclear cells of HAM/TSP patients *(143)*. In addition, α4β1 and α5β1 integrins appear to be overexpressed in HTLV-1-infected T cells of patients with HAM/TSP *(144)*.

After entering the CNS, HTLV-1-infected CD4$^+$ and CD8$^+$ T cells are believed to participate in a number of events, resulting in infection of resident CNS cell populations, activation of astrocytes and microglial cells, induction of proinflammatory cytokine and chemokine synthesis, recruitment of inflammatory infiltrates into the CNS, BBB disruption, dysregulation of oligodendrocyte homeostasis, demyelination, and axonal degradation *(145)*. Within the CNS, astrocytes and microglial cells are susceptible to HTLV-1 infection *(43,146,147)*, presumably serving to promote increased production of proinflammatory cytokines and chemokines and to recruit of antigen-specific CD4$^+$ and CD8$^+$ T cells from the circulation.

7. MECHANISM OF VIRAL PERSISTENCE, DESPITE A STRONG IMMUNE RESPONSE

Among the many characteristics of HTLV-1 that influence viral persistence, one important peculiarity of this virus is its low rate of evolution and low sequence diversity, in contrast to human immunodeficiency virus-1. A number of mechanisms have been postulated to explain how this retrovirus maintains persistence yet elicits a prominent immune response in infected individuals. In this regard, it is important to understand that the virus may be spread either by infectiously (primarily from infected cells) or by mitotic division of infected cells (replication of the integrated provirus during cell division) *(148)*, although based on the relatively lower level of variability in sequence, HTLV-1 is thought to be maintained mainly by mitotic transmission and proliferation of cells harboring the provirus, since this route is associated with a much lower rate of mutation *(17)* than infectious transmission. In support of this hypothesis, clonal expansion of infected CD4$^+$ and CD8$^+$ T-cell populations have been observed in patients with HAM/TSP *(137,148,149)*. In contrast and perhaps not mutually exclusive are observations that some patients form a persistent and vigorous CTL response against HTLV-1 *tax*, and this accounts for reduced proviral loads and protection against HAM/TSP; these studies suggest the existence of active viral gene expression in vivo *(89)*. Based upon positive responses to treatments with the nucleoside analogue lamivudine (3TC), a reverse transcriptase inhibitor, Taylor et al. *(150)* has speculated that HTLV-1 must undergo reverse transcription and maintain *tax* expression to elicit a high frequency of *tax*-specific CD8$^+$ T cells. Recent studies suggest that an elevated proportion of HTLV-1-infected cells (10–80%) express *tax* within 12 h of infection and thus stimulate a high frequency of *tax*-specific CTLs *(17,89)*. These in turn are stimulated to divide rapidly but are made highly susceptible to *tax*-specific CTL-mediated lysis. The virus cannot complete the replication cycle because of limited availability of activated susceptible host cells and the rapid CTL-mediated lysis; thus, mitotic spread might be responsible for the maintenance of the proviral load, possibly accounting for the low rate of mutation and evolution *(17)*. Furthermore, this sequence of events would also account for the immunodominance of *tax* as a target antigen for CTLs, since *tax*-expressing cells appear to be susceptible to CTL lysis before expressing other viral proteins. Since *tax* is essential for the maintenance of proviral load, generation of strong CTL response to *tax* possibly lowers proviral load and susceptibility to HAM/TSP *(89)*. Thus, host factors may determine the strength or efficiency of CTL response to HTLV-1 and an individual's proviral load and their risk of HAM/TSP. Equally likely in this balance is the tenet that CTLs might contribute to the inflammation in HAM/TSP *(90,151)*. The concentration of antigen necessary to elicit IFN-γ secretion by a CD8$^+$ T cell is greater than for target cell lysis. Based upon this immunological principal, it has been suggested that a patients balance between an active CTL response and control of virus replication vs an overactive immune response with IFN-γ secretion that promotes inflammation is a key determinant of whether a patient develops HAM/TSP *(89)*.

8. PROPOSED MECHANISMS OF PATHOGENESIS

Immunologic mechanisms are generally considered to have a significant role in the pathogenesis of HAM/TSP. This belief is strongly supported by studies indicating that patients with HAM/TSP have elevated cellular and humoral anti-HTLV-1 immune responses in comparison to asymptomatic carriers and seronegative controls. The virus predominantly targets CD4$^+$ T cells *(152–155)*, which have increased adhesion activity to endothelial cells, promoting transmigrating activity through basement membranes *(156)* and secreting proinflammatory cytokines, such as IFN-γ and TNF-α *(157)*. Both the peripheral blood and CSF of patients with HAM/TSP contain HTLV-1-specific HLA class I-restricted CD8$^+$ CTLs *(100)*, with activity mostly against pX gene products, especially the *Tax* 11–19 peptide (LLFGYPVYV) *(158)*. With spinal cord lesions, the presence of CD8$^+$ T cells, presumably in response to CD4$^+$ T cells expressing HTLV-1 proteins, suggests a direct involvement of these cells in lesion development *(37,41)*. These HTLV-1-specific CD8$^+$ CTLs most likely mediate target cell destruction through perforin-dependent mechanisms or the production of inflammatory cytokines and chemoattractants *(159,160)*, although the mechanism of maintaining these CD8$^+$ T cells during the prolonged course of infection is not certain. Although IL-15 may have a role in the disease *(161)*, it is also thought that viral antigens continuously drive these cells in vivo *(91)*.

An autoimmune mechanism has also been proposed to be involved in the pathogenesis of HAM/TSP, as in inflammatory neurological diseases, such as multiple sclerosis (MS) and Guillain-Barre syndrome. In support of this hypothesis, researchers have demonstrated that infiltrating lymphocytes in the spinal cord lesions of patients with HAM/TSP have a unique T-cell receptor CDR3 motif, which is also found in brain lesions in patients with MS and experimental autoimmune encephalomyelitis *(162)*. An HTLV-1-infected CD4$^+$ T-cell clone derived from the peripheral blood of a patient with HAM/TSP showed a proliferative response to crude protein extracted from seronegative spinal cord samples but not to proteins from lymph nodes *(11)*, whereas the HTLV-1 *tax*-specific CD8$^+$ CTL clones recognized and lysed self-peptide-pulsed target cells in vitro *(163)*.

Another hypothesis couples infection with autoimmune disease. Molecular mimicry has also been implicated in the pathogenesis of diseases, such as diabetes, lupus, and MS, in which there is little direct evidence linking causative agents to pathogenic immune reactions. Molecular mimicry is characterized by an immune response to an environmental agent that crossreacts with a host antigen, resulting in disease. The clinical presentation of HAM/TSP is often difficult to distinguish from MS. In this regard, serum immunoglobulin (IgG) from HAM/TSP patients reacted to neurons in human CNS not infected with HTLV-1 but not to cells in the peripheral nervous system or other organs, and more importantly, the reactivity could be abrogated by pretreatment with recombinant *tax* protein *(164)*. Interestingly, IgG from patients with HAM/TSP identified hetero-geneous nuclear ribonuclear protein-A1 as the autoantigen *(164)*. It was hypothesized that axons are preferentially damaged by such autoantibodies, which inhibits neuronal firing.

9. TREATMENT AND PREVENTION

To date, effective treatments against the devastating neurological complications of HAM/TSP or preventive measures to stop the development of the disease in HTLV-1-infected patients have had limited success. Interventions with corticosteroids, plasmapheresis, IFN, and antiretroviral drugs have been used as treatments in patients with HAM/TSP with poor or inconsistent results, although virological and clinical improvement has been obtained patients with HAM/TSP who were treated with zidovudine and/or lamivudine *(150)*. Inhibition of HTLV reverse transcriptase, along with the cytostatic effect of some nucleoside analogues, including zidovudine, is thought to reduce the virus' replication, as well as the proviral load; however, the clinical consequences of this need further examination *(165)*. Based on the finding that MMPs, specifically MMP-2 and MMP-9, have important roles in the breakdown of the BBB in the CNS of patients with HAM/TSP, *N*-biphenyl sulphonyl-phenylalanine hydroxamic acid, a selective inhibitor of MMP-2 and MMP-9, was recently used tested as an inhibitor of the migrating activity of CD4$^+$ T cells in patients with HAM/TSP and was found effective, suggesting its therapeutic potential against HAM/TSP *(166)*. In the past, some cases of TSP have responded to steroids, such as prednisone and danazol. These are generally considered useful in the clinical management of patients, partic-ularly females, with HAM/TSP *(167)*. Prednisolone, IFN-α, fosfomycin, high-dose vitamin C, blood purification therapy, heparin, sulfapyridine, thyrotropin-releasing hormone, erythromycin, and mizoribine have been found useful in improving motor disability in patients with HAM/TSP, although success rates vary *(168,169)*. Rolipram, a phosphodiesterase type IV inhibitor was demonstrated to inhibit TNF-α production in HTLV-1-infected cells lines and peripheral blood cells of patients with HAM/TSP, to variable degrees *(168,170)*. Overall, an effective and long-term therapeutic protocol or specific drug that treats HAM/TSP is lacking.

Multiple factors favor development of a vaccine against HTLV-1: the virus displays relatively low antigenic variability, natural immunity occurs in humans, and experimental vaccination with the envelope antigen has been successful in animal models *(171–173)*. There have been sugges-tions that gene therapy to control virus replication may be useful against HAM/TSP *(174)*, although, thus far, there is no successful gene therapy or vaccine for HAM/TSP, owing in part to the lack of animal models that can be used for testing. In addition, the low incidence and unpre-dictability of onset of clinical signs of the disease among those infected with the virus makes clinical trial accrual problematic.

10. CONCLUSION AND FUTURE DIRECTIONS

It is critical that future studies focus on therapeutic and prevention strategies of HTLV-1-associated diseases. Although the clinical symptoms of these diseases are well characterized, the pathogenesis is not clearly understood. Our understanding of the risk factors for HAM/TSP has increased tremendously, and many theories have been proposed concerning pathogenic mecha-nisms of the disease. Many of these theories on pathogenesis and immune response are contradictory, and additional studies are necessary to elucidate this apparent dichotomy in our understanding. Nevertheless, the knowledge of risk factors and possible pathogenesis mechanisms should enable us, in the near future, to predict the risk of progression from asymptomatic carrier stage to HAM/TSP. Future studies directed toward understanding the role of cell-mediated immunity in HTLV-1 infection will likely lead to further clarification of the pathogenesis of HAM/TSP. This knowledge, in turn, will provide valuable directions to develop efficient therapeutic and pre-ventive strategies against HAM/TSP. Recent studies have provided new information about repli-cation strategies used by the virus to regulate its gene expression and will undoubtedly help in the effort to understand the role of viral-mediated events vs immune-mediated damage in HAM/TSP. Additional studies of the transcriptional regulation of the long terminal repeat during cell activation should facilitate the design of therapeutic strategies to prevent the initiation of viral gene expression within the peripheral blood and CNS. Studies of proviral DNA and viral gene expression in the peripheral blood and CNS during clinical latency and HAM/TSP would also provide important information.

There has been great progress in the development of new animal models that exhibit many of the pathological features associated with HAM/TSP and ATLL, and future studies to refine these animal models would clarify the early events that take place after initial exposure of the host to HTLV-1 and the kinetics of viral gene expression in various cell types and stages of disease development.

Gene array studies to identify patterns of gene expression in various stages in asymptomatic carriers and patients with ATLL or HAM/TSP would provide valuable insight into the pathogenesis of these diseases. The ultimate goal of these studies is to prevent the onset of the devastating neurological diseases associated with HTLV-1 infection.

REFERENCES

1. Poiesz BJ, Ruscetti FW, Gazdar AF, Bunn PA, Minna JD, Gallo RC. Detection and isolation of type C retrovirus particles from fresh and cultured lymphocytes of a patient with cutaneous T-cell lymphoma. Proc Natl Acad Sci USA 1980;77:7415–7419.
2. Hinuma Y, Nagata K, Hanaoka M, et al. Adult T Cell Leukemia: antigens in an ATL cell line and detection of antibodies to antigen in human sera. Proc Natl Acad Sci USA 1981;78:6476–6480.
3. Miyoshi I, Kubonishi I, Yoshimoto S, et al. Type C virus particles in a cord T-cell line derived by co-cultivating normal human cord leukocytes and human leukaemic T cells. Nature 1981;294:770–771.
4. Yoshida M, Miyoshi I, Hinuma Y. Isolation and characterization of retrovirus from cell lines of human T-cell leukemia and its implication in the disease. Proc Natl Acad Sci U S A 1982;79:2031–2035.
5. Kalyanaraman VS, Sarngadharan MG, Robert-Guroff M, Miyoshi I, Golde D, Gallo RC. A new subtype of human T-cell leukemia virus (HTLV-II) associated with a T-cell variant of hairy cell leukemia. Science 1982;218:571–573.
6. Osame M, Usuku K, Izumo S, et al. HTLV-I associated myelopathy, a new clinical entity. Lancet 1986;1(8488):1031–1032.
7. Gessain A, Barin F, Vernant J, et al. Antibodies to human T lymphotropic virus type 1 in patients with tropical spastic paresis. Lancet 1985;2:407–410.
8. Zehender G, Colasante C, Santambrogio S, De Maddalena C, Massetto B, Cavalli B et al. Increased risk of developing peripheral neuropathy in patients coinfected with HIV-1 and HTLV-2. J Acquir Immune Defic Syndr 2002;314:440–447.
9. Lowis GW, Sheremata WA, Minagar A. Epidemiologic features of HTLV-II: serologic and molecular evidence. Ann Epidemiol 2002;121:46–66.
10. Edlich RF, Arnette JA, Williams FM. Global epidemic of human T-cell lymphotropic virus type-I (HTLV-I). J Emerg Med 2000;181:109–119.
11. Nagai M, Osame M. Human T-cell lymphotropic virus type I and neurological diseases. J Neurovirol 2003;92:228–235.
12. Courouce AM, Pillonel J, Lemaire JM, Saura C. HTLV testing in blood transfusion. Vox Sang 1998;74(Suppl 2):165–169.
13. Ferreira OC, Planelles V, Rosenblatt JD. Human T-cell leukemia viruses: epidemiology, biology, and pathogenesis. Blood Rev 1997;112:91–104.
14. Murphy EL, Glynn SA, Fridey J, et al. Increased incidence of infectious diseases during prospective follow-up of human T-lymphotropic virus type II- and I-infected blood donors. Arch Intern Med 1999;159:1485–1491.
15. Murphy EL, Busch MP, Tong M, Cornett P, Vyas GN. A prospective study of the risk of transfusion-acquired viral infections. Transfus Med 1998;83:173–178.
16. Schreiber GB, Murphy EL, Horton JA, et al. Risk factors for human T-cell lymphotropic virus types I and II HTLV-I and -II. in blood donors: the Retrovirus Epidemiology Donor Study. NHLBI Retrovirus Epidemiology Donor Study. J Acquir Immune Defic Syndr Hum Retrovirol 1997;143:263–271.
17. Mortreux F, Gabet AS, Wattel E. Molecular and cellular aspects of HTLV-1 associated leukemogenesis in vivo. Leukemia 2003;171:26–38.
18. Barmak K, Harhaj E, Grant C, Alefantis T, Wigdahl B. Human T cell leukemia virus type I-induced disease: pathways to cancer and neurodegeneration. Virology 2003;3081:1–12.
19. Fujino T, Nagata Y. HTLV-I transmission from mother to child. J Reprod Immunol 2000;472:197–206.
20. Adedayo O, Grell G, Bellot P. Hospital admissions for human T-cell lymphotropic virus type-1 (HTLV-1) associated diseases in Dominica. Postgrad Med J 2003;79:341–344.

21. Kasahata N, Shiota J, Miyazawa Y, Nakano I, Murayama S. Acute human T-lymphotropic virus type 1-associated myelopathy: a clinicopathologic study. Arch Neurol 2003;606:873–876.

22. Furukawa Y, Kubota R, Eiraku N, et al. Human T-cell lymphotropic virus type I (HTLV-I)-related clinical and laboratory findings for HTLV-I-infected blood donors. J Acquir Immune Defic Syndr 2003;323:328–334.

23. Kiwaki T, Umehara F, Arimura Y, et al. The clinical and pathological features of peripheral neuropathy accompanied with HTLV-I associated myelopathy. J Neurol Sci 2003;206:17–21.

24. Castillo LC, Gracia F, Roman GC, Levine P, Reeves WC, Kaplan J. Spinocerebellar syndrome in patients infected with human T-lymphotropic virus types I and II (HTLV-I/HTLV-II): report of 3 cases from Panama. Acta Neurol Scand 2000;101:405–412.

25. Alamy AH, Menezes FB, Leite AC, Nascimento OM, Araujo AQ. Dysautonomia in human T-cell lymphotrophic virus type I-associated myelopathy/tropical spastic paraparesis. Ann Neurol 2001;50:681–685.

26. Matsuzaki T, Nakagawa M, Nagai M, et al. HTLV-I proviral load correlates with progression of motor disability in HAM/TSP: analysis of 239 HAM/TSP patients including 64 patients followed up for 10 years. J Neurovirol 2001;7:228–234.

27. Suga R, Tobimatsu S, Kira J, Kato M. Motor and somatosensory evoked potential findings in HTLV-I associated myelopathy. J Neurol Sci 1999;167:102–106.

28. Godoy AJ, Kira J, Hasuo K, Goto I. Characterization of cerebral white matter lesions of HTLV-I-associated myelopathy tropical spastic paraparesis in comparison with multiple sclerosis and collagen-vasculitis: a semiquantitative MRI study. J Neurol Sci 1995;133:102–111.

29. Fukushima T, Ikeda T, Uyama E, Uchino M, Okabe H, Ando M. Cognitive event-related potentials and brain magnetic resonance imaging in HTLV-1 associated myelopathy (HAM). J Neurol Sci 1994;126:30–39.

30. Kira J, Goto I, Otsuka M, Ichiya Y. Chronic progressive spinocerebellar syndrome associated with antibodies to human T-lymphotropic virus type-I—Clinico-virological and magnetic resonance imaging studies. J Neurol Sci 1993;115:111–116.

31. Kira JI, Fujihara K, Itoyama Y, Goto I, Hasuo K. Leukoencephalopathy in HTLV-I-associated mylopathy/tropical spastic paraparesis: MRI analysis and a two year follow up study after corticosteroid therapy. J Neurol Sci 1991;106:41–49.

32. Silva MT, Mattos P, Alfano A, Araujo AQ. Neuropsychological assessment in HTLV-1 infection: a comparative study among TSP/HAM, asymptomatic carriers, and healthy controls. J Neurol Neurosurg Psychiatry 2003;74:1085–1089.

33. Osame M. Pathological mechanisms of human T-cell lymphotropic virus type I-associated myelopathy (HAM/TSP). J Neurovirol 2002;8:359–364.

34. Umehara F, Abe M, Koreeda Y, Izumo S, Osame M. Axonal damage revealed by accumulation of beta-amyloid precursor protein in HTLV-I-associated myelopathy. J Neurol Sci 2000;176:95–101.

35. McKendall RR, Oas J, Lairmore MD. HTLV-I-associated myelopathy endemic in Texas-born residents and isolation of virus from CSF cells. Neurology 1991;41:831–836.

36. Izumo S, Umehara F, Osame M. HTLV-I-associated myelopathy. Neuropathology 2000;20(Suppl):S65–S68.

37. Umehara F, Izumo S, Ronquillo AT, Matsumuro K, Sato E, Osame M. Cytokine expression in the spinal cord lesions in HTLV-I-associated myelopathy. J Neuropathol Exp Neurol 1994;53:72–77.

38. Umehara F, Izumo S, Nakagawa M, et al. Immunocytochemical analysis of the cellular infiltrate in the spinal cord lesions in HTLV-I-Associated myelopathy. J Neuropathol Exp Neurol 1993;52:424–430.

39. Kubota R, Furukawa Y, Izumo S, Usuku K, Osame M. Degenerate specificity of HTLV-1-specific CD8+ T cells during viral replication in patients with HTLV-1-associated myelopathy (HAM/TSP). Blood 2003;101:3074–3081.

40. Abe M, Umehara F, Kubota R, Moritoyo T, Izumo S, Osame M. Activation of macrophages microglia with the calcium-binding proteins MRP14 and MRP8 is related to the lesional activities in the spinal cord of HTLV-I associated myelopathy. J Neurol 1999;246:358–364.

41. Kubota R, Umehara F, Izumo S, Ijichi S, Matsumuro K, Yashiki S et al. HTLV-I proviral DNA amount correlates with infiltrating CD4+ lymphocytes in the spinal cord from patients with HTLV-I-associated myelopathy. J Neuroimmunol 1994;53:23–29.

42. Moritoyo T, Reinhart TA, Moritoyo H, et al. Human T-lymphotropic virus type I-associated myelopathy and tax gene expression in CD4(+) T lymphocytes. Ann Neurol 1996;40:84–90.

43. Lehky TJ, Fox CH, Koenig S, et al. Detection of human T-lymphotropic virus type I (HTLV-I) tax RNA in the central nervous system of HTLV-I-associated myelopathy/tropical spastic paraparesis patients by in situ hybridization. Ann Neurol 1995;37:167–175.

44. Ohta M, Ohta K, Nishimura M, Saida T. Detection of myelin basic protein in cerebrospinal fluid and serum from patients with HTLV-1-associated myelopathy/tropical spastic paraparesis. Ann Clin Biochem 2002;39(Pt 6): 603–605.

45. Akagi T, Takeda I, Oka T, Ohtsuki Y, Yano S, Miyoshi I. Experimental infection of rabbits with human T-cell leukemia virus type 1. Jpn J Cancer Res 1985;76:86–94.

46. Lairmore MD, Roberts B, Frank D, Rovnak J, Weiser MG, Cockerell GL. Comparative biological responses of rabbits infected with human T-lymphotropic virus Type I isolates from patients with lymphoproliferative and neurodegenerative disease. Int J Cancer 1992;50:124–130.

47. Murata N, Hakoda E, Machida H, et al. Prevention of human T cell lymphotropic virus type 1 infection in Japanese macaques by passive immunization. Leukemia 1996;10:1971–1974.

48. Nakamura H, Hayami M, Ohta Y, et al. Protection of cynomolgus monkeys against infection by human T-cell leukemia virus type-1 by immunization with viral env gene products produced in Escerichia coli. Int J Cancer 1987;40:403–407.

49. Suga T, Kameyama T, Shimotohno K, et al. Infection of rats with HTLV-1: a Small-Animal model for HTLV-1 carriers. Int J Cancer 1991;49:764–769.

50. Ibrahim F, Fiette L, Gessain A, Buisson N, Dethe G, Bomford R. Infection of rats with human T-cell leukemia virus type-1: susceptibility of inbred strains, antibody response and provirus location. Int J Cancer 1994;58:446–451.

51. Nitta T, Tanaka M, Sun B, Hanai S, Miwa M. The genetic background as a determinant of human T-cell leukemia virus type 1 proviral load. Biochem Biophys Res Commun 2003;309:161–165.

52. Furuta RA, Sugiura K, Kawakita S, et al. Mouse model for the equilibration interaction between the host immune system and human T-cell leukemia virus type 1 gene expression. J Virol 2002;76:2703–2713.

53. Furuta RA, Sugiura K, Kawakita S, et al. Mouse model for the equilibration interaction between the host immune system and human T-cell leukemia virus type 1 gene expression. J Virol 2002;76:2703–2713.

54. Feng R, Kabayama A, Uchida K, Hoshino H, Miwa M. Cell-free entry of human T-cell leukemia virus type 1 to mouse cells. Jpn J Cancer Res 2001;92:410–416.

55. Fang JH, Kushida S, Feng RQ, et al. Transmission of human T-cell leukemia virus type 1 to mice. J Virol 1998;72:3952–3957.

56. Leendertz FH, Boesch C, Junglen S, Pauli G, Ellerbrook H. Characterization of a new simian T-lymphocyte virus type 1 (STLV-1) in a wild living chimpanzee (Pan troglodytes verus) from Ivory Coast: evidence of a new STLV-1 group? AIDS Res Hum Retroviruses 2003;19:255–258.

57. Niphuis H, Verschoor EJ, Bontjer I, Peeters M, Heeney JL. Reduced transmission and prevalence of simian T-cell lymphotropic virus in a closed breeding colony of chimpanzees (Pan troglodytes verus). J Gen Virol 2003;84(Pt 3):615–620.

58. Gabet AS, Gessain A, Wattel E. High simian T-cell leukemia virus type 1 proviral loads combined with genetic stability as a result of cell-associated provirus replication in naturally infected, asymptomatic monkeys. Int J Cancer 2003;107:74–83.

59. Takemura T, Yamashita M, Shimada MK, et al. High prevalence of simian T-lymphotropic virus type L in wild ethiopian baboons. J Virol 2002;76:1642–1648.

60. Mahieux R, Chappey C, Georgescourbot MC, et al. Simian T-cell lymphotropic virus type 1 from Mandrillus sphinx as a simian counterpart of human T-cell lymphotropic virus type 1 subtype D. J Virol 1998;72:10,316–10,322.

61. Voevodin A, Samilchuk E, Schatzl H, Boeri E, Franchini G. Interspecies transmission of macaque simian T-cell leukemia/lymphoma virus type 1 in baboons resulted in an outbreak of malignant lymphoma. J Virol 1996;70:1633–1639.

62. Gessain A, De TG. Geographic and molecular epidemiology of primate T lymphotropic retroviruses: HTLV-I, HTLV-II, STLV-I, STLV-PP, and PTLV-L. [Review]. Adv Vir Res 1996;47:377–426, 377–426.

63. Mortreux F, Kazanji M, Gabet AS, de Thoisy B, Wattel E. Two-step nature of human T-cell leukemia virus type 1 replication in experimentally infected squirrel monkeys (Saimiri sciureus). J Virol 2001;75:1083–1089.

64. Kazanji M, Tartaglia J, Franchini G, et al. Immunogenicity and protective efficacy of recombinant human T-cell leukemia/lymphoma virus type 1 NYVAC and naked DNA vaccine candidates in squirrel monkeys (Saimiri sciureus). J Virol 2001;75:5939–5948.

65. Kazanji M, Ureta-Vidal A, Ozden S, et al. Lymphoid organs as a major reservoir for human T-cell leukemia virus type 1 in experimentally infected squirrel monkeys (Saimiri sciureus): provirus expression, persistence, and humoral and cellular immune responses. J Virol 2000;74:4860–4867.

66. Kazanji M. HTLV type 1 infection in squirrel monkeys (Saimiri sciureus): a promising animal model for HTLV type 1 human infection. AIDS Res Hum Retroviruses 2000;16:1741–1746.

67. Hakata Y, Yamada M, Shida H. Rat CRM1 is responsible for the poor activity of human T–cell leukemia virus type 1 rex protein in rat cells. J Virol 2001;75:11515–11525.

68. Kasai T, Ikeda H, Tomaru U, et al. A rat model of human T lymphocyte virus type I (HTLV-I) infection: in situ detection of HTLV-I provirus DNA in microglia/macrophages in affected spinal cords of rats with HTLV-1-induced chronic progressive myeloneuropathy. Acta Neuropathol 1999;97:107–112.

69. Sun B, Fang J, Yagami K, et al. Age-dependent paraparesis in WKA rats: evaluation of MHC k-haplotype and HTLV-1 infection. J Neurol Sci 1999;167:16–21.

70. Ishiguro N, Abe M, Seto K, et al. A rat model of human T lymphocyte virus type 1 (HTLV-1) infection. 1. Humoral antibody response, provirus integration, and YTLV-1-associated myelopathy/tropical spastic paraparesis-like myelopathy in seronegative HTLV-1 carrier rats. J Exp Med 1992;176:981–989.

71. Hasegawa A, Ohashi T, Hanabuchi S, et al. Expansion of human T-cell leukemia virus type 1 (HTLV-1) reservoir in orally infected rats: inverse correlation with HTLV-1-specific cellular immune response. J Virol 2003;77:2956–2963.

72. Hanabuchi S, Ohashi T, Koya Y, et al. Development of human T-cell leukemia virus type 1-transformed tumors in rats following suppression of T-cell immunity by CD80 and CD86 blockade. J Virol 2000;74:428–435.

73. Kannagi M, Ohashi T, Hanabuchi S, et al. Immunological aspects of rat models of HTLV type 1-infected T lympho-proliferative disease. AIDS Res Hum Retroviruses 2000;16:1737–1740.

74. Ohya O, Tomaru U, Yamashita I, et al. HTLV-I induced myeloneuropathy in WKAH rats: apoptosis and local activation of the HTLV-I pX and TNF-alpha genes implicated in the pathogenesis. Leukemia 1997;11(Suppl 3):255–7, 255–257.

75. Seto K, Abe M, Ohya O, et al. A rat model of HTLV-I infection: development of chronic progressive myeloneuropathy in seropositive WKAH rats and related apoptosis. Acta Neuropathol 1995;89:483–490.

76. Kushida S, Mizusawa H, Matsumura M, et al. High incidence of HAM/TSP-like symptoms in WKA rats after administration of human T-cell leukemia virus type 1-producing cells. J Virol 1994;68:7221–7226.

77. Yoshiki T. Chronic progressive myeloneuropathy in WKAH rats induced by HTLV-I infection as an animal model for HAM/TSP in humans. Intervirology 1995;38:229–237.

78. Nerenberg M, Xu X, Brown DA. Transgenic models of HTLV-I mediated disease and latency. Curr Top Microbiol Immunol 1996;206:175–196.

79. Nerenberg M, Hinrichs SH, Reynolds RK, Khoury G, Jay G. The tat gene of human T-lymphotropic virus type 1 induces mesenchymal tumors in transgenic mice. Science 1987;237:1324–1329.

80. Xu X, Heidenreich O, Kitajima I, et al. Constitutively activated JNK is associated with HTLV-1 mediated tumorigenesis. Oncogene 1996;13:135–142.

81. Kitajima I, Shinohara T, Bilakovics J, Brown DA, Xu X, Nerenberg M. Ablation of transplanted HTLV-I tax-transformed tumors in mice by antisense inhibition of NF-kappa B. Science 1993;259:1523.

82. Coscoy L, Gonzalez-Dunia D, Chirinian-Swan S, Brahic M, Ozden S. Analysis of the expression directed by two HTLV-I promoters in transgenic mice. J Neurovirol 1996;2:336–344.

83. Green J, Begley C, Wagner D, Waldmann TA, Jay G. Trans-activation of granulocyte macrophage colony-stimulating factor and the interleukin 2 receptor in transgenic mice carrying the HTLV-I tax gene. Mol Cell Biol 1989;9:4731–4737.

84. Green JE. Trans activation of nerve growth factor in transgenic mice containing the human T-cell lymphotropic virus type I tax gene. Mol Cell Biol 1997;11:4635–4641.

85. Iwakura Y. Roles of IL-1 in the development of rheumatoid arthritis: consideration from mouse models. Cytokine Growth Factor Rev 2002;13:341–355.

86. Grossman WJ, Ratner L. Transgenic mouse models for HTLV-I infection. J Acquir Immune Defic Syndr Hum Retrovirol 1996;13(Suppl 1):S162–S169.

87. Ozden S, Coscoy L, Gonzalez-Dunia D. HTLV-I transgenic models: an overview. J Acquir Immune Defic Syndr Hum Retrovirol 1996;13(Suppl 1):S154–S161.

88. Kaplan JE, Osame M, Kubota H, et al. The risk of development of HTLV-I-associated myelopathy/tropical spastic paraparesis among persons infected with HTLV-I. J Acq Immun Defic Synd 1990;3:1096–1101.

89. Bangham CR. Human T-lymphotropic virus type 1 (HTLV-1): persistence and immune control. Int J Hematol 2003;78:297–303.

90. Bangham CR. The immune control and cell-to-cell spread of human T-lymphotropic virus type 1. J Gen Virol 2003;84(Pt 12):3177–3189.

91. Yamano Y, Nagai M, Brennan M, et al. Correlation of human T-cell lymphotropic virus type 1 (HTLV-1). mRNA with proviral DNA load, virus-specific CD8(+) T cells, and disease severity in HTLV-1-associated myelopathy (HAM/TSP). Blood 2002;99:88–94.

92. Kitze B, Usuku K. HTLV-1-mediated immunopathological CNS disease. Curr Top Microbiol Immunol 2002;265:197–211.

93. Hashimoto K, Higuchi I, Osame M, Izumo S. Quantitative in situ PCR assay of HTLV-1 infected cells in peripheral blood lymphocytes of patients with ATL, HAM/TSP and asymptomatic carriers. J Neurol Sci 1998;159:67–72.

94. Albrecht B, Collins ND, Newbound GC, Ratner L, Lairmore MD. Quantification of human T-cell lymphotropic virus type 1 proviral load by quantitative competitive polymerase chain reaction. J Virol Meth 1998;75:123–140.

95. Nagai M, Usuku K, Matsumoto W, et al. Analysis of HTLV-I proviral load in 202 HAM/TSP patients and 243 asymptomatic HTLV-I carriers: high proviral load strongly predisposes to HAM/TSP. J Neurovirol 1998;4:586–593.

96. Jeffery KJ, Usuku K, Hall SE, et al. HLA alleles determine human T-lymphotropic virus-I (HTLV-I) proviral load and the risk of HTLV-I-associated myelopathy. Proc Nat Acad Sci U S A 1999;96:3848–3853.

97. Jeffery KJ, Siddiqui AA, Bunce M, et al. The influence of HLA class I alleles and heterozygosity on the outcome of human T cell lymphotropic virus type I infection. J Immunol 2000;165:7278–7284.

98. Yashiki S, Fujiyoshi T, Arima N, et al. HLA-A*26, HLA-B*4002, HLA-B*4006, and HLA-B*4801 alleles predispose to adult T cell leukemia: the limited recognition of HTLV type 1 tax peptide anchor motifs and epitopes to generate anti-HTLV type 1 tax CD8(+) cytotoxic T lymphocytes. AIDS Res Hum Retroviruses 2001;17:1047–1061.

99. Usuku K, Nishizawa M, Matsuki K, et al. Association of a particular amino acid sequence of the HLA-DR β1 chain with HTLV-I-associated myelopathy. Eur J Immunol 1990;20:1603–1606.

100. Jacobson S, Shida H, Mcfarlin DE, Fauci AS, Koenig S. Circulating CD8+ cytotoxic T lymphocytes specific for HTLV-I pX in patients with HTLV-I associated neurological disease. Nature 1990;348:245–248.

101. Kannagi M, Shida H, Igarashi H, et al. Target epitope in the tax protein of HTLV-I recognized by class I MHC-restricted cytotoxic T cells. J Virol 1992;66:2928–2933.

102. Vine AM, Witkover AD, Lloyd AL, Jeffery KJ, Siddiqui A, Marshall SE et al. Polygenic control of human T lymphotropic virus type I (HTLV-I) provirus load and the risk of HTLV-I-associated myelopathy/tropical spastic paraparesis. J Infect Dis 2002;186:932–939.

103. Daenke S, Nightingale S, Cruickshank JK, Bangham CRM. Sequence variants of human T-cell lymphotropic virus type I from patients with tropical spastic paraparesis and adult T-cell leukemia do not distinguish neurological from leukemic isolates. J Virol 1990;64:1278–1282.

104. Evangelista A, Maroushek S, Minnigan H, et al. Nucleotide sequence analysis of a provirus derived from an individual with tropical spastic paraparesis. Microb Pathog 1990;8:259–278.

105. Gould KG, Bangham CR. Virus variation, escape from cytotoxic T lymphocytes and human retroviral persistence. Semin Cell Dev Biol 1998;9:321–328.

106. Mahieux R, Ibrahim F, Mauclere P, et al. Molecular epidemiology of 58 new African human T-cell leukemia virus type 1 (HTLV-1) strains: identification of a new and distinct HTLV-1 molecular subtype in central Africa and in pygmies. J Virol 1997;71:1317–1333.

107. Saito M, Furukawa Y, Kubota R, et al. Frequent mutation in pX region of HTLV-1 is observed in HAM/TSP patients, but is not specifically associated with the central nervous system lesions. J Neurovirol 1995;1:286–294.

108. Kira JI. The presence of HTLV-I proviral DNA in the central nervous system of patients with HTLV-I-associated myelopathy/tropical spastic paraparesis. Mol Neurobiol 1994;8:139–145.

109. Furukawa Y, Yamashita M, Usuku K, Izumo S, Nakagawa M, Osame M. Phylogenetic subgroups of human T cell lymphotropic virus (HTLV) type I in the tax gene and their association with different risks for HTLV-I-associated myelopathy/tropical spastic paraparesis. J Infect Dis 2000;182(5):1343–1349.

110. Nakane S, Shirabe S, Moriuchi R, et al. Comparative molecular analysis of HTLV-I proviral DNA in HTLV-I infected members of a family with a discordant HTLV-I-associated myelopathy in monozygotic twins. J Neurovirol 2000;6:275–283.

111. Furukawa Y, Kubota R, Tara M, Izumo S, Osame M. Existence of escape mutant in HTLV-I tax during the development of adult T-cell leukemia. Blood 2001;97:987–993.

112. Renjifo B, Borrero I, Essex M. Tax mutation associated with tropical spastic paraparesis human T-cell leukemia virus type I-associated myelopathy. J Virol 1995;69:2611–2616.

113. Mahieux R, de The G, Gessain A. The tax mutation at nucleotide 7959 of human T-cell leukemia virus type 1 (HTLV-1) is not associated with tropical spastic paraparesis/HTLV-1-associated myelopathy but is linked to the cosmopolitan molecular genotype. J Virol 1995;69:5925–5927.

114. Johnson JM, Mulloy JC, Ciminale V, Fullen J, Nicot C, Franchini G. The MHC class I heavy chain is a common target of the small proteins encoded by the 3´ end of HTLV type 1 and HTLV type 2. AIDS Res Hum Retroviruses 2000;16:1777–1781.

115. Johnson JM, Nicot C, Fullen J, et al. Free major histocompatibility complex class I heavy chain is preferentially targeted for degradation by human T-cell leukemia/lymphotropic virus type 1 p12(I) protein. J Virol 2001;75:6086–6094.

116. Dantuma NP, Masucci MG. The ubiquitin/proteasome system in Epstein-Barr virus latency and associated malignancies. Semin Cancer Biol 2003;13:69–76.

117. Laney JD, Hochstrasser M. Substrate targeting in the ubiquitin system. Cell 1999;97:427–430.

118. Varshavsky A. The ubiquitin system. Trends Biochem Sci 1997;22:383–387.

119. Trovato R, Mulloy JC, Johnson JM, Takemoto S, de Oliveira MP, Franchini G. A lysine-to-arginine change found in natural alleles of the human T-cell lymphotropic/leukemia virus type 1 p12(I) protein greatly influences its stability. J Virol 1999;73:6460–6467.

120. Franchini G. Molecular mechanisms of human T-cell leukemia/lymphotropic virus type I infection. Blood 1995;86:3619–3639.

121. Martins ML, Soares BC, Ribas JG, et al. Frequency of p12K and p12R alleles of HTLV type 1 in HAM/TSP patients and in asymptomatic HTLV type 1 carriers. AIDS Res Hum Retroviruses 2002;18:899–902.

122. Kakuda K, Ikematsu H, Chong WL, Hayashi J, Kashiwagi S. Molecular epidemiology of human T lymphotropic virus type 1 transmission in Okinawa, Japan. Am J Trop Med Hyg 2002;66:404–408.

123. Osame M, Janssen R, Kubota H, et al. Nationwide survey of HTLV-I-associated myelopathy in Japan: association with blood transfusion. Ann Neurol 1990;28:50–56.

124. Lin BT, Musset M, Szekely AM, et al. Human T-cell lymphotropic virus-1-positive T-cell leukemia/lymphoma in a child: report of a case and review of the literature. Arch Pathol Lab Med 1997;121:1282–1286.

125. Kato H, Koya Y, Ohashi T, et al. Oral administration of human T-cell leukemia virus type 1 induces immune unresponsiveness with persistent infection in adult rats. J Virol 1998;72:7289–7293.

126. Bangham CR, Hall SE, Jeffery KJ, et al. Genetic control and dynamics of the cellular immune response to the human T-cell leukaemia virus, HTLV-I. Philos Trans R Soc Lond B Biol Sci 1999;354:691–700.

127. Jacobson S. Immunopathogenesis of human T cell lymphotropic virus type I-associated neurologic disease. J Infect Dis 2002;186(Suppl 2):S187–S192.

128. Kuroda Y, Matsui M. Cerebrospinal fluid interferon–gamma is increased in HTLV-I-associated Myelopathy. J Neuroimmunol 1993;42:223–226.

129. Matsui M, Nagumo F, Tadano J, Kuroda Y. Characterization of humoral and cellular immunity in the central nervous system of HAM/TSP. J Neurol Sci 1995;130:183–189.

130. Azimi N, Mariner J, Jacobson S, Waldmann TA. How does interleukin 15 contribute to the pathogenesis of HTLV type 1-associated myelopathy/tropical spastic paraparesis? AIDS Res Hum Retroviruses 2000;16:1717–1722.

131. Kawakami K, Miyazato A, Iwakura Y, Saito A. Induction of lymphocytic inflammatory changes in lung interstitium by human T lymphotropic virus type I. Amer J Respir Crit Care Med 1999;160:995–1000.

132. Sakai JA, Nagai M, Brennan MB, Mora CA, Jacobson S. In vitro spontaneous lymphoproliferation in patients with human T-cell lymphotropic virus type I-associated neurologic disease: predominant expansion of CD8+ T cells. Blood 2001;98:1506–1511.

133. Kubota R, Soldan SS, Martin R, Jacobson S. Selected cytotoxic T lymphocytes with high specificity for HTLV-I in cerebrospinal fluid from a HAM/TSP patient. J Neurovirol 2002;8:53–57.

134. Gessain A. Virological aspects of tropical spastic paraparesis/HTLV-I associated myelopathy and HTLV-I infection. J Neurovirology 1996;2:299–306.

135. Greten TF, Slansky JE, Kubota R, et al. Direct visualization of antigen-specific T cells: HTLV–1 Tax11-19-specific CD8(+) T cells are activated in peripheral blood and accumulate in cerebrospinal fluid from HAM/TSP patients. Proc Natl Acad Sci U S A 1998;95:7568–7573.

136. Nagai M, Jacobson S. Immunopathogenesis of human T cell lymphotropic virus type I-associated myelopathy. Curr Opin Neurol 2001;14:381–386.

137. Cavrois M, Leclercq I, Gout O, Gessain A, Wainhobson S, Wattel E. Persistent oligoclonal expansion of human T-cell leukemia virus type 1 infected circulating cells in patients with tropical spastic paraparesis/HTLV-1 associated myelopathy. Oncogene 1998;17:77–82.

138. Cavrois M, Gessain A, Gout O, Wain-Hobson S, Wattel E. Common human T cell leukemia virus type 1 (HTLV–1) integration sites in cerebrospinal fluid and blood lymphocytes of patients with HTLV-1-associated myelopathy/tropical spastic paraparesis indicate that HTLV–1 crosses the blood-brain barrier via clonal HTLV-1-Infected Cells. J Infect Dis 2000;182:1044–1050.

139. Furuya T, Nakamura T, Fujimoto T, et al. Elevated levels of interleukin-12 and interferon-gamma in patients with human T lymphotropic virus type I associated myelopathy. J Neuroimmunol 1999;95:185–189.

140. Ichinose K, Nakamura T, Nishiura Y, et al. Characterization of T cells transmigrating through human endothelial cells in patients with HTLV-I-associated myelopathy. Immunobiology 1997;196:485–490.

141. Romero IA, Prevost MC, Perret E, et al. Interactions between brain endothelial cells and human T-cell leukemia virus type 1-infected lymphocytes: mechanisms of viral entry into the central nervous system. J Virol 2000;74:6021–6030.

142. Umehara F, Izumo S, Takeya M, Takahashi K, Sato E, Osame M. Expression of adhesion molecules and monocyte chemoattractant protein-1 (MCP-1) in the spinal cord lesions in HTLV-I-associated myelopathy. Acta Neuropathol 1996;91:343–350.

143. Umehara F, Okada Y, Fujimoto N, Abe M, Izumo S, Osame M. Expression of matrix metalloproteinases and tissue inhibitors of metalloproteinases in HTLV-I-associated myelopathy. J Neuropathol Exp Neurol 1998;57:839–849.

144. Dhawan S, Weeks BS, Abbasi F, et al. Increased expression of alpha 4 beta 1 and alpha 5 beta 1 integrins on HTLV-I-infected lymphocytes. Virology 1993;197:778–781.

145. Grant C, Barmak K, Alefantis T, Yao J, Jacobson S, Wigdahl B. Human T cell leukemia virus type I and neurologic disease: events in bone marrow, peripheral blood, and central nervous system during normal immune surveillance and neuroinflammation. J Cell Physiol 2002;190:133–159.

146. Szymocha R, Brisson C, Bernard A, Akaoka H, Belin MF, Giraudon P. Long-term effects of HTLV-1 on brain astrocytes: sustained expression of Tax-1 associated with synthesis of inflammatory mediators. J Neurovirol 2000;6:350–357.

147. Szymocha R, Akaoka H, Brisson C, et al. Astrocytic alterations induced by HTLV type 1-infected T lymphocytes: a role for tax-1 and tumor necrosis factor alpha. AIDS Res Hum Retroviruses 2000;16:1723–1729.

148. Wattel E, Vartanian JP, Pannetier C, Wainhobson S. Clonal expansion of human T-cell leukemia virus type I-infected cells in asymptomatic and symptomatic carriers without malignancy. J Virol 1995;69:2863–2868.

149. Leclercq I, Cavrois M, Mortreux F, et al. Oligoclonal proliferation of human T-cell leukaemia virus type 1 bearing T cells in adult T-cell leukaemia/lymphoma without deletion of the 3′ provirus integration sites. Br J Haematol 1998;101:500–506.

150. Taylor GP, Hall SE, Navarrete S, et al. Effect of lamivudine on human T-cell leukemia virus type 1 (HTLV-1) DNA copy number, T-cell phenotype, and anti-tax cytotoxic T-cell frequency in patients with HTLV-1-associated myelopathy. J Virol 1999;73:10,289–10,295.

151. Bangham CR. The immune response to HTLV-I. Curr Opin Immunol 2000;12:397–402.

152. Alkhatib G, Broder CC, Berger EA. Cell type-specific fusion cofactors determine human immunodeficiency virus type 1 tropism for T-cell lines versus primary macrophages. J Virol 1996;70:5487–5494.

153. Newbound GC, Andrews JM, Orourke J, Brady JN, Lairmore MD. Human T-cell lymphotropic virus type 1 tax mediates enhanced transcription in CD4(+) T lymphocytes. J Virol 1996;70:2101–2106.

154. Richardson JH, Edwards AJ, Cruickshank JK, Rudge P, Dalgleish AG. In vivo cellular tropism of human T-cell leukemia virus type 1. J Virol 1990;64:5682–5687.

155. Ye J, Xie L, Green PL. Tax and overlapping rex sequences do not confer the distinct transformation tropisms of human T-cell leukemia virus types 1 and 2. J Virol 2003;77:7728–7735.

156. Nakamura T. Immunopathogenesis of HTLV-I-associated myelopathy/tropical spastic paraparesis. Ann Med 2000;32:600–607.

157. Hanon E, Goon P, Taylor GP, et al. High production of interferon gamma but not interleukin-2 by human T-lymphotropic virus type I-infected peripheral blood mononuclear cells. Blood 2001;98:721–726.

158. Koenig S, Woods RM, Brewah YA, et al. Characterization of MHC class I restricted cytotoxic T-cell responses to tax in HTLV-I infected patients with neurologic diseases. J Immunol 1993;156:3874–3883.

159. Biddison WE, Kubota R, Kawanishi T, et al. Human T cell leukemia virus type I (HTLV-1)-specific CD8(+) CTL clones from patients with HTLV-I-associated neurologic disease secrete proinflammatory cytokines, chemokines, and matrix metalloproteinase. J Immunol 1997;159:2018–2025.

160. Kubota R, Kawanishi T, Matsubara H, Manns A, Jacobson S. Demonstration of human T lymphotropic virus type I (HTLV-I) tax-specific CD8(+) lymphocytes directly in peripheral blood of HTLV-I-associated myelopathy tropical spastic paraparesis patients by intracellular cytokine detection. J Immunol 1998;161:482–488.

161. Azimi N, Brown K, Bamford RN, Tagaya Y, Siebenlist U, Waldmann TA. Human T cell lymphotropic virus type I Tax protein trans-activates interleukin 15 gene transcription through an NF-kappa B site. Proc Natl Acad Sci U S A 1998;95:2452–2457.

162. Hara H, Morita M, Iwaki T, et al. Detection of human T lymphotrophic virus type I (HTLV-I) proviral DNA and analysis of T cell receptor V beta CDR3 sequences in spinal cord lesions of HTLV-I-associated myelopathy/tropical spastic paraparesis. J Exp Med 1994;180:831–839.

163. Hausmann S, Biddison WE, Smith KJ, et al. Peptide recognition by two HLA-A2/Tax11-19-specific T cell clones in relationship to their MHC/peptide/TCR crystal structures. J Immunol 1999;162:5389–5397.

164. Levin MC, Lee SM, Morcos Y, Brady J, Stuart J. Cross-reactivity between immunodominant human T lymphotropic virus type I tax and neurons: implications for molecular mimicry. J Infect Dis 2002;186:1514–1517.

165. Machuca A, Rodes B, Soriano V. The effect of antiretroviral therapy on HTLV infection. Virus Res 2001;78:93–100.

166. Ikegami M, Umehara F, Ikegami N, Maekawa R, Osame M. Selective matrix metalloproteinase inhibitor, N-biphenyl sulfonyl phenylalanine hydroxamic acid, inhibits the migration of CD4+ T lymphocytes in patients with HTLV-I-associated myelopathy. J Neuroimmunol 2002;127:134–138.

167. Harrington WJ, Ucar A, Gill P, et al. Clinical spectrum of HTLV-I in South Florida. J Acq Immun Defic Synd Hum R 1995;8:466–473.

168. Nakagawa M, Nakahara K, Maruyama Y, et al. Therapeutic trials in 200 patients with HTLV-I-associated myelopathy/tropical spastic paraparesis. J Neurovirology 1996;2:345–355.

169. Nakagawa M, Izumo S, Ijichi S, et al. HTLV-I-associated myelopathy: analysis of 213 patients based on clinical features and laboratory findings. J Neurovirol 1995;1:50–61.

170. Osame M, Arimura K, Nakagawa M, Umehara F, Usuku K, Ijichi S. HTLV-I associated myelopathy (HAM): review and recent studies. Leukemia 1997;11(Suppl 3):63–64.

171. Lairmore MD, Digeorge AM, Conrad SF, Trevino AV, Lal RB, Kaumaya PTP. Human T-lymphotropic virus type 1 peptides in chimeric and multivalent constructs with promiscuous T-cell epitopes enhance immunogenicity and overcome genetic restriction. J Virol 1995;69:6077–6089.

172. Sundaram R, Sun Y, Walker CM, Lemonnier FA, Jacobson S, Kaumaya PT. A novel multivalent human CTL peptide construct elicits robust cellular immune responses in HLA-A*0201 transgenic mice: implications for HTLV-1 vaccine design. Vaccine 2003;21:2767–2781.

173. Frangione-Beebe M, Albrecht B, Dakappagari N, et al. Enhanced immunogenicity of a conformational epitope of human T-lymphotropic virus type 1 using a novel chimeric peptide. Vaccine 2000;19:1068–1081.

174. Essex M, Matsuda Z, Yu X, Lee TH. Gene therapy against retroviral diseases. [Review]. Leukemia 1995;9(Suppl 1): S71–S74.

CME QUESTIONS

1. Which of the following clinical signs is commonly linked to human T-lymphotropic virus (HTLV)-1-associated myelopathy?
   A. Paraparesis and spasticity in the lower extremities
   B. Stroke with loss of cognitive function
   C. Bleeding disorders that lead to thrombosis of the lower extremities
   D. Peripheral neuropathy affecting only the upper limbs

2. Which is *not* a common route of transmission of HTLV-1 and HTLV-2?
   A. Orally via breast milk
   B. Sexual contact
   C. Exposure to plasma of infected persons
   D. Exposure to infected cellular-based blood products

3. Which of the following is characteristic of an HTLV-1 infected subject's immune response to the viral infection?
   A. Viral specific immunoglobulin (Ig)-G1 antibody responses are associated with protection from HTLV-1 infection
   B. Cytotoxic T-cell responses against the *tax* antigen are commonly observed in HTLV-1-infected subjects
   C. Vaccines effectively eliminate HTLV-1 infection if they promote a strong IgA and IgG response
   D. Macrophages most likely mediate target cell destruction through perforin-dependent mechanisms

4. Which of the following pathogenic mechanisms has been proposed to explain the lesions associated with HTLV-1-associated myelopathy?
   A. HTLV-1 predominantly infects macrophages, leading to immune suppression and secondary bacterial meningitis
   B. HTLV-1 predominantly targets T cells, which have increased adhesion activity against endothelial cells that promote inflammation in the brain and spinal cord
   C. Epithelial cells infected with HTLV-1 lose their cilia, leading to invasion by secondary pathogens that infect the spinal cord and brain
   D. The virus causes direct lysis of cells that make up the blood–brain barrier, leading to brain edema and subsequent inflammation

18

West Nile Virus Infection of the Nervous System

Pathogenesis, Immunology, and Clinical Management

Douglas J. Lanska

1. PATHOGENESIS

West Nile virus (WNV) is a flavivirus belonging to the Japanese encephalitis subgroup (1,2). This subgroup also includes the serologically closely related St. Louis encephalitis virus. Flaviviruses are small single-stranded RNA viruses, with spherical (or more precisely, icosahedral) envelopes between 40 and 50 nm in diameter.

1.1. Epidemiology

1.1.1. Descriptive Epidemiology

WNV was first isolated in 1937 from a febrile woman in the West Nile district of Uganda (3). In the 1950s, outbreaks of a nonfatal encephalitic human WNV infection occurred in the Middle East. The first major urban outbreaks occurred in Romania in 1996, where there were 17 deaths among 800 cases (4–7), and in Russia in 1999, where there were 40 deaths among more than 800 cases (8). By the 1990s, WNV was recognized in Africa, Europe, the Middle East, and Asia.

In 1999, an outbreak was identified in New York City, with seven deaths among 62 cases (9–14). The epidemic coincided with the WNV-related deaths of several thousand crows, as well as the deaths of exotic birds at the zoos in the Bronx and Queens (15–17). The viral genome in this epidemic was almost identical to that of a WNV strain identified in Israel in 1998, suggesting that the strain found in New York originated in the Middle East (18,19).

WNV subsequently spread along the east coast and then progressively westward across the entire continental United States (20–26). The 2002 and 2003 US WNV epidemics were the largest arboviral meningoencephalitis epidemics ever documented in the Western hemisphere and the largest WNV meningoencephalitis epidemics ever recorded. In 2002, more than 3587 laboratory-confirmed human cases of WNV infection and 211 deaths were reported, compared with less than 150 for the 3 previous years. In 2003, a total of 8567 laboratory-confirmed cases of WNV infection and 199 deaths were reported. The case-fatality rate among recognized cases was 5.9% in 2002 and 2.3% in 2003. The lower case-fatality rate in 2003 probably reflected greater detection of milder cases, rather than a changing virulence of the virus.

Peak incidence of human WNV infection occurs in late August. The median age of patients with meningoencephalitis is about 60 yr. Approximately 9% of these patients die, and almost all of the deaths occur in people over age 50 yr.

From: Current Clinical Neurology: Inflammatory Disorders of the Nervous System:
Pathogenesis, Immunology, and Clinical Management
Edited by: A. Minagar and J. S. Alexander © Humana Press Inc., Totowa, NJ

1.1.2. Mosquito-Borne Transmission

WNV is usually transmitted by mosquitoes that have bitten infected birds. At least 36 mosquito species can transmit WNV. The different mosquito species have (a) variable lifecycles and habit requirements; (b) are collectively more common, are less localized, and have less specific breeding requirements than species that transmit LaCrosse encephalitis; (c) may bite at different times of the day; and (d) often move into homes. These factors make WNV difficult to control with mosquito management plans.

Based on mosquito life cycles and escalation of bird infections throughout the summer, human WNV encephalitis occurs in temperate regions primarily in the late summer and early fall. The number of human cases decreases with onset of cooler weather in fall as the mosquitoes die off, even though the virus can survive through winter in mosquitoes *(27,28)*. In warmer climates, WNV can be transmitted by mosquitoes year round.

Although more than 115 species of birds have been infected, crows, blue jays, and ravens seem to be most susceptible to the virus. In addition to crows and jays, Canadian geese, mallards, ring-necked pheasants, and various birds of prey have been infected. Birds of prey are thought to have acquired the virus most often from other birds, rather than through a mosquito vector.

Mosquito and bird surveillance has become an important component of WNV monitoring in the United States. Counts of infected mosquitoes and dead birds are important indicators of risk of human infections, and dead bird counts typically increase prior to identification of human cases *(15–17,20,28–32)*. Horse and other mammal deaths are less useful for surveillance, because they are much less common and less often precede identification of human cases.

The first indicator of WNV activity in a county is usually a WNV-infected dead bird. An index human case is uncommon and occurred in only 4% of affected counties. Of US counties reporting human cases, the first human illness is typically preceded by reports of infected animals by a median of 1 mo.

1.1.3. Other Modes of West Nile Virus Transmission

Documented transmission can also occur through blood transfusions *(33–40)*, organ transplantation *(34,36,37,41)*, breastfeeding *(42)*, and through the placenta *(43)*, although the proportion of cases transmitted by these routes is less than 0.5%. There is no information to suggest that ticks or other vectors have any role transmitting the WNV infection identified in the United States, nor is there evidence to suggest that WNV can be transmitted to people by consumption of infected animals.

Twenty-three cases of confirmed transfusion-related WNV transmission were documented in the United States in 2002, compared with just two cases in 2003 *(44)*. Since July 2003, blood-collection agencies in the United States have been using investigational WNV nucleic-acid amplification tests to screen all blood donations and have been quarantining and retrieving potentially infectious blood products. Preliminary data indicate that this approach is successful in preventing most cases of WNV transmission through transfusion of blood and blood products. In both of the 2003 cases of transfusion-associated WNV infection, the WNV-contaminated blood had screened negative during initial minipool testing. Later, a retrospective examination of the individual donations comprising these minipools found that two donations contained low levels of WNV. It is currently not feasible to test individually all blood donations in the United States, but individual-donation testing may be considered in areas with a high incidence of WNV infection. In addition, more sensitive methods of minipool testing should be developed. In the meantime, clinicians should continue to investigate cases of WNV infection in people who have received blood transfusions and report cases with suspected transfusion-associated illness.

1.1.4. Risk Factors for Human West Nile Virus Infection

Risk factors for human WNV infection include standing water (e.g., flooded basements), which can support in-home mosquito breeding *(7)*. WNV is most likely to produce encephalitis or death in those over age 50 yr, as well as those with weakened immune systems, but people of any age can develop severe neurological disease from WNV infection *(23,46)*.

1.1.5. Prevention of West Nile Virus Infection

Prevention efforts are directed at limiting exposure to mosquitoes *(30,47)*. To avoid mosquito bites, adults should apply insect repellant containing no more than 35% of the active ingredient, diethyltoluamide (DEET). Children should use products containing no more than 10% DEET. Adults and children should consider staying indoors at peak mosquito biting times (dawn, dusk, and early evening) and should wear long-sleeved shirts and long pants when outdoors. Window and door screens should be maintained in good repair. Stagnant or standing water should be eliminated around homes to eradicate mosquito egg-laying sites; this includes water in flower pots, buckets, old tires, clogged rain gutters, and bird baths.

Hunters are at greater risk from mosquito bites than from cleaning or eating potentially infected birds. Hunters can minimize their risk by taking precautions to avoid mosquito bites, avoiding shooting or handling sick birds, wearing gloves while handling and cleaning game, and thoroughly cooking any game meat.

1.2. Pathology

1.2.1. West Nile Virus Meningoencephalitis

With WNV meningoencephalitis, the brain may be grossly normal or show evidence of mild cerebral edema *(48,49)*. Histological findings include (a) variable neuronal necrosis in the grey matter with neuron loss, neuronal degeneration, neuronophagia, and microglial and polymorphonuclear leukocytic infiltration; (b) microglial nodules composed primarily of lymphocytes and histiocytes and presenting predominantly in the grey matter; (c) variable mononuclear perivascular inflammation (perivascular cuffing); (d) scattered mononuclear leptomeningeal infiltrates; and (e) focal mononuclear inflammation of the cranial nerve roots, especially in the medulla *(11,48,50–53)*.

The pathological changes in the central nervous system (CNS) result from viral replication in neurons and glia, as well as a cytotoxic immune response to infected cells *(54,55)*. CD8 T-lymphocytes predominate over CD4 lymphoctyes in the microglial nodules, perivascular infiltrates, and meningeal and cranial nerve infiltrates *(55)*. B lymphocytes are found primarily in areas of perivascular inflammation *(55)*.

1.2.2. West Nile Virus Poliomyelitis

Early case reports and case series generally attributed the flaccid paralysis accompanying WNV infection to an inflammatory neuropathy similar to Guillain-Barre syndrome (GBS) *(56,57)*. Most of these initial reports did not have supporting electrophysiological studies, and none reported spinal cord pathology. GBS cannot explain the clinical, laboratory, and electrophysiologic abnormalities in most of these cases. GBS generally presents with symmetric weakness, is frequently accompanied by sensory abnormalities or paresthesias, is associated with elevated cerebrospinal fluid (CSF) protein, but without CSF pleocytosis, and has associated electrophysiological findings that are consistent with a predominantly demyelinating neuropathy.

The clinical, laboratory, and electrophysiological abnormalities in some patients with asymmetric flaccid paralysis result from a polio-like syndrome with involvement of spinal cord anterior horn cells and motor nerve axons. Cases of poliomyelitis in patients with WNV infection have been identified in the United States since July 2002 *(34,49,50,58–63)*. Two previous reports also suggested that the acute flaccid paralysis of WNV infection resulted from myelitis, with electrophysiological support in one case, but without pathologic support in either *(64,65)*. Subsequent reports have supported these findings *(50,51,53,66)* and documented an overlapping spectrum of meningitis, encephalitis, and myeloradiculitis. Pathological findings have included loss of anterior-horn neurons, accompanied by gliosis, macrophages, neuronophagia, microglial nodules, chronic perivascular inflammation, and mild lymphocytic infiltration of anterior horn roots *(49,51,53,67)*. In addition, a polio-like syndrome has been previously reported with Japanese encephalitis virus, a flavivirus closely related to WNV *(68,69)*, and with tick-borne flavivirus infections in continental Europe, including Far Eastern tick-borne encephalitis and Central European encephalitis *(70)*. Moreover, pathological studies in animals have demonstrated lesions of the ventral spinal cord grey matter and the spinal motor neurons, with an absence of peripheral nerve lesions, in birds, horses, and nonhuman primates infected with WNV *(71–73)*.

A few recent studies have suggested an alternative or concomitant mechanism for some cases of acute flaccid paralysis associated with WNV (i.e., acute anterior radiculitis) *(61,62)*. Previous electrophysiological studies have, in fact, localized the abnormality to *either* the anterior horn or the ventral nerve roots. Magnetic resonance imaging (MRI) studies of cases of polio-virus poliomyelitis have shown increased signals in the anterior horn, whereas some cases of WNV-associated flaccid paralysis have instead demonstrated intradural nerve-root enhancement *(61)*.

2. IMMUNOLOGY

2.1. Viral Proteins

Flavivirus structural proteins are now designated E (envelope), C (core), and M (membrane-like), replacing older terminology of V3, V2, and V1, respectively *(74)*.

The E protein is the major constituent of the viral surface and is oriented parallel to the viral surface *(75,76)*. It is a class II viral fusion protein that mediates both the binding of WNV to target-cell receptors and the entry of WNV into target cells *(75,77,78)*. The E protein differs structurally from the spiky projections of class I viral fusion proteins seen in orthomyxoviruses, paramyxoviruses, retroviruses, and filoviruses *(76)*. Also, unlike class I viral fusion proteins, the E protein itself is not proteolytically cleaved for activation but instead requires cleavage of an accessory protein *(76)*. Fusion in WNV and other viruses (e.g., alphaviruses) that use class II fusion proteins is faster and less temperature-dependent than fusion in viruses with class I fusion proteins *(76)*.

Each E protein is folded into three domains:

1. an antigenic domain that carries the N-glycosylation site,
2. a domain responsible for pH-dependent fusion of the E protein to the endosomal membrane during uncoating,
3. a domain important for binding to target cells and postulated to contain the receptor-binding site *(77)*.

2.2. Target Cell Binding, Viral Entry, and Replication

Arboviruses are inoculated directly into the bloodstream or subcutaneous tissue. Initial WNV replication occurs in the skin and regional lymph nodes, followed by a primary viremia that seeds the reticuloendothelial system and a secondary viremia, following replication in the reticuloendothelial system *(54,55)*. Depending on a number of host factors, including the integrity of the blood–brain barrier (BBB), the CNS may be seeded during the secondary viremia *(55)*.

On the other hand, flaviviruses bind to a specific cell-surface protein and then enter target cells by a vesicle-mediated process (i.e., so-called *receptor-mediated endocytosis*) *(54,77,79,80)*. Because of the wide host range of natural WNV transmission, the cell-surface protein target is likely to be highly conserved across different species *(80)*. This target-cell-receptor molecule is not fully characterized, but recent work suggests that it is a 105-kDa plasma membrane-associated glycoprotein *(77)*. Although not absolutely required, cholesterol in the target cell membrane significantly facilitates viral binding *(76)*.

Irreversible conformational changes in the E protein and viral uncoating occurs within the endocytic vacuoles at an acidic pH, after which the viral genome is released into the cytoplasm for replication *(54,77,79)*. Virus assembly takes place in the endoplasmic reticulum *(75)*. Initially, the E protein forms a stable heterodimeric complex with the precursor of the M protein. The precursor M protein is cleaved by a protease in the Golgi system to generate fusion-competent mature infectious virions *(75)*.

2.3. Host Factors

Host factors can influence the ability of viruses to enter the CNS *(81)*. WNV and other arboviruses spread hematogenously and must cross the BBB. Penetration of WNV into the CNS depends heavily on the degree and persistence of viremia *(54)* but is facilitated by altered BBB permeability, as from hypercarbia, hyperosmotic agents, and mechanical breach *(81)*. Animal studies have suggested the coincident Gram-negative bacterial infections can induce WNV to invade the CNS, leading to markedly increased rates of encephalitis and death *(81)*; this effect is apparently caused by endotoxin-stimulated release of various cytokines and secondary changes in the integrity of the BBB *(81)*.

Virus-specific antibodies and cytotoxic T cells are important for the clearance of flaviviruses *(55,80)*. Available evidence suggests that humoral immunity, in particular, protects against WNV infection and severe WNV-related disease *(82,83)*. Furthermore, preliminary studies have suggested that patients with WNV encephalitis may benefit from intravenous immunoglobulin (Ig) from donors who have had a high frequency of WNV exposure *(84–86)*. WNV-specific antibody in the CSF may decrease viral replication by interfering with viral attachment to receptors on the cell surface or by preventing endosomal fusion *(55)*. Little is known about a specific cell-mediated immune response to WNV *(55)*.

2.4. Persistent Infection

Several studies in animals have suggested that WNV may produce persistent infection in the CNS *(87–89)*. The pathophysiological mechanisms of this phenomenon are still poorly understood.

2.5. Vaccines

Previous infection with WNV is believed to confer lifelong immunity. Immunization of experimental animals with heterologous flaviviruses (i.e., Japanese encephalitis virus, St. Louis encephalitis virus, yellow fever virus) reduces the severity of subsequent WNV infection *(90)*; however, protective neutralizing antibodies to WNV have not been identified in human subjects following vaccination with Japanese encephalitis or dengue vaccines *(91)*.

WNV vaccines are in development but are not expected to be available for several years. Kunjin virus, an Australian flavivirus, is an attractive WNV vaccine candidate because it is closely antigenically related to WNV but is less virulent *(92)*. Mice immunized with a plasmid DNA vaccine coding for the full-length infectious Kunjin virus RNA did not develop clinical disease but did develop neutralizing antibodies and were protected against wild-type Kunjin virus and otherwise lethal doses of virulent WNV *(92)*.

Another approach is the use of molecularly engineered live-attenuated chimeric virus vaccines, with the pre-M (membrane precursor) and E (envelope) protein genes of WNV on a backbone of dengue virus *(93)*. A further modification of this chimeric virus vaccine was accomplished by a 30-nucleotide deletion mutation in the 3′ noncoding region of the dengue virus backbone. Such chimeric viruses induced moderate-to-high titers of neutralizing antibodies and prevented viremia in monkeys challenged with WNV *(93)*.

3. CLINICAL MANAGEMENT

3.1. Clinical Manifestations

Most people who have been bitten by WNV-infected mosquitoes have no symptoms or only mild ones. Approximately 20% of infected individuals develop a mild illness resembling the flu. Mild illness is referred to as West Nile fever. Symptoms of mild illness can include sudden onset of fever with malaise, anorexia, nausea, vomiting, diarrhea, headache, photobia, neck pain and stiffness, myalgias, rash, and lymphadenopathy *(4,94–97)*.

Severe illness can occur in individuals of all ages, but only 1 out of every 150 infected individuals develops severe disease. Severe neurologic illness may include encephalitis, meningoencephalitis, or poliomyelitis. Symptoms of severe disease can include high fever; headache; nuchal rigidity; confusion and disorientation; severe muscle weakness; or paralysis, cranial nerve palsies, tremors or other abnormal movements, sensory deficits, and seizures *(4,14,97–100)*. Some patients may develop cerebral edema, aphasia, ataxia, tremor, myoclonus, parkinsonism, cranial neuropathies, dysarthria, breathing difficulties, myocarditis, pancreatitis, or hepatitis *(14,52,99,101–103)*.

Cases of poliomyelitis in patients with WNV infection have been identified since July 2002 *(34,58,59,66)*. Patients were generally admitted to hospital with a 1- to 4-d history of symptoms, including fever, chills, vomiting, headache, fatigue, lethargy, confusion, myalgias, and facial and acute asymmetric painless limb weakness. Physical examination demonstrated asymmetric hyporeflexic or areflexic weakness of various extremities, generally with intact sensation. Several patients developed bladder dysfunction and acute respiratory distress requiring ventilatory support.

3.2. Differential Diagnosis

The differential diagnosis includes stroke, GBS, polyradiculitis, meningoencephaloradiculitis, encephalitis (including other arboviral encephalitises), myelitis, poliomyelitis, meningitis, and postviral demyelination. WNV is now the most common cause of arbovirus encephalitis and meningoencephaloradiculitis in the United States but is not a common cause of GBS, polyradiculitis, myelitis, meningitis, or postviral demyelination. Even in areas of recognized WNV infection in animals, most human cases of aseptic meningitis are caused by enteroviruses and not WNV *(104)*.

3.3. Diagnostic Workup

3.3.1. Clinical Suspicion

WNV or another arbovirus (e.g., St. Louis encephalitis virus) infection should be strongly considered in patients with unexplained encephalitis, meningitis, or poliomyelitis in late summer or early fall, particularly in adults 50 yr or older *(97)*. The local presence of other human cases or documented WNV infection in animals (e.g., mosquitoes, birds, horses) should further raise clinical suspicion.

3.3.2. Diagnostic Studies

Serological testing for WNV can be problematic for several reasons, including crossreactivity between WNV and other flaviviruses, and persistence of IgM antibodies. False-positive results can occur with WNV testing because of exposure to St. Louis encephalitis virus or dengue virus or because of previous vaccination for yellow fever or Japanese encephalitis *(20,90,97)*. Also, WNV IgM antibodies can persist for more than 1 yr, potentially producing confusion regarding whether the antibodies are a marker of current or previous infection *(20,97)*. In the latter case, an increase in WNV-specific neutralizing antibody titer in acute and convalescent serum can confirm acute infection *(97)*. Furthermore, some immunocompromised patients may never make antibodies.

Serum and CSF should be obtained for assay of IgM and IgG antibodies to WNV using enzyme-linked immunosorbent assays (ELISA) *(20,30,97,105)*. Ideally, serologic testing should be performed for both WNV and St. Louis encephalitis virus. Positive ELISA results should be confirmed with the more specific plaque reduction neutralization test, which may take 10 d. If CSF is not obtained, paired acute- and convalescent-phase serum samples should be obtained, with the initial specimen obtained during the acute illness and the subsequent specimen obtained 7 to 14 d later.

Other laboratory findings include variable peripheral blood leukocytosis, lymphocytopenia, anemia, and hyponatremia, particularly in patients with encephalitis *(86)*. Stool cultures and polymerase chain reaction (PCR) studies for enterovirus are negative.

CSF analysis typically shows a lymphocytic pleocytosis, an elevated protein level, and a normal glucose level *(97)*. Because IgM antibody does not cross the BBB, WNV-specific IgM antibody in CSF strongly suggests CNS infection *(20,97)*. CSF should also be cultured and analyzed by PCR

Table 1
Case Definition for Arboviral Encephalitis or Meningitis

Probable WNV encephalitis or meningitis
  Encephalitis or meningitis
  Occurring when WNV transmission is likely (late summer or early fall)
  Supportive serology
- Single or stable (twofold change) elevated titer of WNV-specific serum antibodies; *or*
- Serum IgM antibodies detected by antibody-capture ELISA but with no available confirmatory results from WNV-specific serum IgG antibodies

Confirmed WNV encephalitis or meningitis
  Encephalitis or meningitis
  Laboratory confirmation
- Fourfold or greater increase in WNV-specific serum antibody titer; *or*
- Isolation of WNV or demonstration of WNV-specific antigen or genomic sequences in tissue, blood, CSF, or other body fluid; *or*
- WNV-specific IgM antibodies demonstrated in CSF by ELISA; *or*
- WNV-specific serum IgM antibodies (demonstrated by ELISA) confirmed by WNV-specific IgG antibodies (demonstrated by neutralization or hemagglutination inhibition).

WNV, West Nile virus, Ig, immunoglobulin; ELISA, enzyme-linked immunosorbent assay.

techniques to detect WNV nucleic acid; however, because isolation and PCR testing are relatively insensitive, negative results do not exclude WNV infection *(20,97)*.

Computed tomography of the brain is usually normal but may show evidence of hydrocephalus and subependymal edema *(52)*. T1- and T2-weighted MRI of the brain is also usually normal but may show hydrocephalus, basal ganglia, and deep white-matter edema. T2-weighted images may show petechial hemorrhages, symmetric areas of hyperintensity in the thalami, corticospinal tracts, hippocampi, cerebellum, and substantia nigra, as well as enhancement of the leptomeninges, the periventricular areas, or both *(52,86,97,106)*. Diffusion-weighted MRI imaging may be more sensitive, with early changes evident on apparent diffusion coefficient maps prior to evidence of enhancement on postgadolinium T1-weighted images *(106)*.

In patients with WNV poliomyelitis, electromyogram (EMG) and nerve conduction studies indicate a severe, asymmetric process affecting anterior horn cells, their axons, or both. Sensory amplitudes, motor distal latencies, and conduction velocities are normal. Motor amplitudes are typically 25 to 50% of normal. Recruitment is severely reduced with normal appearing motor units on EMG. Spontaneous activity is profuse 2 wk after onset of illness.

3.3.3. Centers for Disease Control and Prevention Case Classification for WNV Encephalitis and Meningitis

The US Centers for Disease Control and Prevention has published a case definition for arboviral encephalitis or meningitis that is applicable to WNV encephalitis and meningitis (Table 1) *(107)*. There is presently no similar case definition for WNV poliomyelitis, although the criteria are easily modified to include poliomyelitis in the same line with encephalitis and meningitis.

3.4. Prognosis and Complications

Symptoms of mild illness generally last from several days to 1 wk. Symptoms of severe disease can last for weeks and, in some cases, neurologic effects can be permanent *(108)*. Only about one-third of people who develop WNV encephalitis or meningitis are fully recovered after 12 mo. Between 3 and 15% of patients who develop severe illness ultimately die from it, with most deaths reported in those over age 50 yr.

3.5. Treatment

Although there is no specific treatment for WNV infection, patients with symptoms such as high fever, confusion, headaches, or muscle weakness should seek medical attention immediately. Intensive supportive care is sometimes needed and may include hospitalization, intravenous fluids, breathing support with a ventilator, and good nursing care *(105)*. Some preliminary studies have suggested that patients with WNV encephalitis may benefit from intravenous immunoglobulin from donors with a high frequency of WNV exposure *(84,85)*. High-dose ribavirin and interferon α2b have some in vitro activity against WNV, but there are no controlled trials of these drugs in people.

REFERENCES

1. Chamber TJ, Hahn CS, Galler R, Rice CM. Flavivirus genome organization, expression, and replication. Annu Rev Microbiol 1990;44:649–688.
2. Monath TP, Heinz FX. Flaviviruses. In: Fields BN, Knipe DM, Howley PM, et al., eds. Fields Virology. 3rd ed. Philadelphia, Lippincott-Raven, 1996:961–1034.
3. Hayes CG. West Nile virus: Uganda, 1937, to New York City, 1999. Ann N Y Acad Sci 2001;951:25–37.
4. Ceausu E, Erscoiu S, Calistru P, et al. Clinical manifestations in the West Nile virus outbreak. Rom J Virol 1997;48:3–11.
5. Cernescu C, Ruta SM, Tardei G, et al. A high number of severe neurologic clinical forms during an epidemic of West Nile virus infection. Rom J Virol 1997;48:13–25.
6. Tsai TF, Popovici F, Cernescu C, Campbell GL, Nedelcu NI. West Nile encephalitis epidemic in southeastern Romania. Lancet 1988;352:767–771.
7. Han LL, Popovici F, Alexander JP J., et al. Risk factors for West Nile virus infection and meningoencephalitis, Romania, 1996. J Infect Dis 1999;179:230–233.
8. Platonov AE, Shipulin GA, Shipulina OY, et al. Outbreak of West Nile virus infection, Volgograd Region, Russia, 1999. Emerg Infect Dis 2001;7:128–132.
9. Centers for Disease Control and Prevention. Outbreak of West Nile-like viral encephalitis—New York, 1999. MMWR 1999;48:845–849.
10. Centers for Disease Control and Prevention. Update: West Nile-like viral encephalitis—New York, 1999. MMWR 1999;48:890–892.
11. Shieh WJ, Guarner J, Layton M, et al. The role of pathology in an investigation of an outbreak of West Nile encephalitis in New York, 1999. Emerg Infect Dis 2001;6:370–372.
12. Fine A, Layton M. Lessons from the West Nile viral encephalitis outbreak in New York City, 1999: implications for bioterrorism preparedness. Clin Infect Dis 2001;32:277–282.
13. Mostashari F, Bunning ML, Kitsutani PT, et al. Epidemic West Nile encephalitis, New York, 1999: results of a household-based seroepidemiological survey. Lancet 2001;358:261–264.
14. Nash D, Mostashari F, Fine A, et al. The outbreak of West Nile virus infection in the New York City area in 1999. N Engl J Med 2001;344:1807–1814.
15. Eidson M, Komar N, Sorhage F, et al. Crow deaths as a sentinel surveillance system for West Nile virus in the northeastern United States, 1999. Emerg Infect Dis 2001;7:615–620.
16. Eidson M, Kramer L, Stone W, Hagiwara Y, Schmit K. Dead bird surveillance as an early warning system for West Nile virus. Emerg Infect Dis 2001;7:631–635.
17. Eidson M, Miller J, Kramer L, Cherry B, Hagiwara Y. Dead crow densities and human cases of West Nile virus, New York State, 2000. Emerg Infect Dis 2001;7:662–664.
18. Lanciotti RS, Roehrig JT, Deubel V, et al. Origin of the West Nile virus responsible for an outbreak of encephalitis in the northeastern United States. Science 1999;286:2333–2337.
19. Giladi M, Metzkor-Cotter E, Martin DA, et al. West Nile encephalitis in Israel, 1999: the New York connection. Emerg Infect Dis 2001;7:659–661.
20. Craven RB, Roehrig JT. West Nile virus. JAMA 2001;286:651–653.
21. Marfin AA, Petersen LR, Eidson M, et al. Widespread West Nile virus activity, eastern United States, 2000. Emerg Infect Dis 2001;7:730–735.
22. Tyler KL. West Nile virus encephalitis in America. N Engl J Med 2001;344:1858–1859.
23. Weiss D, Carr D, Kellachan J, et al. Clinical findings of West Nile virus infection in hospitalized patients, New York and New Jersey, 2000. Emerg Infect Dis 2001;7:654–658.
24. Centers for Disease Control and Prevention. West Nile virus activity—United States, 2001. MMWR 2002;51:497–501.
25. Johnson R. West Nile virus in the US and abroad. Curr Clin Top Infect Dis 2002;22:52–60.

26. Centers for Disease Control and Prevention. Provisional surveillance summary of the West Nile virus epidemic—United States, January–November, 2002. MMWR 2002;51:1129–1133.

27. Centers for Disease Control and Prevention. Update: surveillance for West Nile virus in overwintering mosquitoes—New York, 2000. MMWR 2000;49:178–179.

28. Kulasekera VL, Kramer L, Nasci RS, et al. West Nile virus infection in mosquitoes, birds, horses, and humans, Staten Island, New York, 2000. Emerg Infect Dis 2001;7:722–725.

29. Anderson JF, Andreadis TG, Vossbinck CR, et al. Isolation of West Nile virus from mosquitoes, crows, and a Cooper's hawk in Connecticut. Science 1999;286:2331–2333.

30. Centers for Disease Control and Prevention. Guidelines for surveillance, prevention, and control of West Nile virus infection—United States. MMWR 2000;49:25–28.

31. Guptill SC, Julian KG, Campbell GL, Price SD, Marfin AA. Early-season avian deaths from West Nile virus as warnings of human infection. Emerg Infect Dis 2003;9:483–484.

32. Mostashari F, Kulldorff M, Hartman JJ, Miller JR, Kulasekera V. Dead bird clusters as an early warning system for West Nile virus activity. Emerg Infect Dis 2003;9:641–646.

33. Centers for Disease Control and Prevention. West Nile virus infection in organ donor and transplant recipients—Georgia and Florida, 2002. MMWR 2002;51:790.

34. Centers for Disease Control and Prevention. Investigation of blood transfusion recipients with West Nile virus infections. MMWR 2002;51:823.

35. Centers for Disease Control and Prevention. Acute flaccid paralysis syndrome associated with West Nile virus infection—Mississippi and Louisiana, July–August 2002. MMWR 2002;51:825–828.

36. Centers for Disease Control and Prevention. Update: investigations of West Nile virus infections in recipients of organ transplantation and blood transfusion. MMWR 2002;51:833–836.

37. Centers for Disease Control and Prevention. Update: investigations of West Nile virus infections in recipients of organ transplantation and blood transfusion—Michigan, 2002. MMWR 2002;51:879.

38. Centers for Disease Control and Prevention. West Nile virus activity—United States, October 10–16, 2002, and update on West Nile virus infections in recipients of blood transfusions. MMWR 2002;51:929–931.

39. Centers for Disease Control and Prevention. Investigations of West Nile virus infections in recipients of blood transfusions. MMWR 2002;973:974.

40. Stephenson J. Investigation probes risk of contracting West Nile virus via blood transfusions. JAMA 2002;288:1573–1574.

41. Iwamoto M, Jernigan DB, Guasch A, et al. Transmission of West Nile virus from an organ donor to four transplant recipients. N Engl J Med 2003;348:2196–2203.

42. Centers for Disease Control and Prevention. Possible West Nile virus transmission to an infant through breast–feeding—Michigan, 2002. MMWR 2002;51:877–878.

43. Centers for Disease Control and Prevention. Intrauterine West Nile virus infection—New York, 2002. MMWR 2002;51:1135–1136.

44. Pealer LN, Marfin AA, Petersen LR, et al. Transmission of West Nile virus through blood transfusion in the United States in 2002. N Engl J Med 2003;349:1236–1245.

45. Centers for Disease Control and Prevention. Detection of West Nile virus in blood donations—United States, 2003. MMWR 2003;52:769–772.

46. Weinberger M, Pitlik SD, Gandacu D, et al. West Nile fever outbreak, Israel, 2000: epidemiologic aspects. Emerg Infect Dis 2001;7:686–691.

47. Centers for Disease Control and Prevention. Epidemic/epizootic West Nile virus in the United States. Guidelines for surveillance, prevention, and control. Fort Collins, CO, U.S. Department of Health and Human Services, 2003.

48. Sampson BA, Armbrustmacher V. West Nile encephalitis: the neuropathology of four fatalities. Ann N Y Acad Sci 2001;951:172–178.

49. Kelley TW, Prayson RA, Isada CM. Spinal cord disease in West Nile virus infection. N Engl J Med 2003;348:564–565.

50. Kelley TW, Prayson RA, Ruiz AI, Isada CM, Gordon SM. The neuropathology of West Nile virus meningoencephalitis. A report of two cases and review of the literature. Am J Clin Pathol 2003;119:749–753.

51. Agamanolis DP, Leslie MJ, Caveny EA, Guarner J, Shieh W-J, Zaki SR. Neuropathological findings in West Nile virus encephalitis: a case report. Ann Neurol 2003;54:547–551.

52. Bosanko CM, Gilroy J, Wang A-M, et al. West Nile virus encephalitis involving the substantia nigra. Arch Neurol 2003;60:1448–1452.

53. Kelley TW, Prayson RA, Ruiz AI, Isada CM, Gordon SM. The neuropathology of West Nile virus meningoencephalitis. Am J Clin Pathol 2003;119:749–753.

54. Gonzalez-Scarano F, Tyler KL. Molecular pathogenesis of neurotropic viral infections. Ann Neurol 1987;22:565–574.

55. Campbell GL, Marfin AA, Lanciotti RS, Gubler DJ. West Nile virus. Lancet Infect Dis 2002;2:519–529.

56. Ahmed S, Libman R, Wesson K, Ahmed F, Einberg K. Guillain-Barre syndrome: an unusual presentation of West Nile virus infection. Neurology 2000;55:144–146.

57. Sampson BA, Ambrosi C, Charcolt A, Reiber K, Veress JF, Armbrustmacher V. The pathology of human West Nile virus infection. Hum Pathol 2000;31:527–531.

58. Glass JD, Samuels O, Rich MM. Poliomyelitis due to West Nile virus. N Engl J Med 2002;347:1280–1281.

59. Leis AA, Stokic DS, Polk JL, Dostow V, Winkelmann M. A poliomyelitis-like syndrome from West Nile virus infection. N Engl J Med 2002;347:1279–1280.

60. Sejvar JJ, Leis AA, Stokic DS, et al. Acute flaccid paralysis and West Nile virus infection. Emerg Infect Dis 2003;9:788–793.

61. Park M, Hui JS, Bartt RE. Acute anterior radiculitis associated with West Nile virus infection. J Neurol Neurosurg Psychiatry 2003;74:823–825.

62. Li J, Loeb JA, Shy ME, et al. Asymmetric flaccid paralysis: a neuromuscular presentation of West Nile virus infection. Ann Neurol 2003;53:703–710.

63. Sampson BA, Nields H, Armbrustmacher V, Asnis DS. Muscle weakness in West Nile encephalitis is due to destruction of motor neurons. Hum Pathol 2003;34:628–629.

64. Gadoth N, Weitzman S, Lehman EE. Acute anterior myelitis complicating West Nile fever. Arch Neurol 1979;36:172–173.

65. Ohry A, Karpin H, Yoeli D, Lazari A, Lerman Y. West Nile virus myelitis. Spinal Cord 2001;39:662–663.

66. Jeha LE, Cila CA, Lederman RJ, Prayson RA, Isada CM, Gordon SM. West Nile virus infection: a new acute paralytic illness. Neurology 2003;61:55–59.

67. Leis AA, Stokic DS, Fratkin J. Spinal cord disease in West Nile virus infection. N Engl J Med 2003;348:565–566.

68. Solomon T, Kneen R, Dung NM, et al. Poliomyelitis-like illness due to Japanese encephalitis virus. Lancet 1998;351:1094–1097.

69. Solomon T. Recent advances in Japanese encephalitis. J Neurovirol 2003;9:274–283.

70. Schelinger PD, Schmutzhard E, Fiebach JB, Pfausler B, Maier H, Schwab S. Poliomyelitis-like illness in central European encephalitis. Neurology 2000;55:299–302.

71. Manuelidis EE. Neuropathology of experimental West Nile virus infection in monkeys. J Neuropathol Exp Neurol 1956;15:448–460.

72. Steele KE, Linn MJ, Schoepp RJ, et al. Pathology of fatal West Nile virus infections in native and exotic birds during the 1999 outbreak in New York City, New York. Vet Pathol 2000;37:208–224.

73. Cantile C, Del Piero F, Di Guardo G, Arispici M. Pathologic and immunohistochemical findings in naturally occurring West Nile virus infection in horses. Vet Pathol 2001;38:414–421.

74. Westaway EG, Schlesinger RW, Dalrymple JM, Trent DW. Nomenclature of flavivirus-specified proteins. Intervirology 1980;14:114–117.

75. Heinz FX, Allison SL. The machinery for flavivirus fusion with host cell membranes. Curr Opin Microbiol 2001;4:450–454.

76. Stiasny K, Koessl C, Heinz FX. Involvement of lipids in different steps of the flavivirus fusion mechanism. J Virol 2003;77:7856–7862.

77. Chu JJH, Ng ML. Characterization of a 105-kDa plasma membrane associated glycoprotein that is involved in West Nile virus binding and infection. Virology 2003;312:458–469.

78. Lee E, Lobigs M. Substitutions at the putative receptor-binding site of an encephalitic flavivirus alter virulence and host cell tropism and reveal a role for glycosaminoglycans in entry. J Virol 2000;74:8867–8875.

79. Heinz FX, Auer G, Stiasny K, et al. The interactions of the flavivirus envelope proteins: implications for virus entry and release. Arch Virol 1994;(Suppl 9):339–348.

80. Brinton MA. Host factors involved in West Nile virus replication. Ann N Y Acad Sci 2001;951:207–219.

81. Lustig BS, Danenberg HD, Kafri Y, Kobiler D, Ben-Nathan D. Viral neuroinvasion and encephalitis induced by lipopolysaccharide and its mediators. J Exp Med 1992;176:707–712.

82. Wang T, Anderson JF, Magnarelli LA, et al. West Nile virus envelope protein: role in diagnosis and immunity. Ann N Y Acad Sci 2001;951:325–327.

83. Wang T, Anderson JF, Magnarelli LA, Wong SJ, Koski RA, Fikrig E. Immunization of mice against West Nile virus with recombinant envelope protein. J Immunol 2001;167:5273–5277.

84. Shimoni Z, Niven MJ, Pitlick S, Bulvik S. Treatment of West Nile virus encephalitis with intravenous immunoglobulin. Emerg Infect Dis 2001;7:759.

85. Hamdan A, Green P, Mendelson E, Kramer MR, Pitlik S, Weinberger M. Possible benefit of intravenous immunoglobulin therapy in a lung transplant recipient with West Nile virus encephalitis. Transpl Infect Dis 2002;4:160–162.

86. Solomon T, Ooi MH, Beasley DWC, Mallewa M. West Nile encephalitis. Br Med J 2003;326:865–869.

87. Pogodina VV, Frolova MP, Malenko GV, et al. Study on West Nile virus persistence in monkeys. Arch Virol 1983;75:71–86.

88. Xiao S-Y, Guzman H, Zhang H, Travvasos da Rosa APA, Tesh RB. West Nile virus infection in the golden hamster (Mesocricetus auratus): a model for West Nile encephalitis. Emerg Infect Dis 2001;7:714–721.

89. Komar N, Langevin S, Hinten S, et al. Experimental infection of North American birds with the New York 1999 strain of West Nile virus. Emerg Infect Dis 2003;9:311–322.

90. Tesh RB, Travassos da Rosa AP, Guzman H, Araujo TP, Xiao SY. Immunization with heterologous flaviviruses protective against fatal West Nile encephalitis. Emerg Infect Dis 2002;8:245–251.

91. Kanesa-Thasan N, Putnak JR, Mangiafica JA, Saluzzo JE, Ludwig GV. Short report: Absence of protective neutralizing antibodies to West Nile virus in subjects following vaccination with Japanese encephalitis or dengue vaccines. Am J Trop Med Hyg 2002;66:115–116.

92. Hall RA, Nisbet DJ, Pham KB, Pyke AT, Smith GA, Khromykh AA. DNA vaccine coding for the full-length infectious Kunjin virus RNA protects mice against the New York strain of West Nile virus. Proc Natl Acad Sci USA 2003;100:10,460–10,464.

93. Pletnev AG, St.Claire M, Elkins R, Speicher J, Murphy BR, Chanock RM. Molecularly engineered live-attenuated chimeric West Nile/dengue virus vaccines protect rhesus monkeys from West Nile virus. Virology 2003;314: 190–195.

94. Flatau E, Kohn D, Daher O, Versano N. West Nile fever encephalitis. Isr J Med Sci 1981;17:1057–1059.

95. Paul SD, Murthy DP, Das M. Isolation of West Nile virus from a human case of febrile illness. Indian J Med Res 1970;58:1177–1179.

96. Klein C, Kimiagar I, Pollak L, et al. Neurological features of West Nile virus infection during the 2000 outbreak in a regional hospital in Israel. J Neurol Sci 2002;200:63–66.

97. Petersen L, Marfin A. West Nile virus: a primer for the clinician. Ann Intern Med 2002;137:173–179.

98. Petersen LR, Marfin AA, Gubler DJ. West Nile virus. JAMA 2003;290:524–528.

99. Sejvar JJ, Haddad MB, Tierney BC, et al. Neurologic manifestations and outcome of West Nile virus infection. JAMA 2003;290:511–515.

100. Hirsch MS, Werner B. Base 17–2003: a 38-year-old woman with fever, headache, and confusion. N Engl J Med 2003;348:2239–2247.

101. Spiegel R, Miron D, Gavriel H, Horovitz Y. West Nile virus meningoencephalitis complicated bymotor aphasia in Hodgkin's lymphoma. Arch Dis Child 2002;86:441–442.

102. Vaispapir V, Blum A, Soboh S, Ashkenazi H. West Nile virus meningoencephalitis with optic neuritis. Arch Intern Med 2002;162:606–607.

103. Gilad R, Lampl Y, Sadeh M, Paul M, Dan M. Optic neuritis complicating West Nile virus meningitis in a young adult. Infection 2003;31:55–56.

104. Julian KG, Mullins JA, Olin A, et al. Aseptic meningitis epidemic during a West Nile virus avian epizootic. Emerg Infect Dis 2003;9:1082–1088.

105. Gordon SM, Isada CM. West Nile fever: lessons from the 2002 season. Cleve Clin J Med 2003;70:449–454.

106. Agid R, Ducreux D, Halliday WC, Kucharczyk W, terBrugge KG, Mikulis DJ. MR diffusion-weighted imaging in a case of West Nile virus encephalitis. Neurology 2003;61:1821–1823.

107. Centers for Disease Control and Prevention. Encephalitis or meningitis, arboviral (includes California serogroup, Eastern equine, St. Louis, Western equine, West Nile, Powassan): 2001 case definition. [Last updated June 27, 2003] Available from: www.cdc.gov/epo/dphsi/casedef/encephalitiscurrent.htm. Last accessed September 9, 2003.

108. Nisenbaum C, Wallis K. Meningo-encephalitis due to West Nile fever. Reports of 2 cases. Helv Paediatr Acta 1965;20:392–402.

CME QUESTIONS

1. West Nile virus is transmitted by which of the following vectors?
   A. Fleas
   B. Flies
   C. Mosquitoes
   D. Ticks

2. Which is *not* an extablished mechanism for West Nile virus transmission?
   A. Blood transfusion
   B. Freast-feeding
   C. Eating infected animals
   D. Organ transplantation

3. Which component of the West Nile virus is responsible for target cell binding?
   A. C protein
   B. E protein
   C. M protein
   D. Class I fusion protein

4. Which of the following is *least* likely to be the presentation of West Nile virus infection?
   A. Aseptic meningitis
   B. Encephalitis
   C. Febrile illness
   D. Poliomyelitis

Index